Tumors of the Prostate Gland, Seminal Vesicles, Male Urethra, and Penis

Atlas

of

Tumor Pathology

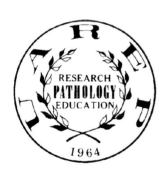

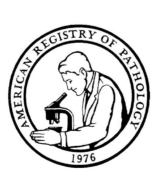

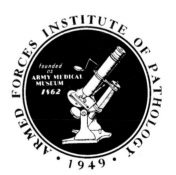

ATLAS OF TUMOR PATHOLOGY

Third Series
Fascicle 28

TUMORS OF THE PROSTATE GLAND, SEMINAL VESICLES, MALE URETHRA, AND PENIS

by

Robert H. Young, M.D., FRCPath
Professor of Pathology, Harvard Medical School
Pathologist and Director of Surgical Pathology
Massachusetts General Hospital
Boston, Massachusetts

John R. Srigley, M.D.
Professor of Pathology and Molecular Medicine
McMaster University, Hamilton, Ontario
Chief, Department of Laboratory Medicine, The Credit Valley Hospital
Mississauga, Ontario

Mahul B. Amin, M.D.
Director of Surgical Pathology, Emory University Hospital
and Associate Professor of Pathology and Urology
Emory University School of Medicine
Atlanta, Georgia

Thomas M. Ulbright, M.D.
Professor of Pathology and Laboratory Medicine
and Director of Anatomic Pathology
Indiana University School of Medicine
Indianapolis, Indiana

Antonio L. Cubilla, M.D.
Professor of Pathology
Facultad de Ciencias Medicas
Director, Instituto de Patologia e Investigacion
Asuncion, Paraguay

Published by the
ARMED FORCES INSTITUTE OF PATHOLOGY
Washington, D.C.

Under the Auspices of
UNIVERSITIES ASSOCIATED FOR RESEARCH AND EDUCATION IN PATHOLOGY, INC.
Bethesda, Maryland
2000

Accepted for Publication
1998

Available from the American Registry of Pathology
Armed Forces Institute of Pathology
Washington, D.C. 20306-6000
www.afip.org
ISSN 0160-6344
ISBN 1-881041-59-X

ATLAS OF TUMOR PATHOLOGY

EDITOR
JUAN ROSAI, M.D.
Dipartimento de Patologia
Instituto Nazionale Tumori
Milano, Italy

ASSOCIATE EDITOR
LESLIE H. SOBIN, M.D.
Armed Forces Institute of Pathology
Washington, D.C. 20306-6000

EDITORIAL ADVISORY BOARD

Jeffrey Cossman, M.D. — Georgetown University School of Medicine
Washington, D.C. 20007

Ronald A. DeLellis, M.D. — Cornell University Medical School
New York, New York 10021

Glauco Frizzera, M.D. — Cornell University Medical School
New York, New York 10021

Leonard B. Kahn, M.D. — Long Island Jewish Hospital/Hillside Medical Center
New Hyde Park, New York 11042

Richard L. Kempson, M.D. — Stanford University Medical School
Stanford, California 94305

Paul Peter Rosen, M.D. — Cornell University Medical School
New York, New York 10021

Robert E. Scully, M.D. — Harvard Medical School and Massachusetts General Hospital
Boston, Massachusetts 02114

Steven G. Silverberg, M.D. — University of Maryland School of Medicine
Baltimore, Maryland 21201

Sharon Weiss, M.D. — Emory University Hospital
Atlanta, Georgia 30322

EDITORS' NOTE

The Atlas of Tumor Pathology has a long and distinguished history. It was first conceived at a Cancer Research Meeting held in St. Louis in September 1947 as an attempt to standardize the nomenclature of neoplastic diseases. The first series was sponsored by the National Academy of Sciences-National Research Council. The organization of this Sisyphean effort was entrusted to the Subcommittee on Oncology of the Committee on Pathology, and Dr. Arthur Purdy Stout was the first editor-in-chief. Many of the illustrations were provided by the Medical Illustration Service of the Armed Forces Institute of Pathology, the type was set by the Government Printing Office, and the final printing was done at the Armed Forces Institute of Pathology (hence the colloquial appellation "AFIP Fascicles"). The American Registry of Pathology purchased the Fascicles from the Government Printing Office and sold them virtually at cost. Over a period of 20 years, approximately 15,000 copies each of nearly 40 Fascicles were produced. The worldwide impact that these publications have had over the years has largely surpassed the original goal. They quickly became among the most influential publications on tumor pathology ever written, primarily because of their overall high quality but also because their low cost made them easily accessible to pathologists and other students of oncology the world over.

Upon completion of the first series, the National Academy of Sciences-National Research Council handed further pursuit of the project over to the newly created Universities Associated for Research and Education in Pathology (UAREP). A second series was started, generously supported by grants from the AFIP, the National Cancer Institute, and the American Cancer Society. Dr. Harlan I. Firminger became the editor-in-chief and was succeeded by Dr. William H. Hartmann. The second series Fascicles were produced as bound volumes instead of loose leaflets. They featured a more comprehensive coverage of the subjects, to the extent that the Fascicles could no longer be regarded as "atlases" but rather as monographs describing and illustrating in detail the tumors and tumor-like conditions of the various organs and systems.

Once the second series was completed, with a success that matched that of the first, UAREP and AFIP decided to embark on a third series. A new editor-in-chief and an associate editor were selected, and a distinguished editorial board was appointed. The mandate for the third series remains the same as for the previous ones, i.e., to oversee the production of an eminently practical publication with surgical pathologists as its primary audience, but also aimed at other workers in oncology. The main purposes of this series are to promote a consistent, unified, and biologically sound nomenclature; to guide the surgical pathologist in the diagnosis of the various tumors and tumor-like lesions; and to provide relevant histogenetic, pathogenetic, and clinicopathologic information on these entities. Just as the second series included data obtained from ultrastructural (and, in the more recent Fascicles, immunohistochemical) examination, the third series will, in addition, incorporate pertinent information obtained with the newer molecular biology techniques. As in the past, a continuous attempt will be made to correlate, whenever possible, the nomenclature used in the Fascicles with that proposed by the World Health Organization's International Histological Classification of Tumors. The format of the third series has been changed in order to incorporate additional items and to ensure a consistency of style throughout. Close cooperation between the various authors and their respective liaisons from the editorial board will be emphasized to minimize unnecessary repetition and discrepancies in the text and illustrations.

To its everlasting credit, the participation and commitment of the AFIP to this venture is even more substantial and encompassing than in previous series. It now extends to virtually all scientific, technical, and financial aspects of the production.

The task confronting the organizations and individuals involved in the third series is even more daunting than in the preceding efforts because of the ever-increasing complexity of the matter at hand. It is hoped that this combined effort—of which, needless to say, that represented by the authors is first and foremost—will result in a series worthy of its two illustrious predecessors and will be a suitable introduction to the tumor pathology of the twenty-first century.

Juan Rosai, M.D.
Leslie H. Sobin, M.D.

ACKNOWLEDGMENTS

This is the second of two Fascicles in the Third Series that are successors to the First Series Fascicle *Tumors of the Male Sex Organs* by Drs. Frank J. Dixon and Robert A. Moore, published in 1952, and the Second Series Fascicle *Tumors of the Male Genital System* by Drs. F. K. Mostofi and Edward B. Price, published in 1973. We are honored to follow in the footsteps of the luminaries who have written the prior male genital Fascicles and hope that our contribution approaches the value of theirs.

Any even casual student of the morphology of male genital disease will be aware of the explosion of interest in many aspects of this area in recent years. Hence the decision to cover the male genital system in two Fascicles rather than one on this occasion was simply a practical one related to the amount of material that needed to be adequately illustrated. As the testis, adnexa, spermatic cord, and scrotum have been previously considered in volume 25 of the Third Series, this contribution deals with the prostate gland, seminal vesicles, male urethra, and penis. Although lesions of the prostate gland, reflecting their frequency, dominate the coverage herein and account for seven of the ten chapters, we have made a particularly strenuous effort to have more detailed coverage of the remaining organs, particularly the penis, as befits the worldwide importance of penile disease.

In the preface to their Fascicle, Drs. Mostofi and Price began as follows: "In preparing this Fascicle for the Atlas of Tumor Pathology, we have been concerned primarily with the pathologic aspects. We have discussed histogenesis, natural history, and prognosis to some extent, but only briefly touched upon treatment, the details of which are beyond the scope of the Atlas." We have carried on the theme of our illustrious predecessors in this work, since therapeutic aspects, if anything, have become even more controversial than in prior times. Furthermore, all the authors are pathologists and felt their greatest contribution could be made by an emphasis on gross and microscopic pathology which form the fundamental framework for the treatment decisions that follow. There is much active investigation of the molecular pathology of prostate cancer but this has yet to impact diagnosis in a significant way and accordingly is not discussed in any depth.

If we have succeeded in our goal of presenting the broad panorama of morphology of the organs considered herein, it is in large measure due to the kindness of numerous individuals who shared material with us over the years, both in consultation and in daily practice at our own hospitals, as well as in response to our specific solicitations for material to depict in this atlas. We are grateful to these investigators, a number of whom are specifically noted in the captions for many of the illustrations, and several of whom deserve particular thanks. It was a great honor for us to communicate during this work with Dr. L. M. Franks whose seminal contributions to prostate pathology are well known. Dr. Franks kindly provided some illustrations from his earlier works which we are delighted to have in these pages. Just as prostatic pathology was well served by those who have written prior Fascicles, study of this area is well served by the current generation of investigators, a number of whom kindly shared material with us, including in some instances prepublication versions of manuscripts which proved very useful. Our sincere thanks are extended to Drs. David G. Bostwick, Jonathan I. Epstein, David J. Grignon, Peter A. Humphrey, Edward C. Jones, and Jae Ro. Dr. Francis W. Chandler kindly read over the section in the chapter on the penis that dealt with infectious diseases and made many helpful suggestions. Drs. Mark A. Weiss and Stacey E. Mills kindly provided a number of illustrations from their *Atlas of Genitourinary Tract Disorders.* Despite the above noted contributions of case material from many sources, the bulk of the illustrative material originates in our own institutions, and we are grateful to our clinical colleagues for this case material and for all we have learned from them over the years about the clinical aspects of the conditions covered. One of us (ALC) is particularly indebted to the late prominent surgeon Professor Manuel Riveros, a pioneer in the study of penile cancer. We also express thanks to Dr. Austin L. Vickery Jr, for over 50 years a stalwart of the Pathology Department of the Massachusetts General Hospital, who kindly donated for our use his extensive collection of photographs of prostatic pathology.

Most of the penile specimens were obtained from two institutions in Paraguay, the Instituto Nacional del Cancer and the "Catedra de Anatomia Patologica" of the medical school. Our thanks are also extended to the following pathologists in Paraguay who have assisted in a number of the studies of penile cancer referred to here: Drs. Enrique Ayala, Gustavo Ayala, Teresa Ayala, Jose Barreto, Carmelo Caballero, Sandra Ocampos, Adriano Piris, Ingrid Rodriguez, and Elsa Velazques. We are grateful to Drs. Juan Rosai and Victor Reuter for their assistance in the review of the penile material from Memorial Hospital, New York City; Mr. Saturnino Sotelo, a gifted artist, did all the drawings in the penile chapter and his contribution is gratefully acknowledged. We thank FUNDUNA and DIPRI, granting agencies in the National University in Asuncion, Paraguay, for the financial support provided to Dr. Cubilla.

The outstanding photographic assistance of Steven Conley and Michelle Forestall of the Pathology Photography Laboratory of the Massachusetts General Hospital is acknowledged with thanks, as is the assistance of Marlene Fairbanks who bore the brunt of the secretarial work involved in this contribution with characteristic efficiency. The additional secretarial assistance of Barbara Jones, Terri Steinke, and Sady Sosa is greatly appreciated. Dr. Pheroze Tamboli kindly assisted in the organization of references. During most of the time this work was being prepared the senior author was fortunate to have the invaluable assistance of Dr. Esther Oliva whose help freed up time for this project. Her generous assistance is acknowledged most sincerely. Our families, particularly our wives, have been most understanding with regard to the demands of this contribution and the necessity for much of the preparation to be done in what otherwise would have been family time.

As is the custom, a draft of our manuscript was read by two anonymous reviewers and we are indebted to them for their numerous helpful suggestions which, almost without exception, were accepted and incorporated into the final manuscript. The editorial staff of the Atlas of Tumor Pathology (Dian Thomas, Andrew Male, and Audrey Kahn) were most helpful throughout the production process and showed more tolerance than we had any right to expect with regard to what must have seemed like a never-ending list of "special requests" to reorient a figure or add a new illustration or reference. This Fascicle, like the previous contribution on the testis and the other male genital structures, was overseen by Dr. Robert E. Scully and his sage advice was generously given to us on numerous occasions. Finally, this work took longer to prepare than we or the Third Series Fascicle editor, Dr. Juan Rosai, ever envisaged and Dr. Rosai's forbearance is something for which we will always be most grateful.

Robert H. Young, M.D., FRCPath
John R. Srigley, M.D.
Mahul B. Amin, M.D.
Thomas M. Ulbright, M.D.
Antonio L. Cubilla, M.D.

WB Saunders:

    Atlas of Surgical Pathology of the Male Reproductive Tract, 1997. For figures 4-3, 5-9, 5-13, 5-22, 5-43, 5-46, 5-52, 5-58, 6-8, 6-16, 7-55, and 10-67.

    Campbell's Urology, 7th ed., 1998. For figure 4-1.

    Hum Pathol 1993;24:298–310. For figure 3-8.

    Pathology of the Prostate, 1998. For figure 3-2.

    A Textbook of Pathology, 1994. For figure 4-4.

Contents

TUMORS OF THE PROSTATE GLAND, SEMINAL VESICLES, MALE URETHRA, AND PENIS

1
THE NORMAL PROSTATE GLAND
CLASSIFICATION OF TUMORS AND TUMOR-LIKE LESIONS

INTRODUCTION

Prostatic hyperplasia and adenocarcinoma are common diseases that account for considerable morbidity and mortality in the aging population. Specimens derived from patients with these conditions account for a large volume of surgical pathologic material, and the pitfalls associated with their evaluation are manifold. In the first seven chapters of this Fascicle the current knowledge in this area is summarized, with emphasis on information that is of practical importance with regard to conventional morphologic analysis. We have highlighted the errors that may lead to the misdiagnosis of a benign process as a malignant neoplasm by continuing the tradition begun in the first series Fascicle (1) of concluding the discussion of the prostate gland with a separate chapter devoted to tumor-like lesions. Description of these processes, many delineated recently, has broadened the differential diagnosis of carcinoma and expanded the list of mimics of neoplasia beyond simple hyperplasia, atrophy, and the changes due to infarction or inflammation that were discussed in the prior Fascicles (1,2).

In the quarter century since the second series Fascicle on the male genital tract (2) was published, there has been steadily increasing interest in prostatic pathology as reflected by numerous publications. Clinical and basic scientific studies have led to a better understanding of previously recognized tumors, and morphologic studies have described many new entities. The histopathologic spectrum of benign prostatic hyperplasia has been broadened with descriptions of several variants, and work done primarily in the last two decades has considerably expanded our knowledge of the pathology and biology of prostatic adenocarcinoma, in particular its possible precursor lesions, special histologic variants, and prognostic factors. Before dealing with specific tumors and tumor-like lesions in subsequent chapters, basic structural and functional aspects of the prostate gland are reviewed. Knowledge of the structure of this gland has particular importance in interpreting pathologic specimens, as the frequency and types of lesions have regional variations (12–15,30,31).

THE NORMAL PROSTATE GLAND

Anatomic Relationships

The prostate gland is situated in the true pelvis between the bladder neck and urogenital diaphragm. It lies behind the inferior aspect of the symphysis pubis and anterior to the rectum. The prostate gland in young adults (fig. 1-1) weighs about 20 g and measures 4 cm in transverse dimension at the base, 3 cm in vertical

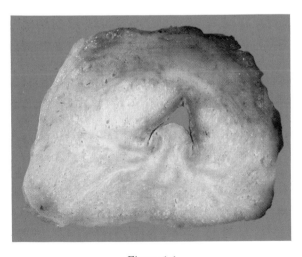

Figure 1-1
NORMAL PROSTATE GLAND
Cross section of prostate from a young adult male at the level of the verumontanum. (Courtesy of Dr. W. A. Sakr, Detroit, MI.)

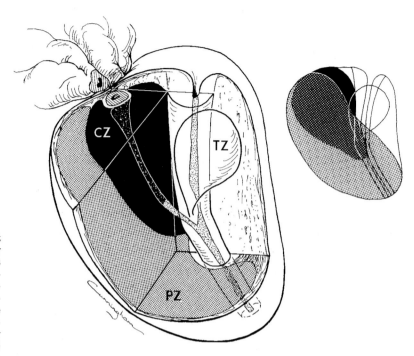

Figure 1-2
ZONAL ANATOMY
OF THE PROSTATE

Top: Artist's representation of a right anterior superolateral view of a partially dissected prostate depicting McNeal's zonal anatomy model. Note the angulation of the prostatic urethra. The transition zone (TZ) wraps around the proximal urethral segment. The central zone (CZ) extends from the base to the verumontanum encircling the ejaculatory duct system. The peripheral zone (PZ) comprises the bulk of the prostatic tissue and virtually all of the prostatic glandular tissue around the distal urethral segment. The small schematic is a mid-sagittal representation of zonal anatomy.

Bottom: Another sagittal section is depicted. (Fig. 4-1A from Kirby RS, Christmas TJ, eds. Benign prostatic hyperplasia. London: Gower Medical Publishers, 1993:18.)

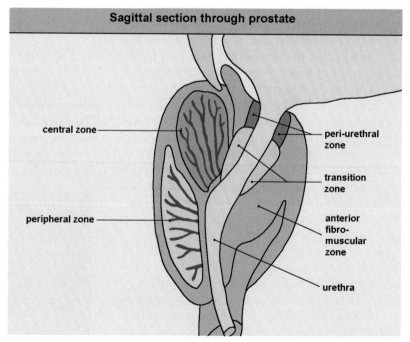

Sagittal section through prostate

central zone

peripheral zone

peri-urethral zone

transition zone

anterior fibro-muscular zone

urethra

dimension, and about 2 cm anteroposteriorly (5,37,38). While the weight of the prostate gland has traditionally been thought to be relatively constant between the ages of 20 and 50, more recent autopsy data suggest a stepwise increase in prostatic weight with each decade of life (6,34). The prostate gland has an inverted conical shape (figs. 1-2, 1-3) with the base, the region of attachment of the seminal vesicles, in direct continuity with the bladder neck and the apex with the urogenital diaphragm (3,5,29,36,37). The prostate is organized around the first part of the urethra (23–25). Two ejaculatory ducts, formed at the junction between the vas deferens and

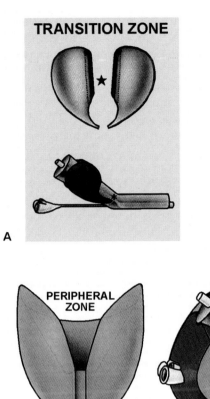

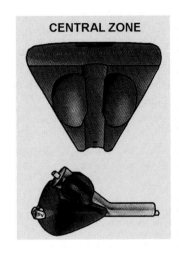

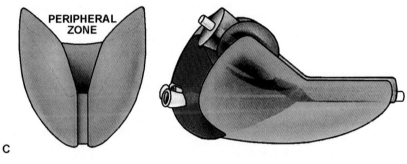

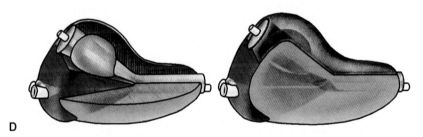

Figure 1-3
SCHEMATIC
REPRESENTATION OF
THE ZONAL ANATOMY
OF THE PROSTATE GLAND

A: Transition zone, showing its relationship to the urethra in the proximal half of the gland.

B: Central zone, demonstrating its relationship to the urethra and ejaculatory ducts.

C: Peripheral zone, with its relationship to the urethra, transition zone, and central zone.

D: Depiction of all three zones with the anterior fibromuscular stroma depicted. Blue to black, transition zone; crimson, central zone; yellow-orange, peripheral zone; green, anterior fibromuscular stroma. (Modified from figs. 2–4 from Lee F, Trop-Pedersen ST, Siders DB, et al. Transrectal ultrasound in the diagnosis and staging of prostate cancer. Radiology 1989; 170: 610–1.)

seminal vesicles on each side, traverse the prostate in an anteroinferior direction to open into the urethra lateral to the verumontanum (colliculus seminalis) (33); the latter is found on the dorsal wall of the prostatic urethra and defines the point of separation between the proximal (preprostatic) and distal (prostatic) segments. On the surface of the verumontanum are openings of several urethral glands, and laterally are orifices of prostatic ducts. In the verumontanum, centrally, is a small depression corresponding to the opening of the utricle. The utricle is a vestigial mullerian structure that is thought to be homologous to the uterus (16), although it is lined by prostatic epithelium.

Anatomic Models

Since the early part of this century several anatomic models of the prostate gland have been proposed (fig. 1-4). In 1912, Lowsley (20,21) suggested that the prostate gland was composed of five lobes (middle, right and left lateral, posterior, anterior) formed by independent groups of tubules fused into a common structure (fig. 1-4A). He also suggested that most carcinomas develop

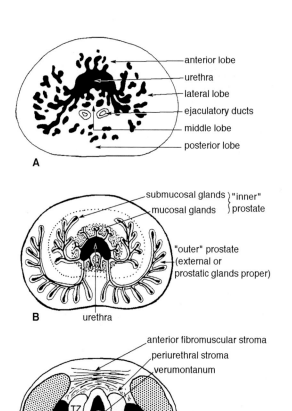

Figure 1-4
CROSS SECTIONS OF THE PROSTATE GLAND
AT THE LEVEL OF THE VERUMONTANUM,
COMPARING THREE ANATOMIC MODELS

A: Lowsley's lobar model. Note location of anterior, posterior, lateral, and middle lobes.

B: Frank's concentric zone model showing mucosal and submucosal glands comprising the "inner" prostate and the peripheral glands comprising the "outer" prostate.

C: McNeal's zonal model displaying the periurethral transition zone (TZ), the central zone (CZ) closely related to ejaculatory ducts, and the peripheral zone (PZ) wrapping around the CZ. In the anterior aspect, stroma predominates and is referred to as the anterior fibromuscular stroma.

in the posterior lobe and that nodular hyperplasia rarely affects that region, a concept now generally accepted (12–14,22,36). The lobar hypothesis was mainly based on studies of the fetal prostate. However, Tisell and Salander (39,40), based on autopsies of 100 adult males, proposed that the prostate gland has six lobes (two dorsal, two lateral, and two median), each with separate ducts. In practice, adult glands do not have a

distinct lobar organization, and the lobar classification has little application to contemporary prostatic pathology (23,26). In 1954, Franks (12–14) suggested that the prostate gland was composed of concentrically arranged groups of glands (fig. 1-4B). The inner region, consisting of mucosal and submucosal glands derived from urogenital sinus endoderm with some mesonephric and paramesonephric structures, was thought to be an estrogen-sensitive zone that could give rise to nodular hyperplasia (17). The outer layers of glands, correlating with the lateral and posterior lobes of Lowsley, originated only from urogenital sinus endoderm and formed the region where most carcinomas develop.

The anatomic constructs of Lowsley, Tisell and Salander, and Franks have now been largely replaced by the McNeal paradigm (figs. 1-2, 1-3, 1-4C) (23–26). In McNeal's model, the key reference point is the prostatic urethra which has a 35° angulation in the mid-portion creating proximal and distal segments of about equal length (figs. 1-2, 1-3). The verumontanum is part of the distal urethral segment and consists of a bulge at the point of angulation. Glandular zones, as defined by McNeal, are arranged in relation to the prostatic urethra and ejaculatory ducts. McNeal's model divides the prostate into three zones, the transition zone, peripheral zone, and central zone, each of which has a different glandular organization and proclivity for disease. A series of small abortive glands immediately around the proximal urethra and lying within the confines of the preprostatic sphincter are considered a separate compartment by McNeal, the periurethral gland region (23).

The transition zone (fig. 1-2) accounts for about 5 percent of normal prostatic volume, and its glands are the chief source of benign prostatic hyperplasia. This zone is located around the proximal prostatic urethra and consists of two small lobes which are normally lateral to the urethra. Transition zone ducts exit in the posterolateral wall of the urethra, proximal to the urethral angulation. About 15 to 20 percent of prostatic carcinomas arise in the transition zone.

The central zone (fig. 1-2) accounts for about 25 percent of normal prostatic volume and is an inverted conical portion of tissue wrapping around the ejaculatory ducts and extending from the prostatic base to an apex at the verumontanum.

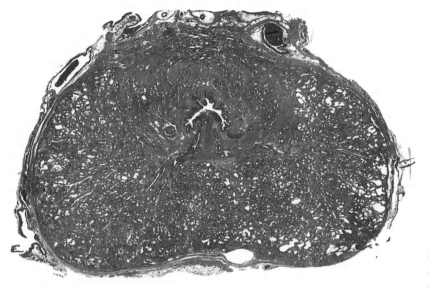

Figure 1-5
NORMAL
VERUMONTANUM
A whole mount cross section of the prostate gland of a 24-year-old at the level of the verumontanum. The inverted U-shaped structure in the middle is the verumontanum. The anterior region (top) is formed predominantly by fibromuscular stroma. The paired ejaculatory ducts are seen better in the lower figure, which shows them running almost vertically from the verumontanum towards the subjacent transition zone.

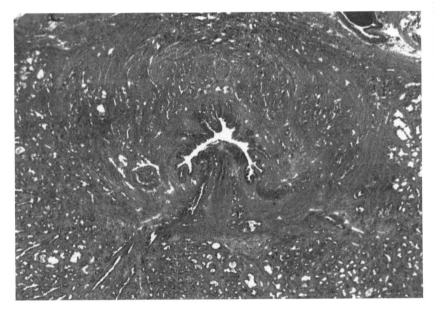

Central zone ducts exit in the convexity of the verumontanum adjacent to the ejaculatory duct orifices. Only about 10 percent of carcinomas arise in the central zone, although peripheral zone cancers frequently spread to involve this zone.

The peripheral zone (figs. 1-2, 1-3) represents the bulk (approximately 70 percent) of normal prostatic tissue. It wraps around both central and transition zones in the basal portion of the gland and accounts for virtually all glandular tissue surrounding the distal prostatic urethra. Peripheral acini empty into ducts that arch through the pe-

ripheral zone to exit in the posterolateral recesses of the distal urethra as a double row, extending from the verumontanum (figs. 1-5, bottom, 1-6) to the prostatic apex. The majority (70 to 75 percent) of carcinomas arise in the peripheral zone, which is accordingly also a common site of prostatic intraepithelial neoplasia. Chronic inflammation and glandular atrophy are common in this zone; it is only an occasional site of hyperplasia (30) (see page 38).

In addition to the glandular zones, the prostate has distinct areas of specialized prostatic stroma

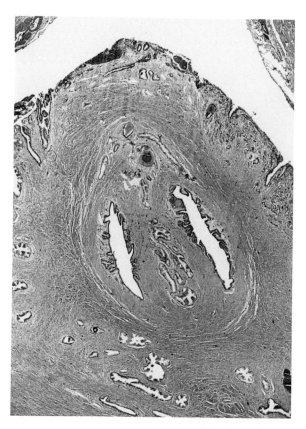

Figure 1-6
NORMAL VERUMONTANUM
Note the dome-shaped elevation, with the two ejaculatory ducts in the center and the utricular glands between the ejaculatory ducts.

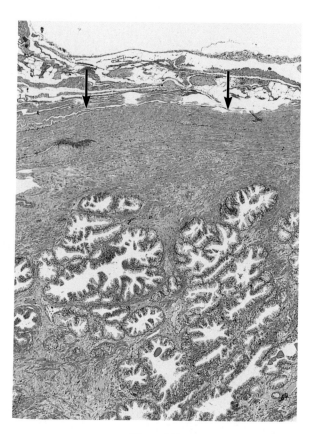

Figure 1-7
PROSTATIC "CAPSULE"
This low-power view shows the condensed fibromuscular stroma (top) bordering the most peripheral glands of the prostate and represents what, for practical purposes, is considered the capsule of the prostate. Spread of tumor beyond this region, the peripheral portion of which is indicated by arrows, is deemed extraprostatic extension.

and other important nonglandular elements, namely, the preprostatic sphincter, striated sphincter, anterior fibromuscular stroma, and prostatic "capsule" (see below) (4,23,35). The prostatic urethra is encircled by a sheath of sphincteric muscle. The proximal (preprostatic) sphincter consists of a sleeve of smooth muscle fibers organized around the proximal urethral segment. It maintains closure of the proximal segment during ejaculation, thus preventing retrograde flow of seminal fluid. Distal to the verumontanum is a sphincter composed of compactly arranged, striated muscle fibers which is continuous with the external urethral sphincter inferior to the prostatic apex (28a). The anterior fibromuscular stroma accounts for much of the tissue anterior to the prostatic urethra (fig. 1-5, top). It is composed of compact smooth muscle bundles similar to those of the bladder neck into

which it blends superiorly at the prostatic base; anteriorly it merges with the pelvic musculature. Distally the anterior fibromuscular stroma contains admixed smooth and skeletal muscle bundles which blend into the external sphincter.

Capsule

The prostatic "capsule" is not a true capsule but a peripheral condensation of fibromuscular stroma (fig. 1-7) (4,28,35); as a matter of convenience, it is referred to as a capsule by eminent authorities (23) and in most of the literature. The capsule covers most of the posterior and lateral surfaces of the prostate. The terminal acini of the peripheral and central zones reach the capsule while the terminal acini of the transition zone impinge on the anterior fibromuscular stroma;

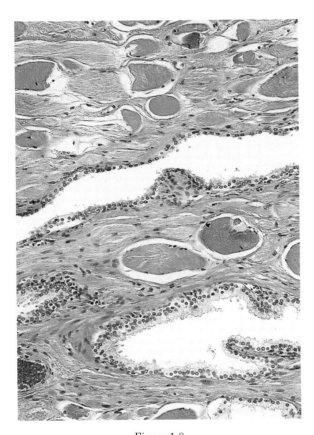

Figure 1-8
NORMAL PROSTATE GLAND
Benign prostatic acini are interspersed between striated muscle of the anterior fibromuscular stroma.

occasionally, nodules of hyperplastic tissue of transition zone origin compress the peripheral zone and reach the prostatic capsule. Anteriorly, the capsular stroma blends with the anterior fibromuscular stroma. At the prostatic apex the capsule is indistinct or absent over the antero-lateral aspect. At this point, glandular tissue intermingles with striated muscle (fig. 1-8) including that of the external sphincter (see chapter 7). No capsule is present at the bladder neck since the prostatic stroma blends seamlessly into bladder neck smooth muscle. The capsular stroma also blends imperceptibly with intraprostatic stroma and with thin bands of extraprostatic connective tissue that are randomly arranged with adipose tissue, forming the usually relatively scant amount of periprostatic connective tissue. Although adipose tissue in a tissue fragment usually indicates that it is extraprostatic, rarely fat is

present within the prostate (9). The capsule forms an important landmark with respect to evaluating extraprostatic extension of carcinoma (see chapter 4) in regions other than those just noted in which it is absent or indistinct.

Urologists have used the term "surgical capsule" to indicate the plane of tissue separating hyperplastic transition zone tissue from the outer peripheral zone tissue (see fig. 2-6, top).

Blood Supply

The prostate gland is supplied by branches of the internal iliac arteries (8,11). The arteries enter the gland through the neurovascular pedicles located on the superolateral aspect of the gland bilaterally. The arterial branches ramify within the capsule and extend inward towards the prostatic urethra. Major arterial branches extend toward the verumontanum parallel to the proximal prostatic urethra and supply the periurethral region and transition zone (11). Prostatic veins drain into the prostatic plexus (8). There is an extensive venous network in the capsule and pericapsular connective tissue. The veins eventually drain into the internal iliac veins.

Lymphatic Drainage

There is a network of intraprostatic lymphatics (10), and they are also prominent in the capsule and the periprostatic connective tissue. These lymphatics drain mainly into the internal iliac lymph nodes, although some drain directly to the external iliac and sacral lymph nodes (10). The internal iliac lymph nodes are usually the first site of lymphatic spread of prostatic carcinoma and are commonly removed as a staging procedure.

Nerve Supply

The prostate is supplied by a rich neural plexus (18,41). The main nerves are located in the neurovascular bundles on the superior-lateral borders of the prostate (fig. 1-9). Numerous autonomic ganglia are present near the capsule in the region of the neurovascular bundles (fig. 1-10) or, less commonly, in the outermost prostatic stroma. The latter circumstance indicates that involvement of ganglia by carcinoma in a needle biopsy does not necessarily connote extraprostatic spread. Small nerve branches penetrate the capsule,

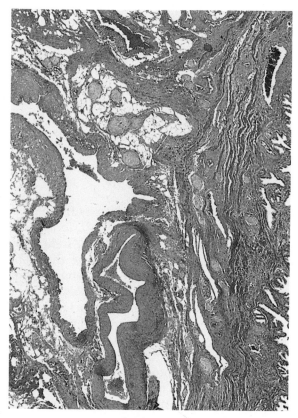

Figure 1-9
POSTERIOR NEUROVASCULAR BUNDLE
Note the large caliber blood vessels and nerve bundles.

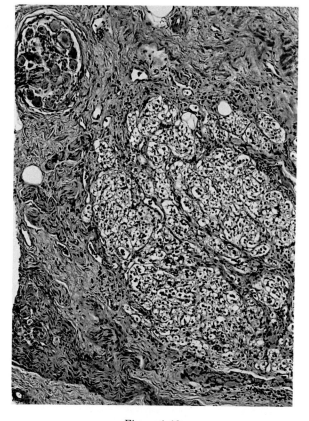

Figure 1-10
PERIPROSTATIC CONNECTIVE TISSUE
A ganglion (upper left) and paraganglion (center) are present.

where they may be found in close proximity to peripheral acini. Adenocarcinoma commonly spreads along the perineural spaces, which is the pathway of least resistance (42). Since benign glands may be closely apposed to nerves and impinge on them, an overdiagnosis of carcinoma based on the presence of this mimic of perineural invasion by cancer should be avoided (see chapter 7) (7). Islands of paraganglionic tissue may also be found in the immediate periprostatic connective tissue (fig. 1-10); these may occasionally be confused with carcinoma (see chapter 7) (15,32).

Developmental Anatomy

During the 12th week of gestation the prostate gland develops under the influence of androgenic hormones produced by the fetal testis (3,29). The earliest prostatic ducts originate as epithelial outgrowths of urogenital sinus endoderm. These epithelial buds are associated with primitive mesenchyme which differentiates into fibromuscular elements. The glands proximal to the verumontanum are relatively short and simple while the distal glands are longer and more complex. The latter glands arch into the peripheral posterolateral region of the gland and successively branch to end in acinar units. Although it is clear that glands of the peripheral and transition zones develop from endoderm of the urogenital sinus, the embryologic origin of central zone glands is more controversial (22,26). There is some evidence from comparative anatomic studies that the central zone is homologous to the cranial accessory glands in primates and other higher mammals (22). These accessory glands are closely related to wolffian duct structures such as the seminal vesicles and ejaculatory ducts, and there are some morphologic, biochemical, and histochemical observations suggesting that the central zone is actually of wolffian duct origin (19,27).

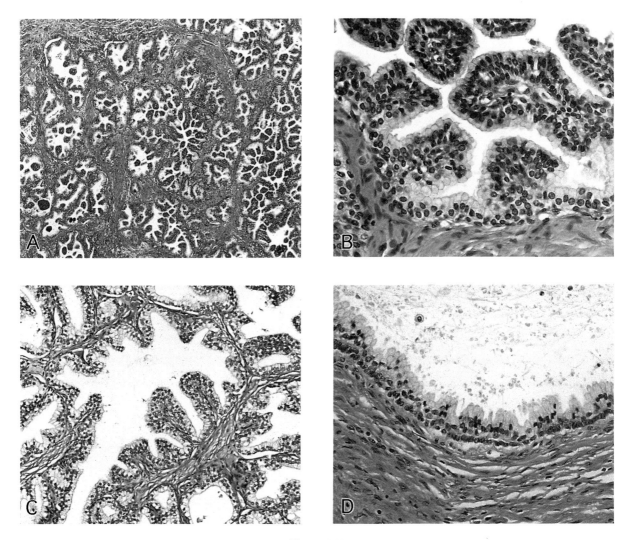

Figure 1-11
HISTOLOGY OF PROSTATE GLAND

A: Complex normal histology of the central zone of the gland from a 37-year-old.

B: Prostatic acinus from same case showing cuboidal to columnar secretory cells with abundant, finely granular, lightly eosinophilic cytoplasm. Basal cells are appreciable focally.

C: Papillary infoldings and well-displayed secretory cells from another case.

D: Dilated acinus from an older man showing clearly delineated basal and secretory cells.

Histology

The prostate gland has a compound tubulo-alveolar organization (fig. 1-11) (44,68,76), with some variations in histology in the three zones (fig. 1-12) (see below). The acinar units responsible for prostatic secretion open into a series of ramifying ducts which empty into large (primary) ducts (fig. 1-13). The primary prostatic ducts in turn open into the prostatic urethra; they are often lined by transitional epithelium near their entry points into the urethra. The prostatic acini and ducts, except for the immediate periurethral segments, are lined by a double-layered epithelium consisting of secretory and basal cells (fig. 1-11B,D). It is often difficult to distinguish between acini and ducts although the ducts tend to have less complex infolding. Sometimes long straight or arching ducts leading from peripheral acini and reaching the prostatic urethra are observed. The smaller ducts and acini are functionally and histologically similar. Unlike salivary and other

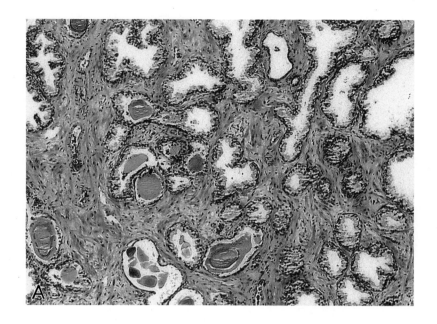

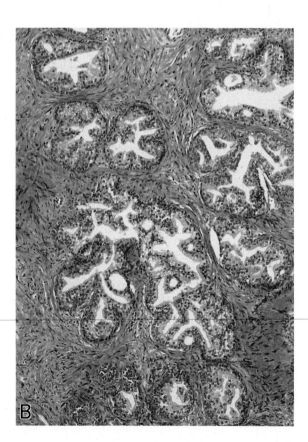
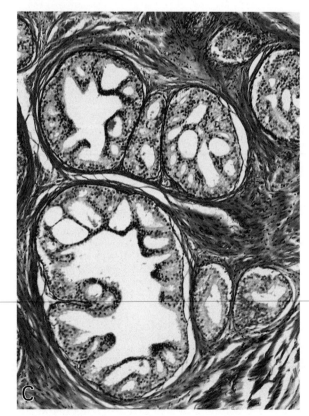

Figure 1-12
HISTOLOGIC COMPARISON BETWEEN NORMAL PERIPHERAL AND CENTRAL ZONES

A: Glands of the peripheral zone have a simpler architecture and are surrounded by loose fibromuscular connective tissue.

B: Glands of the central zone are architecturally more complex than those of the peripheral zone.

C: Papillations and epithelial arches are prominent in the central zone. The fibromuscular stroma is more compact than that of the peripheral zone.

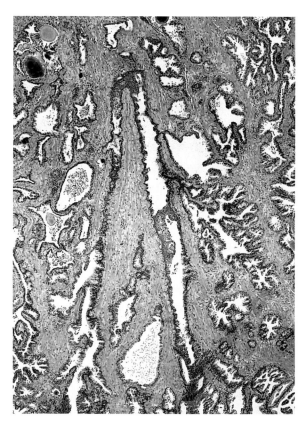

Figure 1-13
NORMAL PROSTATE GLAND
Ramifying ducts lead to groups of acini. The latter show more complex infolding of epithelium than the former.

exocrine glands, the ducts do not have a myoepithelial layer but, like prostatic acini, have an outer layer of basal cells. The inner secretory cells produce prostate-specific antigen and prostatic acid phosphatase like their counterparts in the acini.

The secretory cells are cuboidal to columnar and may appear multilayered depending on the plane of section (fig. 1-11B). They generally have basally located, uniform nuclei and abundant apical cytoplasm, which is pale and granular or rarely, vacuolated. In the central zone the cytoplasm tends to be darker and more granular than in other zones (76). The secretory cells are responsible for the production and release of biochemical products such as citric acid and acid phosphatase (51,66,74). The secretory cells rest on a basal cell layer which consists of cuboidal to, more usually, flattened, attenuated cells with relatively high nuclear to cytoplasmic ratios, round to oval nuclei, and occasional visible small

basophilic nucleoli. Commonly, a single basal cell will subtend several overlying secretory cells. In many instances basal cells are difficult to discern by routine light microscopy. The basal cells rest on a delicate basement membrane which is not usually visualized with routine stains.

The role of the prostatic basal cells is poorly understood. There is little experimental evidence that basal cells serve as continuous or facultative stem cells, although some authors have identified transitional forms of basal cells expressing some secretory or neuroendocrine differentiation, implying that basal cells can differentiate along these lines (49,50,53). It is likely that a population of stem cells resides within the basal cell compartment (78). Basal cells do not normally display a myoepithelial phenotype (87). They are negative for S-100 protein and smooth muscle actin and lack the ultrastructural features of myoepithelial cells (62,87).

In addition to secretory and basal epithelial cells, the prostate contains transitional cells which are usually confined, in conspicuous number, to the main prostatic ducts close to the prostatic urethra. A stratified layer of transitional cells with the typical oval to fusiform nuclei and nuclear grooves is usually covered by a layer of secretory cells. Transitional cells may be seen distant from the main ducts, presumably on a metaplastic basis, and may cause some diagnostic confusion, particularly if hyperplastic (see chapter 7).

Prostatic secretion is commonly present, at least focally, within the lumens of normal prostatic glands and has a light eosinophilic color in hematoxylin and eosin–stained specimens. It is periodic acid–Schiff (PAS) positive, diastase resistant, indicating that it contains neutral mucopolysaccharides (55,63). Neutral mucin may also be seen in prostatic adenocarcinoma and is not specific for benign glands. Acidic mucins (alcian blue positive, colloidal iron positive) are not usually found in normal or hyperplastic glands but are commonly found, at least focally, in prostatic adenocarcinoma (see chapter 4).

Corpora amylacea (fig. 1-14) are laminated luminal concretions that are commonly present in prostatic glands and increase in prevalence with advancing age (75,80,81). They are present in 25 percent of men as early as the third to fifth decades

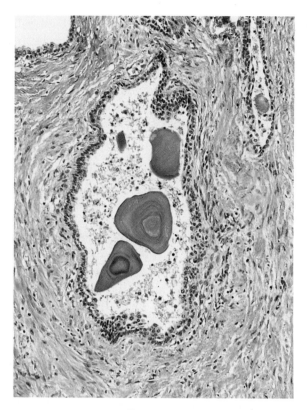

Figure 1-14
CORPORA AMYLACEA
Note the laminations.

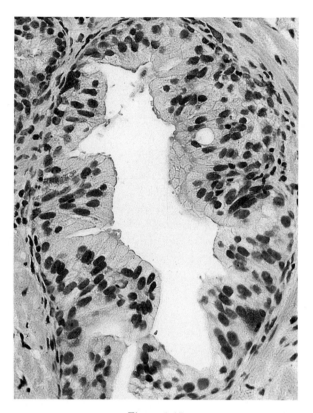

Figure 1-15
ARGENTAFFIN CELLS IN
NORMAL PROSTATE GLAND
The characteristic basal bright red cytoplasmic granules are evident in a few cells.

of life and are thought to be related to epithelial cell desquamation and degeneration (75).

The normal prostate gland contains a population of neuroendocrine cells that are occasionally visualized on routine light microscopy (fig. 1-15) (46,65). These argentaffin cells have a finely granular eosinophilic cytoplasm, the granularity being especially prominent in the basal aspect of the cell, and stain with silver stains. Argentaffin cells should be distinguished from a second cell type with granular eosinophilic cytoplasm that may be seen in the normal prostate and resembles the Paneth cells of the intestinal tract (fig. 1-16). Because of this resemblance, this phenomenon has been referred to as Paneth cell–like metaplasia (89,90). This change may be seen in hyperplastic and neoplastic, as well as normal, tissue. The Paneth-like cells differ from typical argentaffin cells by their large granule size, more intense eosinophilia, and often apical (juxtaluminal) distribution of the granules within individual cells (figs. 1-15, 1-16).

It is now recognized that prostatic epithelium commonly contains lipofuscin pigment (43,52,70). Lipofuscin pigment, which is characteristically found in wolffian duct derivatives including vas deferens, seminal vesicle, and ejaculatory duct (fig. 1-17) (45), usually has a granular, golden yellow appearance and may be present in the cytoplasm of prostatic epithelial cells (fig. 1-18, left) (see page 324). Some authors have found it more common in the central zone (70), but others have not (43). The amount of pigment is variable, but occasionally, large amounts are present in the epithelium similar to that seen in the seminal vesicles (see chapter 9). Accordingly, lipofuscin in glandular epithelium cannot be used as a criterion for origin from the seminal vesicle rather than the prostate. The pigment may be highlighted by special stains such as PAS, Masson Fontana, and modified Ziehl-Neelsen (fig. 1-18, right) and by fluorescence microscopy because of its autofluorescent nature (70). In some

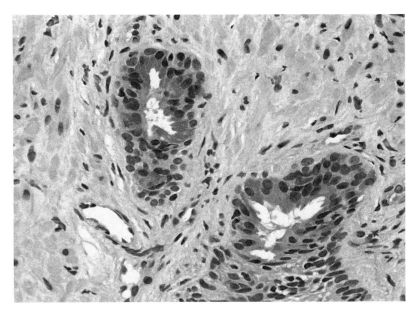

Figure 1-16
PANETH CELL-LIKE CHANGE
IN NORMAL PROSTATE
Two atrophic acini have abundant, slightly granular, eosinophilic cytoplasm.

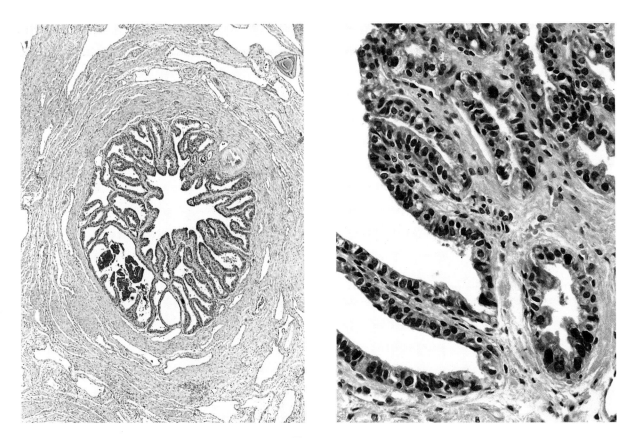

Figure 1-17
EJACULATORY DUCT
Ejaculatory duct in transverse section (left) and at high-power (right) magnification showing nuclear atypia of degenerative type and intracytoplasmic lipofuscin pigment.

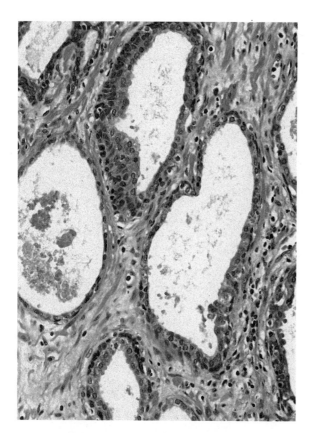 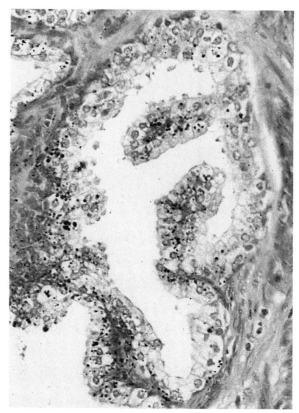

Figure 1-18
LIPOFUSCIN PIGMENT IN PROSTATIC EPITHELIUM
Left: Peripheral zone glands with yellow-brown pigment within the secretory cells in a hematoxylin and eosin–stained specimen. (Fig. 1 from Amin MB, Bostwick DG. Pigment in prostatic epithelium and adenocarcinoma: a potential source of diagnostic confusion with seminal vesicular epithelium. Mod Pathol 1996;9:791–5.)
Right: Prominent red pigmentation within the secretory cells of the prostatic central zone is seen with a modified Ziehl-Neelsen stain.

cases, the granules are gray-brown with a dark blue rim (52). Previous reports of epithelial melanosis in the prostate probably represent examples of lipofuscin in prostatic epithelium (57,58,69,84,85). Sometimes, aggregates of cells which contain melanin-like pigment may be seen within the prostatic stroma; these actually represent collections of lipofuscin-containing macrophages (fig. 1-19) (52).

True melanin pigment has been rarely documented in the prostate gland. It may be seen in spindled melanocytes and free in the stroma. This process has been referred to as prostatic blue nevus (48,64,72,88) (see chapter 7).

The prostatic ducts and acini are surrounded by stroma consisting of smooth muscle cells, fibroblasts, and undifferentiated spindle cells embedded in a matrix consisting of collagen and ground substance. Elastin fibers may also be found in this matrix and in the prostatic capsule. An extensive capillary network is present in the interstitium. Scattered lymphatics and nerve twigs may also be noted. Skeletal muscle is commonly found in the prostate gland, especially in the anterior fibromuscular stroma and apex (61, 67,73,77). Normal or hyperplastic glands may be intermingled with this skeletal muscle (fig. 1-8) and should not lead to their misinterpretation as neoplastic (see page 332).

Zonal Variations in Histology

There is variation in normal histology among the prostatic zones as described by McNeal (fig. 1-12) (76). Glands of the transition and peripheral zones have simple, rounded contours, with some gentle undulation of the luminal borders.

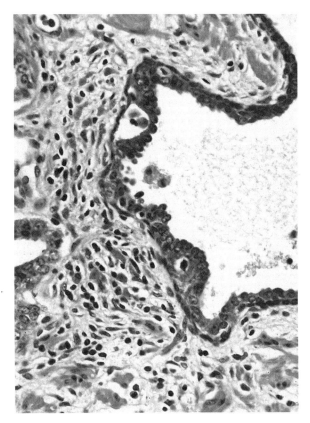

Figure 1-19
LIPOFUSCIN PIGMENT WITHIN
PROSTATIC STROMAL MACROPHAGES
(Fig. 2 from Amin MB, Bostwick DG. Pigment in prostatic epithelium and adenocarcinoma: a potential source of diagnostic confusion with seminal vesicular epithelium. Mod Pathol 1996;9:791–5.)

Glands of the central zone are larger and are often arranged in lobules around central ducts. Intraluminal ridges, epithelial arches, and papillary infoldings are common (fig. 1-12 B,C). The epithelium is often pseudostratified and frequently has granular rather than pale cytoplasm in contrast to secretory cells of other zones. The pseudostratification and intraluminal bridges with papillary infoldings are features of the central zone that overlap with those of benign hyperplasia (chapter 2) and prostatic intraepithelial neoplasia (chapter 3). Accordingly, central zone glands may be mistaken for hyperplasia or prostatic intraepithelial neoplasia, particularly the cribriform patterns thereof, especially in needle biopsies.

The stroma of the peripheral zone is loosely woven with randomly arranged smooth muscle bundles. Transition zone stroma consists of more compact, interlacing smooth muscle bundles which blend into the preprostatic sphincter and the anterior fibromuscular stroma (82). The stroma in the central zone is less abundant than in the other zones and is composed of compact smooth muscle fibers.

Histology of the Aging Prostate Gland

With advancing age the prostate gland is commonly involved by both atrophy and hyperplasia (54,71,79,81). The latter is discussed in chapter 2 and pseudoneoplastic aspects of the former in chapter 7.

Atrophy (figs. 1-20–1-22) is usually seen after the sixth decade of life but may be present, at least focally, from the third decade on (54,56). Atrophy associated with aging is generally diffuse and involves the peripheral zone. Focal atrophy involving the peripheral and transition zones may also be seen. The focal nature of atrophy relates to the lobular arrangement of the prostatic gland. Atrophy is characterized primarily by shrinkage of distal (terminal) ductules, acini, and surrounding stroma. This common pattern has been referred to as *simple* or *lobular atrophy* (fig. 1-20). The acini are typically small with narrow caliber lumens (fig. 1-21B,C) but may be dilated to varying degrees, with striking examples designated as *cystic atrophy* (fig. 1-22). Frequently, the stroma around the atrophic glands becomes fibrotic, and the glands appear more angulated and irregular (*sclerotic atrophy*) (fig. 1-21). This form of atrophy may represent the end result of chronic inflammation (fig. 1-21D) (76). In one study it was suggested that the atrophy of aging may be related to ischemia (47). Atrophy may also result from hormonal or radiation therapy. Diffuse atrophy affecting the peripheral zone often results in a marked reduction in the amount of peripheral tissue and may be characterized by a striking cystic appearance. Prominent cysts of the peripheral zone may, in some cases at least, result from obstruction due to nodular hyperplasia (see chapter 2). Distinction between this process and cystic atrophy is only of academic interest. Atrophy accounts for many of the cases in which a hypoechoic lesion on transrectal ultrasound is suspicious for carcinoma but is actually due to a benign process (60). Franks (54) and others have used the term

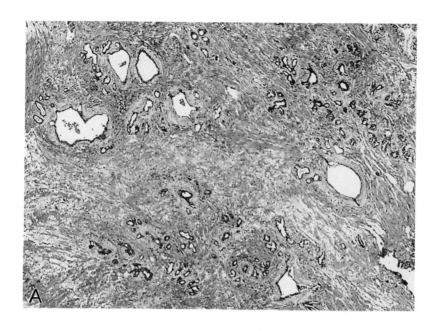

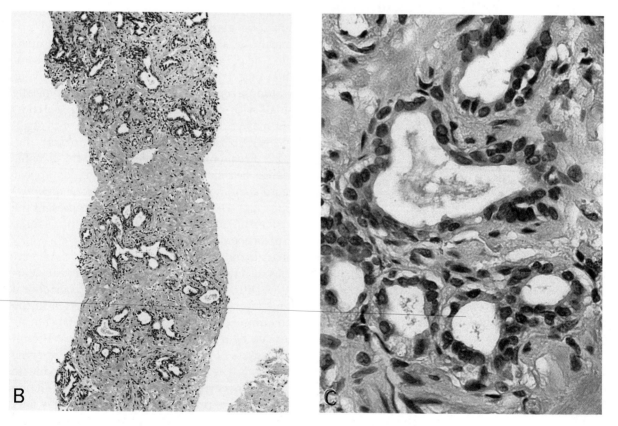

Figure 1-20
LOBULAR (SIMPLE) ATROPHY

Low-power views of prostatectomy (A) and needle biopsy (B) specimens show the typical lobular arrangement of atrophic acini, the narrow caliber of most of them, and dilatation of a minority. (C) A high-power view of the process in B shows the characteristic cuboidal cells of atrophy with scant cytoplasm and bland cytologic features.

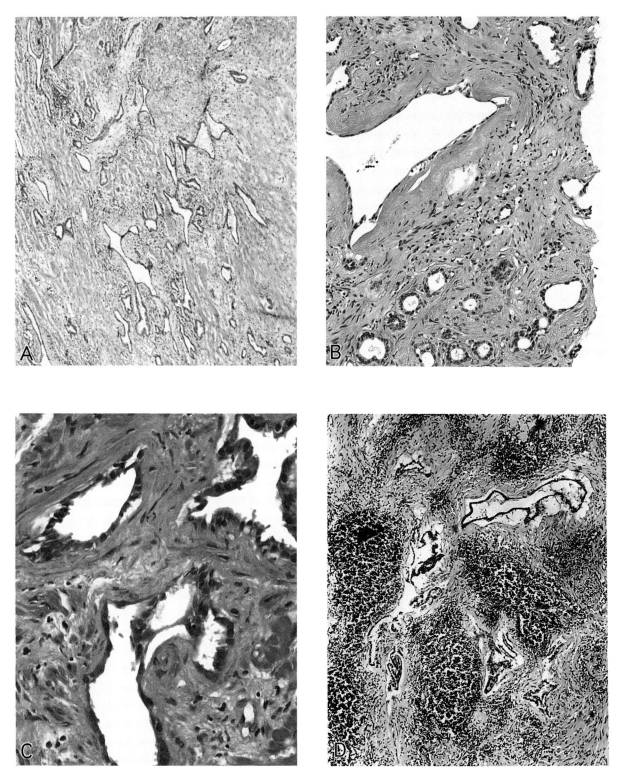

Figure 1-21
SCLEROTIC ATROPHY
Sharply angulated, hyperchromatic glands are lined by cells with scant cytoplasm and separated by a variably sclerotic stroma. Intense inflammation with lymphoid aggregates is present in D. (D: Fig. 5 from Franks LM. Atrophy and hyperplasia in the prostate proper. J Pathol Bacteriol 1954;68:617–21.)

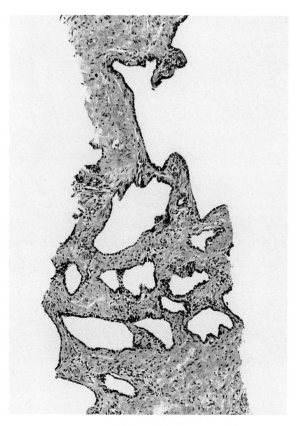

Figure 1-22
CYSTIC ATROPHY IN A NEEDLE BIOPSY

periglandular and intralobular stroma is shrunken, and intralobular smooth muscle cells may be inconspicuous. The amount of fibrous connective tissue is variable but may be excessive and dominate the histologic picture in cases of sclerotic atrophy. The resultant pattern often results in irregular glands, with cytologic features similar to simple atrophy, embedded in a sclerotic matrix. In large tissue sections, the diagnoses of simple and sclerotic atrophy, specifically their distinction from carcinoma, is usually straightforward. However in small biopsies, especially thin-core (18 gauge) samples, a lobular organization of the atrophic tissue may be inapparent, and the pathologist must rely on the character of individual glands and cells to distinguish atrophy from small acinar carcinoma (see chapter 7). With age the glands of the central zone also exhibit atrophic features, becoming less complex architecturally, somewhat stellate, and shrunken (76).

Immunohistochemical Features

The secretory cells lining ducts and acini stain with a variety of keratin antibodies including those directed at low molecular weight and broad spectrum cytokeratins (97,135,148,149). The staining pattern is usually intense and diffuse within the cytoplasm. The secretory cells are negative for high molecular weight cytokeratin (clone 34βE12) (see below).

The basal cells also stain with broad spectrum and low molecular weight keratins but, in addition, demonstrate positivity with antibodies against high molecular weight keratins, including cytokeratins 1, 5, 10, and 12 of the Moll catalogue. The antibody designated 34βE12 has specificity for high molecular weight cytokeratins and has been widely used to demonstrate prostatic basal cells (fig. 1-23) (97,112,132). Since the secretory cells are negative for these cytokeratins, basal cell–specific keratin staining with this antibody is important diagnostically (112,132). The complete absence of basal cells in an acinar proliferation is an important criterion of malignancy and useful in separating small acinar patterns of carcinoma from mimics such as atrophy, postatrophic hyperplasia, radiation-induced atypia, and atypical adenomatous hyperplasia. In many cases, the absence of basal cells is determined on routine

postatrophic hyperplasia to describe a form of atrophy with a component of hyperplasia (see chapters 2 and 7). More recently, others have used the terms "partial atrophy" (83) or "hyperplastic atrophy" (47) for lesions that, in our opinion, are essentially identical to postatrophic hyperplasia.

On low-power microscopy, atrophic glands usually appear organized, and even when somewhat crowded, there is a regular distribution of glands and stroma. The secretory cells of terminal ductules and acini are shrunken and display increased nuclear to cytoplasmic ratios and hyperchromasia. The basal cell layer is maintained. There is a lack of significant nuclear atypia, and nucleoli are inconspicuous. The lumens are usually empty but exceptionally contain a small amount of mucinous material. Very rarely, atrophic glands exhibit mucinous metaplasia (59,86). Occasionally, atrophic acini may show Paneth cell–like features (fig. 1-16). The

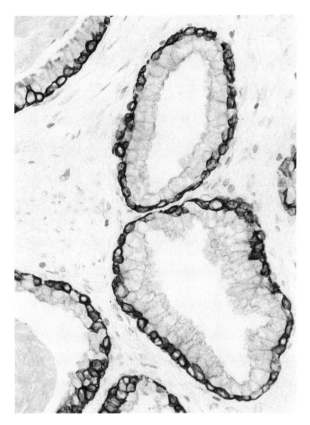

Figure 1-23
IMMUNOHISTOCHEMISTRY OF NORMAL PROSTATE
Basal cells stain with a basal cell–specific, high molecular weight cytokeratin (clone 34βE12). The secretory cells are negative.

microscopy, but in difficult interpretations a high molecular weight cytokeratin stain may be required. The basal cell staining may be widespread and continuous as one often sees in atrophy, or patchy and discontinuous, the usual pattern in atypical adenomatous hyperplasia.

The normal prostatic epithelium may also show focal staining for vimentin (149). The prostatic stromal cells may be highlighted with antibodies against vimentin, desmin, pan-muscle actin, and smooth muscle actin.

Prostate-Specific Antigen

Following the historic discovery in 1979 of a glycoprotein specific to the prostate, the serum ranges (131) and tissue distribution of prostate-specific antigen (PSA) have been extensively studied (91,109,128,133,141,145,149). PSA is absent in prepubertal prostatic glands and appears at the

time of puberty (109). Polyclonal and monoclonal antibodies directed against this antigen usually reveal diffuse and strong positivity in the secretory cells of normal and hyperplastic glands. The basal cells show little or no PSA staining. Glandular epithelia from all prostatic zones stain with PSA. Most adenocarcinomas display positivity with PSA antibodies, although there is considerable intertumoral and intratumoral variation in extent and intensity (see chapter 4). The epithelium of seminal vesicles and ejaculatory ducts and the transitional epithelium of the prostatic urethra and periurethral ducts are negative for PSA. PSA staining has been noted in the periurethral glands in both males and females, the anal glands in males, urachal remnants, and cystitis cystica and glandularis of the urinary bladder (102,107,110,114,130,134,143). Furthermore, extraprostatic tumors including urethral and bladder adenocarcinoma, extramammary Paget's disease of the penis, some gastrointestinal adenocarcinomas, mature teratomas, and salivary gland pleomorphic adenomas and carcinomas in males may be PSA positive (99,137,139,144).

Prostatic Acid Phosphatase

The clinical importance of prostatic acid phosphatase in the diagnosis and follow-up of patients with metastatic adenocarcinoma of the prostate gland was established in 1938 (111), but has been supplanted by serum PSA as a prostatic tumor marker (122). The histochemical assessment of prostatic acid phosphatase is limited because it is identified in a variety of normal tissues and neoplasms of nonprostatic origin (95,117). An isoenzyme of acid phosphatase specific to the prostate gland was discovered in 1970 (126). Subsequent developments in immunohistochemistry allowed this marker, prostatic-specific acid phosphatase (PAP), to be studied in formalin-fixed, paraffin-embedded tissues (127). PAP is found in normal and hyperplastic prostate glands and also in most prostatic adenocarcinomas (127). Antibodies to PAP and PSA are useful in the investigation of adenocarcinomas of unknown origin and in poorly differentiated carcinomas of the lower genitourinary tract where the differential diagnosis includes prostatic adenocarcinoma and urothelial carcinoma (113,119–121,129,142). PAP is not

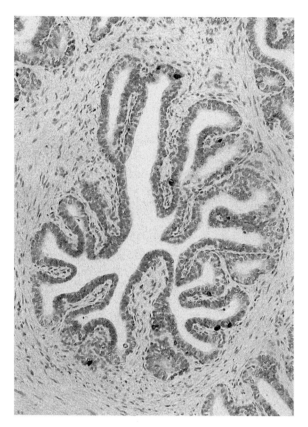

Figure 1-24
NORMAL PROSTATE GLAND SHOWING
SCATTERED CHROMOGRANIN-POSITIVE CELLS

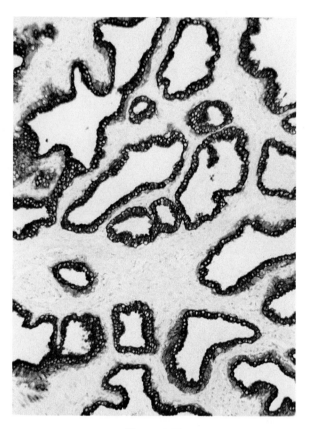

Figure 1-25
CD57 (LEU-7) POSITIVITY IN PROSTATE GLAND
Note the strong staining of secretory cells similar to that seen with prostate-specific antigen and prostatic acid phosphatase immunostains.

entirely specific for prostatic tissue and may be detected in pancreatic islet cells, parietal cells of stomach, hepatocytes, and some renal tubular cells. Furthermore, pancreatic islet cell tumor, mammary carcinoma, adenocarcinoma of the bladder, cloacogenic carcinoma of the anus, mature teratoma, gastrointestinal carcinoid tumor, and pleomorphic adenoma and carcinoma of the salivary glands in males may display PAP staining (98,99,103–105,116,138,144).

Neuroendocrine and Other Immunohistochemical Markers

The neuroendocrine nature of the argentaffin cells of the normal prostate (see page 12) that are recognizable on routine preparations is confirmed if immunohistochemical stains such as neuron-specific enolase, chromogranin, and synaptophysin are performed; they also often demonstrate a more plentiful number of neuroendocrine cells than is appreciable by routine light micros-

copy (fig. 1-24). A variety of specific hormones have been identified in these cells including serotonin and calcitonin- and bombesin-like proteins (101). Neuroendocrine cells likely arise through differentiation of the prostate epithelium rather than migration of cells of neural crest origin (94). They probably serve a regulatory role in prostate growth and function through both neuroendocrine and paracrine mechanisms (100,101).

The Paneth-like cells in the non-neoplastic prostate do not usually stain with neuroendocrine markers, in contrast to what is seen in cancer (92) (see page 153), but do stain for lysosomal markers (146,147).

In 1985 it was recognized that the anti-CD57 antibody (Leu-7), a marker of natural killer lymphocytes, stains both normal and hyperplastic prostate tissue (fig. 1-25) (136). Subsequently, CD57 was identified in most prostatic adenocarcinomas

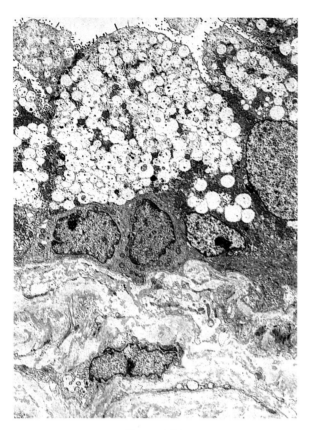

Figure 1-26
WALL OF PROSTATIC ACINUS

Note the secretory cells with abundant apical vacuoles and granules. These are surrounded by smaller and darker basal cells with cytoplasm containing tonofilaments. At the bottom, prostatic stromal cells lie within ground substance and collagen.

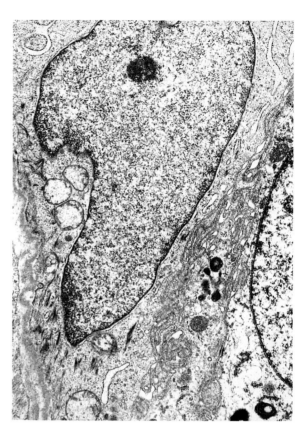

Figure 1-27
PROSTATIC BASAL CELL RESTING ON DELICATE BASAL LAMINA

Note the collections of tonofilaments within the cytoplasm of the basal cell. Part of a secretory cell is seen at the right. Note the occasional cytoplasmic granules.

and, like PSA and PAP, it often shows considerable intratumoral heterogeneity. Anti-CD57 is of value in a panel of prostatic markers, especially when the others yield negative or equivocal results (125). Prostatic secretory cells stain with antibodies against epithelial membrane antigen and carcinoembryonic antigen (93,108). The latter marker is usually found along the luminal aspect of the secretory cells and also within the luminal contents.

Ultrastructural Features

The secretory compartment of the prostatic acinus consists of columnar cells with abundant apical cytoplasm joined together by tight junctional complexes and desmosomes (fig. 1-26) (96,106, 115,140). The basally located nuclei are round and oval, and have evenly distributed euchroma-

tin with occasional chromocenters. The cytoplasm contains a variety of organelles including mitochondria, endoplasmic reticulum, and Golgi apparatus. There are usually abundant secretory type vacuoles within the apical cytoplasm in addition to lysosomes and lipid droplets. Some vacuoles contain electron dense bodies. Electron dense bodies containing acid phosphatase activity have been noted using immunoultrastructural techniques (124). The luminal surfaces of secretory cells contain small microvilli, and small subplasmalemmal vesicles may be found.

The secretory cells rest on a basal cell layer which is generally, but not always, continuous (fig. 1-27) (123). The basal cells sit directly on a delicate, electron dense basement membrane, 0.07 to 0.10 μm thick. They are usually oval and attenuated but may be cuboidal, and are oriented

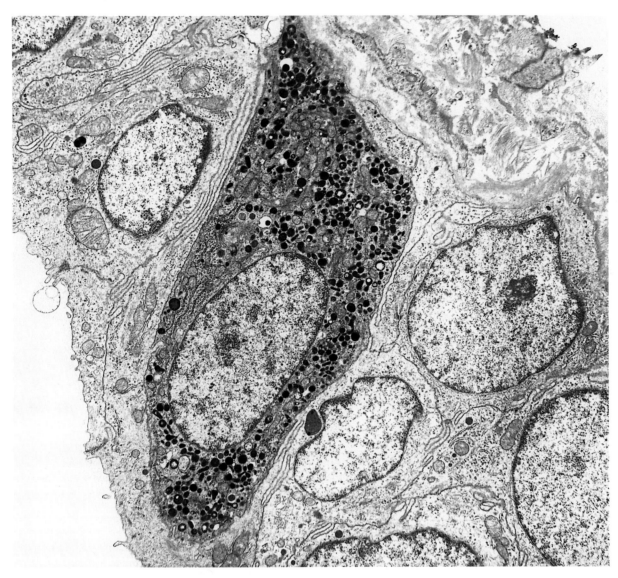

Figure 1-28
NORMAL PROSTATIC NEUROENDOCRINE CELL
Note abundant, darkly staining dense core granules within the cytoplasm of the cell in the center. Adjacent basal and secretory cells are seen. (Courtesy of Dr. P.A. di Sant'Agnese, Rochester, NY.)

perpendicular to the long axis of the secretory cells. The basal cells embrace a number of overlying secretory cells to which they are joined by small desmosomes. Their nuclei are round to oval and have evenly distributed, fine chromatin and usually inconspicuous nucleoli. The cytoplasm contains some mitochondria, rough endoplasmic reticulum, and ribosomes. Tonofilament-like collections of intermediate filaments may occasionally be seen, correlating with the high molecular weight keratin staining noted by immunohisto-

chemistry. Neuroendocrine cells, containing dense core granules of various sizes and shapes, are closely apposed to adjacent secretory and basal cells and usually rest on the basement membrane (fig. 1-28).

The normal prostatic stroma consists mainly of smooth muscle cells with typical ultrastructural morphology including serrated nuclei, abundant cytoplasmic thin filaments (6 to 8 nm), dense bodies, subplasmalemmal attachment plaques, and occasional micropinocytotic vesicles. Typical fibroblasts with well-developed rough endoplasmic reticulum and uncommitted mesenchymal cells are also seen. The stromal cells lie in a matrix of ground substance and collagen bundles. Skeletal muscle cells with a typical sarcomeric structure may also be seen, especially in tissue from the apical and anterior portions of the gland.

Physiology

The prostatic exocrine secretion forms a significant component of seminal fluid (153,160,164). Several biochemical components of prostatic fluid have been identified, but their specific roles in the maintenance of spermatozoa and fertilization are not well understood (154,164). There is a continuous basal flow of prostatic fluid even in the absence of ejaculation (157). This output has been estimated at 0.5 to 2.0 ml per day and during ejaculation an additional volume of 0.5 to 1.0 ml is produced (156). Prostatic secretion is partly apocrine in nature. Among its main components are acid phosphatase and citric acid (153,154,158,160,164). A number of proteolytic enzymes have also been identified including fibrinolysin, fibrinogenase, and aminopeptidase (154, 162). These enzymes may be involved in the liquification of coagulated human semen. Additionally, prostaglandin F2α, produced by prostate epithelium, is found in the seminal plasma (154). Prostaglandin F2α increases the binding of testosterone in vitro and stimulates cyclic adenosine monophosphate (AMP)-dependent secretion of some intracellular material. It increases motility of the fibromuscular stroma, thus facilitating the excretion of acinar fluid into the seminal pool (154). Prostatic secretion is controlled in part by sympathetic and parasympathetic stimulation resulting in contraction of stromal smooth muscle fibers (154).

Zinc has been found in very high concentrations in the human prostate gland (152,159,160). The overall zinc content, uptake, and excretion appear to be under hormonal regulation (155). The specific role of zinc in the physiology and pathology of the prostate gland is not understood.

The prostate gland is under complex hormonal regulation involving the hypothalamic-hypophyseal-testicular axis (fig. 1-29) (153,162). It is widely believed that both normal and abnormal growth of prostatic tissue is dependant upon testicular hormones (160). Prepubertal orchiectomy prevents the development of both hyperplasia and carcinoma (160,162). Testicular androgens control the differentiation of the prostate gland during embryogenesis and its maturation at puberty. Androgens are responsible for the maintenance of the integrity of the adult gland (160).

Although, the main circulating androgen is testosterone, the active intracellular hormone is dihydrotestosterone (DHT) (151). About 90 percent of the free testosterone is metabolized to DHT by the action of the enzyme 5-α-reductase (150,163). This enzyme is located in the endoplasmic reticulum and the nuclear membrane of prostatic secretory cells. After binding to a cytosolic androgen receptor, DHT is transported to the nucleus where the DHT receptor complex interacts with nucleic acid to induce RNA, protein synthesis, and cell replication (154). Although the testis is the main source of androgens, the adrenal gland also produces androgens, although these are thought to play little role in human prostatic growth (159a,160,161).

There are alterations in hormonal production with advancing age (160,162,163). These changes may be responsible for creating an abnormal milieu resulting in the development of proliferative diseases such as hyperplasia and carcinoma (160). The following hormonal changes have been noted with advancing age: 1) decrease in the total and free testosterone level; 2) increase in levels of luteinizing hormone; and 3) increase in estradiol levels (160).

The interrelations among the hypothalamus, pituitary gland, testis, adrenal gland, and prostate are complex, and a number of pharmacologic agents have been used to interfere with various pathways. Steroidal and nonsteroidal antiandrogens and 5-α-reductase inhibitors have been used to treat benign prostatic hyperplasia. Antiestrogen drugs have also been used in treating hyperplasia since estrogens are known to stimulate prolactin secretion which increases prostate growth. Furthermore, a variety of antiandrogens have also been used to treat advanced-stage adenocarcinoma and more recently as neoadjuvants prior to radiotherapy and radical prostatectomy for localized disease. Their effects on neoplastic tissue are described in chapter 4.

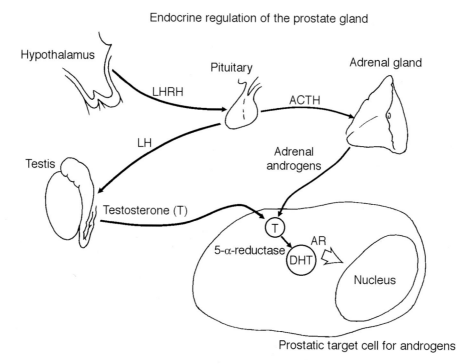

Figure 1-29
ENDOCRINE REGULATION OF THE PROSTATE GLAND
Note the hypothalamic and pituitary control over testicular and adrenal androgens. Testosterone is converted into dihydro-testosterone within the prostatic cell by 5-α-reductase. Dihyrotestosterone binds to the androgen receptor which is transported into the nucleus. (LHRH - Luteinizing hormone releasing hormone; ACTH - adrenal corticotrophic hormone; LH - luteinizing hormone, T - testosterone; DHT - dihydrotestosterone; AR - androgen receptor.)

CLASSIFICATION OF PROSTATIC HYPERPLASIA, TUMORS, AND TUMOR-LIKE LESIONS

The surgical pathology of the prostate gland primarily concerns the diagnosis of carcinoma and its distinction from the various processes that may mimic it, and additionally, the recognition of possible or probable premalignant lesions. Knowledge of the spectrum of prostatic hyperplasia is important because some of the patterns that may mimic neoplasia occur within this category. Benign neoplasms are rare and are usually of mesenchymal origin. True papillomas and adenomas of glandular epithelial origin are almost unheard of. Occasional dominant hyperplastic nodules, composed mainly of secretory or basal epithelium, have been referred to as giant adenoma and basal cell adenoma, respectively. These lesions are usually found in the setting of ordinary nodular hyperplasia or basal cell hyperplasia and probably do not represent true adenomas in the traditional sense of the word. In view of the rarity of benign neoplasms and the frequency and importance of hyperplasias and atypical proliferations of the prostate, these latter processes will be discussed first. Most prostatic neoplasms are derived from glandular epithelium. Some uncommon cancers, such as transitional cell and squamous cell carcinoma of the prostate, likely arise from epithelia of larger ducts. Tumors may potentially derive from the neuroendocrine cells of the prostate, although it is usually not possible in these situations to determine whether the neoplasm actually arose primarily from a neuroendocrine cell population or simply exhibits neuroendocrine differentiation. Mesenchymal tumors often exhibit a muscle phenotype reflecting the high content of muscle cells in the prostatic stroma. Other primary and secondary neoplasms are distinctly uncommon. The classification of prostatic hyperplasia, tumors, and tumor-like lesions used in this Fascicle is shown in Table 1-1. Expanded subclassifications of certain entities are presented in the subsequent chapters.

Table 1-1

CLASSIFICATION OF PROSTATIC HYPERPLASIA, TUMORS, AND TUMOR-LIKE LESIONS

Hyperplasia
Benign nodular hyperplasia
Basal cell hyperplasia
Postatrophic hyperplasia
Atypical adenomatous hyperplasia (adenosis)

Benign Epithelial Tumors
Adenoma
Multilocular cystadenoma

Prostatic Intraepithelial Neoplasia

Conventional Adenocarcinoma

Special Variants of Adenocarcinoma and Other Carcinomas
Prostatic duct adenocarcinoma
Mucinous (colloid) adenocarcinoma
Signet ring cell carcinoma
Adenosquamous carcinoma
Squamous cell carcinoma
Basaloid and adenoid cystic carcinoma
Transitional cell carcinoma
Small cell carcinoma
Sarcomatoid carcinoma
Lymphoepithelioma-like carcinoma
Undifferentiated carcinoma, not otherwise specified

Mixed Tumors
Epithelial-stromal tumor, not otherwise specified (phyllodes tumor)
Carcinosarcoma

Mesenchymal Tumors
Benign
Leiomyoma
Fibroma
Hemangioma
Other
Malignant
Rhabdomyosarcoma
Leiomyosarcoma
Stromal sarcoma
Other

Other Tumors
Hematolymphoid neoplasms
Lymphoma
Leukemia
Plasmacytoma
Paraganglioma
Germ cell tumors
Wilms' tumor

Secondary Tumors

Tumor-Like Lesions*
Atrophy
Postatrophic hyperplasia
Sclerosing adenosis**
Cribriform hyperplasia**
Mesonephric remnant hyperplasia
Nephrogenic adenoma of prostatic urethra
Squamous metaplasia
Transitional cell metaplasia/hyperplasia
Basal cell hyperplasia and variants
Prostatitis
Malakoplakia
Reactive atypia
Radiation atypia
Postoperative spindle cell nodule
Inflammatory pseudotumor (pseudosarcomatous fibromyxoid tumor)
Atypical stromal cells
Melanosis (including blue nevus)
Endometriosis
Seminal vesicle/ejaculatory duct, Cowper's glands, and paraganglia in prostate samples
Verumontanum mucosal gland hyperplasia
Mucinous metaplasia
Benign glands adjacent to nerves and in skeletal muscle
Cysts
Amyloidosis
Calculi/Calcification/Cartilage
(Ectopic prostatic tissue)

*Processes categorized under hyperplasia may also be tumor-like.
**These processes occur in the context of nodular hyperplasia but have particular tumor-like aspects.

REFERENCES

Introduction

1. Dixon FJ, Moore RA. Tumors of the male sex organs. Atlas of Tumor Pathology, 1st Series, Fascicle. Washington D.C.: Armed Forces Institute of Pathology, 1952.

2. Mostofi FK, Price EB Jr. Tumors of the male genital system. Atlas of Tumor Pathology, 2nd series, Fascicle 8. Washington, D.C.: Armed Forces Institute of Pathology, 1973.

Anatomy

3. Arey LB. Developmental anatomy. A textbook and laboratory manual of embryology. 7th ed. Philadelphia: WB Saunders, 1974:328.

4. Ayala AG, Ro JY, Babaian R, Troncoso P, Grignon DJ. The prostatic capsule: does it exist? Its importance in the staging and treatment of prostatic carcinoma. Am J Surg Pathol 1989;13:21–7.

5. Bannister LH, Dyson M. Reproductive system. In: Williams PL, Bannister LH, Berry MM, et al, eds. Gray's anatomy. The anatomical basis of medicine and surgery, 38th ed. New York: Churchill Livingstone, 1995:1847–80.

6. Berry SJ, Coffey DS, Walsh PC, Ewing LL. Human benign prostatic hyperplasia with age. J Urol 1984;132:474–9.

7. Carstens PH. Perineural glands in normal and hyperplastic prostates. J Urol 1980;123:686–8.

8. Clegg EJ. The vascular arrangements within the human prostate gland. Br J Urol 1956;28:428–35.

9. Cohen RJ, Stables S. Intraprostatic fat [Letter]. Hum Pathol 1998;29:424–5.

10. Connolly JG, Thomson A, Jewett MA, Hartman N, Webber M. Intraprostatic lymphatics. Invest Urol 1968;5:371–8.

11. Flocks RH. Arterial distribution within the prostate gland: its role in transurethral prostatic resection. In: Nesbit RM, ed. Transurethral prostatectomy. Springfield, IL: Charles C Thomas, Springfield, Illinois, 1943:3.

12. Franks LM. Atrophy and hyperplasia in the prostate proper. J Pathol Bacteriol 1954;68:627–31.

13. Franks LM. Benign nodular hyperplasia of the prostate: a review. Ann R Coll Surg Engl 1954;14:92–106.

14. Franks LM. Benign prostatic hyperplasia: gross and microscopic anatomy. In: Grayhack JT, Wilson JD, Scherbenske MJ, eds. Benign prostatic hyperplasia. Department of Health, Education and Welfare (NIH) Publication #76-1113 1976:63–89.

15. Freedman SR, Goldman RL. Normal paraganglia in the human prostate. J Urol 1975;113:874–5.

16. Glenister TW. The development of the utricle and of the so-called "middle" or "median" lobe of the human prostate. J Anat 1962;96:443–55.

17. Huggins C, Webster WO. Duality of the human prostate in response to oestrogens. J Urol 1948;59:258.

18. Lepor H, Gregerman M, Crosby R, Mostofi FK, Walsh PC. Precise localization of the autonomic nerves from the pelvic plexus to the corpora cavernosa: a detailed anatomical study of the adult male pelvis. J Urol 1985;133:207–12.

19. Leung CS, Srigley JR. Distribution of lipochrome pigment in the prostate gland: biological and diagnostic implications. Hum Pathol 1995;26:1302–7.

20. Lowsley OS. The development of the human prostate gland with reference to the development of other structures at the neck of the urinary bladder. Am J Anat 1912;13:299–346.

21. Lowsley OS. The prostate gland. In: Lowsley OS, Hinman F, Smith DR, Gutierrez R, eds. The sexual glands of the male. New York: Oxford University Press, 1942.

22. McNeal JE. Development and comparative anatomy of the prostate. In: Grayhack J, Wilson J, Schereenske M, eds. Benign prostatic hyperplasia. DHEW (NIH) #76-1113, Washington, DC. 1976.

23. McNeal JE. Normal histology of the prostate. Am J Surg Pathol 1988;12:619–33.

24. McNeal JE. The prostate and prostatic urethra: a morphologic synthesis. J Urol 1972;107:1008–16.

25. McNeal JE. Regional morphology and pathology of the prostate. Am J Clin Pathol 1968;49:347–57.

26. McNeal JE. The zonal anatomy of the prostate. Prostate 1981;2:35–49.

27. McNeal JE, Leav I, Alroy J, Skutelsky E. Differential lectin staining of central and peripheral zones of the prostate and alterations in dysplasia. Am J Clin Pathol 1988;89:41–8.

28. McNeal JE, Villers AA, Redwine ER, Freiha FS, Stamey TA. Capsular penetration in prostate cancer. Significance for natural history and treatment. Am J Surg Pathol 1990;14:240–7.

28a. Myers RP, Goellner JR, Cahill DR. Prostate shape, external striated urethral sphincter and radical prostatectomy: the apical dissection. J Urol 1987;138:543–50.

29. Narbaitz R. Embryology, anatomy and histology of the male accessory gland. In: Brandes D, ed. Male accessory sex organs: structure and function in mammals. New York: Academic Press, 1974:3.

30. Ohori M, Egawa S, Wheeler TM. Nodules resembling nodular hyperplasia in the peripheral zone of the prostate gland. J Urol Pathol 1994;2:223–34.

31. Oppenheimer JR, Wills ML, Epstein JI. Partial atrophy in prostate needle cores: another diagnostic pitfall for the surgical pathologist. Am J Surg Pathol 1998;22:440–5.

32. Ostrowski ML, Wheeler TM. Paraganglia of the prostate. Location, frequency and differentiation from prostatic adenocarcinoma. Am J Surg Pathol 1994;18:412–20.

33. Rytina AG. The verumontanum, with special reference to the sinus pocularis: its anatomy, histology, and physiology. J Urol 1917;1:231–43.

34. Sakr WA, Haas GP, Cassin BF, Pontes JE, Crissman JD. The frequency of carcinoma and intraepithelial neoplasia of the prostate in young male patients. J Urol 1993;150:379–85.

35. Sattar AA, Noel JC, Vanderhaeghen JJ, Schulman CC, Wespes E. Prostate capsule: computerized morphometric analysis of its components. Urology 1995;46:178–81.

36. Spring-Mills E, Krall A. Functional anatomy of the prostate. In: Hafez ES, Spring-Mills E, eds. Prostate carcinoma, biology and diagnosis. The Hague: Martinus Nijhoff, 1981:5.

37. Tanagho EA. Anatomy of the lower urinary tract. In: Walsh PC, Retik AB, Stamey TA, Vaughan ED Jr, eds. Campbell's urology, 6th ed., Philadelphia: WB Saunders, 1992:40–69.

38. Teem MV. Size and weight of the normal and of the pathologic prostate gland. Arch Pathol 1936;22:817–22.

39. Tisell LE, Salander H. The lobes of the human prostate. Scand J Urol Nephrol 1975;9:185–91.

40. Tisell LE, Salander H. Anatomy of the human prostate and its three paired lobes. In: New approaches to the study of benign prostatic hyperplasia. New York: Alan R. Liss Inc, 1984:55–65.

41. Vaalasti A, Hervonen A. Autonomic innervation of the human prostate. Invest Urol 1980;17:293–7.

42. Warren S, Harris PN, Graves RC. Osseous metastasis of carcinoma of the prostate with specific reference to the perineural lymphatics. Arch Pathol 1936;22:139–60.

Histology

43. Amin MB, Bostwick DG. Pigment in prostatic epithelium and adenocarcinoma: a potential source of diagnostic confusion with seminal vesicular epithelium. Mod Pathol 1996;9:791–5.

44. Andrews GS. The histology of the human, foetal and prepubertal prostates. J Anat 1951;85:44–54.

45. Arias-Stella J, Takano-Moron J. Atypical epithelial changes in the seminal vesicles. Arch Pathol 1958;66:761–6.

46. Azzopardi JG, Evans DJ. Argentaffin cells in prostatic carcinoma: differentiation from lipofuscin and melanin in prostatic epithelium. J Pathol 1971;104:247–51.

47. Billis A. Prostatic atrophy: an autopsy study of a histologic mimic of adenocarcinoma. Mod Pathol 1998;11:47–54.

48. Block NL, Weber D, Schinella R. Blue nevi and other melanotic lesions of the prostate: report of 3 cases and review of the literature. J Urol 1972;107:85–7.

49. Bonkhoff H, Stein U, Remberger K. Multidirectional differentiation in the normal, hyperplastic and neoplastic prostate. Simultaneous demonstration of cell-specific epithelial markers. Hum Pathol 1994;25:42–6.

50. Bonkhoff H, Stein U, Remberger K. The proliferative function of basal cells in the normal and hyperplastic human prostate. Prostate 1994; 24:114–8.

51. Brandes D, Bourne GH. Histochemistry of the human prostate gland: normal and neoplastic. J Pathol Bacteriol 1956;71:33–6.

52. Brennick JB, O'Connell JX, Dickersin GR, Pilch BZ, Young RH. Lipofuscin pigmentation (so-called "melanosis") of the prostate. Am J Surg Pathol 1994;18:446–54.

53. Evans GS, Chandler JA. Cell proliferation studies in the rat prostate. I. The proliferative role of basal and secretory epithelial cells during normal growth. Prostate 1987;10:163–78.

54. Franks LM. Atrophy and hyperplasia in the prostate proper. J Pathol Bacteriol 1954;68:617.

55. Franks LM, O'Shea JD, Thomson AE. Mucin in the prostate: a histochemical study in normal glands, latent, clinical and colloid cancers. Cancer 1964;17:983–91.

56. Gardner WA Jr, Culberson DE. Atrophy and proliferation in the young adult prostate. J Urol 1987;137:53–6.

57. Gardner WA Jr, Spitz WU. Melanosis of the prostate gland. Am J Clin Pathol 1971;56:762-4.

58. Goldman RL. Melanogenic epithelium in the prostate gland. Am J Clin Pathol 1968;80:49:75–8.

59. Grignon DJ, O'Malley FP. Mucinous metaplasia in the prostate gland. Am J Surg Pathol 1993;17:287–90.

60. Hampers UM, Sheth S, Walsh PC, Holtz PM, Epstein JI. Stage B adenocarcinoma of the prostate: transrectal US and pathologic correlation of nonmalignant hypoechoic peripheral zone lesions. Radiology 1991;180:101–4.

61. Hasui Y, Shinkawa T, Osada Y, Sumiyoshi A. Striated muscle in the biopsy specimen of the prostate. Prostate 1989;14:65–9.

62. Howat AJ, Mills PM, Lyons TJ, Stephenson TJ. Absence of S-100 protein in prostatic glands. Histopathology 1988;13:468–70.

63. Hukill PB, Vidone RA. Histochemistry of mucus and other polysaccharides in tumors: II. Carcinoma of the prostate. Lab Invest 1967;16:395–406.

64. Jao W, Fretzin DF, Christ ML, Prinz LM. Blue nevus of the prostate gland. Arch Pathol 1971;91:187–91.

65. Kazzaz BA. Argentaffin and argyrophil cells in the prostate. J Pathol 1974;112:189–93.

66. Kircheim D, Gyorkey F, Brandes D, Scott WW. Histochemistry of the normal, hyperplastic and neoplastic human prostate. Invest Urol 1964;1:403–21.

67. Kost LV, Evans GW. Occurrence and significance of striated muscle within the prostate. J Urol 1964;92:703–4.

68. Kovi J. Surgical pathology of prostate and seminal vesicles. Boca Raton: CRC Press, 1989:5–7.

69. Langley JW, Weitzner S. Blue nevus and melanosis of prostate. J Urol 1974;112:359–61.

70. Leung CS, Srigley JR. Distribution of lipochrome pigment in the prostate gland: biological and diagnostic implications. Hum Pathol 1995;26:1302–7.

71. Liavag I. Atrophy and regeneration in the pathogenesis of prostatic carcinoma. Acta Pathol Microbiol Scand 1968;73:338–50.

72. Lippert MC, Bensimon H, Javadpour N. Immunoperoxidase staining of acid phosphatase in human prostatic tissue. J Urol 1982;128:1114–6.

73. Manley CB Jr. The striated muscle of the prostate. J Urol 1966;95:234–40.

74. Mann T. Biochemistry of semen. In: Greep RO, Astwood EB, eds. Handbook of physiology. Male reproductive system, Vol 5. Baltimore: Williams & Wilkins, 1975:461.

75. Marx AJ, Gueft B, Moskal JF. Prostatic corpora amylacea. A study with the electron microscope and electron probe. Arch Pathol 1965;80:487–94.

76. McNeal JE. Normal histology of the prostate. Am J Surg Pathol 1988;12:619–33.

77. McNeal JE. The prostate and prostatic urethra: a morphologic synthesis. J Urol 1972;107:1008–16.

78. Montironi R, Bostwick DG, Bonkhoff H, et al. Origins of prostate cancer. Cancer 1996;78:362–5.

79. Moore RA. The evolution and involution of the prostate gland. J Urol 1948;60:599–624.

80. Moore RA. Morphology of prostatic corpora amylacea and calculi. Arch Pathol 1936;22:24–40.

81. Moore RA, Hanzel RF. Chemical composition of prostatic corpora amylacea and calculi. Arch Pathol 1936;22:41–54.

82. Myers RP, Goellner JR, Cahill DR. Prostate shape, external striated urethral sphincter and radical prostatectomy: the apical dissection. J Urol 1987;138:543–50.

83. Oppenheimer JR, Wills ML, Epstein JI. Partial atrophy in prostate needle cores: another diagnostic pitfall for the surgical pathologist. Am J Surg Pathol 1998;22:440–5.

84. Rios CN, Wright JR. Melanosis of the prostate gland: report of a case with neoplastic epithelium involvement. J Urol 1976;115:616–7.

85. Ro JY, Grignon DJ, Ayala AG, Hogan SF, Tetu B, Ordonez NG. Blue nevus and melanosis of the prostate. Electron-microscopic and immunohistochemical studies. Am J Clin Pathol 1988;90:530–5.

86. Shiraishi T, Kusano I, Watanabe M, Yatani R, Liu PI. Mucous gland metaplasia of the prostate. Am J Surg Pathol 1993;17:618–22.

87. Srigley JR, Dardick I, Hartwick RW, Klotz L. Basal epithelial cells of human prostate gland are not myoepithelial cells. A comparative immunohistochemical and ultrastructural study with human salivary gland. Am J Pathol 1990;136:957–66.

88. Tannenbaum M. Differential diagnosis in uropathology. III. Melanotic lesions of the prostate: blue nevus and prostatic epithelial melanosis. Urology 1974;4:617–21.

89. Weaver MG, Abdul-Karim FW, Srigley JR. Paneth cell-like change and small cell carcinoma of the prostate. Two divergent forms of prostatic neuroendocrine differentiation. Am J Surg Pathol 1992;16:1013–6.

90. Weaver MG, Abdul-Karim FW, Srigley JR, Bostwick DG, Ro JY, Ayala AG. Paneth cell-like change of the prostate gland: a histological, immunohistochemical and electron microscopic study. Am J Surg Pathol 1992;16:62–8.

Immunohistochemical and Ultrastructural Studies

91. Allhoff EP, Proppe KH, Chapman CM, Lin CW, Prout GR Jr. Evaluation of prostate specific acid phosphatase and prostate specific antigen in identification of prostatic cancer. J Urol 1983;129:315–8.

92. Almagro UA, Tieu TM, Remeniuk E, Kueck B, Strumpf K. Argyrophilic, "carcinoid-like" prostatic carcinoma. An immunocytochemical study. Arch Pathol Lab Med 1986;110:916–9.

93. Aumuller G, Krause W, Bischof W, Seitz J. Carcinoembryonic antigen-like substance is a marker of prostatic secretory function. Andrologia 1983;15(2):159–63.

94. Azumi N, Shibuya H, Ishikura M. Primary prostatic carcinoid tumor with intracytoplasmic prostatic acid phosphatase and prostate-specific antigen. Am J Surg Pathol 1984;8:545–50.

95. Brandes D, Bourne GH. Histochemistry of the human prostate gland: normal and neoplastic. J Pathol Bacteriol 1956;71:33–6.

96. Brandes D, Kirchheim D, Scott WW. Ultrastructure of the human prostate: normal and neoplastic. Lab Invest 1964;13:1541–60.

97. Brawer MK, Peehl DM, Stamey TA, Bostwick DG. Keratin immunoreactivity in the benign and neoplastic human prostate. Cancer Res 1985;45:3663–7.

98. Choe BK, Pontes EJ, Rose NR, Henderson MD. Expression of human prostatic acid phosphatase in a pancreatic islet cell carcinoma. Invest Urol 1978;15:312–8.

99. Cote RJ, Taylor CR. Prostate, bladder and kidney. In: Taylor CR, Cote RJ, eds. Immunomicroscopy: a diagnostic tool for the surgical pathologist, 2nd ed. Philadelphia: WB Saunders, 1994.

100. di Sant'Agnese PA. Calcitonin like immunoreactive and bombesin like immunoreactive endocrine-paracrine cells of the human prostate. Arch Pathol Lab Med 1986;110:412–5.

101. di Sant'Agnese PA, De Mesy Jensen KL. Endocrine-paracrine cells of the prostate and prostatic urethra: an ultrastructural study. Hum Pathol 1984;15:1034–41.

102. Elgamal AA, Van de Voorde W, Van Poppel H, Lauweryns J, Baert L. Immunohistochemical localization of prostate-specific markers within the accessory male sex glands of Cowper, Littre, and Morgagni. Urology 1994;44:84–90.

103. Epstein JI, Kuhajda FP, Lieberman PH. Prostate-specific acid phosphatase immunoreactivity in adenocarcinomas of the urinary bladder. Hum Pathol 1986;17:939–42.

104. Fernandez PL, Gomez M, Caballero T, Alfaro P, Aguilar D. Prostatic acid phosphatase in cloacogenic carcinoma. Acta Oncologica 1990;29:776–7.

105. Filmus JE, Podhajcer OL, Mareso E, Guman N, Mordoh J. Acid phosphatase in human breast cancer tissue. Cancer 1984;53:301–5.

106. Fisher ER, Sieracki JC. Ultrastructure of human normal and neoplastic prostate. Pathol Annu 1970;5:1–26.

107. Frazier HA, Humphrey PA, Burchette JL, Paulson DF. Immunoreative prostatic specific antigen in male periurethral glands. J Urol 1992;147:246–8.

108. Ghazizadeh M, Kagawa S, Izumi K, et al. Immunohistochemical detection of carcinoembryonic antigen in benign hyperplasia and adenocarcinoma of the prostate with monoclonal antibody. J Urol 1984;131:501–3.

109. Goldfarb DA, Stein BS, Shamszadeh M, Petersen RO. Age-related changes in tissue levels of prostatic acid phosphatase and prostate specific antigen. J Urol 1986;136:1266–9.

110. Golz R, Schubert GE. Prostatic specific antigen: immunoreactivity in urachal remnants. J Urol 1989;141:1480–2.

111. Gutman AB, Gutman ED. An "acid" phosphatase occurring in the serum of patients with metastasizing carcinoma of the prostate gland. J Clin Invest 1938;17:473–8.

112. Hedrick L, Epstein JI. Use of keratin 903 as an adjunct in the diagnosis of prostate carcinoma. Am J Surg Pathol 1989;13:389–96.

113. Jobsis AC, DeVries GP, Anholt RR, Sanders GT. Demonstration of the prostatic origin of metastasis. An immunohistochemical method for formalin-fixed embedded tissue. Cancer 1978;41:1788–93.

114. Kamoshida S, Tsutsumi Y. Extraprostatic localization of prostatic acid phosphatase and prostate-specific antigen. Distribution in cloacogenic glandular epithelium and sex-dependent expression in human anal gland. Hum Pathol 1990;21:1108–11.

115. Kastendieck H. Ultrastructural pathology of the human prostatic gland. Cyto- and histomorphogenesis of atrophy, hyperplasia, metaplasia, dysplasia, and carcinoma. Veroffentlichungen aus der pathologie 1977;106:1–16.

116. Kimura N, Sasano N. Prostate-specific acid phosphatase in carcinoid tumors. Virchows Arch A Pathol Anat Histopathol 1986;410:247–51.

117. Kircheim D, Gyorkey F, Brandes D, Scott WW. Histochemistry of the normal, hyperplastic and neoplastic human prostate. Invest Urol 1964;1:403–21.

118. Kovi J, Jackson AG, Jackson MA. Blue nevus of the prostate. ultrastructural study. Urology 1977;9:576–8.

119. Lam KW, Li CY, Yam LT, Sun T, Lee G, Ziesmer S. Improved immunohistochemical detection of prostatic acid phosphatase by a monoclonal antibody. Prostate 1989;15:13–21.

120. Li CY, Lam WK, Yam LT. Immunohistochemical diagnosis of prostatic cancer with metastasis. Cancer 1980;46:706–12.

121. Lippert MC, Bensimon H, Javadpour N. Immunoperoxidase staining of acid phosphatase in human prostatic tissue. J Urol 1982;128:1114–6.

122. Lowe FC, Trauzzi SJ. Prostatic acid phosphatase in 1993. Its limited clinical utility. Urol Clin N Am 1993;20:589–95.

123. Mao P, Angrist A. The fine structure of the basal cell of human prostate. Lab Invest 1966;15:1768–82.

124. Mao P, Nakao K, Angrist A. Acid phosphatase and 5-nucleotidase activities of human nodular prostatic hyperplasia as revealed by electron microscopy. Lab Invest 1966;15:422–34.

125. May EE, Perentes E. Anti-Leu 7 immunoreactivity with human tumours: its value in the diagnosis of prostatic adenocarcinoma. Histopathology 1987;11:295–304.

126. Moncure CW, Prout GR Jr. Antigenicity of human prostatic acid phosphatase. Cancer 1970;25:463–7.

127. Nadji M, Morales AR. Immunohistochemical markers for prostatic cancer. Ann NY Acad Sci 1983;420:134–9.

128. Nadji M, Tabei SZ, Castro A, et al. Prostatic specific antigen: an immunohistologic marker for prostatic neoplasms. Cancer 1981;48:1229–32.

129. Najdi M, Tabei SZ, Castro A, Chu TM, Morales AR. Prostatic origin of tumors. An immunohistochemical study. Am J Clin Pathol 1980;73.735–9.

130. Nowels K, Kent E, Rinsho K, Oyasu R. Prostate specific antigen and acid phosphatase–reactive cells in cystitis cystica and glandularis. Arch Pathol Lab Med 1988;112.734–7.

131. Oesterling JE, Jacobsen SJ, Chute CG, et al. Serum prostate-specific antigen in a community-based population of healthy men: establishment of age-specific reference ranges. JAMA 1993;270:860–4.

132. O'Malley FP, Grignon DJ, Shum DT. Usefulness of immunoperoxidase staining with high-molecular-weight cytokeratin in the differential diagnosis of small-acinar lesions of the prostate gland. Virchows Arch [A] 1990;417:191–6.

133. Papsidero LD, Kuriyama M, Wang MC, et al. Prostate antigen: a marker for human prostate epithelial cells. JNCI 1981;66:37–42.

134. Pollen JJ, Dreilinger A. Immunohistochemical identification of prostatic acid phosphatase and prostate specific antigen in female periurethral glands. Urology 1984;23:303–4.

135. Purnell DM, Heatfield BM, Anthony RL, Trump BF. Immunohistochemistry of the cytoskeleton of human prostatic epithelium. Evidence for disturbed organization in neoplasia. Am J Pathol 1987;126:384–95.

136. Rusthoven JJ, Robinson JB, Kolin A, Pinkerton PH. The natural-killer cell–associated HNK-1 (Leu-7) antibody reacts with hypertrophic and malignant prostatic epithelium. Cancer 1985;56:289–93.

137. Sleater JP, Ford MJ, Beers BB. Extramammary Paget's disease associated with prostate adenocarcinoma. Hum Pathol 1994;25:615–7.

138. Sobin LH, Hjermstad BM, Sesterhenn IA, Helwig EB. Prostatic acid phosphatase activity in carcinoid tumors. Cancer 1986;58:136–8.

139. Spencer JR, Brodin AG, Ignatoff JM. Clear cell adenocarcinoma of the urethra. Evidence for origin within paraurethral ducts. J Urol 1990;143:122–5.

140. Srigley JR, Hartwick WJ, Edwards V, Dettarven E. Selected ultrastructural aspects of urothelial and prostatic tumors. Ultrastruct Pathol 1988;12:49–65.

141. Stein BS, Vangore S, Petersen RO. Immunoperoxidase localization of prostatic antigens. Comparison of primary and metastatic sites. Urology 1984;24:146–52.

142. Stein BS, Vangore S, Petersen RO, Kendall AR. Immunoperoxidase localization of prostate-specific antigen. Am J Surg Pathol 1982;6:553–7.

143. Tepper SL, Jagirdar J, Heath D, Geller SA. Homology between the female paraurethral (Skene's) gland and the prostate. Immunohistochemical demonstration. Arch Pathol Lab Med 1984;108:423–5.

144. Van Krieken JH. Prostate marker immunoreactivity in salivary gland neoplasms. A rare pitfall in immunohistochemistry. Am J Surg Pathol 1993;17:410–4.

145. Wang MC, Valenzuela LA, Murphy GP, Chu TM. Purification of a human prostate specific antigen. Invest Urol 1979;17:159–63.

146. Weaver MG, Abdul-Karim FW, Srigley JR. Paneth cell-like change and small cell carcinoma of the prostate. Two divergent forms of prostatic neuroendocrine differentiation. Am J Surg Pathol 1992;16:1013–16.

147. Weaver MG, Abdul-Karim FW, Srigley JR, Bostwick DG, Ro JY, Ayala AG. Paneth cell-like change of the prostate gland: a histological, immunohistochemical and electron microscopic study. Am J Surg Pathol 1992;16:62–8.

148. Wernert N, Kern L, Heitz P, et al. Morphological and immunohistochemical investigations of the utriculus prostaticus from the fetal period up to adulthood. Prostate 1990;17:19–30

149. Wernert N, Seitz G, Achtstatter T. Immunohistochemical investigation of different cytokeratins and vimentin in the prostate from the fetal period up to adulthood and in prostate carcinoma. Path Res Pract 1987;182.617–26.

Physiology

150. Bruchovsky N, Wilson JD. The conversion of testosterone to 5-alpha-androstan-17 beta-ol-3-one by rat prostate in vivo and in vitro. J Biol Chem 1968;243:2012–21.

151. Bruchovsky N, Wilson JD. The intranuclear binding of testosterone and 5-alpha-androstan-17 beta-ol-3-one by rat prostate. J Biol Chem 1968;243:5953–60.

152. Byar DP. Zinc in male sex accessory organs: distribution and hormonal response. In: Brandes D, ed. Male accessory sex organs. Structure and function in mammals. New York: Academic Press, 1974.

153. Coffey DS. Physiological control of prostatic growth: an overview. In: Coffey DS, Isaacs JT, eds. Prostate cancer. Vol. 48. Geneva: UICC technical report series, 1979.

154. Farnsworth WE. Physiology and biochemistry of prostatic secretion. In: Chisholm GD, Williams DI, eds. Scientific foundation of urology, 2nd ed. Portsmouth, NH: W. Heineman Medical Book Publications, 1982:485.

155. Gunn SA, Gould TC, Anderson WA. The effect of growth hormone and prolactin preparations on the control of intestinal cell-stimulating hormone of uptake of 65Zn by the rat dorsolateral prostate. J Endocrinol 1965;32:205.

156. Huggins C, Scott WW, Heimen JH. Chemical composition of human semen and of the secretions of the prostate and seminal vesicle. Am J Physiol 1941;136:467.

157. Isaacs JT. Prostatic structure and function in relation to the etiology of prostatic cancer. Prostate 1983;4:351–66.

158. Lundquist F. Aspects of the biochemistry of human semen. Acta Physiol Scan 1949;19:66.

159. Mann T. Biochemistry of semen. In: Greep RO, Astwood EB, eds. Handbook of physiology: endocrinology: male reproductive system. Vol 5. Baltimore: Williams & Wilkins, 1975:461–71.

159a.Oesterling JE, Epstein JI, Walsh PC. The inability of adrenal androgens to stimulate the adult prostate: an autopsy evaluation of men with hypogonadotropic hypogonadism and panhypopituitarism. J Urol 1986;136:103–4.

160. Partin AW, Coffey DS. The molecular biology, endocrinology, and physiology of the prostate and seminal vesicles. In: Walsh PC, Retik AB, Darracott VE Jr, eds. Campbell's urology, 7th ed, vol 2. Philadelphia: WB Saunders, 1998.

161. Pollen JJ, Dreilinger A. Immunohistochemical identification of prostatic acid phosphatase and prostate specific antigen in female periurethral glands. Urology 1984;23:303–4.

162. Vermeulen A, Van Camp A, Mattelaer J, DeSy W. Hormonal factors related to abnormal growth of the prostate. In: Coffey DS, Isaacs JT, eds. Prostate cancer. Vol. 48. Geneva: UICC Technical Report Series, 1979.

163. Wilson JD. The pathogenesis of benign prostatic hyperplasia. Am J Med 1980;68:745–56.

164. Zaneveld LJ, Tauber PF. Contribution of prostatic fluid components to the ejaculation. In: Murphy GP, Sandberg AA, Karr JP, eds. The prostatic cell: structure and function. Part A. New York: Alan R. Liss, 1981.

2
PROSTATIC HYPERPLASIA

Benign prostatic hyperplasia is a widely used clinical term (1,2) which histologically correlates in most cases with nodular hyperplasia of the transition zone. Interpreted more broadly, it has been used to include other benign proliferations of the prostate gland, such as postatrophic hyperplasia, which bear little or no relation to nodular hyperplasia. For this reason we use "benign nodular hyperplasia" to denote the specific pathologic lesion that correlates with, in most cases, the clinical entity "benign prostatic hyperplasia" and that is, by far, the most common form of prostatic hyperplasia (3). In this chapter, benign nodular hyperplasia and its histologic variants, and other forms of benign hyperplasia (except atypical adenomatous hyperplasia) are reviewed (Table 2-1). Particularly exuberant examples of some of them are also considered in chapter 7 with specific regard to their tumor-like

Table 2-1

CLASSIFICATION OF PROSTATIC HYPERPLASIA

I. **Benign nodular hyperplasia**

Usual patterns:
  Glandular
  Stromal
  Mixed

Special patterns:
  Epithelial predominant
    small glandular
    cribriform
    basal cell
  Stromal
    leiomyomatous
  Mixed glandular-stromal
    fibroadenoma-like
    phyllodes-like

II. **Atrophy-associated hyperplasia**

Basal cell hyperplasia
Postatrophic hyperplasia

III. **Atypical adenomatous hyperplasia— Adenosis** (see chapter 3)

manifestations and potential for misdiagnosis as carcinoma. Atypical adenomatous hyperplasia (adenosis) is excluded from this presentation and is discussed in chapter 3, along with prostatic intraepithelial neoplasia, because some evidence suggests that atypical adenomatous hyperplasia may possibly be associated with carcinoma, although the evidence for this is much less convincing than it is for prostatic intraepithelial neoplasia.

BENIGN NODULAR HYPERPLASIA

Definition. Benign nodular hyperplasia represents nodular expansion of prostatic glandular elements, stromal elements, or both.

General Features. The prevalence of nodular hyperplasia in autopsy series increases with advancing age from about 8 percent in the fourth decade to almost 90 percent at 80 years (8,20,27, 37,45,49,58,67,70,73). About 50 percent of men in the sixth decade have pathologic evidence of it, and the peak age of clinical presentation is in the seventh decade (29); it is very rare under the age of 30 years (8,20,67). In one series of over 700 consecutive autopsies on males, no examples were seen before the fourth decade (68). In a clinical series of 1,000 cases of prostatic hyperplasia, the youngest patient was 40 years of age, and 98 percent were over 50 years (29). We have, however, seen a striking example in a 15-year-old, and there is another similar case in a 16-year-old who, like our patient, underwent suprapubic prostatectomy (10). The data on the autopsy prevalence of nodular hyperplasia are paralleled by clinical studies of prostatic enlargement and by weights of surgically removed glands (9,24,41,43,67,73).

Mortality data for patients with nodular hyperplasia show considerable worldwide variation (63,78). The data from developing countries are weaker because of bias introduced by premature deaths from infectious and nutritional diseases (63). In more developed countries death rates due to uremia caused by nodular hyperplasia vary; higher mortality rates are found in several European countries including Iceland, Germany, Austria, Romania, Norway, and Denmark.

Lower death rates are found in the Philippines, Taiwan, Hong Kong, Japan, Mexico, the United States, Canada, and Israel. Countries with intermediate rates include Sweden, Belgium, Finland, Great Britain, and France (62,63).

There are racial differences in the prevalence of nodular hyperplasia. Orientals in China, Hong Kong, and Japan are infrequently affected (13,49,78), whereas significant numbers of cases are documented in some studies from Africa, although it has been suggested that nodular hyperplasia is rare to nonexistent in certain African countries such as Sudan (36). Some data suggest that nodular hyperplasia develops more often in American blacks than whites and that symptoms occur at an earlier age (35,42,49,62).

The etiology and pathogenesis of nodular hyperplasia remain poorly understood (33). A number of factors, including marital status, socioeconomic status, and libido, and diseases such as diabetes mellitus, hypertension, and cirrhosis, have been investigated and are not thought to be etiologically related to nodular hyperplasia (6,49,61-63). Age is clearly an important factor as evidenced by its strong correlation with the prevalence of nodular hyperplasia (8,54). Some studies have suggested that certain families are predisposed to develop clinical manifestations of the disease at a young age; histologic studies in such cases have shown a stromal predominant pattern (19,56,64). Testicular androgen production is necessary for the development of nodular hyperplasia (6) which has not been described in eunuchs and is only rarely found in patients castrated in adolescence or early adulthood (69,77,79).

Early studies on castration as a treatment of nodular hyperplasia suggested that patients improved clinically, but in later studies it was shown that the shrinkage was mainly in the peripheral prostate and not in the periurethral regions (12,17,28,76,79). In a classic study by Huggins and Stevens (28), patients had serial biopsies after castration, and it was demonstrated that the epithelial compartment underwent atrophy after 86 days. In a study of patients with prostate cancer treated with orchiectomy and estrogens, the degree of nodular hyperplasia in these prostatic specimens was lower than in controls (75); once again the atrophy was mainly epithelial.

The principal androgenic hormones are testosterone and dihydrotestosterone (DHT) (55). After age 50 there is a progressive decrease in the level of serum testosterone, but there is no consensus on significant differences in testosterone levels between patients with nodular hyperplasia and "normal controls" (7,26,72). The common presence of subclinical nodular hyperplasia in the population weakens any conclusion drawn from such studies. DHT is the active metabolite of testosterone which many authors believe is related to the development of nodular hyperplasia (11,66). The DHT level is elevated in tissues with nodular hyperplasia compared to normal tissues in some studies (22,32,38,48); others find no significant difference in tissue levels of DHT between normal and nodular hyperplasia and suggest that low DHT levels in the control tissues are spurious since they were obtained at autopsy (73,74). There is no clear relationship between plasma DHT levels and the clinical presence of nodular hyperplasia (7,22,25,26,52,57,71).

Some authors have suggested that the development of nodular hyperplasia is related to estrogen metabolism (52). With increasing age there are elevations in estrogenic compounds, principally 17-β-estradiol and estrone, which are produced by peripheral conversion of testosterone and androstenedione, respectively (57). The conversion occurs mainly in adipose tissue. While some investigators have noted elevated estradiol levels with advancing age, others have not found significant changes in the levels of the estrogen metabolites (80). It is clear, however, that the estrogen/androgen ratio increases with age (23).

Nodular hyperplasia preferentially involves the proximal periurethral tissues (the so called estrogen sensitive zone) (20,49,58). In the anatomic model of McNeal (see chapter 1), the tissues surrounding the proximal urethral segment include the submucosal compartment, the specialized mesenchyme of the preprostatic sphincter, and the transition zone (44–47). The true periurethral (submucosal) tissue contains relatively few glands. The small hyperplastic nodules occurring in this region usually have a pure stromal morphology and are thought to be of little clinical significance (45). The transition zone expands with advancing age, resulting in a nodular gross appearance due to the lobar structure of this zone; most clinically significant nodules develop here. This usual location for nodular hyperplasia was pointed out by Morgagni over 200 years ago (50). Franks (21) summarized the evolution of understanding of the histogenesis of nodular hyperplasia, and provided references from the old non-English language literature to which the interested reader is referred (4,5,34,53,60).

The earliest lesion of nodular hyperplasia in the transition zone consists of epithelial budding (46). The signal for this epithelial proliferation may be delivered from stromal cells, and the bulk of evidence suggests that stromal proliferation is of paramount importance in the development of nodular hyperplasia (18,40,49). Some evidence suggests that hyperplasia with stromal predominance is seen more often in patients with symptomatic disease compared to those who are asymptomatic (65). The elegant experiments of Cunha and others have documented the inductive capacity of mesenchyme on the urogenital sinus epithelium (14–16). These studies have shown that during embryogenesis the development of prostatic epithelium is dependent on the inductive forces of the stroma. It has been suggested that in human nodular hyperplasia there is a "reawakening" of the embryonic interactions between glands and stroma, leading to the nodular combinations of glandular and stromal elements that typify this condition. Growth factors such as basic fibroblastic growth factor may play an important role in this process (53). More recently it has been suggested that nodular hyperplasia develops as a result of increased prostatic stem cell activity (6,31). The number of prostatic stem cells may be programmed or imprinted in utero or in infancy (31,51,59).

It is likely that the pathogenesis of nodular hyperplasia is multifactorial and involves hormonal alterations, stromal-epithelial communication, and fundamental changes in proliferative cellular compartments. Current experimental work is looking at the exact roles of hormone growth factors and their respective receptors. There is also considerable interest in the role of programmed cell death (apoptosis) in the development of nodular hyperplasia (30,39).

Clinical Features. About 50 percent of patients with histologic evidence of nodular hyperplasia have grossly detectable disease on digital rectal examination (86,92). About 50 percent of patients with grossly enlarged glands develop prostatism (86). During the 1980s, it was estimated that one in four men in the United States required surgery for relief of symptoms of prostatic hyperplasia by age 80 (82). In recent years, however, many men are opting for medical therapy such as finasteride (87) and α-blockers or minimally invasive treatments such as microwave and laser ablation (88). This trend is reflected in surgical pathology practice as fewer transurethral resection specimens are processed than in the past.

The symptoms of prostatism may be categorized as either obstructive or irritative (85,91,92). Obstructive symptoms include hesitancy, weak stream, and terminal dribbling. Irritative symptoms include urgency, frequency, dysuria, and nocturia. Irritative symptoms often suggest the possibility of superimposed infection. Symptoms usually gradually progress although they may either stabilize or, uncommonly, regress. The severity of symptoms does not necessarily correlate with gland size, and, indeed, cases of small volume nodular hyperplasia may result in significant symptoms, especially if there is interference with the urinary flow at the proximal urethral sphincter.

In severe cases, the bladder incompletely drains leading to stagnant residual urine and cystitis; longstanding bladder neck obstruction results in bladder dilatation, hypertrophy, and trabeculation. This may be complicated by hydroureter and hydronephrosis and eventually chronic pyelonephritis and renal insufficiency. Patients may present with acute urinary retention resulting from a complete blockage of flow at the level of the proximal prostatic urethra. Sometimes this complication results from a prominent "median lobe" or "bar" (fig. 2-1) (90) which can result in a ball-valve phenomenon. This situation presents a urologic emergency necessitating catheterization or, in some cases, suprapubic cystostomy.

On digital rectal examination, the prostatic gland is typically large and may have a nodular contour. The enlargement is often symmetric, and the texture is rubbery. Tenderness may be present, especially if there is superimposed prostatitis.

Patients with benign prostatic hyperplasia may have elevations in their serum prostate-specific antigen (PSA) level in the absence of prostatic adenocarcinoma. Since the prevalence of benign hyperplasia increases with advancing age, some investigators have developed age-specific PSA

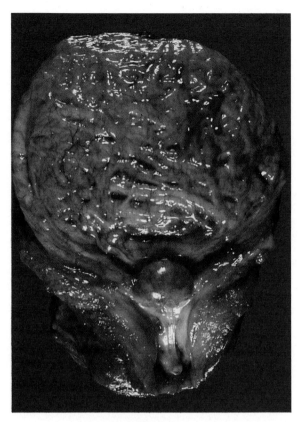

Figure 2-1

BENIGN NODULAR HYPERPLASIA

The prostate gland and urinary bladder have been opened anteriorly to disclose a prominent median lobe (bar) of the prostate. Obstruction of the prostatic urethra has resulted in bladder dilatation and trabeculation. (Courtesy of Dr. K. Barwick, Jacksonville, FL.)

Table 2-2

**AGE-SPECIFIC REFERENCE RANGE
FOR SERUM PROSTATE-SPECIFIC
ANTIGEN (PSA)***

Age (year)	PSA Range (ng/mL)**	Age (year)	PSA Range (ng/mL)**
40	2.0	60	3.8
41	2.1	61	4.0
42	2.2	62	4.1
43	2.3	63	4.2
44	2.3	64	4.4
45	2.4	65	4.5
46	2.5	66	4.6
47	2.6	67	4.7
48	2.6	68	4.9
49	2.7	69	5.1
50	2.8	70	5.3
51	2.9	71	5.4
52	3.0	72	5.6
53	3.1	73	5.8
54	3.2	74	6.0
55	3.3	75	6.2
56	3.4	76	6.4
57	3.5	77	6.6
58	3.6	78	6.8
59	3.7	79	7.0

*From Oesterling JE, Jacobsen SJ, Chute CG, et al: Serum prostate-specific antigen in a community-based population of healthy men: establishment of age specific reference ranges. JAMA 1993;270:860–6.
**From 0.0 to the specified value.

values for the general population (Table 2-2) (84,89). The confounding influence of hyperplasia on PSA levels has prompted the development of measurements such as PSA density which takes into account total serum PSA value and prostatic volume (81). Other approaches include the determination of the ratio of free to total PSA, with higher ratios found in benign cases (83).

Imaging studies using ultrasound, computerized tomography, and magnetic resonance imaging may demonstrate nodular hyperplasia. Postvoiding residual urine with bladder dilatation and trabeculation may be detected radiographically. In advanced cases, radiologic evidence of hydroureter, hydronephrosis, and chronic pyelonephritis may be noted.

Gross Findings. Gross abnormalities associated with nodular hyperplasia may sometimes

be identified in prostatic chips but are much more readily seen in prostatectomy specimens (figs. 2-2A,B,C, 2-3, 2-4), or at autopsy (fig. 2-2D). Multinodular masses of variable sizes that are occasionally massive are seen (fig. 2-2A) (103,130). Sectioning shows nodules that may be bulging (fig. 2-2C), are often numerous, and range in size from millimeters to several centimeters (fig. 2-2B). They are usually tan-white and firm (fig. 2-4) but may be spongy and honeycomb-like due to interspersed cysts (fig. 2-3), or occasionally predominantly cystic (fig. 2-2B).

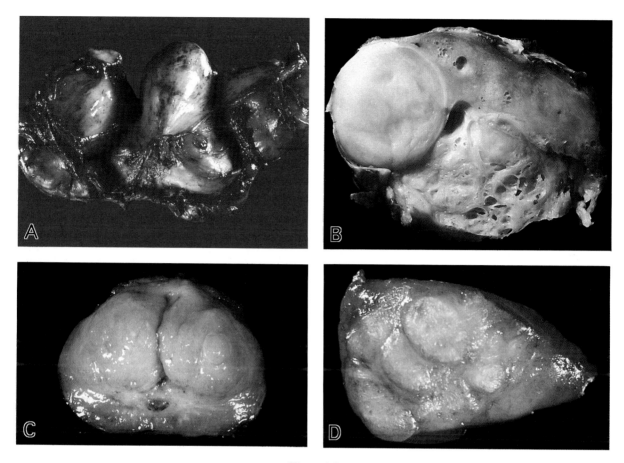

Figure 2-2
BENIGN NODULAR HYPERPLASIA

A: A suprapubic prostatectomy specimen shows multiple nodules.

B: Cut section of another case shows nodules that are variably solid, solid and cystic, and predominantly cystic.

C: Cross section from a radical prostatectomy specimen shows bulging tan-white nodules punctuated by yellow areas; the urethra is narrowed and there is compression of the peripheral zone. (Courtesy of Dr. E.C. Jones, Vancouver, BC, Canada.)

D: An autopsy case shows uniformly solid, relatively discrete, yellow nodules.

The location of nodular hyperplasia in most cases is often strikingly apparent in radical prostatectomy specimens when the nodularity within the transition zone is in marked contrast to the peripheral zone, which lacks nodules and may have a normal tan-brown appearance (fig. 2-2C), or shows cysts that may in part be related to obstruction (figs. 2-3, 2-4). Pure stromal nodules may have a tan-gray to white whorled appearance similar to uterine leiomyomas. Secondary infarction may be present and is characteristically either yellow or red depending on the amount of blood (fig. 2-5). In the older literature nodular hyperplasia was sometimes classified according to the location of the nodules: middle (median), anterior, and right and left lateral

(138). This approach has generally been abandoned, although one can sometimes see a prominent median lobe (bar) which protrudes as a polypoid nodule into the posterior aspect of the bladder neck (fig. 2-1) (137).

The nodules are centered around the proximal prostatic urethra; they typically involve the submucosal stroma and transition zone (96,99,124, 126,127). With increasing growth they encroach on the lumen of the urethra, resulting in partial obstruction (fig. 2-3). The nodules also expand outward to compress the peripheral zone, which may be attenuated or show cystic dilatation of its acini. The interface between the expanding nodular tissue and the compressed peripheral zone represents the so-called surgical capsule which

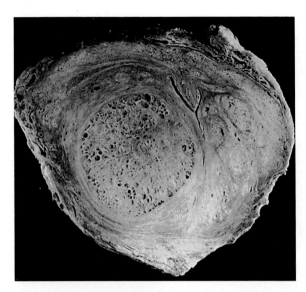

Figure 2-3
BENIGN
NODULAR HYPERPLASIA

A cross section of prostate gland at the level of the verumontanum shows pronounced hyperplasia with one dominant, large nodule with a spongy appearance (left center). Note the compression and distortion of the prostatic urethra. (Fig. 29 from Fascicle 31b and 32, 1st Series.)

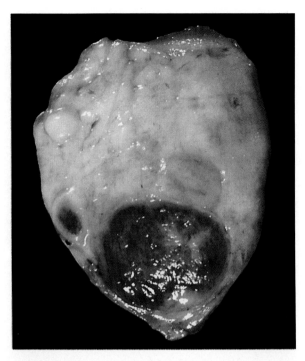

Figure 2-5
BENIGN NODULAR HYPERPLASIA WITH INFARCTION

One large nodule shows extensive hemorrhagic infarction, and there is focal hemorrhagic infarction of a smaller nodule. Many noninfarcted yellow nodules are also appreciable.

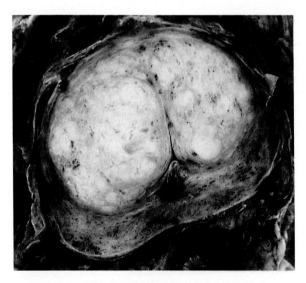

Figure 2-4
BENIGN NODULAR HYPERPLASIA

The hyperplasia of the transition zone contrasts markedly with the peripheral zone which shows no evidence of hyperplasia but only scattered small cysts due to cystic atrophy or cystic dilatation of acini secondary to obstruction. (Fig. 9 from Franks LM. Benign nodular hyperplasia of the prostate. A review. Ann Roy Coll Surg Engl 1954;14:92–106.)

comprises the dissection plane used by the urologist during a suprapubic prostatectomy (fig. 2-2C) (140,147).

From 2 to 15 percent of prostatectomy specimens contain foci of nodular hyperplasia that are of peripheral zone origin (131,132,145) and hypoechoic on transrectal ultrasonography, suggesting the diagnosis of carcinoma (118,131). These nodules rarely attain the sometimes massive size of transition zone nodules but may result in a palpable mass on digital rectal examination (118). In contrast to transition zone nodules, these are more often solitary (145). The relatively uncommon nodular hyperplasia of the peripheral zone should be distinguished from cysts in the peripheral zone, cystic atrophy, and cystic dilatation of peripheral zone acini possibly due to obstruction. The latter explanation for peripheral zone cysts has been suggested by animal experiments (111), although their occasional occurrence in early life suggests other possible etiologies (145). Although this phenomenon has sometimes been referred to in the literature as

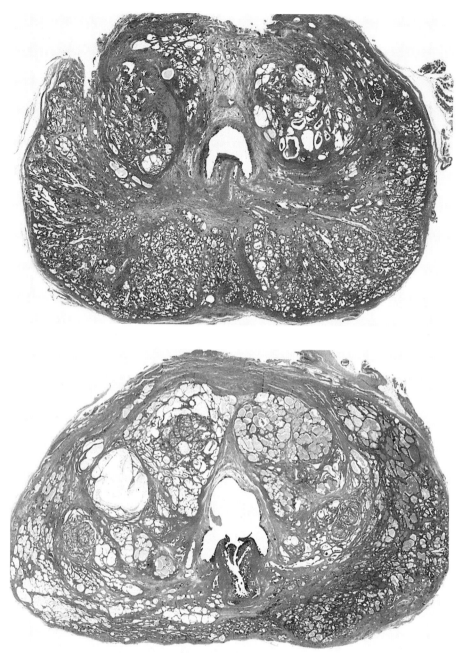

Figure 2-6
BENIGN
NODULAR HYPERPLASIA
Whole mount sections of prostate show nodular hyperplasia of the transition zone.

Top: A nodule at the top left shows solid areas correlating with a prominent stromal proliferation; most other areas contain cysts and have scant stroma. The peripheral zone is not involved. Note the connective tissue band, the "surgical capsule," separating the transition and peripheral zones.

Bottom: The peripheral zone is more compressed than in the top figure with cystic dilatation of some acini.

"cystic hyperplasia" (142), in our opinion it is preferably referred to descriptively as "cystic dilatation" as it is not hyperplasia in the usual sense of the term, and in one study was found not to correlate with nodular hyperplasia (142).

Microscopic Findings. The microscopic appearance of nodular hyperplasia is varied (figs. 2-6–2-23, 2-25–2-36). In order to accommodate this diversity, various classification systems have been devised that are highly descriptive but generally have little biologic or clinical significance (105, 106,136). The approach used in this Fascicle is also descriptive and reflects the spectrum of cell types in the normal prostate gland that gives rise to nodular hyperplasia (Table 2-1; fig. 2-9); it is derived in part from the 1954 classification of Franks (Table 2-3). Stromal cells, including primitive (undifferentiated) mesenchyme, fibroblasts, and

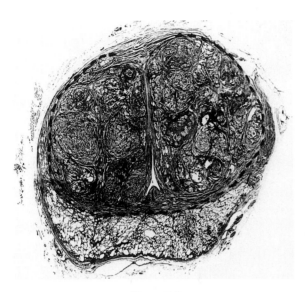

Figure 2-7
BENIGN NODULAR HYPERPLASIA
The prostatic hyperplasia involves the transition zone (dashed line around the upper two thirds of the illustration) and is separated by connective tissue, the surgical capsule, from the peripheral zone (bottom) which shows cystic dilatation of almost all the acini. (Fig. 9 from Franks LM. Benign nodular hyperplasia of the prostate. A review. Ann Royal Col Surg Engl 1954;14:92–106.)

Table 2-3

FRANKS' CLASSIFICATION OF HYPERPLASTIC NODULES*

1. The stromal (fibrous or fibrovascular) nodule.

2. The fibromuscular nodule.

3. The muscular nodule ("leiomyoma").

4. The fibroadenomatous nodule.

5. The fibromyoadenomatous nodule.

*Data from reference 105.

smooth muscle cells, as well as epithelial cells (secretory and basal), may take part in the hyperplastic process (96). Common patterns of nodular hyperplasia are epithelial predominant, stromal predominant, and mixed (Tables 2-1, 2-3). In addition, there are special morphologic variants in which one component is preferentially involved resulting in a distinctive histologic pattern. These are small glandular, cribriform, basal cell, and leiomyomatous hyperplasias. Rare mixed patterns of fibroadenoma-like and phyllodes-like hyperplasia may be seen (Table 2-1).

The earliest manifestation of nodular hyperplasia consists of tiny nodules of often pale staining, primitive fibrovascular stroma located in submucosal connective tissue around the proximal prostatic urethra (fig. 2-10A) (105,106,128). Capillary-like blood vessels (fig. 2-10B) are surrounded by small, bland spindle cells with tapered nuclei and little cytoplasm. The spindle cells appear similar to uncommitted mesenchyme or primitive fibroblasts (fig. 2-10B); their plump nuclei with open chromatin contrast with the smaller,

denser nuclei of the surrounding stroma (128). Sometimes the nodules are very cellular (fig. 2-10C) or there is dense collagen around the capillaries (fig. 2-10D). These stromal nodules often blend into the adjacent submucosal connective tissue and sphincteric muscle. Similar nodules may also be seen within the transition zone (see below) (125). It has been shown that these nodules are usually devoid of elastic fibers, unlike the normal prostatic stroma (105,128). With increasing size, focal or widely distributed smooth muscle cells are often admixed with the fibrovascular elements (see page 42). As noted earlier, some evidence suggests that stromal-predominant nodules may be more symptomatic than those of other types (141).

The predominantly epithelial pattern of nodular hyperplasia is usually identified within the transition zone tissue, as characterized by McNeal (figs. 2-11, 2-12) (124,125), but may also involve the periurethral gland region (fig. 2-11B). Relatively discrete epithelial nodules may be identified on low-power microscopy (figs. 2-11A, 2-12A), but in other instances nodular growth is less conspicuous. The nodules consist of branching and converging duct-acinar elements. Within a given case, some nodules are mainly glandular, others are purely stromal, and others have a uniform admixture of glandular and stromal elements within the nodule (fig. 2-13). In some, a central mass of proliferating stroma with peripheral glandular elements suggests possible gland recruitment from adjacent duct-acinar units (fig. 2-13, right). The rare nodular hyperplasia of the peripheral zone (fig. 2-8) does not differ microscopically from that of the transition zone.

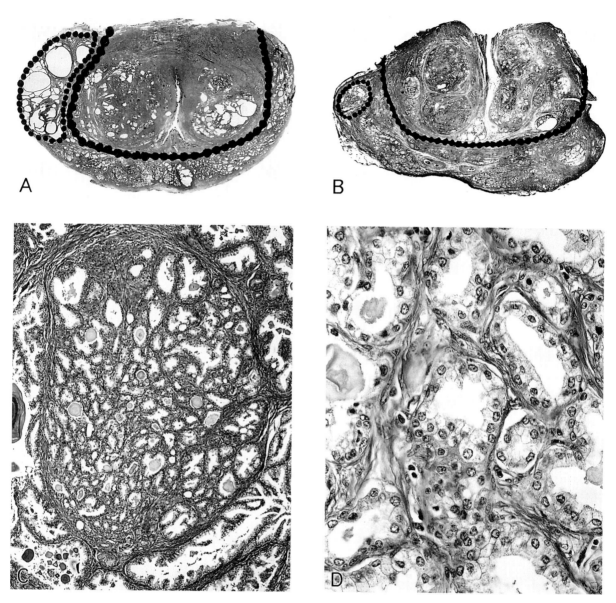

Figure 2-8
BENIGN NODULAR HYPERPLASIA IN PERIPHERAL ZONE

A,B: In these two whole mount sections there is hyperplasia in the peripheral zone as well as in the transition zone. The larger dotted line in each illustration outlines the boundary between the transition and peripheral zones and the smaller dotted lines draw attention to foci of nodular hyperplasia in the peripheral zone.

C: A discrete epithelial dominant nodule of nodular hyperplasia is seen in the peripheral zone.

D: A higher power magnification of such an area shows benign cytologic features. (A–D: Figs. 1A,B and 2A,B from Kerley SW, Corica FA, Qian J, Myers RP, Bostwick DG. Peripheral zone involvement by prostatic hyperplasia. J Urol Pathol 1997;6:87–94.)

The glands of nodular hyperplasia are usually medium to large, sometimes cystic (fig. 2-14), and may show architectural complexity and papillary infoldings (figs. 2-15, 2-16). The epithelium usually has a distinct double layer of secretory and basal cells, but the basal cells are not always conspicuous (figs. 2-16, 2-17). The basal cell layer can be identified as dark, elongated, cuboidal to oval cells which often underlie more than one secretory cell (fig. 2-17). The secretory cells are usually tall and columnar (figs. 2-16, 2-17), although in cystic glands they are often attenuated.

Benign Nodular Hyperplasia
Morphologic Patterns

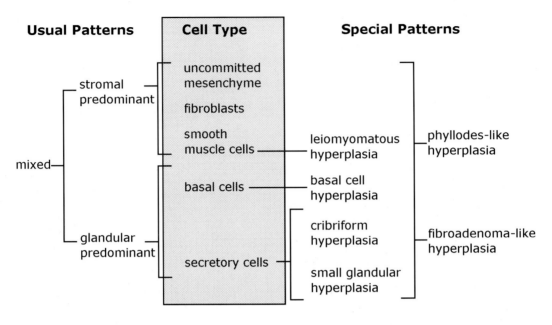

Figure 2-9
BENIGN NODULAR HYPERPLASIA: MORPHOLOGIC PATTERNS
Conceptual schematic showing usual and special patterns of benign nodular hyperplasia in relationship to cell types.

The cells are often thrown into papillary folds with some stratification, although the nuclei are usually aligned in a single row (fig. 2-16). This contrasts with the appearance of prostatic intraepithelial neoplasia in which the nuclei are irregularly arranged within stratified layers. The bridges and arches commonly present in normal prostatic central zone glands are generally lacking in nodular hyperplasia. The cytoplasm is abundant and clear to lightly eosinophilic and sometimes has a granular appearance. The nuclei are uniform, and nucleoli are inconspicuous; mitoses are rare. In general, there is reduced luminal secretion and smaller and less numerous corpora amylacea in hyperplastic glands compared to normal ones (128). Occasionally, however, eosinophilic secretion is prominent and corpora amylacea common. The stroma of mixed nodules usually consists of fibroblasts and smooth muscle cells. Rarely, the stromal cells exhibit hyperchromatic bizarre nuclei of degenerative type (see chapter 7), but this phenomenon should be carefully distinguished from

the neoplastic atypia that may be seen in epithelial-stromal tumors (see chapter 6).

Special Histologic Patterns. The special patterns that may be seen under the overall spectrum of nodular hyperplasia are listed in Table 2-1 and figure 2-9. Basal cell hyperplasia is considered separately later because of its unique features; since it may be a component of nodular hyperplasia or associated with atrophy, it is listed in two places in Table 2-1.

Small Glandular Hyperplasia. This is a variant of the epithelial-dominant pattern of nodular hyperplasia in which there is a circumscribed proliferation of relatively small glands in a fibromuscular stroma (figs. 2-18, 2-19) (120). The secretory cells are often less columnar than in typical nodular hyperplasia (fig. 2-19). The basal cells may be increased, suggesting that this pattern overlaps with incomplete basal cell hyperplasia (fig. 2-19). The small glandular variant of nodular hyperplasia is distinguished from atypical adenomatous hyperplasia (adenosis) by its more uniform appearance, more commonly associated stromal hyperplasia, and absence of "parent" ducts.

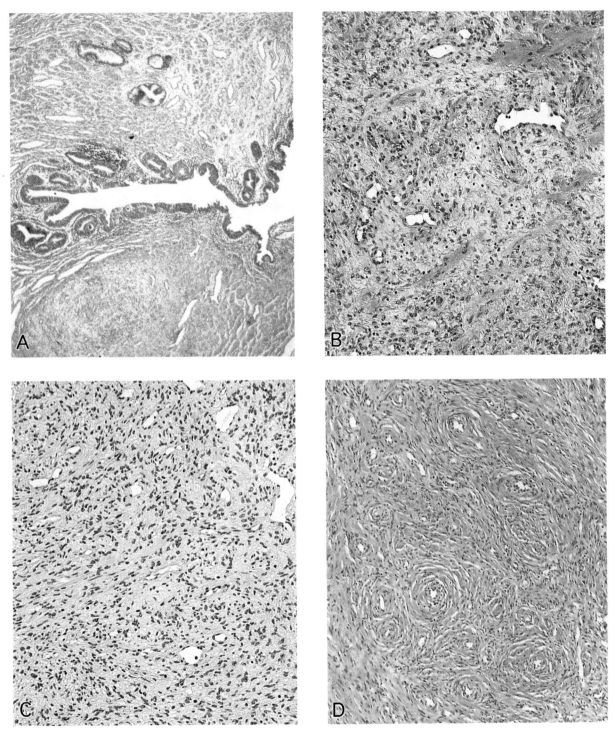

Figure 2-10
BENIGN NODULAR HYPERPLASIA—STROMAL PREDOMINANT

A: A low-power photomicrograph shows the prostatic urethra with an early stromal nodule arising in the submucosal connective tissue (bottom).

B: A high-power photomicrograph of the stromal nodule shows small spindle cells around capillaries. A small amount of loose ground substance is seen between the spindle cells.

C: An intensely cellular stromal nodule is present.

D: This is a more collagenous stromal nodule.

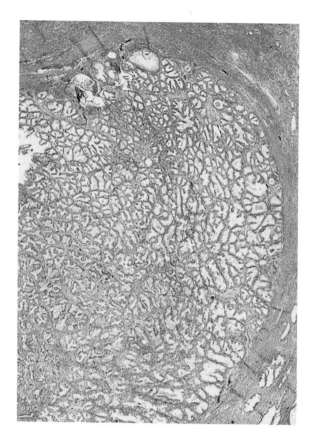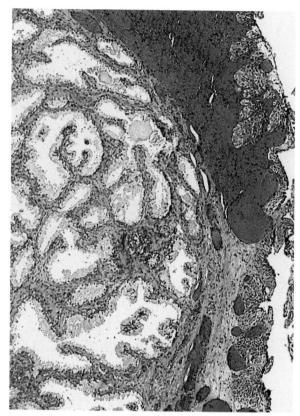

Figure 2-11
BENIGN NODULAR HYPERPLASIA
Note the sharp circumscription of the nodule on the left and the suburethral location on the right, with prominent ectasia of subepithelial blood vessels.

Cribriform Hyperplasia. This is an uncommon variant of nodular hyperplasia in which part of the epithelial component consists of medium to large glands with a cribriform architecture (fig. 2-20) (95,110). The low-power microscopic pattern is generally nodular, as in typical nodular hyperplasia, and there is usually architectural and cytologic uniformity with distinct separation of the cribriform units from one another in most instances. Rounded cribriform aggregates are surrounded by a distinct, and sometimes prominent, basal cell layer (95,108). The cells comprising the cribriform glands may have abundant clear cytoplasm ("clear cell cribriform hyperplasia") (fig. 2-20) (95), but clarity of the cytoplasm is not always conspicuous and is not distinctive for this variant of hyperplasia. The cells lining the glands have uniform nuclei with fine chromatin and inconspicuous nucleoli. The glands of cribriform hyperplasia usually have a smooth luminal aspect, but rarely, small papillae are noted. The stroma around the cribriform glands is usually similar in appearance to that of other mixed hyperplastic nodules. Florid cases that may cause particular diagnostic difficulty are considered on page 297.

Leiomyomatous Nodules. Occasionally, nodular hyperplasia is characterized by stromal nodules with prominent smooth muscle differentiation (fig. 2-21) (105,106,117,135). Leiomyomatous hyperplasia is often cellular, with mild nuclear variability and, rarely, occasional mitoses; atypical mitoses, however, are not seen. Infarction may be present and mimic tumor necrosis. This process may be difficult to distinguish from a smooth muscle neoplasm, especially in transurethral resectates (fig. 2-22) where the interface between the myoma-like nodule and normal prostate may not be readily identified (110,120), and hence the criteria separating the two are

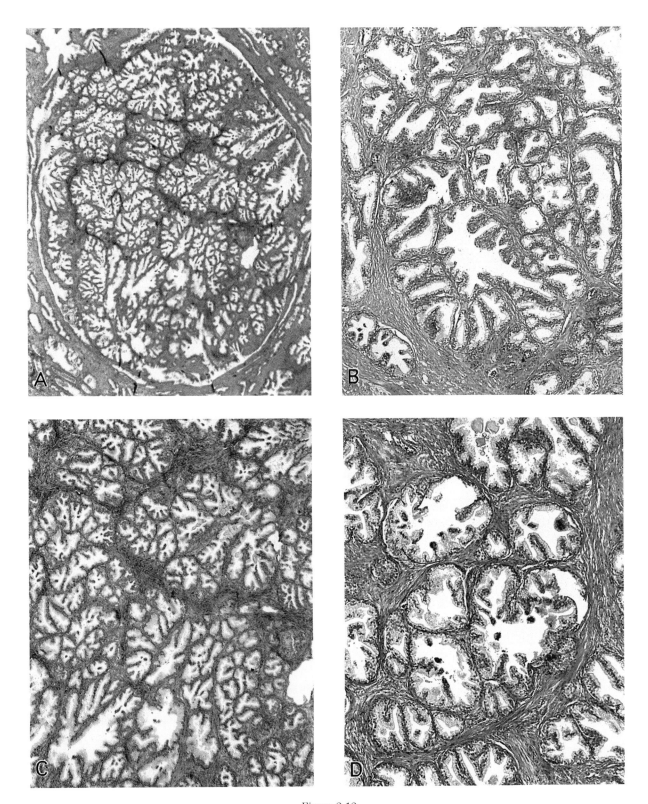

Figure 2-12

BENIGN NODULAR HYPERPLASIA—EPITHELIAL PREDOMINANT

Four views of epithelial dominant nodules within the transition zone. Note the overall nodular configuration and papillary infoldings.

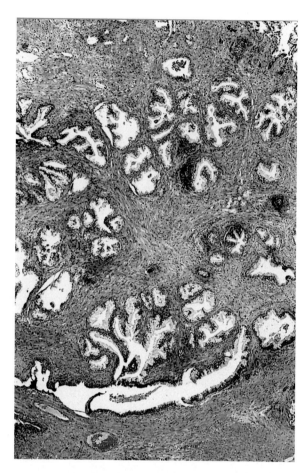
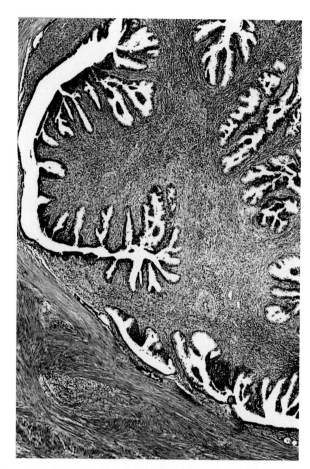

Figure 2-13
BENIGN NODULAR HYPERPLASIA—MIXED EPITHELIAL-STROMAL
On the right, the cellular proliferating stroma is intimately associated with peripheral glands, suggesting recruitment of epithelial elements by a stromal signal.

arbitrary (115). It is important to recognize that the process is multinodular and that there is a spectrum of change from typical stromal nodules to those predominantly composed of smooth muscle. In leiomyomatous hyperplasia, the nodules tend to blend into the adjacent stroma (fig. 2-21, left), whereas smooth muscle neoplasms have a discrete interface. We restrict the diagnosis of leiomyoma to circumscribed lesions greater than 1 cm, composed purely of smooth muscle elements, and lacking an admixed fibroblastic proliferation or prominent thin-walled vessels.

Fibroadenoma-Like Hyperplasia. Hyperplastic patterns in which the glands and cellular fibrovascular stroma are organized in a fashion similar to fibroadenoma of the breast may be encountered (fig. 2-23, left) but are rare, being noted in only 1 percent

of cases of nodular hyperplasia in one study (113). This pattern has no special significance.

Phyllodes-Type Hyperplasia. An exuberant, sometimes myxoid, stromal proliferation, usually associated with cleft-like spaces with intraluminal polypoid projections, imparts a pattern similar to a phyllodes tumor of the breast (93,94,121,139). Phyllodes-like hyperplasia is very rare and typically associated with usual nodular hyperplasia (fig. 2-23, right). This variant must be distinguished from an epithelial-stromal tumor (so-called phyllodes tumor) of the prostate, an issue not easily resolvable in limited tissue samples (see chapter 6). We diagnose a neoplasm in cases that form a distinct mass and show marked stromal hypercellularity or atypia that is not acceptable as degenerative in nature.

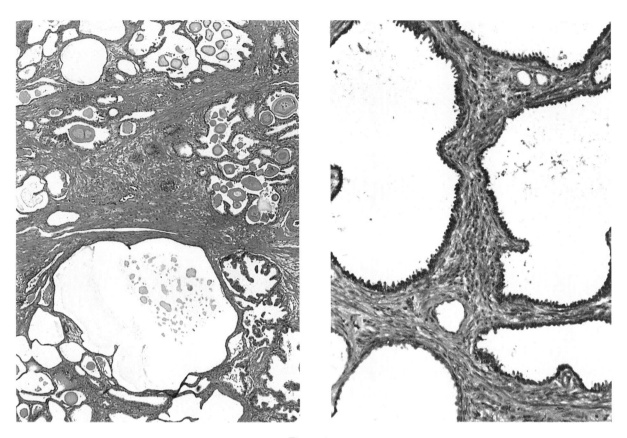

Figure 2-14
BENIGN NODULAR HYPERPLASIA
Cysts are prominent and a small focus of prostatic intraepithelial neoplasia is seen on the left (bottom right). The lining is attenuated in the large cyst on the left and characterized by cuboidal cells on the right.

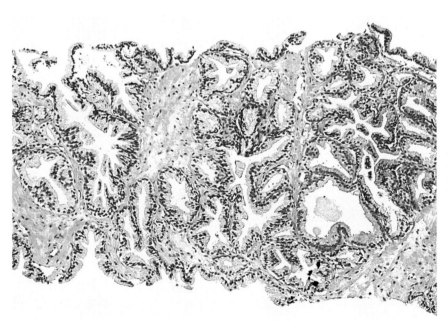

Figure 2-15
BENIGN NODULAR
HYPERPLASIA

A needle biopsy specimen shows the typical picture of glands of varying sizes and shapes, some of them dilated, imparting a picture that is, paradoxically, more "complex" than needle biopsy specimens of many carcinomas.

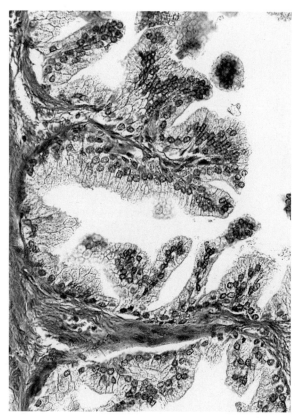

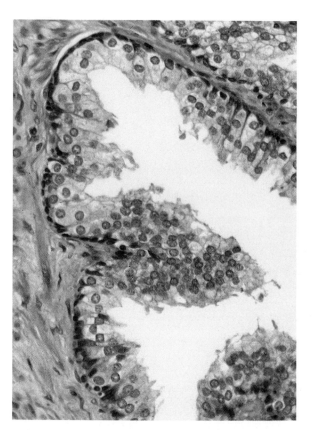

Figure 2-16
BENIGN NODULAR HYPERPLASIA
The typical columnar to cuboidal epithelium lines the glands. The basal cells are relatively inconspicuous.

Figure 2-17
BENIGN NODULAR HYPERPLASIA
Basal cells are conspicuous.

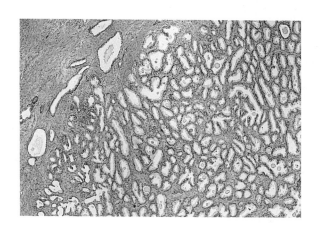

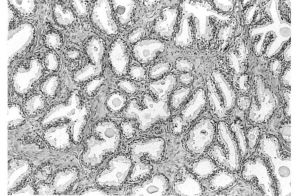

Figure 2-18
BENIGN NODULAR HYPERPLASIA, SMALL GLANDULAR VARIANT
Left: There is a nodule composed of small to medium-sized, closely packed glands evenly distributed in the stroma.
Right: There are small glands with well-preserved basal cells. Small amounts of cellular stroma separate the glandular elements.

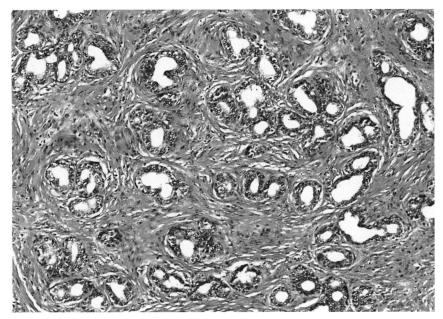

Figure 2-19
BENIGN NODULAR
HYPERPLASIA, SMALL
GLANDULAR VARIANT
The secretory cells are cuboidal, and the stroma is prominent.

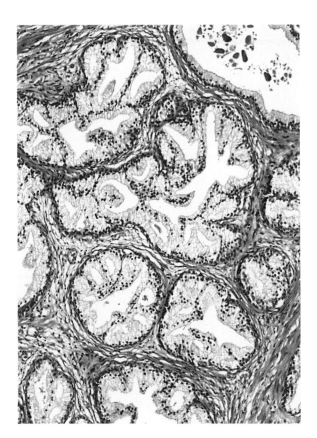
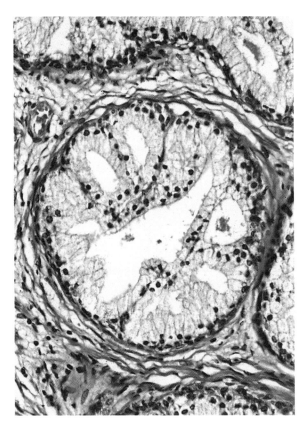

Figure 2-20
BENIGN NODULAR HYPERPLASIA WITH FOCAL CRIBRIFORM PATTERN
Left: Note the uniform distribution of glands and stroma.
Right: The cytology is bland, and basal cells are present.

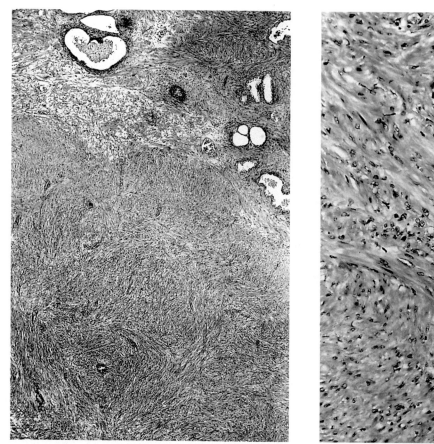
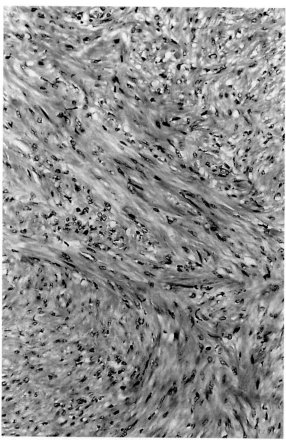

Figure 2-21
LEIOMYOMATOUS HYPERPLASIA
Left: Note the nodular configuration of proliferating smooth muscle cells and ill-defined interface with adjacent tissue.
Right: A high-power view shows interlacing fascicles of smooth muscle cells.

Figure 2-22
LEIOMYOMATOUS NODULE
The pure muscular nodule (right) in this transurethral resection specimen cannot be reliably distinguished from a leiomyoma.

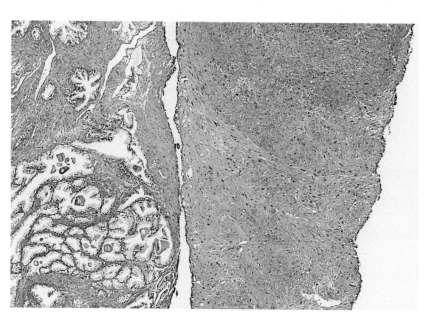

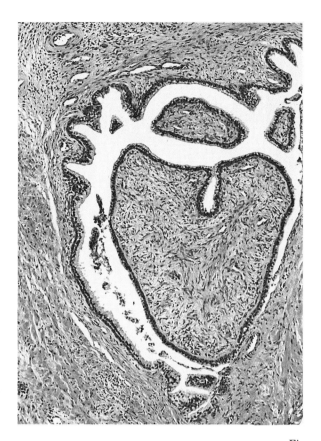 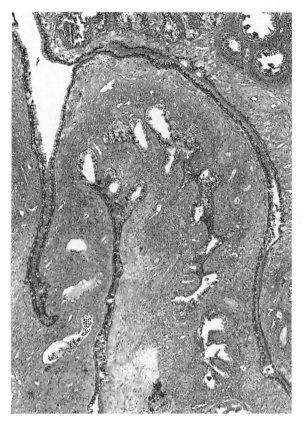

Figure 2-23
BENIGN NODULAR HYPERPLASIA
The proliferation of glands and stroma has produced a pattern reminiscent of a mammary fibroadenoma (left) and a mammary phyllodes tumor (right). Note the cleft-like spaces. (Right figure courtesy of Dr. D.G. Bostwick, Rochester, MN.)

Secondary Changes and Other Associated Findings in Nodular Hyperplasia. A rare but important associated pattern is sclerosing adenosis. The significance of this lesion is almost entirely its potential for misdiagnosis as cancer and accordingly it is considered in chapter 7. Nodular hyperplasia may undergo a number of other secondary changes or be associated with miscellaneous other findings, some relatively common, such as cystic dilatation and irregular branching of peripheral zone acini (figs. 2-7, 2-24) or corpora amylacea (fig. 2-25). Rare findings include psammomatous calcification (fig. 2-26), oncocytic (fig. 2-27) or mucinous metaplasia of the epithelium (fig. 2-28). The number of corpora amylacea is less than usually seen in nonhyperplastic tissue (136). Focal epithelial atrophy, with low cuboidal cells rather than the usual tall columnar cells, may be seen (fig. 2-14, right) (136). The glands may undergo marked and extensive cystic dilatation with attenuation of the epithelium (fig. 2-14, left). Acute and chronic inflammation are common accompaniments of nodular hyperplasia. In one study, inflammatory changes were noted in 98 percent of surgically removed glands with nodular hyperplasia (119). Suppurative, chronic lymphocytic and granulomatous inflammation may be seen, the latter sometimes associated with duct rupture and release of contents into the stroma, mimicking idiopathic nonspecific granulomatous prostatitis (see chapter 7). Basal cell hyperplasia (see below) and transitional cell metaplasia, at least in minor amounts, may be noted in some nodules and are uncommonly striking (see chapter 7).

Infarction of hyperplastic nodules is relatively common, and is seen in up to 25 percent of large nodules (fig. 2-4) (128). Although the precise mechanism is unknown, it is thought to result from interference with the blood supply of the nodule, perhaps by compression from adjacent

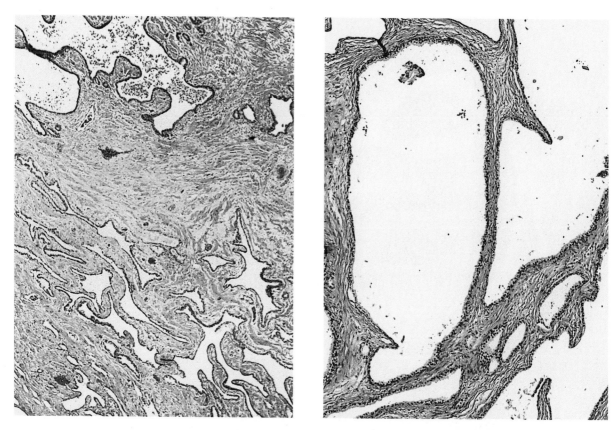

Figure 2-24
PERIPHERAL ZONE CHANGES SECONDARY TO BENIGN NODULAR HYPERPLASIA
There are irregular branching glands that are focally cystic in the peripheral zone. This abnormality is probably secondary to obstruction related to the hyperplasia and should be distinguished from the uncommon nodular hyperplasia of the peripheral zone.

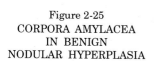

Figure 2-25
CORPORA AMYLACEA
IN BENIGN
NODULAR HYPERPLASIA

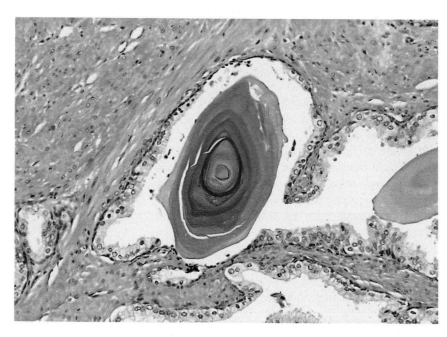

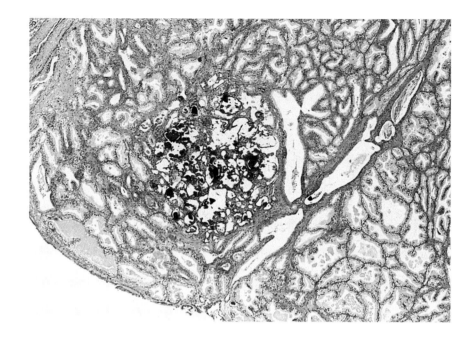

Figure 2-26
BENIGN NODULAR
HYPERPLASIA WITH
CALCIFICATION

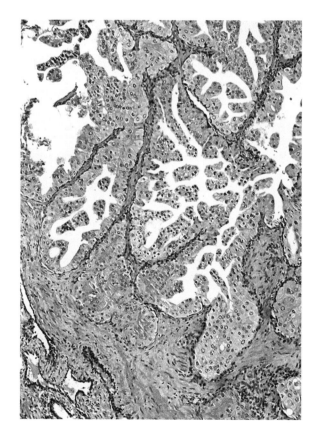

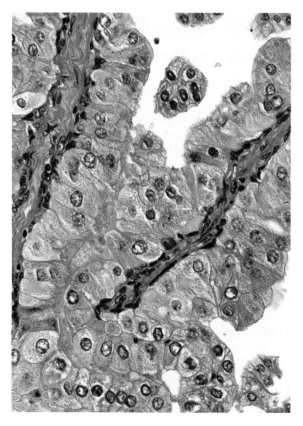

Figure 2-27
BENIGN NODULAR HYPERPLASIA
Oncocytic metaplasia of the epithelial cells is present.

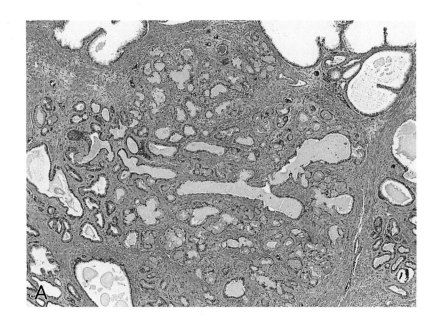

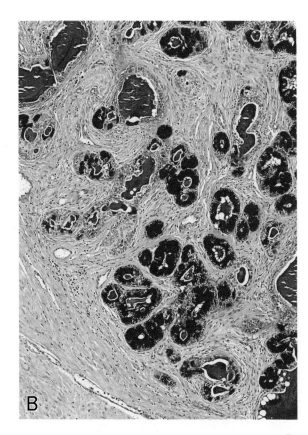

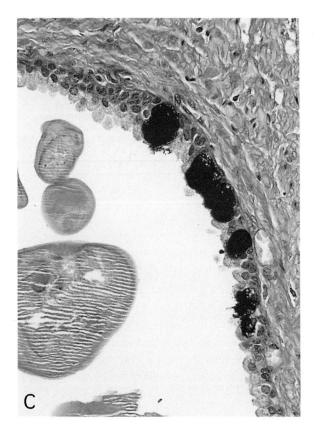

Figure 2-28
BENIGN NODULAR HYPERPLASIA WITH MUCINOUS METAPLASIA
A: The typical nodular configuration is present.
B: The mucinous nature of the epithelium is highlighted by a periodic acid–Schiff (PAS) stain.
C: Goblet cells lining some of the acini are demonstrated by the PAS stain.

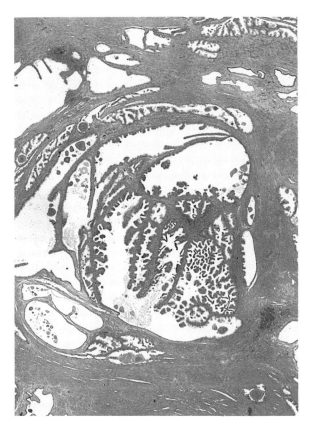

Figure 2-29
BENIGN NODULAR HYPERPLASIA WITH
ASSOCIATED HIGH-GRADE PROSTATIC
INTRAEPITHELIAL NEOPLASIA
Note the hyperplastic nodule in which numerous cystically dilated glands are apparent. Several spaces are lined by architecturally complex structures with hyperchromatic epithelium, making this area stand out on low-power evaluation.

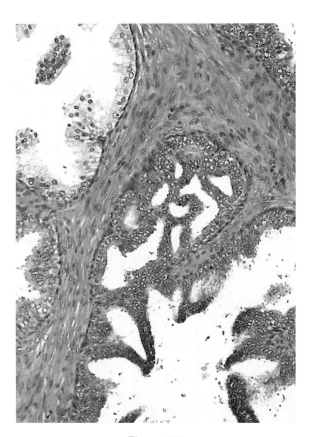

Figure 2-30
BENIGN NODULAR HYPERPLASIA WITH
ASSOCIATED HIGH-GRADE PROSTATIC
INTRAEPITHELIAL NEOPLASIA
A high-power view shows tufted, micropapillary, and cribriform patterns (lower right) in comparison to a routine hyperplastic gland (upper left).

nodules. Squamous metaplasia is commonly seen at the edge of the infarcted tissue and may also be seen within the infarct (see chapter 7).

Prostatic intraepithelial neoplasia (figs. 2-29, 2-30) (see page 73) and atypical adenomatous hyperplasia (see page 96) may be seen in association with nodular hyperplasia. Adenocarcinoma is found in up to 20 percent of transurethral resectates performed for clinical hyperplasia (101,109,133). Many of these tumors are small volume lesions that are frequently well differentiated (see chapter 4).

The lumens of the glands in nodular hyperplasia often contain eosinophilic material that has a more homogeneous dense appearance than the flocculent eosinophilic material often seen in the lumens of neoplastic glands (see page 146). The wispy basophilic mucin seen in many neoplastic acini is also, for practical purposes, absent in the lumens of hyperplastic glands. The luminal secretions of hyperplastic glands may be periodic acid–Schiff (PAS)-positive, diastase resistant, indicative of neutral mucins. In contrast to many adenocarcinomas, the luminal contents are usually negative for acid mucosubstances (alcian blue negative) (107,112).

Lipofuscin (see chapter 1) may occasionally be observed in areas of nodular hyperplasia (122). Rare scattered neuroendocrine (argentaffin) cells can be seen on routine hematoxylin and eosin stains and confirmed or highlighted using silver stains; they are more readily demonstrated using immunohistochemistry for neuron-specific enolase, chromogranin, and synaptophysin (100, 116). Various peptide hormones are identifiable in

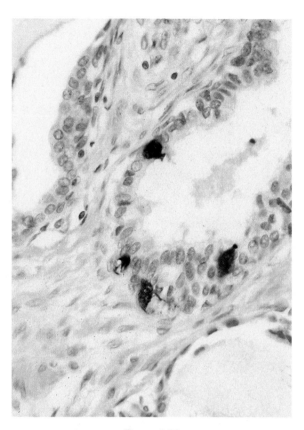

Figure 2-31
BENIGN NODULAR HYPERPLASIA WITH
SEROTONIN-POSITIVE CELLS

Table 2-4

CLASSIFICATION OF PROSTATIC BASAL CELL LESIONS

Basal cell hyperplasia
    complete
    incomplete
    atypical basal cell hyperplasia
    adenoid cystic-like basal cell hyperplasia
    atrophy-associated basal cell hyperplasia

Adenoid cystic carcinoma (see chapter 5)

Basaloid carcinoma (see chapter 5)

In some studies, the ultrastructural features of nodular hyperplasia are indistinguishable from those of the normal gland (102). Others have noted a reduction in the number of tall secretory cells and an increase in cuboidal cells, correlating with reduced secretory activity (114,123).

Most DNA flow cytometric studies performed on nodular hyperplasia tissue have yielded diploid results (98,104,144). Occasional examples of aneuploid stem lines, however, have been found (104).

BASAL CELL HYPERPLASIA

A classification of basal cell proliferations of the prostate gland is presented in Table 2-4. Since basal cell hyperplasia is usually seen in cases of nodular hyperplasia, the clinical features are essentially the same as those of that condition (152,156). The only different significant clinical association is with antiandrogen therapy (see page 59). Basal cell hyperplasia is typically found in the transition zone and is therefore usually identified in transurethral resection or prostatectomy specimens, but it may be encountered, infrequently, in needle biopsies. It has no specific gross features. Basal cell hyperplasia may also be atrophy-associated and found in the peripheral zone in contrast to usual basal cell hyperplasia.

Microscopic Findings. The normal prostatic ducts and acini have a well-defined basal cell layer which may undergo proliferation that varies from minor, not warranting a specific diagnosis, to florid basal cell hyperplasia (figs. 2-33, 2-34) (152,153,156). The latter, particularly if cytologically atypical (154,155), may cause confusion

these cells including calcitonin-like proteins and serotonin (fig. 2-31). Paneth cell-like metaplasia (see chapter 1) may also be seen.

Immunohistochemical studies of nodular hyperplasia using the prostatic-specific markers, PSA and PAP, show strong diffuse cytoplasmic staining of secretory cells as seen in the normal prostate (fig. 2-32, left) (129,134,143,146). A positive carcinoembryonic antigen (CEA) reaction is often present in the apical cytoplasm of the secretory cells and along the luminal border.

Both secretory and basal cell compartments stain strongly with broad spectrum and low molecular weight cytokeratins while the basal cells are specifically decorated with high molecular weight cytokeratin (clone 34βE12) (fig. 2-32, right). This pattern of filament expression is similar to that of normal glands (97,148). Furthermore, the secretory cells, like those of the normal prostate, may exhibit focal paranuclear vimentin positivity (148).

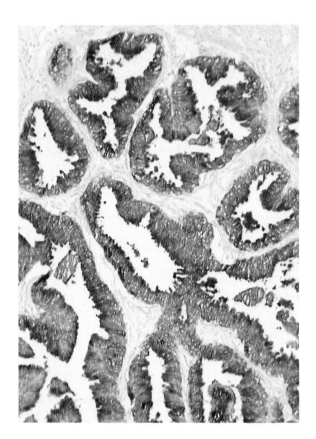 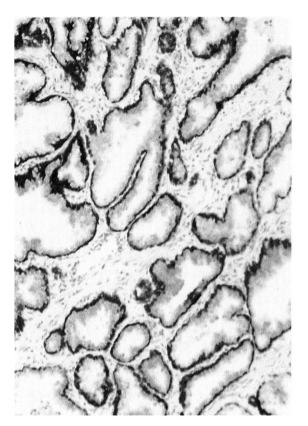

Figure 2-32
BENIGN NODULAR HYPERPLASIA
Left: There is intense immunoreactivity in the secretory cells for prostate-specific antigen.
Right: The basal cell–specific high molecular weight cytokeratin stain (clone 34βE12) intensely stains the basal cells.

with carcinoma, including the rare basaloid carcinoma (see page 230). On low-power microscopy, a nodule of nodular hyperplasia may be partially or completely involved. The edge of the nodule is usually relatively smooth and pushing, but on occasion may have a pseudoinfiltrative appearance. When well delineated, the term basal cell adenoma has been used (158) but is not indicated for what, in our opinion, is a hyperplastic rather than a benign neoplastic process. The basaloid nests and cords are often solid (complete basal cell hyperplasia) (fig. 2-33F), but tubules, occasionally lined by secretory cells, may be seen (incomplete basal cell hyperplasia) (fig. 2-33E). The basal cells are multilayered and relatively uniform, with a high nuclear to cytoplasmic ratio. The nuclear chromatin is evenly distributed, and small chromocenters may be seen. Small amounts of pale eosinophilic cytoplasm are ap-

parent; rarely, the cytoplasm is more conspicuous and clear. When tubules are present, they are lined by cuboidal or low columnar cells with basally located, round, uniform nuclei and apical, clear to lightly eosinophilic cytoplasm. These juxtaluminal cells are surrounded by the multiple layers of basal cells. The lumens are usually central but may be eccentric within the nests (fig. 2-33B). A cribriform secretory cell pattern, as noted in the cribriform variant of benign nodular hyperplasia, may also be present (see page 309). However, the glandular structures are usually smaller than in cribriform hyperplasia and are, by definition, surrounded by more conspicuous basal cells. The lumens within basal cell hyperplasia may be empty or contain an eosinophilic secretion; sometimes calcification and psammoma body–like structures may be noted. Rarely, wispy basophilic mucin is seen. Occasionally, the glandular pattern of basal cell

Figure 2-33
SCHEMATIC REPRESENTATION
OF THE SPECTRUM OF BENIGN
BASAL CELL PROLIFERATIONS
IN THE PROSTATE

The proliferations range from limited (B,C) to florid examples of incomplete (E) or complete (F) basal cell hyperplasia.

A: This is a normal gland with a thin peripheral layer of basal cells underlying the cuboidal to columnar secretory layer that abuts the lumen.

B: There is a focal eccentric proliferation of basal cells causing mild distortion of the lumen.

C: There is symmetric proliferation of basal cells of limited degree.

D: Eccentric proliferation of basal cells with prominent nucleoli.

E: There is loss of the secretory cell layer due to the prominent basal cell proliferation but with retention of the lumen.

F: There is complete obliteration of the lumen with formation of solid nests of basal cells. (A–F: Fig. 1 from Devaraj LT, Bostwick DG. Atypical basal cell hyperplasia of the prostate. Immunophenotypic profile and proposed classification of basal cell proliferations. Am J Surg Pathol 1993;17:645–59.)

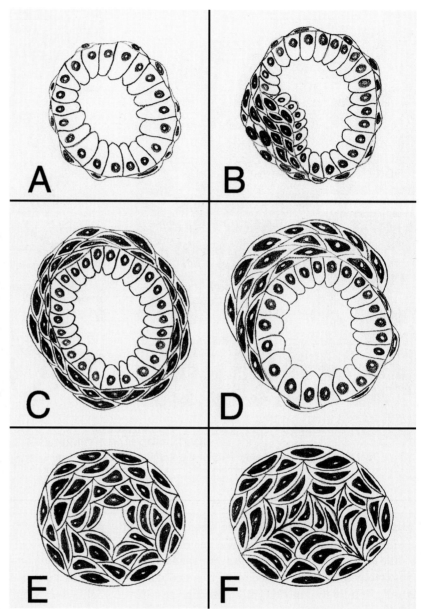

hyperplasia has an adenoid cystic-like appearance (see page 309) (162,167). Focal keratinizing or nonkeratinizing squamous metaplasia may also be present (fig. 2-35).

The stroma of basal cell hyperplasia usually resembles the fibroblastic or fibromuscular stroma of ordinary nodular hyperplasia but may be more cellular and, occasionally, myxoid ("embryonal hyperplasia") (149). In some cases the stroma resembles that of sclerosing adenosis, and rarely, foci of sclerosing adenosis coexist with basal cell hyperplasia (163).

The nuclei of the hyperplastic basal cells are typically small, round to oval, and uniform, and lack prominent nucleoli or pleomorphism (152, 156). In some cases, small basophilic nucleoli are seen without associated pleomorphism or mitoses. When nuclear enlargement, nucleolar prominence (fig. 2-36), hyperchromasia, and mitoses are identified, the term "atypical basal cell hyperplasia" has been used (see chapter 7) (154,155). Prominent nucleoli are occasionally seen in the basal cells in the absence of basal cell hyperplasia.

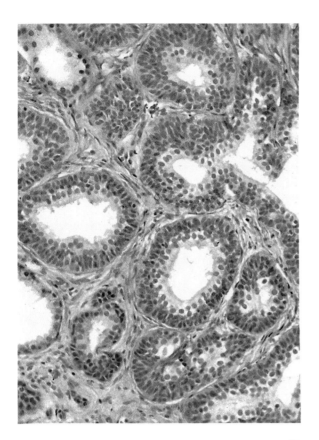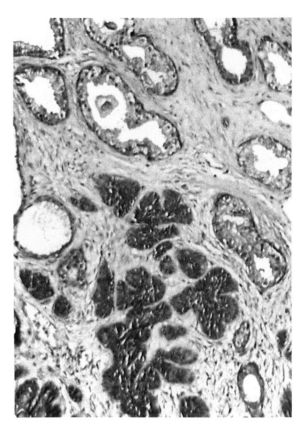

Figure 2-34
BASAL CELL HYPERPLASIA
Left: The process is limited, with preservation of the secretory cell layer ("incomplete" basal cell hyperplasia).
Right: There is striking basal cell hyperplasia with a solid appearance ("complete" basal cell hyperplasia).

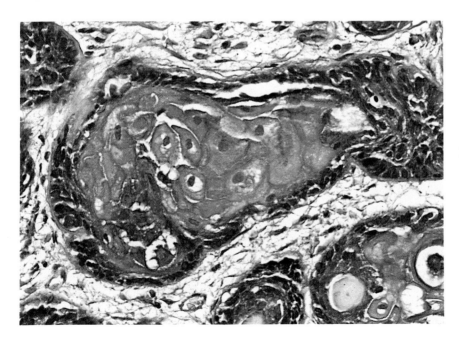

Figure 2-35
BASAL CELL HYPERPLASIA
WITH
SQUAMOUS METAPLASIA

Foci of basal cell hyperplasia may occasionally be seen in atrophic glands, especially in the peripheral zone (atrophy-associated basal cell hyperplasia). With androgen ablation therapy, the basal cell layer surrounding non-neoplastic glands is often prominent (fig. 2-37, left), and areas of basal cell hyperplasia are common (fig. 2-37, right) (151,157,160,165). This change may also be present in transition zone nodules and may be striking.

The basal cells stain with antibodies against broad spectrum keratins and basal cell–specific high molecular weight cytokeratin (clone 34βE12) (fig. 2-38) (150,159,161,164,166). Stains for vimentin and actin are usually negative. Positivity for PSA and PAP is usually found in areas containing secretory cells but may also be seen in some basal cells. S-100 protein is usually negative, although occasionally positive in basal cell hyperplasia (154). Occasional neuroendocrine cells have also been demonstrated with the neuron-specific enolase and chromogranin stains (154). The basaloid cells in basal cell hyperplasia resemble normal basal cells at the ultrastructural level (fig. 2-39) (153).

Differential Diagnosis. Basal cell hyperplasia may be confused with several metaplastic, preneoplastic, and neoplastic entities, specifically, transitional cell metaplasia, prostatic intraepithelial neoplasia, conventional adenocarcinoma, and basaloid carcinoma.

Transitional cell metaplasia (see page 301) may occur in peripheral ducts and acini, and is sometimes associated with prostatitis and reactive atypia. It is usually focal and not necessarily related to areas of nodular hyperplasia. The transitional cells generally have a lower nuclear to cytoplasmic ratio than that seen in basal cell hyperplasia due to their more abundant cytoplasm. They have elongated nuclei, rather than the round ones of basal cell hyperplasia, and frequently exhibit nuclear grooves. There is evidence of basal to luminal maturation. In contrast, basal cell hyperplasia is usually seen in relationship to nodular hyperplasia and consists of piled up, smaller, round, and more basophilic cells with higher nuclear to cytoplasmic ratios. Overlapping features do occur, however, in some cases.

Basal cell hyperplasia, particularly when there are enlarged nucleoli, may be confused with high-grade prostatic intraepithelial neopla-

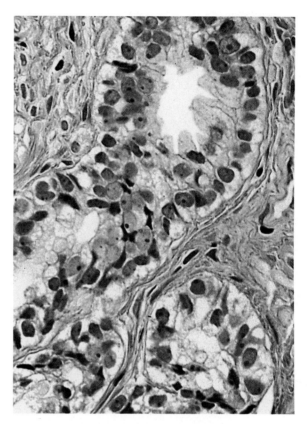

Figure 2-36
ATYPICAL BASAL CELL HYPERPLASIA
Note the nucleolar prominence.

sia with a "flat" architecture (see chapter 3). In the latter the secretory cells usually show other architectural patterns, specifically tufted and micropapillary, which are not features of basal cell hyperplasia. The atypical nuclear features of high-grade prostatic intraepithelial neoplasia occur in secretory cells, not basal cells. Furthermore, in basal cell hyperplasia, positive immunostaining for basal cell–specific high molecular weight cytokeratin (clone 34βE12) is identified in most of the proliferating cells, while this marker is negative in the proliferating secretory cells of prostatic intraepithelial neoplasia but highlights a continuous or disrupted basal cell layer around the proliferating secretory cells.

Basal cell hyperplasia and atypical basal cell hyperplasia have a nodular configuration due to their usual occurrence within foci of nodular hyperplasia, and the distinction from conventional adenocarcinoma should not be a problem. Furthermore, basal cells are almost invariably

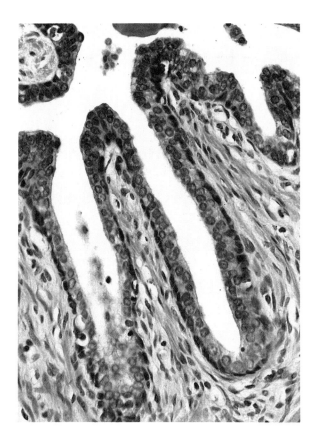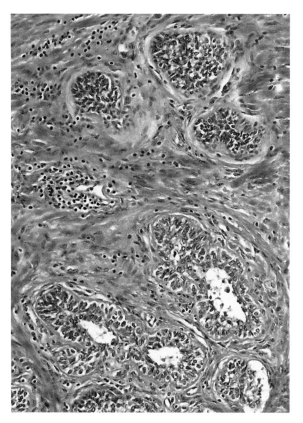

Figure 2-37
BASAL CELL CHANGES ASSOCIATED WITH ANDROGEN ABLATION THERAPY
Left: Note the shrinkage of secretory cells and basal cell prominence.
Right: Note the focal obliteration of the secretory cells by hyperplastic basal cells.

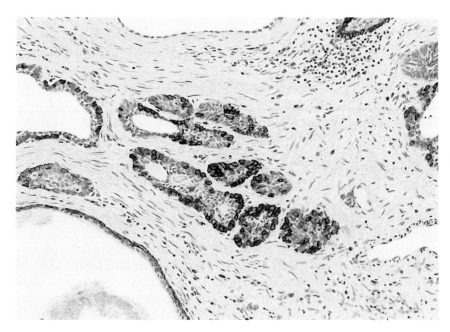

Figure 2-38
BASAL CELL HYPERPLASIA
There is positivity for high molecular weight cytokeratin (34βE12).

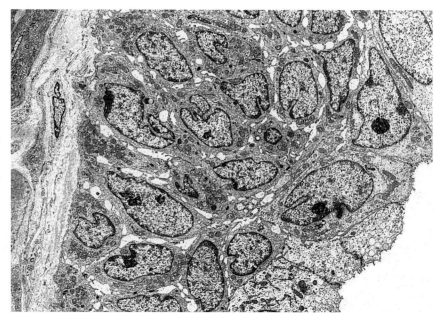

Figure 2-39
BASAL CELL HYPERPLASIA
Note the proliferation of oval to polygonal basal cells with nuclear irregularity. Occasional tonofilament-like bundles are seen in the cytoplasm.

absent in adenocarcinoma with negative high molecular weight cytokeratin stains (clone 34βE12). Basal cell hyperplasia may mimic both adenoid cystic and basaloid carcinomas (see chapter 5). The diagnosis of a carcinoma of these types, however, is only tenable in cases with infiltrative growth, marked cytologic atypia, perineural invasion, extraprostatic spread, or areas of necrosis. Immunohistochemistry is not helpful in distinguishing basal cell hyperplasia from basaloid carcinoma.

ATROPHY-ASSOCIATED HYPERPLASIA

Basal Cell Hyperplasia

This variant of basal cell hyperplasia (fig. 2-37) has been discussed above (see page 58).

Postatrophic Hyperplasia

General Features and Historical Background. Epithelial and acinar proliferations in the setting of atrophy have been referred to most commonly as postatrophic hyperplasia (168, 170,173,174,181). Knowledge of this process is clouded by varied nomenclature in the literature and a relative dearth of morphologic studies. To place this lesion in context with other lesions it is necessary to review the development of the nomenclature in this area.

Franks (173) introduced the term postatrophic hyperplasia and described two patterns depending on whether the preexisting (or associated) atrophy was simple (lobular) or sclerotic. Hyperplasia occurring in the setting of simple (lobular) atrophy was referred to as "lobular hyperplasia" (fig. 2-40) (173), and he likened it to the breast process of the same name. The characteristic appearance is that of a lobule containing closely packed acini, some of them dilated and most having empty lumens. The acini are lined by cells with scant cytoplasm for the most part (fig. 2-40, right). The process has the regular appearance of typical atrophy and, in our experience, does not provide diagnostic difficulty, in contrast to the second pattern of postatrophic hyperplasia that Franks referred to as "sclerotic atrophy with hyperplasia" or "postsclerotic hyperplasia" (see below).

Further nosological confusion results from the fact that the term "secondary hyperplasia" has apparently been used synonymously for postatrophic hyperplasia by some recent workers (171) and, on the basis of his description, seemingly by Moore in one of his classic studies (178). However, Franks appears to have considered secondary hyperplasia a separate process. Furthermore, Totten et al. (182) previously used the term "lobular hyperplasia" to connote the second pattern of Franks (his first pattern being

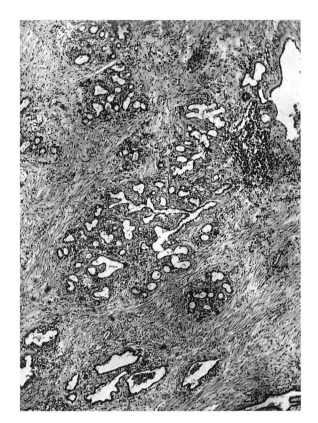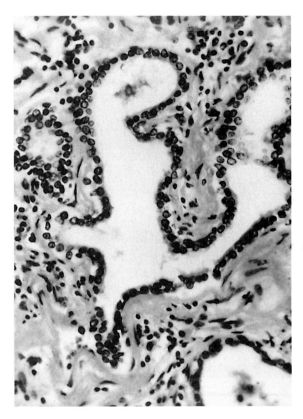

Figure 2-40
POSTATROPHIC HYPERPLASIA
Low (left) and higher power (right) views of the pattern that has been subtyped as lobular hyperplasia. (Figs. 8 and 9 from Franks LM. Atrophy and hyperplasia in the prostate proper. J Path Bact 1954;68:617–21.)

"lobular hyperplasia"). Because of this varied usage of these terms we do not use the designations "secondary hyperplasia" or "lobular hyperplasia," although some do (177). We use the term "postatrophic hyperplasia" primarily in cases that would qualify as the second pattern of Franks, in which he emphasized stromal sclerosis. However, in our experience, sclerosis is not an invariable feature of the lesion and that has also been the experience of others. Additionally, there is overlap between the two patterns.

The exact nature of postatrophic hyperplasia is unknown. It is unsettled whether it represents atrophy that is undergoing secondary hyperplasia or glands that are becoming atrophic but some of whose cells still retain appreciable cytoplasm. The term "partial atrophy" has been used to describe this process by some who favor the second hypothesis (172,179), and others favor the designation "hyperplastic atrophy" (169). Due to

the apparent neoacinar formation in some cases, suggesting proliferation, this pattern is included in the classification of hyperplasia here. Furthermore, a recent kinetic study using the MIB-1 antibody showed that the small glands of postatrophic hyperplasia exhibit greater proliferative activity than benign nonatrophic glands (179a). Postatrophic hyperplasia is typically, but not invariably, seen in the peripheral zone.

Microscopic Findings. This process is characterized by glands that usually exhibit some architectural abnormality, often appearing irregular, elongated, or stellate with, in some instances, an uneven distribution of glands and stroma (figs. 2-41, 2-42). Small glands may appear to "bud-off" larger dilated acini. Stromal sclerosis may accentuate the architectural irregularity (176,180). However, despite what may initially be a disconcerting picture suggesting a possibility of carcinoma, lobulation is usually still

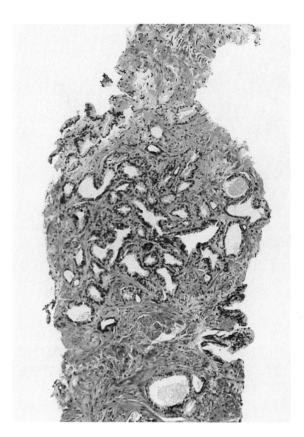
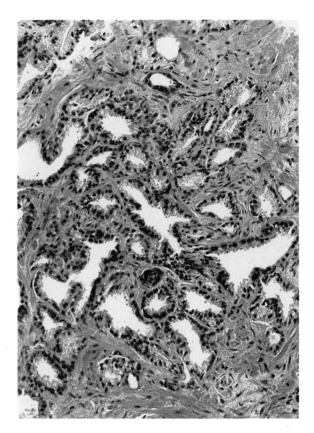

Figure 2-41
POSTATROPHIC HYPERPLASIA: NEEDLE BIOPSY
Left: The low-power appearance may raise some concern for carcinoma.
Right: Note the closely packed acini lined by cells, most of which have appreciable pale cytoplasm but a few of which have scant cytoplasm.

apparent (figs. 2-41, 2-42). The glands are lined by cuboidal cells with scant or appreciable cytoplasm, most often the former. The resultant variable nuclear-cytoplasmic ratio creates an irregular luminal contour and apical cytoplasmic apocrine-like blebs may also be seen. The nuclei may display minor nuclear abnormalities including slight enlargement, mild pleomorphism, and hyperchromasia (fig. 2-41, right). Nucleoli may be seen but are not as prominent as in carcinoma. The acini very rarely have acid mucin in their lumens, a finding more commonly associated with adenocarcinoma (173,175,181), but frequently contain amorphous eosinophilic debris in the experience of one group (179). Although the pattern is irregular, basal cells are usually visualized, at least focally, in our experience (fig. 2-43). However, in one study they were not identified in almost 30 percent of the cases

(179). Superimposed mucinous metaplasia of the epithelium has been described in two cases of postatrophic hyperplasia (170).

Differential Diagnosis. Postatrophic hyperplasia may simulate small acinar carcinoma as first emphasized by Totten et al. (182) (see page 293). The key points in this differential diagnosis are: 1) postatrophic hyperplasia is characterized by hyperplastic glands intermingled with atrophic ones; overall there is scant cytoplasm in contrast to most moderate to well-differentiated carcinomas; 2) the degree of nuclear atypia is less in postatrophic hyperplasia than in most carcinomas. Some slight nuclear pleomorphism may be present but the large nucleoli that typify most prostatic adenocarcinomas are not seen; 3) the slit-like acini and apical blebs of some cases of postatrophic hyperplasia are not features of most carcinomas; 4) the dense fibrotic stroma and shrunken smooth muscle cells

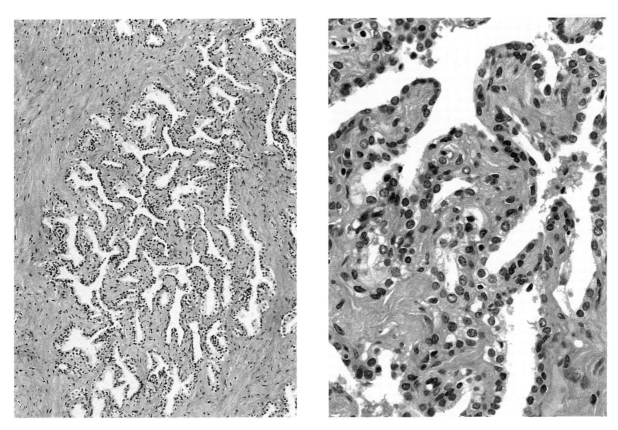

Figure 2-42
POSTATROPHIC HYPERPLASIA: PROSTATECTOMY SPECIMEN
Left: Branching elongated acini are lined by cuboidal cells with generally scant cytoplasm.
Right: Note the bland cytologic features.

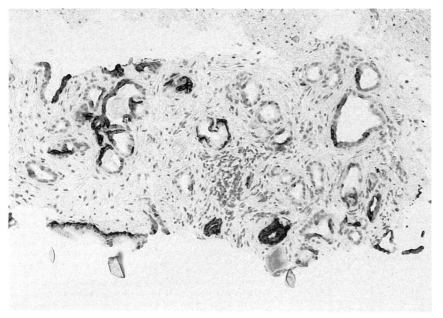

Figure 2-43
POSTATROPHIC
HYPERPLASIA
Patchy and discontinuous stain-
ing for high molecular weight
cytokeratin (clone 34βE12).

of some cases of postatrophic hyperplasia are uncommon in prostatic adenocarcinoma; 5) an obvious infiltrative pattern is not seen in postatrophic hyperplasia and lobulation is a typical helpful architectural feature; 6) adjacent typical atrophy may be a clue to the diagnosis; and

7) the basal cell layer is typically present, although it may be difficult to appreciate in some cases. Immunohistochemistry using high molecular weight cytokeratin (clone 34βE12) may be invaluable in this regard (fig. 2-43).

REFERENCES

Benign Nodular Hyperplasia

General References

1. Kirby RS, Christmas TJ. Benign prostatic hyperplasia. London: Gower Medical Publishing, 1993.
2. Kirby R, McConnell J, Fitzpatrick J, Roehrborn C, Boyle P, eds. Textbook of benign prostatic hyperplasia. UK: Isis Medical Media, 1996.

3. Moore RA. Benign hypertrophy of the prostate. A morphologic study. J Urol 1943;50:680–710.

General Features

4. Albarran J, Hallé N. Hypertrophie et néoplasies épithéliales de la prostate. Ann Mal Org Génitourin 1900;18:113–147, 225–261.
5. Albarran J, Motz B. Contribution à l'étude de l'anatomie macroscopique de la prostate hypertrophiée. Ann Mal Org Génitourin 1902;20:769–817.
6. Barry MJ. Epidemiology and natural history of benign prostatic hyperplasia. Urol Clin North Am 1990; 17:495–507.
7. Bartsch W, Becker H, Pinkenburg FA, Krieg M. Hormone blood levels and their interrelationships in normal men and men with benign prostatic hyperplasia. Acta Endocrinol 1979;90:727–36.
8. Berry SJ, Coffey DS, Walsh PC, Ewing LL. The development of human benign prostatic hyperplasia with age. J Urol 1984:132:474–9.
9. Birkhoff JD. Natural history of benign prostatic hypertrophy. In: Benign prostatic hypertrophy. Hinman F Jr, Boyarsky S, eds. New York: Springer-Verlag, 1983:5–9.
10. Bostwick DG. Pathology of benign prostatic hyperplasia. In: Kirby R, McConnell J, Fitzpatrick J, Roehrborn C, Boyle P, eds. Textbook of benign hyperplasia. UK: Isis Medical Media, 1996:91–104.
11. Bruchovsky N, Wilson JD. The conversion of testosterone to 5-alpha-androstan-17-beta-ol-3-one by rat prostate in vivo and in vitro. J Biol Chem 1968;243:2012–21.
12. Cabot AT. The question of castration for enlarged prostate. Ann Surg 1896;24:265–309.
13. Chang HL, Char GY. Benign hypertrophy of prostate. Chin Med J 1936;50:1707–22.
14. Cunha GR. Tissue interactions between epithelium and mesenchyme of urogenital and integumental origin. Anat Rec 1972;172:529–41.
15. Cunha GR, Chung LW, Shannon JM, Reese BA. Stromal-epithelial interactions in sex differentiation. Biol Reprod 1980;22:19–42.

16. Cunha GR, Fujii H, Neubauer BL, Shannon JM, Sawyer L, Reese BA. Epithelial-mesenchymal interactions in prostatic development. I. Morphological observations of prostatic induction by urogenital sinus mesenchyme in epithelium of the adult rodent urinary bladder. J Cell Biol 1983;96:1662–70.
17. Deming CL. The effect of castration on benign hypertrophy of the prostate in man. J Urol 1935;33:388–99.
18. Deming CL, Neumann C. Early phases of prostatic hyperplasia. Surg Gynec Obst 1939;68:155–60.
19. Doehring CB, Sandra MG, Partin AW, et al. Histologic characterization of hereditary benign prostatic hyperplasia. Urology 1996;48:650–3.
20. Franks LM. Benign nodular hyperplasia of the prostate: a review. Ann R Coll Surg Engl 1954;14:92–106.
21. Franks LM. Benign prostatic hyperplasia. Gross and microscopic anatomy. In: Grayhack JT, Wilson JD, Scherbenske MJ, eds., Benign prostatic hyperplasia, DHEW #NIH 76–113, Washington, D.C.: US Government Printing Office, 1976:63.
22. Geller J, Albert J, Lopez D, Geller S, Niwayama G. Comparison of androgen metabolites in benign prostatic hypertrophy (BPH) and normal prostate. J Clin Endocrinol Metab 1976;43:686–8.
23. Ghanadian R. Hormonal environment of the normal prostate. In: Ghanadian R, ed. The endocrinology of prostate tumours. Lancaster, England: TP Press, 1983:35.
24. Gover M. A statistical study of the etiology of benign hypertrophy of the prostate gland. Johns Hopkins Hosp Rep 1923;21:231–95.
25. Habib FK, Lee IR, Stitch SR, Smith PH. Androgen levels in the plasma and prostatic tissues of patients with benign hypertrophy and carcinoma of the prostate. J Endocrinol 1976;71:99–107.

26. Hammond GL, Kontturi M, Vihko P, Vihko R. Serum steroids in normal males and patients with prostatic diseases. Clin Endocrinol 1978;9:113–21.

27. Harbitz TB, Haugen OA. Histology of the prostate in elderly men. A study in an autopsy series. Acta Path Microbiol Scand [A] 1972;80:756–68.

28. Huggins C, Stevens R. The effect of castration on benign hypertrophy of the prostate in man. J Urol 1940;43:705–14.

29. Hunt VC. Benign prostatic hypertrophy. Surg Gynecol Obstet 1928;46:769–73.

30. Isaacs JT. Antagonistic effect of androgen on prostatic cell death. Prostate 1984;5:545–57.

31. Isaacs JT. Control of cell proliferation and cell death in the normal and neoplastic prostate: a stem cell model. In: Rogers CH, Coffey DS, Cunha G, Grayhack JT, Hinman F Jr, Horton R, eds. Benign prostatic hyperplasia. Washington, DC: US Department of Health and Human Services, NIH Publication #87–2881, 1987:85–94.

32. Isaacs JT, Brendler CB, Walsh PC. Changes in the metabolism of dihydrotestosterone in the hyperplastic human prostate. J Clin Endocrin Metab 1983; 56:139–45.

33. Isaacs JT, Coffey DS. Etiology and disease process of benign prostatic hyperplasia. Prostate [Suppl.] 1989;2:33–50.

34. Jores L. Ueber die hypertrophie des sogenannten mittleren lappens der prostata. Archiv Pathol Anat Physiol Klinische 1894;135:224–47.

35. Kahle PJ, Beacham HT. Review of prostatic operations of Charity Hospital, New Orleans, Louisiana. Urol Cutaneous Rev 1936;40:769–74.

36. Kambal A. Prostatic obstruction in Sudan. Br J Urol 1977;49:139–41.

37. Kovi J. Surgical pathology of prostate and seminal vesicles, Boca Raton, FL: CRC Press, 1989:101–2.

38. Krieg M, Bartsch W, Janssen W, Voigt KD. A comparative study of binding, metabolism and endogenous levels of androgen in normal, hyperplastic and carcinomatous human prostate. J Steroid Biochem 1979;11:615–24.

39. Kyprianou N, Isaacs JT. Activation of programmed cell death in the rat ventral prostate after castration. Endocrinology 1988;122:552–62.

40. Leduc IE. The anatomy of the prostate and the pathology of early benign hypertrophy. J Urol 1939;43:1217–41.

41. Leissner KH, Tisell LE. The weight of the human prostate. Scan J Urol Nephrol 1979;13:137–42.

42. Lytton B. Interracial incidence of benign prostatic hypertrophy. In: Hinman F Jr, Boyarsky S, eds. Benign prostatic hypertrophy. New York: Springer-Verlag, 1983:22.

43. Lytton B, Emery JM, Harvard BM. The incidence of benign prostatic obstruction. J Urol 1968;90:639–45.

44. McNeal JE. Normal histology of the prostate. Am J Surg Pathol 1988;12:619–33.

45. McNeal JE. Origin and evolution of benign prostatic enlargement. Invest Urol 1978;15:340–5.

46. McNeal JE. The prostate and prostatic urethra: a morphologic synthesis. J Urol 1972;107:1008–16.

47. McNeal JE. Regional morphology and pathology of the prostate. Am J Clin Pathol 1968;49:347–57.

48. Meikle AW, Stringham JD, Olsen DC. Subnormal tissue 3-alpha-androstanediol and androsterone in prostatic hyperplasia. J Clin Endocrinol Metab 1978;47:909–13.

49. Moore RA. Benign hypertrophy of the prostate. A morphologic study. J Urol 1943;50:680–710.

50. Morgagni G. The seats and causes of disease investigated by anatomy. Miller A, Cadell T, eds. London: Johnson and Payne, 1769:460–2.

51. Naslund MJ, Coffey DS. The hormonal imprinting of the prostate and the regulation of stem cells in prostatic growth. In: Rogers CH, Coffey DS, Cunha G, Grayhack JT, Hinman F Jr, Horton R, eds. Benign prostatic hyperplasia, Washington, DC: US Department of Health and Human Services, NIH Publication #87–2881, 1987:73–83.

52. Neubauer BL. Endocrine and cellular inductive factors in the development of human benign prostatic hypertrophy. In: Hinman F Jr, Boyarsky S, eds. Benign prostatic hypertrophy. New York: Springer-Verlag, 1983:179.

53. Oberndorfer S. Die inneren mäännlichen gerschlectsorgane. In: Henke F, Lubarsch O, eds. Handbuch der speziellen pathologischen anatomie und histologie, Berlin: Verlag von Julius Springer, 1931:427–825.

54. Oesterling JE. The origin and development of benign prostatic hyperplasia. An age-dependent process. J Androl 1991;12:348–55.

55. Partin AW, Coffey DS. The molecular biology, endocrinology, and physiology of the prostate and seminal vesicles. In: Walsh PC, Retik AB, Vaughan ED Jr, Wein AJ, eds. Campbell's urology, 7th ed. Philadelphia: WB Saunders, 1998:1381–428.

56. Partin AW, Page WF, Lee BR, Sanda MG, Miller RN, Walsh PC. Concordance rates for benign prostatic disease among twins suggest hereditary influence. Urology 1994;44:646–50.

57. Pirke KM, Doerr P. Age-related changes in free plasma testosterone, dihydrotestosterone and oestradiol. Acta Endocrinol 1975;80:171–8.

58. Pradhan BK, Chandra K. Morphogenesis of nodular hyperplasia-prostate. J Urol 1975;113:210–3.

59. Rajfer J, Coffey DS. Sex steroid imprinting of the immature prostate: long-term effects. Invest Urol 1978;16:186–90.

60. Reischauer F. Die entsehung der sogenannten prostatahypertrophie. Virchows Arch [A] 1925;256:357–89.

61. Robson MC. The incidence of benign prostatic hyperplasia and prostatic carcinoma in cirrhosis of the liver. J Urol 1964;92:307–10.

62. Rotkin ID. Epidemiology of benign prostatic hypertrophy: review and speculations. In: Grayhack JT, Wilson JD, Sherbenske MJ, eds. Benign prostatic hyperplasia. DHEW (NIH) #76–1113, Washington, D.C.: US Government Printing Office, 1976:105–7.

63. Rotkin ID. Origins, distribution, and risk of benign prostatic hypertrophy. In: Hinman F Jr, Boyarsky S, eds. Benign prostatic hypertrophy. New York: Springer-Verlag, 1983:10.

64. Sanda MG, Beaty TH, Stuzman RE, Childs B, Walsh PC. Genetic susceptibility of benign prostatic hyperplasia. J Urol 1994;152:115–9.

65. Shapiro E, Becich MJ, Hartanto V, Lepor H. The relative proportion of stromal and epithelial hyperplasia is related to the development of symptomatic benign prostate hyperplasia. J Urol 1992;147:1293–7.

66. Siiteri PK, Wilson JD. Dihydrotestosterone in prostatic hypertrophy. I. The formation and content of dihydrotestosterone in the hypertrophic prostate of man. J Clin Invest 1970;49:1737–45.

67. Swyer GI. Post-natal growth changes in the human prostate. J Anat 1944;78:130–45.

68. Teem MV. The relation of the interstitial cells of the testis to prostatic hypertrophy. J Urol 1935;34:692–713.

69. Tveter KJ. Some aspects of the pathogenesis of prostatic hyperplasia. Acta Pathol Microbiol Scand [Suppl] 1974;248:167–74.

70. van Duzen RE, Looney WW, Duncan CN. Development of prostate: anatomical and histological studies. J Urol 1939;41:473–81.

71. Vermeulen A, De Sy W. Androgens in patients with benign prostatic hyperplasia before and after prostatectomy. J Clin Endocrinol Metab 1976;43:1250–4.

72. Vermeulen A, Rubens R, Verdonck L. Testosterone secretion and metabolism in male senescence. J Clin Endocrinol Metab 1972;34:730–5.

73. Walsh PC. Benign prostatic hyperplasia. In: Walsh PC, Retik AB, Stamey TA, Vaughan ED Jr, eds. Campbell's urology, 6th ed. Philadelphia: WB Saunders Co, 1992:1009.

74. Walsh PC, Hutchins GM, Ewing LL. The tissue content of dihydrotestosterone in human prostatic hyperplasia is not supranormal. J Clin Invest 1983;72:1772–7.

75. Wendel EF, Brannen GE, Putong PB, Grayhack JT. The effect of orchiectomy and estrogens on benign prostatic hyperplasia. J Urol 1972;108:116–9.

76. White JW. The results of double castration in hypertrophy of the prostate. Ann Surg 1895;22:1–80.

77. Wilson JD. The pathogenesis of benign prostatic hyperplasia. Am J Med 1980;68:745–56.

78. World Health Statistics Annual. Geneva: World Health Organization, 1985.

79. Yokoyama M, Seki N, Tamai M, Takeuchi M. Benign prostatic hyperplasia in a patient castrated in his youth. J Urol 1989;142:134–5.

80. Zumoff B, Strain GW, Kream J, et al. Age variation of the 24-hour mean plasma concentrations of androgens, estrogens and gonadotropins in normal adult men. J Clin Endocrinol Metab 1982;54:534–8.

Clinical Features

81. Benson MC, Whang IS, Pantuck A, et al. Prostate specific antigen density: a means of distinguishing benign prostatic hypertrophy and prostate cancer. J Urol 1992;147:815–6.

82. Birkhoff JD. Natural history of benign prostatic hypertrophy. In: Hinman F Jr, Boyarsky S, eds. Benign prostatic hypertrophy. New York: Springer-Verlag, 1983:5–9.

83. Catalona WJ, Smith DS, Ornstein DK. Prostate cancer detection in men with serum PSA concentrations of 2.6 to 4.0 mg/ml and benign prostate examination. Enhancement of specificity with free PSA measurements. JAMA 1997;277:1452–5.

84. DeAntoni EP, Crawford ED, Oesterling JE, et al. Age- and race-specific reference ranges from prostate-specific antigen from a large community-based study. Urology 1996;48:234–9.

85. Du Beau CE, Resnick NM. Controversies in the diagnosis and management of benign prostatic hypertrophy. Adv Int Med 1992;37:55–83.

86. Isaacs JT, Coffey DS. Etiology and disease process of benign prostatic hyperplasia. Prostate (Suppl.) 1989;2:33–50.

87. McConnell JD, Bruskewitz R, Walsh P, et al. The effect of finasteride on the risk of acute urinary retention and the need for surgical treatment among men with benign prostatic hyperplasia. N Engl J Med 1998;338:557–63.

88. Oesterling JE. Benign prostatic hyperplasia. Medical and minimally invasive treatment options. N Engl J Med 1995;332:99–109.

89. Oesterling JE, Jacobsen SJ, Chute CG, et al. Serum prostate-specific antigen in a community-based population of healthy men: establishment of age-specific reference ranges. JAMA 1993;270:860–4.

90. Randall A. Median bars as found at autopsy. J Urol 1917;1:383–403.

91. Stimson JB, Fihn SD. Benign prostatic hyperplasia and its treatment. J Gen Int Med 1990;5:153–65.

92. Walsh PC. Benign prostatic hyperplasia. In: Walsh PC, Retik AB, Stamey TA, Vaughan ED Jr, eds. Campbell's urology, 6th ed. Philadelphia: WB Saunders Co, 1992:1009.

Pathology of Nodular Hyperplasia

93. Attah EB, Nkposong EO. Phyllodes type of atypical prostatic hyperplasia. J Urol 1976;115:762–4.

94. Attah EB, Powell ME. Atypical stromal hyperplasia of the prostate gland. Am J Clin Pathol 1977;67:324–7.

95. Ayala AG, Srigley JR, Ro JY, Abdul-Karim FW, Johnson DE. Clear cell cribriform hyperplasia of prostate. Report of 10 cases. Am J Surg Pathol 1986;10:665–71.

96. Bostwick DG. Pathology of benign prostatic hyperplasia. In: Kirby R, McConnell J, Fitzpatrick J, Roehrborn C, Boyle P, eds. Benign prostatic hyperplasia. UK: Isis Medical Media, 1996:91–104.

97. Brawer MK, Peehl DM, Stamey TA, Bostwick DG. Keratin immunoreactivity in the benign and neoplastic human prostate. Cancer Res 1985;45:3663–7.

98. Dejter SW Jr, Cunningham RE, Noguchi PD, et al. Prognostic significance of DNA ploidy in carcinoma of prostate. Urology 1989;33:361–6.

99. Deming CL, Wolf JS. The anatomical origin of benign prostatic enlargement. J Urol 1939;42:566–80.

100. di Sant'Agnese PA, De Mesy Jensen KL. Endocrine–paracrine cells of the prostate and prostatic urethra. An ultrastructural study. Hum Pathol 1984;15:1034–41.

101. Eble JN, Epstein JI. Stage A carcinoma of the prostate. In: Bostwick DG, ed. Pathology of the prostate. New York: Churchill Livingstone, 1990:61–82.

102. Fisher ER, Sieracki JC. Ultrastructure of human normal and neoplastic prostate. Pathol Annu 1970;5:1–26.

103. Fishman JR, Merrill DC. A case of giant prostatic hyperplasia. Urology 1993;42:336–7.

104. Frankfurt OS, Chin JL, Englander LS, Greco WR, Pontes JE, Rustum YM. Relationship between DNA ploidy, glandular differentiation and tumor spread in human prostate cancer. Cancer Res 1985;45:1418–23.

105. Franks LM. Benign nodular hyperplasia of the prostate: a review. Ann R Coll Surg Engl 1954;14:92–106.

106. Franks LM. Benign prostatic hyperplasia. Gross and microscopic anatomy. In: Grayhack JT, Wilson JD, Scherbenske MJ, eds. Benign prostatic hyperplasia. DHEW #NIH 76–113, Washington, D.C.: US Government Printing Office, 1976:63.

107. Franks LM, O'Shea JD, Thomson AE. Mucin in the prostate: a histochemical study in normal glands, latent, clinical and colloid cancers. Cancer 1964;17:983–91.

108. Frauenhoffer EE, Ro JY, El-Naggar AK, Ordonez NG, Ayala AG. Clear cell cribriform hyperplasia of the prostate. Immunohistochemical and DNA flow cytometric study. Am J Clin Pathol 1991:95:446–53.

109. Gaudin PB, Sesterhenn IA, Wojno KJ, Mostofi FK, Epstein JI. Incidence and clinical significance of high-grade prostatic intraepithelial neoplasia in TURP specimens. Urology 1997:49:558–63.

110. Gleason DF. Atypical hyperplasia, benign hyperplasia and well-differentiated adenocarcinoma of the prostate. Am J Surg Pathol [Suppl] 1985;9:53–65.

111. Huggins C, Clark PJ. Effect on the prostate gland of occlusion of its ducts. Arch Pathol 1940;30:1178–83.

112. Hukill PB, Vidone RA. Histochemistry of mucus and other polysaccharides in tumors. II. Carcinoma of the prostate. Lab Invest 1967;16:395–406.

113. Kafandaris PM, Polyzonis MB. Fibroadenoma-like foci in human prostatic nodular hyperplasia. Prostate 1983;4:33–6.

114. Kastendieck H. Ultrastructural pathology of the human prostatic gland. Cyto- and histomorphogenesis of atrophy, hyperplasia, metaplasia, dysplasia and carcinoma (author's transl) [German] Veroffentlichungen aus der Pathologie 1977;106:1–163.

115. Kaufman JJ, Berneike RR. Leiomyoma of the prostate. J Urol 1951;65:297–310.

116. Kazzaz BA. Argentaffin and argyrophil cells in the prostate. J Pathol 1974;112:189–93.

117. Keen MR. The leiomyomatous prostate. J Urol 1939;42:158–69.

118. Kerley SW, Corica FA, Qian J, Myers RP, Bostwick DG. Peripheral zone involvement by prostatic hyperplasia. J Urol Pathol 1997;6:87–94.

119. Kohnen PW, Drach GW. Patterns of inflammation in prostatic hyperplasia: a histologic and bacteriologic study. J Urol 1979;121:755–60.

120. Kovi J. Microscopic differential diagnosis of small acinar adenocarcinoma of prostate. Pathol Annu 1985;20:157–96.

121. Kovi J. Surgical pathology of prostate and seminal vesicles. Boca Raton, FL: CRC Press Inc, 1989:101–2.

122. Leung CS, Srigley JR. Distribution of lipochrome pigment in the prostate gland: biological and diagnostic implications. Hum Pathol 1995;26:1302–7.

123. Mao P, Angrist A. The fine structure of the basal cell of human prostate. Lab Invest 1966;15:1768–82.

124. McNeal JE. Normal histology of the prostate. Am J Surg Pathol 1988;12:619–33.

125. McNeal JE. Origin and evolution of benign prostatic enlargement. Invest Urol 1978;15:340–5.

126. McNeal JE. The prostate and prostatic urethra: a morphologic synthesis. J Urol 1972;107:1008–16.

127. McNeal JE. Regional morphology and pathology of the prostate. Am J Clin Pathol 1968;49:347–57.

128. Moore RA. Benign hypertrophy of the prostate. A morphologic study. J Urol 1943;50:680–710.

129. Nadji M, Tabei SZ, Castro A, et al. Prostate-specific antigen: an immunohistologic marker for prostatic neoplasms. Cancer 1981;48:1229–32.

130. Ockerblad NF. Giant prostate: the largest recorded. J Urol 1946;56:81–2.

131. Ohori M, Egawa S, Wheeler TM. Nodules resembling nodular hyperplasia in the peripheral zone of the prostate gland. J Urol Pathol 1994;2:223–33.

132. Oyen RH, Van de Voorde WM, Van Poppel HP, et al. Benign hyperplastic nodules that originate in the peripheral zone of the prostate gland. Radiology 1993;189:707–11.

133. Pacelli A, Bostwick DG. Clinical significance of high-grade prostatic intraepithelial neoplasia in transurethral resection specimens. Urology 1997;50:355–9.

134. Papsidero LD, Kuriyama M, Wang MC, et al. Prostate antigen: a marker for human prostate epithelial cells. JNCI 1981;66:37–42.

135. Patch FS, Rhea LJ. Leiomyoma of the prostate gland. Br J Urol 1935;7:213–28.

136. Pradham BK, Chandra K. Morphogenesis of nodular hyperplasia–prostate. J Urol 1975;113:710–3.

137. Randall A. Median bars as found at autopsy. J Urol 1917;1:383–403.

138. Randall A. Surgical pathology of prostatic obstruction. Baltimore: Williams & Wilkins Co., 1931.

139. Reese JH, Lombard CM, Krone K, Stamey TA. Phyllodes type of atypical prostatic hyperplasia: report of 3 new cases. J Urol 1987;138:623–6.

140. Semple JE. Surgical capsule of the benign enlargement of the prostate. Its development and action. Br Med J 1963;1:1640–3.

141. Shapiro E, Beeich MJ, Hartanto V, Lepor H. The relative proportion of stromal and epithelial hyperplasia is related to the development of symptomatic benign prostatic hyperplasia. J Urol 1992;147:1293–7.

142. Sondergaard G, Vetner M, Christensen PO. Peripheral cystic hyperplasia of the prostate gland. Acta Path Microbiol Immunol Scand [A] 1987;95:137–9.

143. Stein BS, Vangore S, Petersen RO, Kendall AR. Immunoperoxidase localization of prostate-specific antigen. Am J Surg Pathol 1982;6:553–7.

144. Stephenson RA, James BC, Gay H, Fair WR, Whitmore WF Jr, Melamed MR. Flow cytometry of prostate cancer: relationship of DNA content to survival. Cancer Res 1987;47:2504–7.

145. Van de Voorde WM, Oyen RH, van Poppel HP, Wouters K, Baert LV, Lauweryns JM. Peripherally localized benign hyperplastic nodules of the prostate. Mod Pathol 1995;8:46–50.

146. Wang MC, Valenzuela LA, Murphy GP, Chu TM. Purification of a human prostate specific antigen. Invest Urol 1979;17:159–63.

147. Weinerth JL. The male genital system. In: Sabiston DC Jr, ed. Textbook of surgery: the biologic basis of modern surgical practice, 13th ed., Philadelphia: WB Saunders, 1986:1670.

148. Wernert N, Seitz G, Achtstatter T. Immunohistochemical investigation of different cytokeratins and vimentin in the prostate from the fetal period up to adulthood and in prostate carcinoma. Path Res Pract 1987;182:617–26.

Basal Cell Hyperplasia

149. Bennett BD, Gardner WA Jr. Embryonal hyperplasia of prostate. Prostate 1985;7:411–7.
150. Brawer MK, Peehl DM, Stamey TA, Bostwick DG. Keratin immunoreactivity in the benign and neoplastic human prostate. Cancer Res 1985;45:3663–7.
151. Civantos F, Marcial MA, Banks ER, et al. Pathology of androgen deprivation therapy in prostate carcinoma. A comparative study of 173 patients. Cancer 1995;75:1634–41.
152. Cleary KR, Choi HY, Ayala AG. Basal cell hyperplasia of the prostate. Am J Clin Pathol 1983;80:850–4.
153. Dermer GB. Basal cell proliferation in benign prostatic hyperplasia. Cancer 1978;41:1857–62.
154. Devaraj LT, Bostwick DG. Atypical basal cell hyperplasia of the prostate. Immunophenotypic profile and proposed classification of basal cell proliferations. Am J Surg Pathol 1993;17:645–59.
155. Epstein JI, Armas OA. Atypical basal cell hyperplasia of the prostate. Am J Surg Pathol 1992;16:1205–14.
156. Grignon DJ, Ro JY, Ordonez NG, Ayala AG, Cleary KR. Basal cell hyperplasia, adenoid basal cell tumor, and adenoid cystic carcinoma of the prostate gland: an immunohistochemical study. Hum Pathol 1988;19:1425–33.
157. Hellstrom M, Haggman M, Brandstedt S, et al. Histopathological changes in androgen-deprived localized prostatic cancer. A study in total prostatectomy specimens. Eur Urol 1993;24:461–5.
158. Lin JI, Cohen EL, Villacin AB, Garcia MB, Tseng CH. Basal cell adenoma of prostate. Urology 1978;11:409–10.
159. Molinolo AA, Meiss RP, Leo P, Sens AI. Demonstration of cytokeratins by immunoperoxidase staining in prostatic tissue. J Urol 1985;134:1037–40.
160. Murphy WM, Soloway MS, Barrows GH. Pathologic changes associated with androgen deprivation therapy for prostate cancer. Cancer 1991;68:821–8.
161. Nagle RB, Ahmann FR, McDaniel KM, Paquin ML, Clark VA, Celniker A. Cytokeratin characterization of human prostatic carcinoma and its derived cell lines. Cancer Res 1987;47:281–6.
162. Reed RJ. Consultation case. Am J Surg Pathol 1984;8:699–704.
163. Ronnett BM, Epstein JI. A case showing sclerosing adenosis and an unusual form of basal cell hyperplasia of the prostate. Am J Surg Pathol 1989;13:866–72.
164. Srigley JR, Dardick I, Hartwick RW, Klotz L. Basal epithelial cells of human prostate glands are not myoepithelial cells. A comparative immunohistochemical and ultrastructural study with the human salivary gland. Am J Pathol 1990;136:957–66.
165. Tetu B, Srigley JR, Boivin JC, et al. Effect of combination endocrine therapy (LHRH agonist and flutamide) on normal prostate and prostatic adenocarcinoma. A histopathologic and immunohistochemical study. Am J Surg Pathol 1991;15:111–20.
166. Wernert N, Seitz G, Achtstatter T. Immunohistochemical investigation of different cytokeratins and vimentin in the prostate from the fetal period up to adulthood and in prostate carcinoma. Path Res Pract 1987;182:617–26.
167. Young RH, Frierson HF Jr, Mills SE, Kaiser JS, Talbot WH, Bahn AK. Adenoid cystic-like tumor of the prostate gland. A report of two cases and review of the literature on "adenoid cystic carcinoma" of the prostate. Am J Clin Pathol 1988;89:49–56.

Postatrophic Hyperplasia

168. Amin MB, Tamboli P, Varma M, Srigley JR. Postatrophic hyperplasia of prostate: a detailed analysis of its morphology in needle biopsy specimens. Am J Surg Pathol 1999;8:925–31.
169. Billis A. Prostatic atrophy: an autopsy study of a histologic mimic of adenocarcinoma. Mod Pathol 1998;11:47–54.
170. Cheville JC, Bostwick DG. Postatrophic hyperplasia of the prostate. A histologic mimic of prostatic adenocarcinoma. Am J Surg Pathol 1995;19:1068–76.
171. Elbadawi A. Benign proliferative lesions of the prostate gland. In Spring-Mills E, Haeez ES, eds. Male accessory sex glands. Elsevier: North Holland Biomedical Press, 1980.
172. Epstein JI. Differential diagnosis in pathology: urologic disorders. New York: Igaku-Shoin, 1992:104–5.
173. Franks LM. Atrophy and hyperplasia in the prostate problem. J Pathol Bacteriol 1954;68:617–21.
174. Franks LM. Latent carcinoma of prostate. J Pathol Bacteriol 1954;60:603–16.
175. Helpap B. The biological significance of atypical hyperplasia of the prostate. Virchows Arch [A] 1980;387:307–17.
176. Kovi J. Microscopic differential diagnosis of small acinar adenocarcinoma of the prostate. Pathol Annu 1985;20:157–96.
177. Kovi J. Postatrophic hyperplasia. In: Kovi J. Surgical pathology of prostate and seminal vesicles. Boca Raton: CRC Press, 1989:35–8.
178. Moore RA. The evolution and involution of the prostate gland. Am J Pathol 1936;12:599–624.
179. Oppenheimer JR, Epstein JI. Partial atrophy in prostate needle cores. Another diagnostic pitfall for the surgical pathologist. Am J Surg Pathol 1998;22:440–5.
179a. Ruska KM, Sauvageot J, Epstein JI. Histology and cellular kinetics of prostatic atrophy. Am J Surg Pathol 1998;22:1073–7.
180. Srigley JR. Small acinar patterns in the prostate gland with emphasis on atypical adenomatous hyperplasia and small acinar carcinoma. Semin Diagn Pathol 1988;5:254–72.
181. Srigley JR, Bullock M, Amin M. Small glandular patterns in the prostate: differential diagnosis of small acinar carcinoma. In: Foster CS, Bostwick DG, eds. Pathology of the prostate. Philadelphia: WB Saunders Co, 1997:126–55.
182. Totten RS, Heineman MW, Hudson PB, Sproul EE, Stout AP. Microscopic differential diagnosis of latent carcinoma of prostate. Arch Pathol 1953;55:131–41.

3

PRECURSORS AND POSSIBLE PRECURSORS OF PROSTATIC ADENOCARCINOMA: PROSTATIC INTRAEPITHELIAL NEOPLASIA AND ATYPICAL ADENOMATOUS HYPERPLASIA–ADENOSIS

HISTORICAL PERSPECTIVE

The role of benign conditions, including nodular hyperplasia and atrophy, in the development of adenocarcinoma of the prostate has been the subject of much study. Currently there is no convincing evidence to suggest a causal relationship for nodular hyperplasia (4,5,8,19). Atrophy and postatrophic hyperplasia have been considered to play a role in the pathogenesis of carcinoma by some (16,17,25). Both these processes occur mainly in the peripheral zone which is also the site of development of most carcinomas, and, indeed, they may be intimately admixed with carcinoma. Although the labeling index of postatrophic hyperplasia may be high (20,31a) and in the range of some carcinomas (20), the majority of prostatic cancers are not histologically related to postatrophic hyperplasia, and there is little scientific support for a preneoplastic role of the latter (3a,12).

The first English language paper that discussed precancerous conditions of the prostate was that of Oertel in 1926 (30) who pointed out similarities between the prostate and breast, and the prior description by German workers of "atypical epithelial change and beginning cancer" in the senile prostate. Four years later Cheatle and Wale (11) described a case of prostatic carcinoma in which the resected gland exhibited changes that they likened to the spectrum of benign-atypical-carcinoma observed in the breast. In a paper on latent carcinoma of the prostate in 1949, Andrews (3) discussed and illustrated precancerous conditions which he found in 12 of 17 glands with carcinoma compared to 33 of 125 glands without carcinoma. The atypical foci were characterized by cellular stratification, papillae, nuclear enlargement, and mitotic activity. He proposed that these cases provided a link between benign hyperplasia and carcinoma. In 1965, McNeal (27) described and illustrated "a sequence of alterations in the duct epithelium passing through stages of progressively greater anaplasia to frank carcinoma in situ to invasive carcinoma." He later described and illustrated carcinoma originating from foci that he interpreted as atypical hyperplasia and concluded that "the antecedents of prostatic carcinoma are morphologically diagnosable years before the emergence of invasive carcinoma" (26). In 1971, Miller and Seljelid (29) suggested that cases of hyperplasia that they considered markedly atypical represented a premalignant phase of prostatic carcinoma, and in 1974 Tannenbaum (32) illustrated and briefly discussed several examples of atypical hyperplasia.

Detailed studies from Germany provided a significant stimulus to investigation in this area by others in the late 1970s and early 1980s (1,13, 20). Kastendieck (22) found atypical hyperplasia associated with 59 percent of carcinomas, and Helpap (20) found it in 49 percent of carcinomas, in contrast to only 2.8 percent of those without carcinoma. McNeal and Bostwick (28) subsequently found atypical intraductal lesions (intraductal dysplasia) in carcinomatous prostates almost twice as often as in benign prostates. The degree of the atypicality was graded, and the most severe forms were found eight times more frequently in prostates with carcinoma than in those without. These authors noted that the lesions with severe atypia superficially resembled invasive cribriform carcinoma. In another study, large acinar atypical hyperplasia (apparently similar to the intraductal dysplasia of McNeal) was found in 87 percent of prostate carcinoma cases compared to 38 percent of benign glands (24). The last 15 years has seen a veritable explosion of interest in this topic, with numerous papers on both the pathology and clinical features, which are referenced selectively in the subsequent sections.

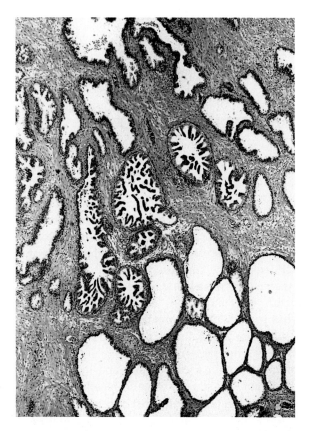 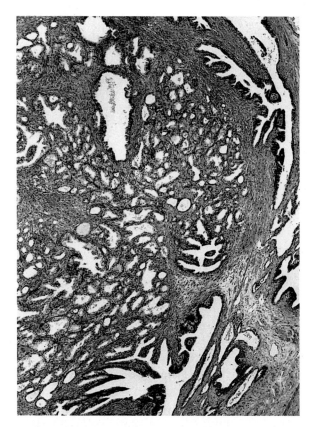

Figure 3-1
POSSIBLE PRECURSORS TO PROSTATIC CARCINOMA

Left: Prostatic intraepithelial neoplasia involves peripheral zone glands. Note the micropapillary, intraluminal proliferation of atypical secretory cells.

Right: Atypical adenomatous hyperplasia forms a nodule in the transition zone. Note the proliferation of crowded, irregular, small acini.

A review of the illustrations and descriptions in the many papers on this subject indicates that the atypical lesions referred to, in some instances at least, are of differing types. In our opinion and that of most investigators these can be considered in two general categories: one characterized, definitionally, by cytologic atypia and usually also showing architectural abnormalities (fig. 3-1, left), and the other characterized, definitionally, by architectural abnormalities and occasionally showing limited cytologic atypia (fig. 3-1, right). Several terms have been used for these lesions over the years, but for the purpose of this Fascicle, the terms *prostatic intraepithelial neoplasia* and *atypical adenomatous hyperplasia* are used (6,9, 10,14). The former term is more or less uniformly accepted now. Some prefer the term *adenosis* for the latter, and it is quite widely used (15,18).

Prostatic intraepithelial neoplasia is characterized by cytologic atypia within preexisting duct-acinar units. McNeal and Bostwick (28) used the term intraductal dysplasia for lesions in this category. However, problems with the definition of "dysplasia" and with the precise histologic location of this lesion, i.e., duct or acinus, led to "prostatic intraepithelial neoplasia" (7) being proposed to encompass this group of atypical patterns. This term was endorsed at a consensus conference on premalignant lesions of the prostate gland (14). Numerous other terms have been used including, atypical primary hyperplasia, hyperplasia with malignant change, large acinar atypical hyperplasia, and duct-acinar dysplasia (2,23,24,31). In contrast, atypical adenomatous hyperplasia is an architectural abnormality (with, at most, limited cytologic atypia) characterized by new gland formation; small acini often bud into the surrounding stroma from adjacent larger glands of conventional nodular hyperplasia (fig. 3-1, right) (21).

Other processes in the prostate gland may be architecturally complex, such as cribriform hyperplasia (see page 297), but are not known to be precursors of adenocarcinoma. Appreciable cytologic atypicality may be seen in cases of basal cell hyperplasia (see page 308), but although it is theoretically possible that such cases may represent a stage in the evolution of the rare basal cell carcinoma of the prostate, proof of this is lacking. Similarly, rare cases of transitional cell metaplasia may be associated with some perceptible cytologic atypia (10). Cytologic atypicality in other settings may be attributable to inflammation, ischemia, radiation therapy, or represent the atypicality that may be present normally in the epithelium of the seminal vesicles and ejaculatory ducts.

PROSTATIC INTRAEPITHELIAL NEOPLASIA

Definition. Prostatic intraepithelial neoplasia (PIN) is usually characterized by an intraluminal proliferation of secretory epithelium that displays a spectrum of cytologic changes culminating in those that are indistinguishable from carcinoma. Occasionally, there is cytologic atypia without increased cellularity. High-grade PIN is strongly associated with invasive adenocarcinoma, particularly of the peripheral zone.

General Features. There is much evidence supporting a preneoplastic role for PIN (36,37, 47,48,56,78,83,84,111,113,140). The prevalence of PIN increases with age, peaking in the sixth decade and predating the onset of most carcinomas by more than 5 years (86,122,123). PIN is much more common in prostates with carcinoma than in benign glands (51,86,95,131) and is more often multifocal, more extensive, and of higher grade in the former (117,135). Like carcinoma, PIN is mainly identified in the peripheral zone and is often adjacent to carcinoma (47,118,135). The prevalence of PIN in the transition zone is less than 5 percent (132) as supported by two large series in which high-grade PIN was seen in 2.3 and 4.2 percent of transurethral resection specimens (72,112). Patients with high-grade PIN in

resectates appear to be at increased risk for developing prostate cancer, although not to the same degree as those with high-grade PIN in needle biopsies (55,62,63,72,85,87,112), reflecting the difference in the significance of PIN in the genesis of transition zone as opposed to peripheral zone carcinomas (69,118). The extent of PIN is inversely related to the tumor stage; this may be related to replacement of areas of PIN by invasive tumor (36, 69,89,118). As in carcinoma, increased production of acid mucin has been documented (79,127).

The cytologic appearances of the cells of high-grade PIN are similar to those seen in invasive carcinoma (95). Increased numbers of mitoses and apoptotic bodies, compared to benign glands, have been identified (73,105), although in general there is a paucity of mitotic figures in PIN. Similarities between high-grade PIN and carcinoma have also been noted at the ultrastructural level (54). In high-grade PIN there is a partial loss of the basal cell layer while in carcinoma there is a complete loss (fig. 3-2) (51). On occasion, carcinoma may be seen arising directly from an area of high-grade PIN, a phenomenon that led McNeal (98) to propose the concept of microinvasion in association with high-grade PIN. The invasive acini are thought to arise through an intermediate morphologic phase he has referred to as the "small transitive gland system" (see page 87).

Additional support for a pathogenetic relationship between PIN and carcinoma comes from phenotypic and genotypic studies. PIN shares many immunophenotypic features with carcinoma. Both stain strongly for cytokeratin KA4; vimentin immunoreactivity is usually absent in both, in contrast to normal and hyperplastic glands where focal paranuclear staining is commonly noted (109). PIN and carcinoma show a similar pattern of staining with *Ulex europaeus* (94,109). In PIN and carcinoma, there is a loss of basement membrane–associated type IV collagen and expression of type IV collagenase (44,126). Expression of A, B, and Lewis blood group antigens is absent in both (114). Some lectin binding studies have shown defective glycosylation of proteins in areas of high-grade PIN (96). An increase in metalloproteinase and matrilysin expression has been noted in both high-grade PIN and carcinoma (110). There is increased expression of the proliferation markers PCNA, Ki-67, and MIB-1 in PIN (45,103, 125,133). Epidermal growth factor receptors are

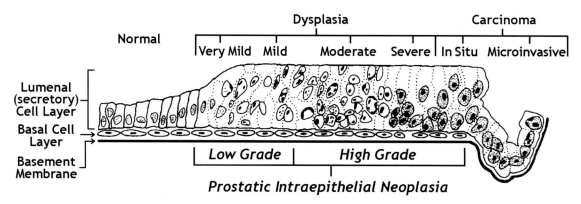

Figure 3-2
PROSTATIC INTRAEPITHELIAL NEOPLASIA
Schematic drawing showing increasing cytologic atypia of secretory epithelial cells corresponding to increasing grades of prostatic intraepithelial neoplasia. Note putative association with the development of carcinoma (right). (Fig. 6-10 from Bostwick DG, Sakr W. Prostatic intraepithelial neoplasia. In: Foster CS, Bostwick DG, eds. Pathology of the prostate. Philadelphia: WB Saunders Co, 1998:105).

reduced in both PIN and carcinoma (80,93,136). Alterations in microvascular density have also been documented in PIN and carcinoma (104).

Nuclear morphometric studies in PIN have shown increases in nuclear area, DNA content, chromatin content and distribution, nuclear perimeter, nuclear diameter, nuclear roundness, nuclear eccentricity, nuclear number, and nucleolar organizer regions (AgNORs) (38,42,64,77, 88,100,102,106,115,128). These morphometric features are similar to those of carcinoma or intermediate between those seen in carcinoma and the normal prostate.

DNA is aneuploid in 32 to 58 percent of cases of high-grade PIN (38,42,62,139). A strong correlation between ploidy abnormalities in PIN and corresponding carcinomas has been found in several studies (38,42,62,139). The DNA index of high-grade PIN appears to be intermediate between that of the normal prostate gland and carcinoma. Several chromosomal and molecular genetic studies reaffirm the close relationship of PIN to cancer (75): numeric alterations of chromosomes 7, 8, 10, 12, and Y have been reported with equal frequency in both, the most common of which is a gain of chromosome 8 (90,116,124). However, the mean number of extra chromosomes is higher in foci of cancer than in PIN. The most common allelic losses reported in prostate cancer have been on the short arm of chromosome 8 (8p) and the long arms of chromosomes 10 (10q) and 16 (16q) (43). Deletions of chromosome 8p have also been

noted in PIN, suggesting its role in early carcinogenesis and possibly the presence of a tumor suppressor gene in this region (68,91).

The role of tumor suppressor genes in prostatic carcinoma and PIN has generated considerable interest (53). p53 mutations have been reported in both and have been shown to be significantly increased compared to benign prostatic epithelium (101,134). The nm23-H1 protein is present in PIN and cancer but absent in benign prostatic epithelium (107a). Mutations of the retinoblastoma suppressor gene have not been found in PIN (134). Of the numerous oncogene studies, c-*erb*B-2 has consistently shown increased expression in PIN and prostate cancer compared to expression in benign prostatic cells (107,108). *Bcl*-2, another oncogene, has been reported to be present in PIN (61).

The above pieces of evidence strongly link but do not prove conclusively that high-grade PIN has a precursor role in the development of carcinoma. It can still be argued that high-grade PIN is an epiphenomenon, possibly with a similar etiology to carcinoma, but that it is neither necessary nor sufficient for its development. Some carcinomas unassociated with high-grade PIN are identified in the third and fourth decades, suggesting that high-grade PIN is not a requirement for the development of all carcinomas. Furthermore, in cases with early cancer and high-grade PIN, the cancer is often not in close proximity to the PIN (122,123).

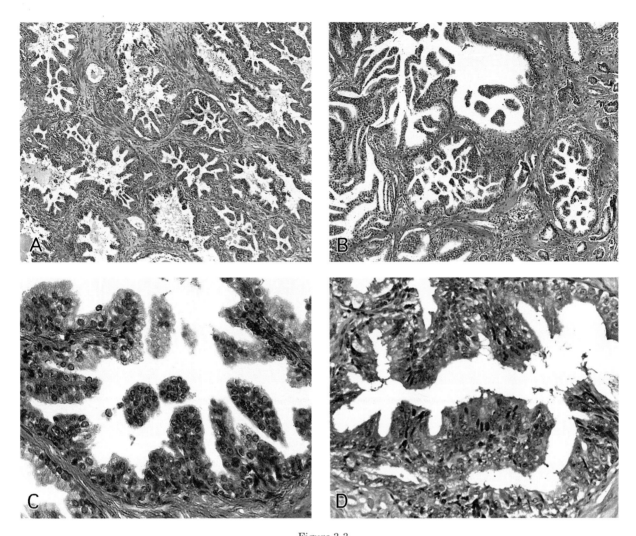

Figure 3-3

HIGH-GRADE PROSTATIC INTRAEPITHELIAL NEOPLASIA INVOLVING THE PERIPHERAL ZONE

A,B: Note the intraluminal proliferation of atypical epithelium with tufted and micropapillary patterns which results in a striking abnormality on low-power examination. There is an associated carcinoma in B (right).

C,D: Note the cytologic abnormalities. The nuclear changes in C would be grade 2 using the initial three-grade system, and those in D, grade 3.

Clinical Features. The frequency of high-grade PIN in recent biopsy series is 4 to 16 percent (40,55,87). There are no specific associated clinical features. Some patients present with elevated prostate-specific antigen (PSA) levels, but this is likely often due to undetected invasive carcinoma (33,59,121). It has been postulated that the attenuation and partial loss of basal cells and the increased neovascularity around PIN may contribute to elevated PSA levels not associated with cancer (58,59). PIN may also present as a hypoechoic peripheral zone lesion (60); 4 to 11 percent of such lesions show isolated high-grade

PIN (66,89). The possibility of concomitant carcinoma, however, cannot be excluded in these cases since the gland was not removed. PIN does not cause a gross abnormality.

Microscopic Findings. PIN is usually found in the peripheral zone where it is frequently multifocal and, when high grade, often associated with adenocarcinoma (fig. 3-3). Occasionally, hyperplastic transition zone epithelium may be affected by PIN. McNeal and Bostwick (95) initially proposed a three-grade system based on progressive abnormalities in architecture and cytology. At the consensus meeting that endorsed the term

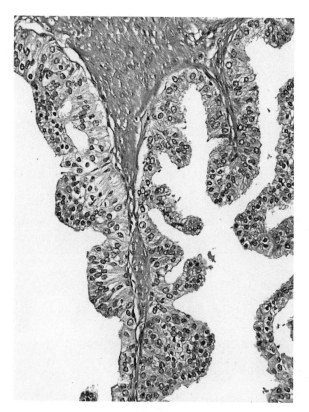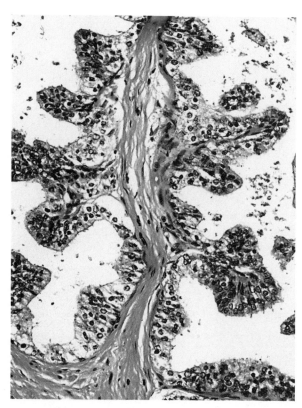

Figure 3-4
LOW-GRADE PROSTATIC INTRAEPITHELIAL NEOPLASIA

Left: Note the tufted and micropapillary patterns. The nuclei show mild nuclear enlargement and anisonucleosis. Prominent nucleoli are lacking.

Right: Note the micropapillary pattern with crowding and stratification of nuclei. There is more cytologic atypia than in the figure on the left but not enough nucleolar prominence to place the lesion in the high-grade category.

PIN, it was agreed to divide the process into two grades, low and high; PIN 1 is now considered low grade and PIN 2 and 3, high grade (67).

Low-Grade PIN. Low-grade PIN may show a tufted or micropapillary pattern, with crowding, stratification, and irregular spacing of secretory cells (fig. 3-4). The nuclei are generally slightly enlarged and there is anisonucleosis (fig. 3-5). Nucleoli are infrequently observed and are not prominent. The nuclear abnormalities do not reach the threshold required for a high-grade lesion.

Reproducibility studies have shown that it is difficult to distinguish low-grade PIN from normal and hyperplastic glands, particularly if there is mild basal cell hyperplasia or transitional cell metaplasia which may mimic PIN (34,70). It is important to compare clearly normal glands to questionably abnormal ones, using the former as an internal control when evaluat-

ing cytologic observations in cases of suspected low-grade PIN (fig. 3-5).

High-Grade PIN. On low-power magnification, high-grade PIN is usually readily recognized as a cellular proliferation within medium to large glands characterized additionally by cytologic atypia (see page 81). The resulting basophilic or amphophilic appearance usually causes the involved glands to stand out from adjacent normal ones (figs. 3-3A,B, 3-6). Four major architectural patterns, in order of decreasing frequency, have been described: tufted, micropapillary, cribriform, and flat (figs. 3-7, 3-8) (50). One or more of these architectural patterns commonly coexist in an individual case, in an individual field, or even in an individual gland, and the patterns often merge (50,120). Similarities to precancerous changes of the breast are evident from the descriptions that follow and from some of the terms

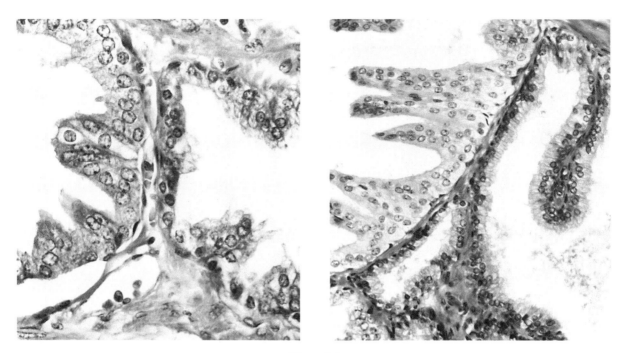

Figure 3-5
LOW-GRADE PROSTATIC INTRAEPITHELIAL NEOPLASIA
Left: There is slight tufting with mild nuclear enlargement, stratification, and crowding.
Right: A micropapillary pattern shows nuclear enlargement and cellular stratification. Normal glands are seen for comparison (right) in each illustration.

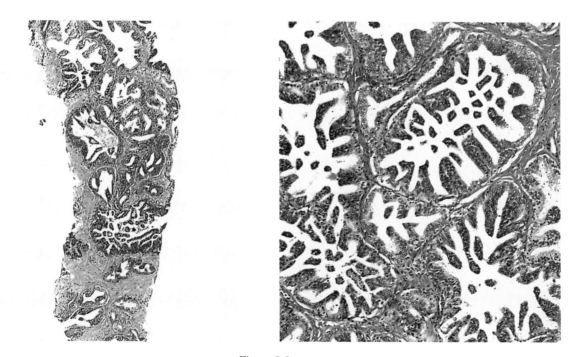

Figure 3-6
HIGH-GRADE PROSTATIC INTRAEPITHELIAL NEOPLASIA
Left: Prostatic intraepithelial neoplasia with tufted and micropapillary patterns is present in a needle biopsy specimen.
Right: A micropapillary pattern is seen.

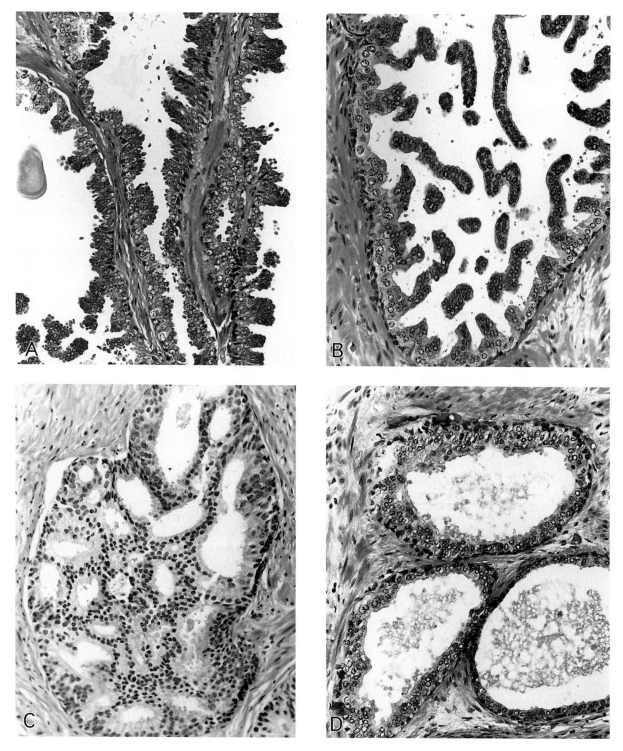

Figure 3-7
ARCHITECTURAL PATTERNS OF HIGH-GRADE PROSTATIC INTRAEPITHELIAL NEOPLASIA

A: Tufted pattern. Note the crowding and stratification of nuclei. Prominent nucleoli are evident in most nuclei.

B: Micropapillary pattern. Note the slender, filiform papillae composed of atypical secretory cells.

C: Cribriform pattern. Note the residual basal cell layer and maturation of cells towards the lumen.

D: Flat pattern. Medium-sized glands are lined by one to several layers of atypical secretory cells without a significant intraluminal proliferation. Residual basal cells are identified.

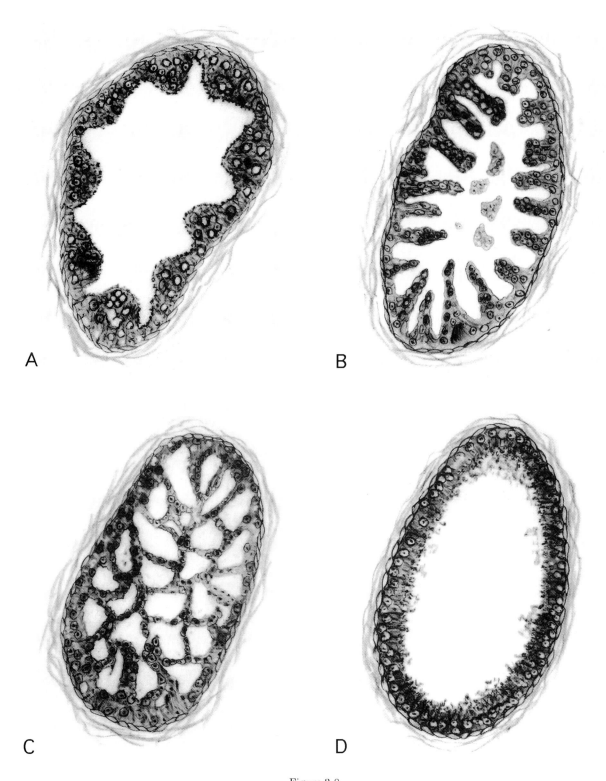

Figure 3-8
ARCHITECTURAL PATTERNS OF HIGH-GRADE PROSTATIC INTRAEPITHELIAL NEOPLASIA
Artistic representation of patterns of prostatic intraepithelial neoplasia including tufted (A), micropapillary (B), cribriform (C), and flat (D). (Fig. 1 from Bostwick DG, Amin MB, Dundore P, Marsh W, Shultz DS. Architectural patterns of high grade prostatic intraepithelial neoplasia. Hum Pathol 1993;24:298–310.)

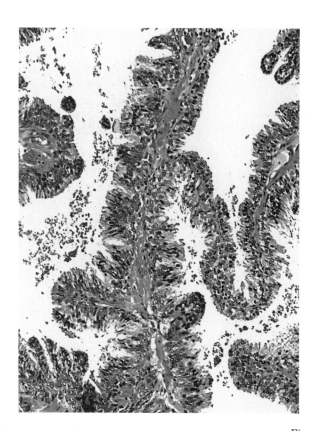 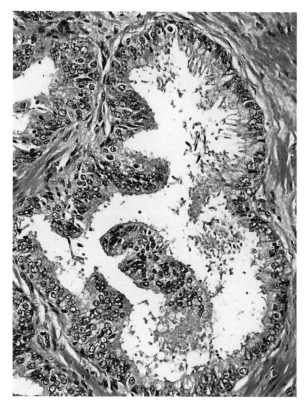

Figure 3-9
TUFTED PATTERN OF HIGH-GRADE PROSTATIC INTRAEPITHELIAL NEOPLASIA
Left: Note the stratification of atypical secretory cells imparting an undulating appearance to the luminal lining.
Right: A high-power photomicrograph of another case shows stratification, crowding, and atypia of the secretory layer. Nucleoli are prominent in many nuclei.

used, such as micropapillary and cribriform. There is no apparent clinicopathologic significance to these different architectural patterns, but familiarity with the spectrum may facilitate recognition of the lesion.

Histologic Subtypes of PIN. *Tufted.* In this pattern, stratified groups of secretory cells protrude into the gland lumens (fig. 3-9). The tufts usually consist of no more than five cell layers. This stratification imparts an undulating appearance to the luminal profile (fig. 3-9).

Micropapillary. This pattern is characterized by slender filiform structures, sometimes with bulbous tips, projecting into lumens (fig. 3-10); the height of the papillae can be quite variable (as seen in the contrast between figures 3-10A, B, and C, and 3-7B). Fibrovascular cores are usually absent but are occasionally identified. Some degeneration and dropping off of cells near the tips may be seen, and sometimes this is conspicuous, resulting in striking cellular budding (figs. 3-6, right, 3-10D).

Cribriform. This pattern is the most diagnostically difficult, particularly in needle biopsies, because of problems that arise in its reliable distinction from cribriform adenocarcinoma (see page 137). Distinction from ductal carcinoma in transurethral resectates may also be a challenge. Cribriform PIN consists of a complex intraluminal proliferation in which multiple fenestrae impart a sieve-like pattern to the gland (fig. 3-11A). The lumens may be round and regular or irregular and oval to elongated. The spaces are often more elongated than in carcinoma, where they are more often round and "punched out" (39,50). The juxtaluminal cells of the cribriform glands may display "maturation" when compared to the more peripheral cells. Maturation is a term that has been used to describe the phenomenon in which the cells at the periphery of an atypical or neoplastic gland have larger nuclei and more prominent nucleoli than those close to or at the luminal aspect (fig. 3-12) (74). Necrotic material is only rarely seen

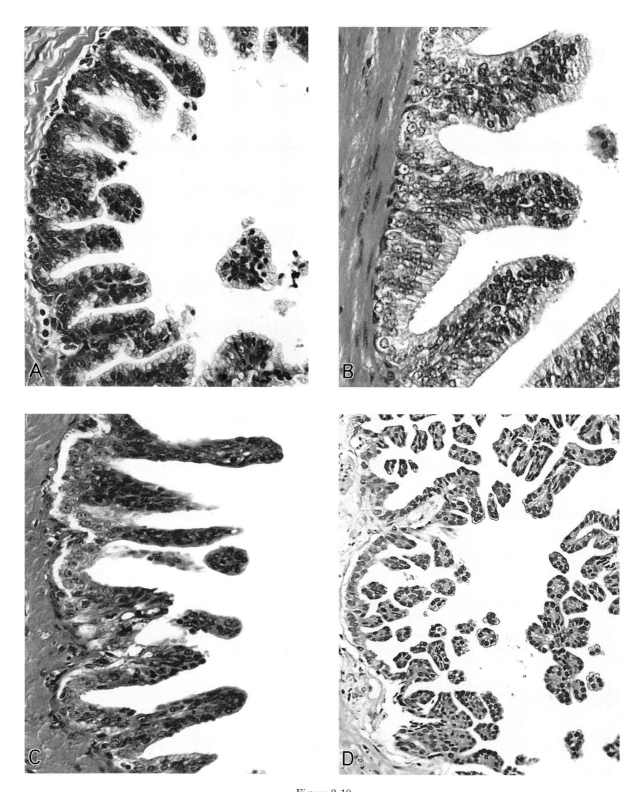

Figure 3-10
MICROPAPILLARY PATTERN OF HIGH-GRADE PROSTATIC INTRAEPITHELIAL NEOPLASIA
A: Note the slender papillae composed of crowded atypical secretory cells, some with prominent nucleoli.
B,C: Nucleoli are more easily identified in two other cases.
D: A particularly exuberant appearance with prominent cellular budding was associated with adjacent carcinoma.

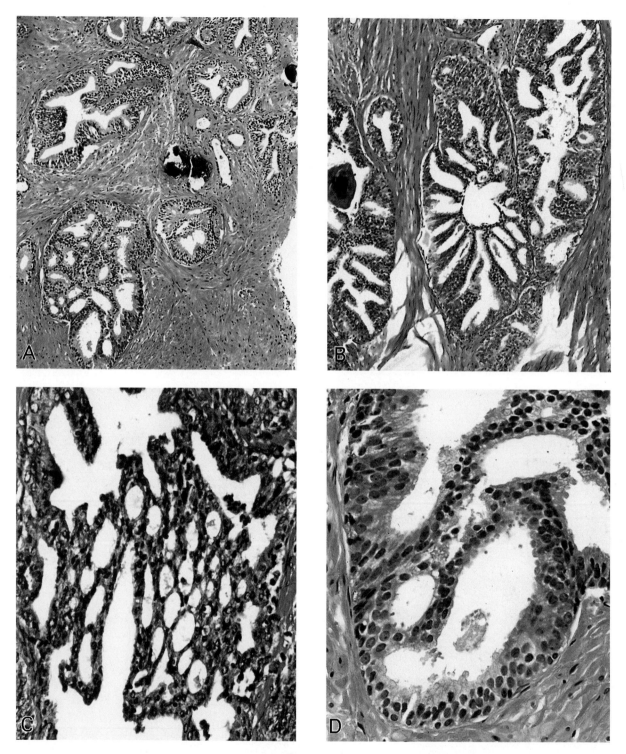

Figure 3-11
CRIBRIFORM PATTERN OF HIGH-GRADE PROSTATIC INTRAEPITHELIAL NEOPLASIA

A: A single cribriform unit (bottom left) in a needle biopsy specimen stands out in sharp contrast to the other glands.

B: Several glands are involved by the atypical cribriform proliferation.

C: There is irregularity in size and shape of the spaces, some of which are elongated.

D: There is high-grade cytologic atypia of the secretory cells with easily recognized, darkly staining bland basal cells (higher power view of abnormal focus in A).

in very small amounts within gland lumens in cases of cribriform PIN.

Flat. This pattern is the least common and is characterized by an absence of significant stratification, with only one or two layers of secretory cells exhibiting the cytologic atypia that is the hallmark of PIN (fig. 3-13). The glands involved by flat PIN are often small to medium in size in contrast to those involved in other patterns (50).

Other Uncommon Patterns. In addition to the above common patterns, which are often admixed (fig. 3-14), other less common to rare architectural features of high-grade PIN include epithelial arches, trabecular bars, "Roman bridges," solid patterns, and involvement of large cystic glands (fig. 3-15) (50). These patterns are composed of proliferating secretory cells similar to those of the more common patterns of PIN and may be associated with carcinoma of the conventional type. Rare forms of PIN include those with cells having mucinous cytoplasm (fig. 3-16A), including signet ring forms, and small cell undifferentiated (neuroendocrine) features (fig. 3-16B,C) (120).

Nuclear Features of High-Grade PIN. Regardless of the architectural pattern, nuclear changes are the hallmark of high-grade PIN. In addition to nuclear enlargement (also seen with low-grade PIN), there is usually hyperchromasia with irregularity of chromatin, parachromatin clearing, nuclear membrane irregularity, and nucleolar enlargement (fig. 3-17). The nuclei of high-grade PIN are relatively monomorphic compared to the anisonucleosis found in low-grade PIN. Nucleoli are large, irregular, often multiple, and may be focal (grade 2 PIN) (fig. 3-17, left) or more extensive (grade 3 PIN) (fig. 3-17, right). Because the juxtaluminal cells may be less atypical than those at the base (maturation), cytologic atypicality should be assessed primarily by evaluating the juxtabasal secretory cells, taking care not to misinterpret atypia which may be present in basal cells as PIN. In some cases there is striking hyperchromasia, identified on low-power magnification, and unquestionable nucleomegaly, but nucleoli may be difficult to see and may require diligent search (70), particularly in needle biopsy specimens.

Other Histologic Features of High-Grade PIN. The basal cell layer is often readily identified on routine slides but may be difficult to appreciate in some cases and is frequently discontinuous (39,51, 113). On occasion, especially in needle biopsy spec-

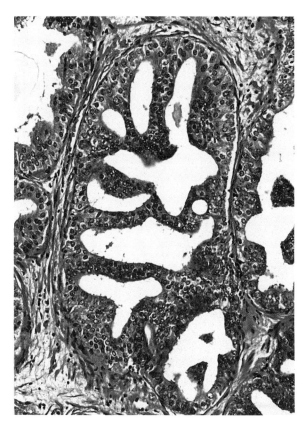

Figure 3-12
CRIBRIFORM PATTERN OF HIGH-GRADE
PROSTATIC INTRAEPITHELIAL NEOPLASIA
Note the irregular shape of the spaces and the maturation of cells towards the lumen in several areas.

imens, basal cell–specific high molecular weight cytokeratin (clone 34βE12) may be needed to positively identify basal cells (fig. 3-18) (137).

A variety of cytoplasmic and luminal features may be seen. Amorphous eosinophilic secretions and discrete needle- or rhomboid-shaped, sharp-edged eosinophilic crystalloids (fig. 3-19A) and corpora amylacea (fig. 3-19B) may be seen. Luminal mucin, sometimes similar to the basophilic wispy material seen in adenocarcinoma, is occasionally striking (fig. 3-19C) (79,127). Mucinous metaplasia of the cells lining glands involved by PIN has also been documented, and apical cytoplasmic blebs suggestive of apocrine secretion are quite common (fig. 3-20) (50). Although the cytoplasm is usually slightly amphophilic and granular, it is occasionally eosinophilic or clear. Rarely, a Paneth cell–like change is seen (fig. 3-21) (52,138). Cytoplasmic lipofuscin pigment (fig. 3-22) is

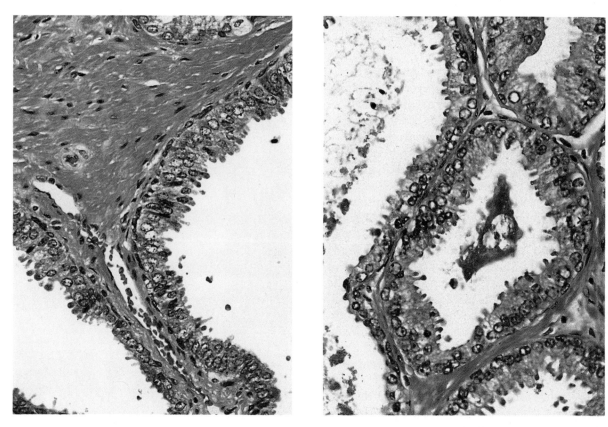

Figure 3-13
FLAT PATTERN OF HIGH-GRADE PROSTATIC INTRAEPITHELIAL NEOPLASIA
Left: Medium-sized glands are lined by one to three layers of atypical secretory cells. Note the apocrine snouting.
Right: Several small glands are involved by high-grade prostatic intraepithelial neoplasia. Note the parachromatin clearing and prominent nucleoli. In both these illustrations it can be determined that the atypia is in the secretory cells, not the basal cells. Normal forms of the latter are readily seen in the left figure.

Figure 3-14
HIGH-GRADE PROSTATIC
INTRAEPITHELIAL
NEOPLASIA

This case has tufted, micropapillary, cribriform, and flat patterns.

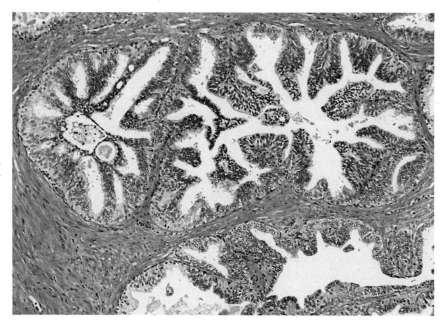

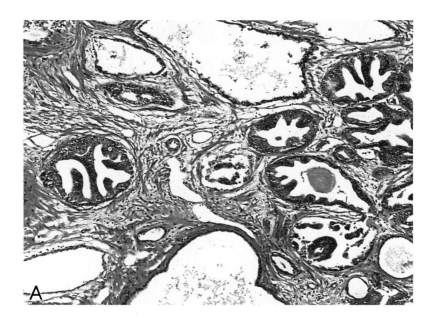

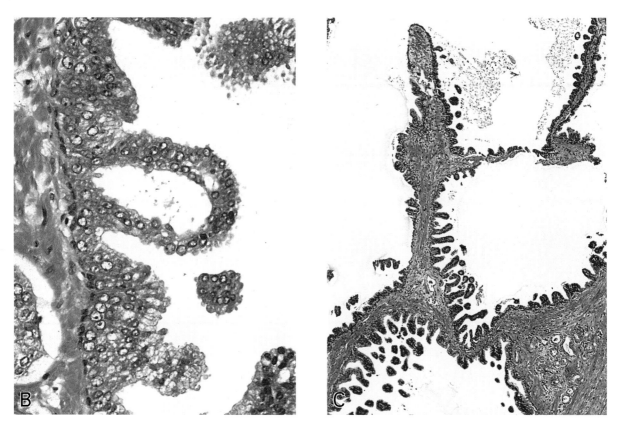

Figure 3-15
HIGH-GRADE PROSTATIC INTRAEPITHELIAL NEOPLASIA

A: A trabecular bar is present (left).

B: A Roman arch is present. Note the nuclear atypia with prominent nucleoli and amphophilic cytoplasm. Residual basal cells are conspicuous.

C: A low-power photomicrograph shows involvement of cystically dilated glands. Flat, tufted, and micropapillary patterns are identified. A small focus of carcinoma is seen at the bottom right.

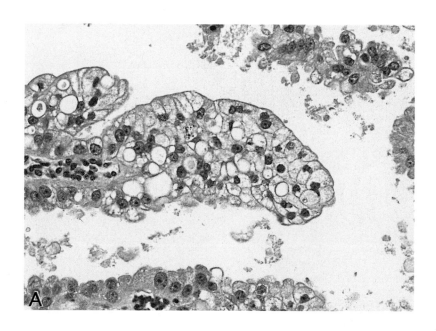

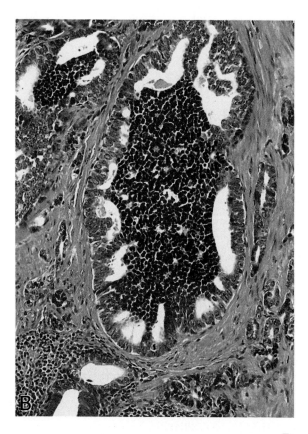

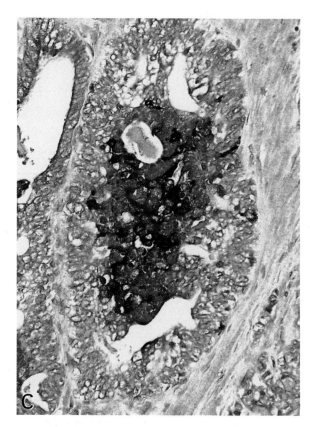

Figure 3-16
PROSTATIC INTRAEPITHELIAL NEOPLASIA, UNUSUAL FEATURES

A: There are cells with mucin-rich cytoplasm.
B: A cribriform aggregate merges centrally with a malignant small cell component.
C: The small cell component seen in B stains for chromogranin. (Courtesy of Dr. P.A. Humphrey, St. Louis, MO.)

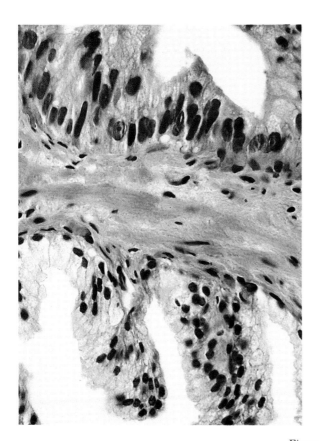 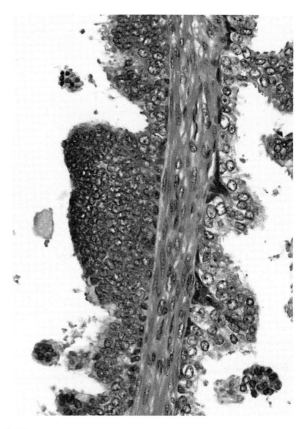

Figure 3-17
HIGH-GRADE PROSTATIC INTRAEPITHELIAL NEOPLASIA
Left: There is nuclear enlargement, parachromatin clearing, and prominent nucleoli. A normal gland is seen below for comparison.
Right: Two glands are lined by atypical cells.

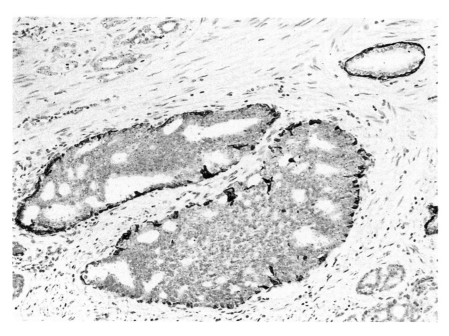

Figure 3-18
HIGH-GRADE PROSTATIC INTRAEPITHELIAL NEOPLASIA WITH CRIBRIFORM PATTERN
Note the rich investment of basal cells. Invasive microacinar carcinoma is seen at top left and bottom right. Note the absence of basal cells in the carcinoma (high molecular weight keratin 34βE12 stain).

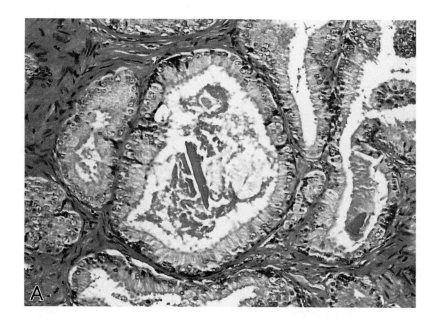

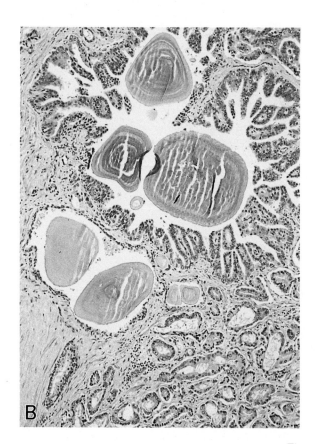

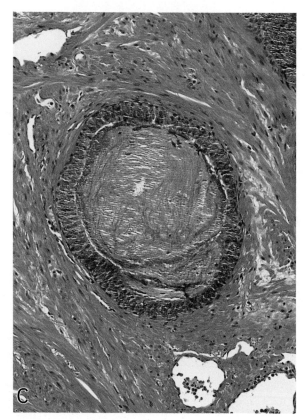

Figure 3-19
HIGH-GRADE PROSTATIC INTRAEPITHELIAL NEOPLASIA

A: A flat pattern has luminal eosinophilic secretion and rod-shaped crystalloids.

B: Corpora amylacea are present in another case with a micropapillary pattern and adjacent carcinoma (bottom right).

C: Prominent mucin is seen within the lumen of a gland exhibiting flat prostatic intraepithelial neoplasia. (Courtesy of Dr. P.A. Humphrey, St. Louis, MO.)

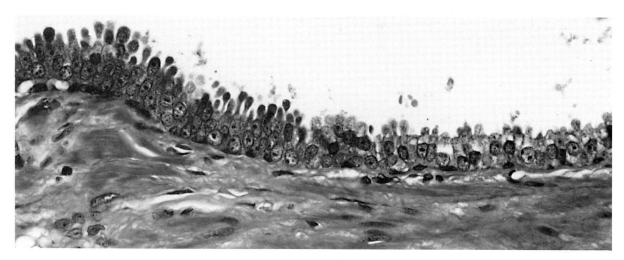

Figure 3-20
HIGH-GRADE PROSTATIC INTRAEPITHELIAL NEOPLASIA
This is a flat pattern with apocrine snouting. Note the prominent nucleoli.

sometimes identified, and, rarely, cytoplasmic microcalcifications are present (35,50).

Occasionally, high-grade PIN is immediately adjacent to microacini showing features of adenocarcinoma (fig. 3-23), and a transition may be seen in which neoplastic acini (so-called transitive glands) appear to bud from glands of high-grade PIN (fig. 3-23, left) (50,98). Transitive glands represent incomplete neoacini that maintain basal cells in a discontinuous pattern. Although abnormal, they do not qualify as invasive carcinoma until there is a complete loss of basal cells and acquisition of the typical nuclear features of carcinoma. In many cases, however, foci of high-grade PIN and carcinoma are close together but distinct and without an apparent transition (fig. 3-23, right) (98).

Immunohistochemical Findings. The secretory cells of PIN stain for both pan and low molecular weight keratins. The basal cell–specific, high molecular weight keratin (34βE12) demonstrates a complete or discontinuous layer of basal cells, a feature important in the differential diagnosis with prostatic carcinoma (fig. 3-18) (76,129,137). There is often a reduction in the intensity of staining with antibodies against PSA, prostatic acid phosphatase (PAP), and CD57 (94). Vimentin stains are usually negative in PIN. A spectrum of neuroendocrine differentiation can be detected as

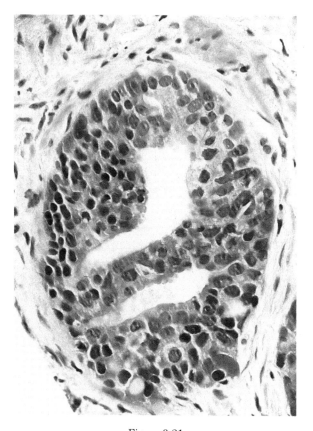

Figure 3-21
HIGH-GRADE PROSTATIC
INTRAEPITHELIAL NEOPLASIA
There is Paneth cell–like change.

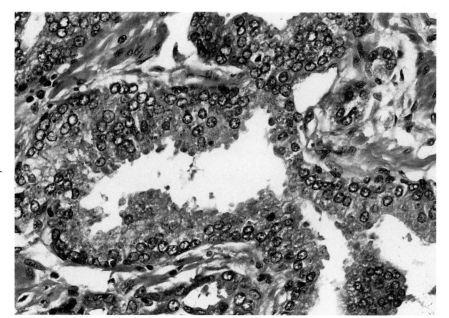

Figure 3-22
HIGH-GRADE PROSTATIC
INTRAEPITHELIAL
NEOPLASIA
Cytoplasmic lipofuscin pigment is present.

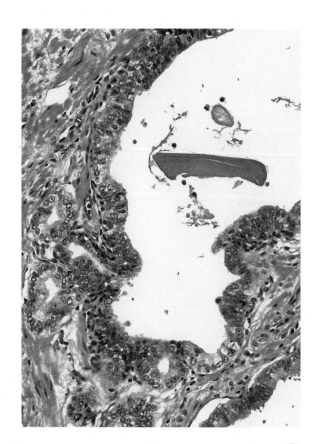
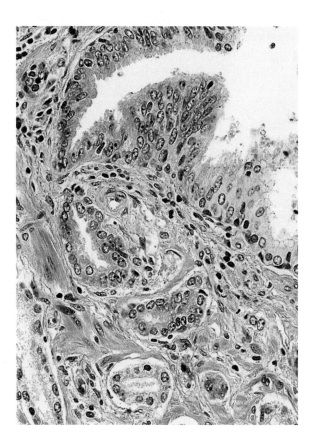

Figure 3-23
HIGH-GRADE PROSTATIC INTRAEPITHELIAL NEOPLASIA

Left: Budding of atypical acini is present (left) (so-called transitive glands).

Right: The small focus of invasive carcinoma that was present (bottom) was adjacent to prostatic intraepithelial neoplasia but not attached to it as are the acini in the left figure.

manifested by focal immunoreactivity for markers such as neuron-specific enolase, chromogranin, and synaptophysin (fig. 3-16C) (52,109). A variety of other immunohistochemical findings in PIN have been published (37,75) but are not of diagnostic importance.

Differential Diagnosis. The differential diagnosis of high-grade PIN is presented in Table 3-1. This list includes normal structures, reactive conditions, metaplasias, hyperplasias, and carcinomas (36,37,81,113). The glands of the prostatic central zone, because of their architectural complexity, may suggest PIN on low-power microscopy, but the typical nuclear changes of high-grade PIN are absent (fig. 3-24) (see page 15). This phenomenon illustrates that while architectural features often suggest PIN, cytologic confirmation is mandatory.

Seminal vesicle or ejaculatory duct epithelium may have a complex papillary-glandular pattern. This architecture, when coupled with the atypical cells that develop with advancing age, may suggest PIN. Seminal vesicle and ejaculatory duct epithelium, however, does not show the characteristic nuclear changes, in particular the prominent nucleoli, characteristic of high-grade PIN. The pleomorphic, hyperchromatic nuclei of ejaculatory duct and seminal vesicle are usually scattered among normal-appearing ones. Nuclear pseudoinclusions are frequent, and the atypicality appears degenerative. The atypical nuclei of high-grade PIN display irregular chromatin, parachromatin clearing, and prominent nucleoli. Lipofuscin pigment in PIN is usually finer, more granular, and less extensive than that in seminal vesicle or ejaculatory duct epithelium (see chapter 7) (35).

Duct-acinar epithelium adjacent to areas of inflammation or infarction may show nuclear atypia, including enlarged nucleoli (fig. 3-25) (37). A diagnosis of PIN should be made with great caution if infarction or inflammation, particularly acute, is seen in the vicinity. Usually, the glands affected by reactive atypia do not demonstrate the prominent architectural changes typical of high-grade PIN.

The atypia of secretory cells seen in irradiated prostates may also be marked but, as with reactive atypia, the architectural complexity of PIN is absent. Furthermore, the nuclei of PIN have open chromatin and prominent nucleoli. Radia-

Table 3-1

**DIFFERENTIAL DIAGNOSIS
OF PROSTATIC
INTRAEPITHELIAL NEOPLASIA**

Prostatic central zone glands

Seminal vesicle/ejaculatory duct

Reactive atypia
    Inflammation
    Infarction
    Radiation

Metaplasia
    Transitional cell
    Squamous cell

Hyperplasia
    Nodular hyperplasia with papillae
    Cribriform hyperplasia
    Atypical basal cell hyperplasia

Carcinoma
    Conventional adenocarcinoma with cribriform pattern
    Ductal adenocarcinoma
    Adenoid cystic carcinoma
    Transitional cell carcinoma

tion is associated with smudgy chromatin, low nuclear to cytoplasmic ratios, and cytoplasmic vacuolation (see chapter 7). In radiation atypia, nuclear pleomorphism is usually pronounced and variable from cell to cell compared to the monomorphic atypical nuclei of high-grade PIN. Furthermore, basal cells are often prominent, unlike in high-grade PIN, and squamous metaplasia is common. In most cases, the clinical history, characteristic atrophic background, and stromal and other changes of radiation point to the correct diagnosis (see page 319).

Transitional metaplasia (see chapter 7) may result in a tufted or even micropapillary pattern which on low-power microscopy can suggest PIN. The nuclei, however, lack the atypical features of PIN: they are frequently oval to slightly elongated, euchromatic and, importantly, display at least focal nuclear grooves (141).

Squamous metaplasia is usually easily separated from PIN, but when the metaplasia is associated with infarction there may be significant nuclear atypia and nucleolar enlargement raising the possibility of PIN. The solid architecture, polygonal eosinophilic squamous cells, and,

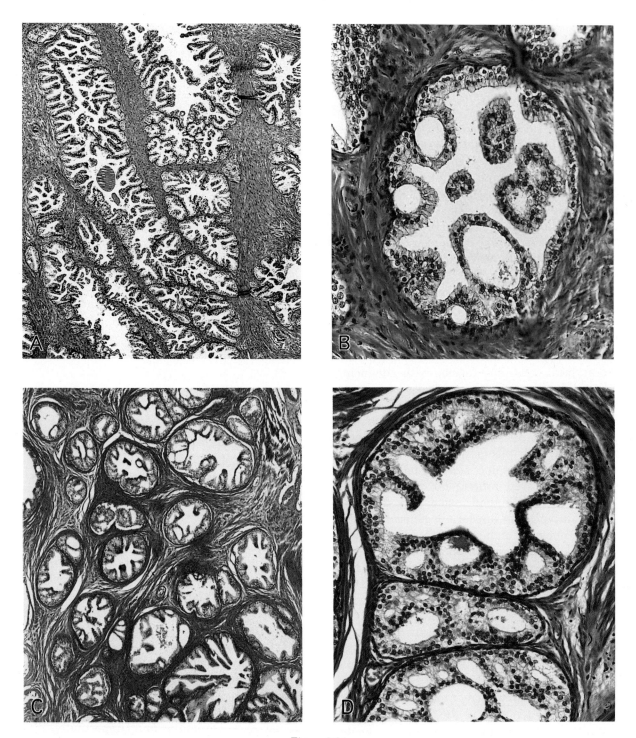

Figure 3-24
PROSTATIC CENTRAL ZONE GLANDS

Note the architectural features that may lead to a misdiagnosis of prostatic intraepithelial neoplasia.

A: A low-power view shows a prominent micropapillary pattern.

B: A high-power view demonstrates prominent epithelial arches. The secretory cells have bland nuclear features and abundant clear cytoplasm.

C: Another example shows architectural complexity.

D: A high-power view of central zone glands from the case illustrated in C shows arches (top) and a well-developed cribriform pattern (bottom) but lacks cytologic atypia, precluding a diagnosis of prostatic intraepithelial neoplasia.

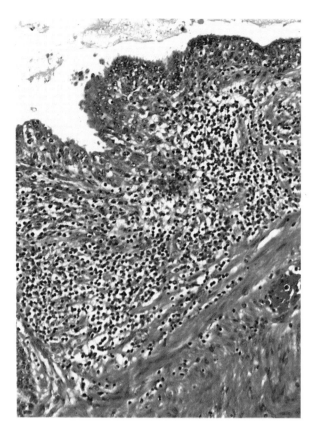

Figure 3-25
PROSTATITIS

There is mild inflammatory atypia and amphophilia of the cytoplasm. Note the striking inflammation. Cytologic atypia should be interpreted cautiously in this setting, particularly in the absence of tufted, micropapillary, and cribriform patterns.

in some cases, evidence of an infarct in the vicinity should facilitate the diagnosis.

Pronounced basal cell hyperplasia has a nodular appearance of overt basaloid nests, sometimes with retained lumens, that is distinctly different from that of PIN. Mild basal cell hyperplasia (fig. 3-26, left) may be more problematic because of the lack of a striking basaloid picture and the presence, in some cases, of easily visible nucleoli (fig. 3-26, right); however, careful examination shows that the nucleoli are in the basal rather than the secretory cells. Atypical basal cell hyperplasia may cause particular diagnostic problems but the solid nested pattern is again helpful (65). The proliferative, at times myxoid, stroma sometimes associated with basal cell hyperplasia (see page 303) is absent in PIN. Secretory cells may be noted in predominantly

basaloid nests in cases of atypical basal cell hyperplasia, but the secretory cells are not atypical. In general, atypical basal cell hyperplasia consists of a proliferation of small to medium caliber nests and glands. In contrast, PIN is an intraluminal proliferation of atypical secretory cells affecting medium to large glands. Rarely, a high molecular weight cytokeratin stain (clone $34\beta E12$) may be needed to resolve this important differential: the proliferating cells with enlarged nucleoli of atypical basal cell hyperplasia are positive while in PIN the atypical secretory cells are not, but a continuous or interrupted peripheral basal cell layer is seen.

Florid papillary nodular hyperplasia and cribriform hyperplasia involve medium to large ducts and acini and have a complex low-power microscopic appearance, hence suggesting PIN from the architectural viewpoint (41). However, the nuclear features that characterize PIN are not found in either form of hyperplasia (fig. 3-27C).

Cribriform adenocarcinoma may be confused with high-grade PIN with a striking cribriform pattern (39,97,99). When a cribriform pattern is associated with comedonecrosis or solid areas (Gleason grade 5A), carcinoma is likely. Papillary-cribriform adenocarcinomas that typify Gleason grade 3C are particularly problematic (39). In general, florid papillarity with extensive budding strongly favors carcinoma, particularly when high-grade cytologic atypia is present (see page 139). Widely distributed high-grade nuclear changes are typical of carcinoma, and, in such cases, there is little or no maturation of nuclei and nucleoli, a feature seen more commonly in high-grade PIN (see page 78), although it may be rarely seen in carcinoma and is not diagnostic by itself. Confluence of cribriform aggregates indicates stromal invasion and, therefore, carcinoma. Cribriform glands around a nerve rule out a diagnosis of PIN. A basal cell layer typically is not identified with routine stains in cribriform carcinoma and is usually absent with the high molecular weight keratin stain (clone $34\beta E12$). Sometimes, however, invasive cribriform adenocarcinoma is associated with spread into nearby glands (99); residual basal cells may be present in such cases as the secretory compartment is replaced by adenocarcinoma. This intraglandular process may be difficult if not impossible to separate from the highest degrees of PIN in limited material.

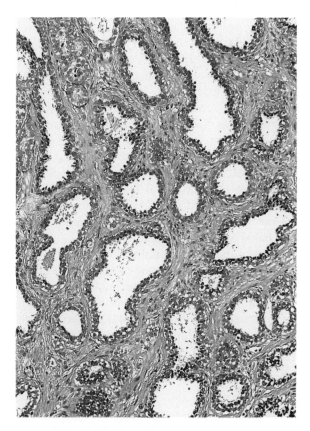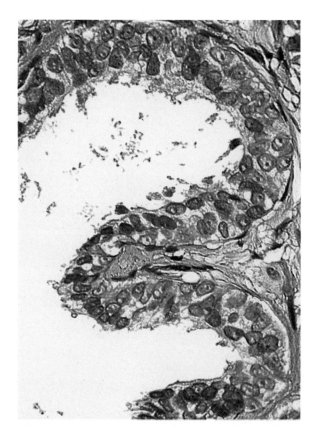

Figure 3-26
BASAL CELL HYPERPLASIA

Left: The low-power picture suggests the possibility of the flat pattern of prostatic intraepithelial neoplasia with a focal component of the tufted pattern.

Right: A high-power view shows that the atypical cells with prominent nucleoli are basal cells.

Adenocarcinomas with ductal features (see chapter 5) may be confused with micropapillary or cribriform PIN, particularly when ductal carcinoma extends to the peripheral zone (fig. 3-27E). Ductal carcinoma, however, typically involves the prostatic urethra and verumontanum and extends into periurethral ducts; these sites are uncommonly involved by PIN. In duct adenocarcinoma the patterns are usually more extensive and irregular than in PIN, such that a diagnosis of carcinoma is usually obvious, especially in transurethral resectates or radical prostatectomy specimens, but may be a problem in needle biopsies. The features helpful in the diagnosis of PIN with cribriform conventional carcinoma are applicable in this circumstance also. Ductal carcinoma may show marked nuclear pleomorphism with markedly enlarged nucleoli, and frequently has a high mitotic rate, features

unusual in high-grade PIN. The papillae in ductal carcinoma often have a fibrovascular stalk in contrast to those of most cases of PIN.

Transitional cell carcinoma involving prostatic ducts and acini (see chapter 5) may superficially resemble PIN (37) but is generally characterized by the replacement of duct-acinar epithelium by predominantly solid, usually highly atypical, mitotically active epithelium often displaying central necrosis and indicating an overt carcinoma (fig. 3-28). Occasionally, replacement of the native prostatic epithelium may be focal, and secretory epithelium and intraluminal corpora amylacea may be seen. Transitional cell carcinoma of prostatic ducts is usually composed of polygonal cells showing a greater degree of pleomorphism and more angular nuclei than seen in PIN. The cells typically have more dense eosinophilic cytoplasm and may have a squamoid

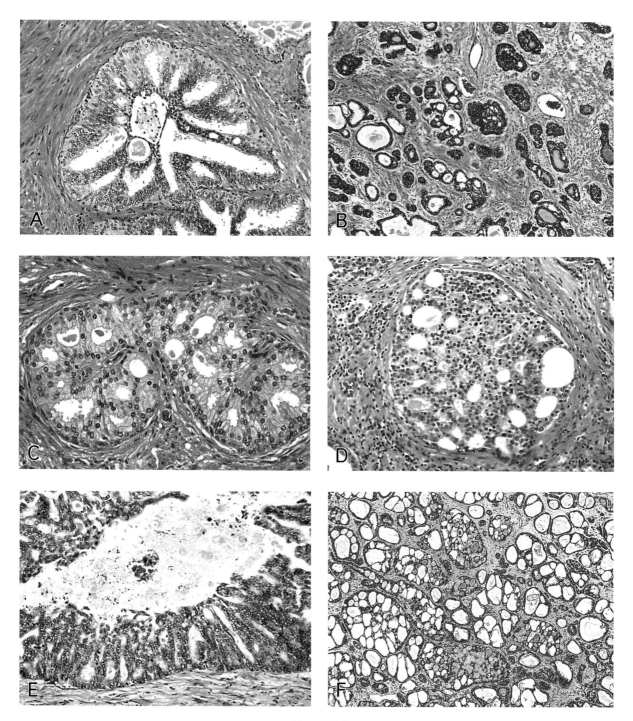

Figure 3-27
CRIBRIFORM PATTERNS IN THE DIFFERENTIAL DIAGNOSIS OF
HIGH-GRADE PROSTATIC INTRAEPITHELIAL NEOPLASIA

A: Cribriform high-grade prostatic intraepithelial neoplasia with a small amount of necrotic luminal material. Note the prominent nucleoli. Maturation of cells towards the lumens is also seen.

B: Basal cell hyperplasia with a cribriform pattern. Note the association with characteristic basaloid nests.

C: Cribriform hyperplasia. Note the presence of residual basal cells. No significant cytologic atypia is apparent.

D: Cribriform carcinoma. Note the absence of a basal cell layer, punched out lumina, and the presence of cytologic atypia.

E: Ductal carcinoma with a cribriform pattern. Note the marked cytologic atypia and central necrosis.

F: Adenoid cystic carcinoma. Note the confluent infiltrative growth.

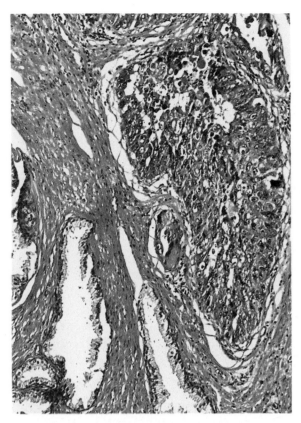

Figure 3-28
TRANSITIONAL CELL CARCINOMA
INVOLVING PROSTATE
The degree of cytologic atypicality, focal necrosis, and resemblance to transitional cell carcinoma all argue strongly against prostatic intraepithelial neoplasia.

appearance. Sometimes, transitional cell carcinoma in situ may spread in a pagetoid fashion, an appearance not characteristic of PIN. Transitional cell carcinoma of the prostate does not usually have the typical architectural diversity of high-grade PIN in the form of tufted, micropapillary, or cribriform patterns and is negative for PSA and PAP but often positive for high molecular weight cytokeratin (clone 34βE12). In contrast, the secretory cells of high-grade PIN are positive for PSA and PAP and negative for high molecular weight cytokeratin.

Clinical Significance of PIN. The finding of low-grade PIN should not prompt further investigation or particular concern; it is easily confused with normal and hyperplastic epithelium and reactive atypias, is not reproducibly recognized, and its relationship with carcinoma is not clearly established. Therefore, in our opinion, a diagnosis of low-grade PIN should not be rendered (34,36,70,113,119).

In contrast, high-grade PIN is an important diagnosis, but it should be made with care, especially in view of the broad differential diagnosis. That there is considerable interobserver variation in the diagnosis is suggested by the varied frequency of PIN reported in the literature (49). If high-grade PIN is encountered in a needle biopsy specimen, additional levels should be considered to rule out carcinoma, if the needle biopsy has not already been examined at multiple levels. In transurethral resection specimens, all of the tissue should be processed.

The reporting of high-grade PIN in association with carcinoma is not mandatory but may be indicated in some clinical situations and for academic reasons. A diagnosis of high-grade PIN without concurrent carcinoma should prompt careful clinical follow-up and further biopsies, especially if the serum PSA is elevated or abnormalities are noted on rectal or ultrasound examination (46,75,130). About 50 percent of patients with high-grade PIN without carcinoma in needle biopsies have had carcinoma detected in subsequent biopsies (57,63,71,82,85,119,140). These studies indicate that high-grade PIN is an important marker for invasive carcinoma. Similar results have been found in follow-up studies of PIN detected by fine needle aspiration biopsy (92). Although there is strong evidence that high-grade PIN is a preneoplastic lesion, aggressive treatment is not warranted in the absence of a diagnosis of adenocarcinoma.

ATYPICAL ADENOMATOUS HYPERPLASIA (ADENOSIS)

Definition. Atypical adenomatous hyperplasia (AAH) is characterized by proliferating small to medium-sized acini that usually form a well-circumscribed nodule but occasionally extend into the adjacent prostatic stroma. In some cases the process closely simulates small acinar carcinoma but does not fulfill all the architectural and cytologic criteria for carcinoma.

General Features. In an autopsy series, McNeal (168) recognized AAH as an atypical small glandular lesion that was associated with transition zone carcinoma. Other terms for similar lesions have included *carcinoma in situ, adenosis, atypical adenosis, small acinar atypical hyperplasia, atypical hyperplasia,* and *atypical primary hyperplasia* (147,160,161,163,165,170). A recent consensus statement has advocated the term, "atypical adenomatous hyperplasia" (143). Some prominent investigators prefer the term "adenosis" (150,153,154). Brawn (147) noted that 6.4 percent of patients with adenosis (AAH) developed carcinoma, compared to 3.7 percent of patients with nodular hyperplasia in a follow-up of 5 to 15 years. This association with carcinoma is in agreement with McNeal's work, however some of Brawn's illustrations have been questioned as representing carcinoma by several experts (142,146,154,156,164).

AAH has been identified in 1.5 to 19.6 percent of transurethral resectates and in up to 33 percent of radical prostatectomies (145,147,171, 177). In autopsy series of men aged 20 to 40 years, it has been detected in about 24 percent of prostates (146,147a). It is uncommon in needle biopsy specimens (less than 2 percent) except when they are directed at the transition zone (153). Although the transition zone is the usual site of involvement, AAH may be found on occasion in the peripheral zone (162,168). It is sometimes multifocal and usually associated with benign nodular hyperplasia (171,175).

The evidence associating AAH and carcinoma is mainly circumstantial. Besides the predilection for the transition zone and morphologic similarities between AAH and low-grade adenocarcinoma (Gleason grades 1 and 2), which may be the strongest argument linking the two (157a), other observations suggest a weak pathogenetic link (146,169,175). The age of patients with AAH is usually 5 to 10 years less than that of patients with carcinoma (142,146,175). As noted previously, AAH reportedly occurs more commonly in glands harboring cancer than in benign ones, although this observation has been questioned. Examples of small glandular carcinoma arising in relationship to AAH have been rarely reported (168).

The basal cell–specific high molecular weight keratin stain (clone 34βE12) usually shows a discontinuous pattern in AAH (172); this pattern is intermediate between a more or less continuous staining pattern for basal cells in normal prostate and benign nodular hyperplasia and the absence of basal cells in carcinoma (142,146, 153,173). Glands of AAH demonstrate increased silver nucleolar-organizer region counts and increased mean nuclear diameters and areas compared to the normal prostate (146,155). Labeling studies using tritiated thymidine have shown that small acinar lesions probably representing AAH have indices higher than those of benign glands and similar to indices found in some carcinomas (161). The interpretation of these early studies, however, is difficult since both PIN and AAH have been included in the "atypical hyperplasia" category (173). More recent studies utilizing tritiated thymidine autoradiography, immunohistochemistry for proliferation markers (Ki-67/MIB-1, PCNA), and silver staining of nucleolar-organizer regions, suggest that AAH has a proliferation rate between benign prostatic hyperplasia and low-grade adenocarcinoma (160,167). In contrast, PIN displays a proliferation rate similar to intermediate-grade carcinoma. One recent molecular genetic study demonstrated an 8p22 allelic loss in 1 of 18 cases of AAH in contrast to 9 of 16 cases of carcinoma (152). Another study using polymorphic microsatellite markers on chromosomes 7q, 8p, 8q, and 18q demonstrated allelic imbalance in 7 of 15 (47 percent) AAH cases. Similar genetic changes have been noted in early carcinogenesis, and this study suggests a genetic link between some cases of AAH and carcinoma (148).

Despite the above observations, there is no compelling evidence linking AAH and carcinoma (149,158). Validation of the hypothesis that some examples of AAH represent incipient carcinoma requires documentation of the evolution of carcinoma from AAH under clinical observation. This is not possible since there is no imaging study or other marker specific for AAH. Since AAH is often seen in transition zone material, it has been suggested that it may be related to adenocarcinoma developing at this site. Many of these tumors are small volume, low-grade lesions, and it is conceivable that AAH may be a precursor of some transition zone carcinomas. The lack of a significantly increased prevalence of AAH in prostate glands with transition zone carcinoma, however, argues against this hypothesis. In summary, the evidence linking AAH and adenocarcinoma is considerably weaker than that relating PIN and cancer. Prospective longitudinal studies

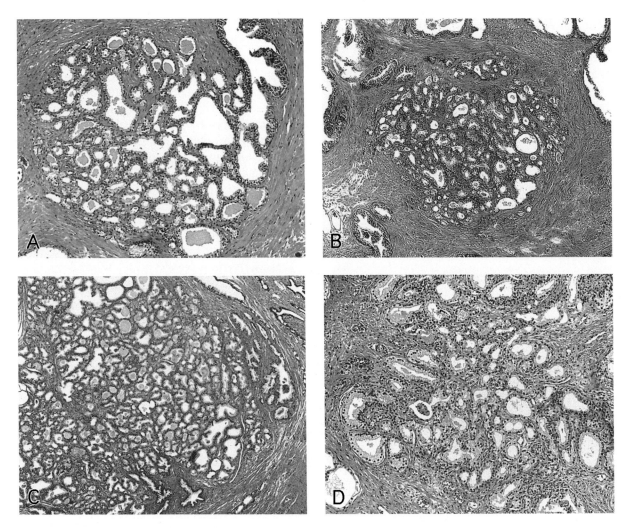

Figure 3-29
ATYPICAL ADENOMATOUS HYPERPLASIA
Note the well-circumscribed proliferation of small to medium-sized glands (predominantly the former) in the four separate examples. Note the relationship to a hyperplastic parent gland (right) in A.

of prostate cancer prevalence in patients with AAH and additional molecular genetic investigations are needed to help resolve this issue.

Clinical Features. AAH has no specific clinical features and is usually detected microscopically in prostatic tissue obtained in the course of investigating and treating prostatic hyperplasia and cancer.

Microscopic Findings. Foci of AAH are usually less than 1 cm and commonly in the 1 to 3 mm range (146,154,161a). On low-power magnification crowded, small to medium-sized acini disturb the uniform distribution of glands and stroma of the normal and hyperplastic prostate (fig. 3-29). The process often has a lobular growth pattern and is frequently found within or adjacent to typical hyperplastic nodules. In some cases there is a striking perinodular distribution (figs. 3-30, 3-31). The low-power architecture of AAH usually conforms to a Gleason grade 1 or 2 carcinoma (146,156). It usually has a "pushing" rather than infiltrating border with the adjacent stroma. A "parent" benign gland from which the small acini appear to arise may be found (fig. 3-29A) (146). In some cases, however, there is more stroma between individual glands, and the edge of the lesion shows limited infiltration (153).

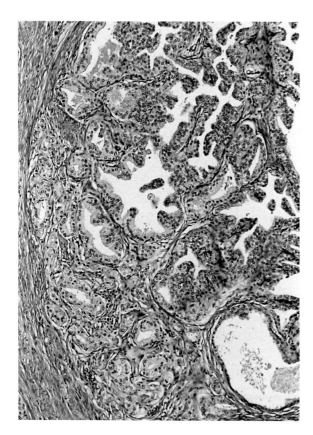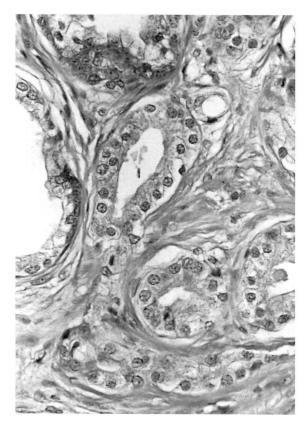

Figure 3-30
ATYPICAL ADENOMATOUS HYPERPLASIA
Left: Benign nodular hyperplasia has a peripheral focus of crowded small glands of atypical adenomatous hyperplasia.
Right: A high-power photomicrograph of the left figure shows small acini lined by bland cuboidal cells with innocuous nuclei lacking prominent nucleoli.

Individual glands of AAH, although closely packed, are separate, round to oval structures showing no tendency to fuse (fig. 3-29). They usually vary in size and shape, with some glands twice or more the size of others (fig. 3-32 A,B,D), although they may also be relatively uniform (fig. 3-32C). The acini are lined by cuboidal to low columnar cells resembling normal secretory cells (figs. 3-33, 3-34). They have basally located nuclei and moderately abundant apical cytoplasm which is often clear, although it may be lightly eosinophilic and granular. Basal cells may be conspicuous (fig. 3-33) or inconspicuous (fig. 3-34). They are often seen as a discontinuous layer when a basal cell–specific high molecular weight cytokeratin stain (clone 34βE12) is employed (fig. 3-35) (159, 174). The luminal borders in AAH are more often irregular and serrated than those of carcinoma which are usually smooth and more rigid (146,153,156,164).

In AAH the lumens are often empty, but corpora amylacea may be present (fig. 3-36B), being seen in 43 percent of AAH foci in one series (153). Luminal crystalloids have been noted in 16 to 40 percent of foci in three large series (fig. 3-36C), but are more common in carcinoma (146,153, 164). Basophilic mucin is rare (151) but when present is positive with the alcian blue stain (146,153,157,164). There is usually no stromal response, but exceptionally a cellular stroma consisting mainly of fibroblasts is noted; in such cases there is histologic overlap with sclerosing adenosis (see page 293).

The nuclei of AAH are usually round to oval and have uniform chromatin usually without parachromatin clearing. The nuclear membranes are smooth. There may be some mild variation in nuclear size and shape (fig. 3-36). Nucleoli are generally inconspicuous and less than 1 μm in

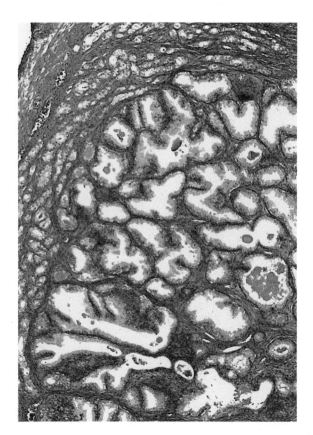 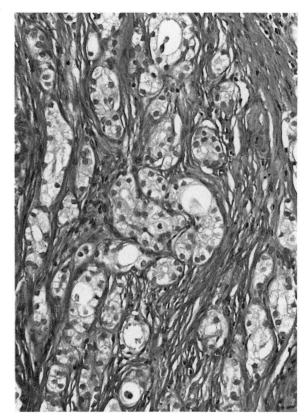

Figure 3-31
ATYPICAL ADENOMATOUS HYPERPLASIA

Left: A focus of atypical adenomatous hyperplasia forms a crescent-shaped band at the periphery of a focus of nodular hyperplasia.

Right: A higher power view shows bland cytologic features including an absence of prominent nucleoli. Basal cells are inconspicuous, a finding that may lead to a misinterpretation of adenocarcinoma.

diameter; occasional nucleoli greater than 1 μm were encountered in 18 percent of the cases in one series (146), and in another, prominent nucleoli (defined as greater than 1.6 μm) were occasional or frequent in 41 percent of the cases and rare in an additional 26 percent (166).

AAH is uncommon in needle biopsies, but may be seen when the transition zone is sampled intentionally or inadvertently (fig. 3-36) (153). The diagnosis of AAH is often particularly challenging in these cases since the typical lobular arrangement and associated "parent" glands may not be present. Areas of stromal hyperplasia suggesting a transition zone site are a clue to consider AAH in the differential diagnosis. A high molecular weight cytokeratin stain may be of particular use in difficult needle biopsy cases (figs. 3-37, 3-38).

Special Studies. Mucin histochemical studies show the occasional presence of acid mucosubstances in the lumens of AAH. In one study, acidic mucin was noted in 54 percent of AAH foci, a figure similar to that reported for carcinoma, although in our experience blue-tinged mucin as identified in hematoxylin and eosin–stained sections is uncommon in AAH. Mucin stains have little diagnostic value in supporting or refuting a diagnosis of AAH (151). The glands of AAH are strongly immunoreactive to antibodies for PSA, PAP, and Leu-7. Secretory cells are positive for pan and low molecular weight keratins. A discontinuous pattern of basal cell staining is noted with high molecular weight keratin markers (clone 34βE12) (fig. 3-35) (142).

Differential Diagnosis. The differential diagnosis of AAH is complex and includes many of

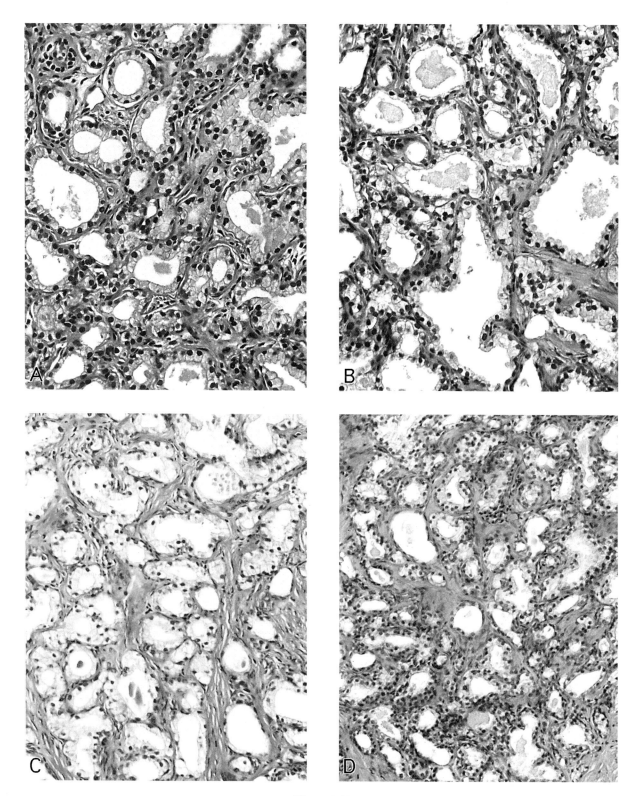

Figure 3-32
ATYPICAL ADENOMATOUS HYPERPLASIA
Intermediate- to high-power views of four separate cases. Note variations in size and shape of individual glands in A, B, and D, and the bland cytology and sporadic basal cells on close scrutiny. Some glands contain eosinophilic luminal secretion.

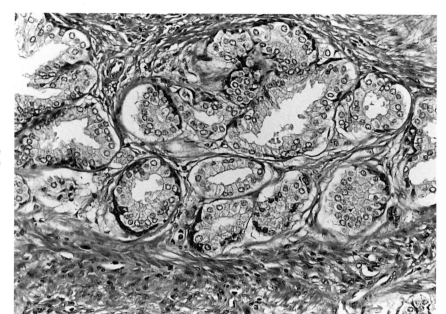

Figure 3-33
ATYPICAL ADENOMATOUS
HYPERPLASIA
The darkly staining cells at the
periphery of some of the acini are
basal cells.

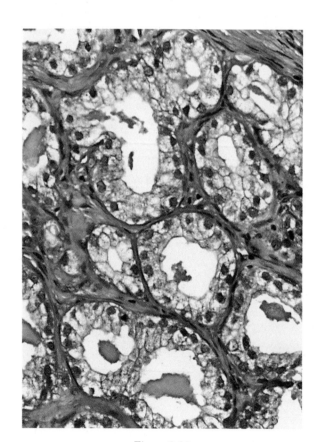

Figure 3-34
ATYPICAL ADENOMATOUS HYPERPLASIA
Note the bland nuclear features. Basal cells are incon-
spicuous.

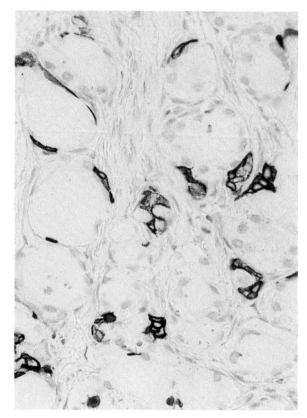

Figure 3-35
ATYPICAL ADENOMATOUS HYPERPLASIA
A discontinuous basal cell layer is demonstrated by the
high molecular weight cytokeratin (34βE12) stain.

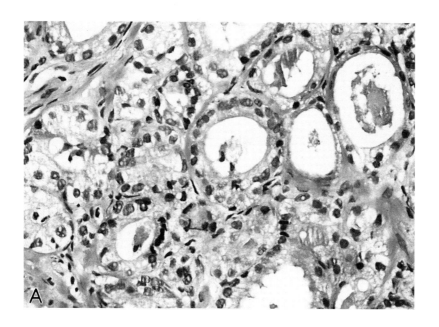

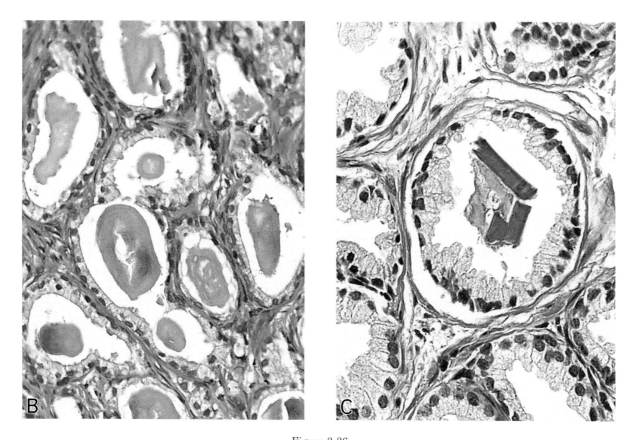

Figure 3-36
ATYPICAL ADENOMATOUS HYPERPLASIA
Atypical adenomatous hyperplasia with intraluminal eosinophilic material (A), corpora amylacea (B), and crystalloids (C).

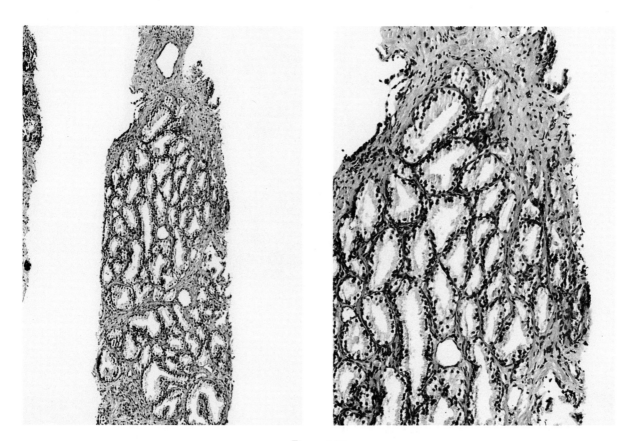

Figure 3-37
ATYPICAL ADENOMATOUS HYPERPLASIA IN A NEEDLE BIOPSY
Note the small acini with minimal variation in size and shape. Bland cytologic characteristics are seen on the right.

the small glandular patterns that one may encounter in the prostate gland (Table 3-2); these are discussed in detail in chapters 4 and 7. Only the histologic differentiation of AAH and well-differentiated carcinoma is considered here (142,146, 153,154,175,176). This sometimes difficult distinction is of considerable practical importance because, although treatment philosophies vary, some urologists take an aggressive approach to even incidentally detected low-grade tumors, especially those identified in young patients.

Both AAH and low-grade carcinoma (Gleason grades 1 and 2) are completely or relatively circumscribed on low-power microscopy. The acini of low-grade carcinoma tend to be more uniform in size and shape than those of AAH and often have a more regular luminal border. Furthermore, the lumen to gland diameter ratios are generally lower in carcinoma than in AAH. In the latter, a benign "parent" gland is often closely

related to the proliferating acini, which often appear to arise as an outgrowth from the clearly benign gland. In AAH the cytoplasm is usually clear, while in small acinar carcinoma it may be clear, eosinophilic, or amphophilic. In both small acinar carcinoma and AAH, the amount of cytoplasm is variable and may be abundant.

The nuclei of both AAH and well-differentiated carcinoma are round to oval and relatively uniform (142). Some variation in nuclear size may be seen in both conditions but is more common in carcinoma. This criterion, however, is subjective and difficult to analyze in the absence of morphometry. The chromatin pattern of AAH is uniform and usually granular; in small acinar carcinoma, it may also be uniform and granular but much more often shows areas of parachromatin clearing. Nuclear membrane irregularity is also more prominent in small acinar carcinoma than AAH, although the changes are subtle.

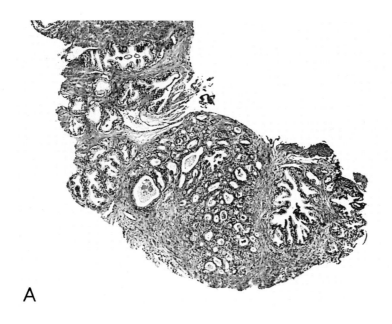

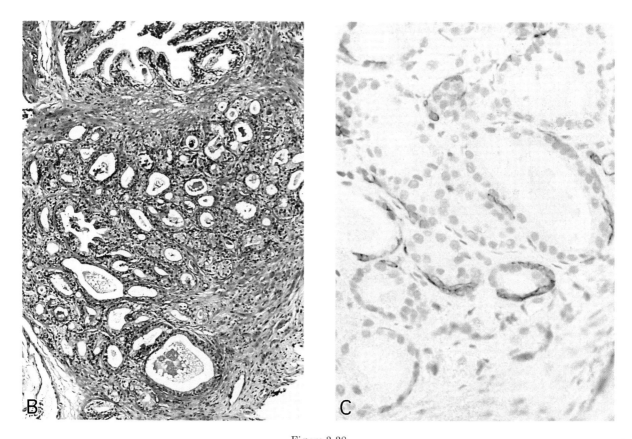

Figure 3-38
ATYPICAL ADENOMATOUS HYPERPLASIA IN A NEEDLE BIOPSY
A,B: There are crowded, irregular, predominantly small acini with associated "parent" glands.
C: Discontinuous basal cells are identified with a high molecular weight cytokeratin (34βE12) stain.

Table 3-2

DIFFERENTIAL DIAGNOSIS OF SMALL GLANDULAR PATTERNS IN THE PROSTATE GLAND

Normal or vestigial structures
    Seminal vesicle/ejaculatory ducts
    Cowper's gland
    Paraganglionic tissue
    Mesonephric remnants

Atrophy
    Simple (lobular) atrophy
    Sclerotic atrophy

Hyperplasia
    Small glandular pattern of benign nodular
        hyperplasia
    Basal cell hyperplasia
    Postatrophic hyperplasia
    Sclerosing adenosis
    Verumontanum mucosal gland hyperplasia
    Mesonephric remnant hyperplasia

Atypical adenomatous hyperplasia (adenosis)

Nephrogenic adenoma of prostatic urethra

Treatment effects
    Radiation effects
    Antiandrogen effects

Small acinar carcinoma

An important criterion in distinguishing AAH and carcinoma is the presence of "significantly" enlarged nucleoli (146,156,160a,176). In general, nucleoli are prominent in small acinar carcinoma, even in low-grade examples, and inconspicuous in AAH. Prominent nucleoli are usually greater than 1 to 1.5 mm in diameter and in carcinoma are often present in many nuclei. They are sometimes irregular and have an eosinophilic hue (146). Occasional prominent nucleoli may be present in AAH, but most are basophilic and usually measure less than 1 µm (146). In general, the nucleoli of AAH are very similar to those of adjacent, clearly benign glands while those of small acinar carcinoma are distinctly different. When judging the significance of nucleoli in a small acinar proliferation it is useful to compare the nucleoli in the atypical area with those in the unequivocally benign glands. If they are similar in both sites, their significance in indicating a diagnosis of carcinoma is much reduced.

Corpora amylacea are more commonly identified in AAH compared to carcinoma, although a small percentage of low-grade carcinomas contain them. Luminal eosinophilic crystalloids and basophilic luminal mucin are commonly found in small acinar carcinoma and are less frequent in AAH (153,154). If both eosinophilic crystalloids and basophilic mucin are present in a lesion, the index of suspicion for carcinoma should be high.

Basal cells are absent in carcinoma and often inconspicuous in AAH with routine stains; the high molecular weight keratin stain (clone 34βE12) is of value in identifying basal cells in AAH (142,153,154,159). This stain usually delineates basal cells with a discontinuous pattern. Caution is warranted in interpreting this staining reaction, as the diagnosis of cancer is based on a negative staining reaction (unlike most immunohistochemical stains), and hence one must check for appropriate staining in internal and external controls, and evaluate the findings within the overall histologic context.

There is overlap in the architectural, cytological, and ancillary features (mucin, crystalloids) of AAH and carcinoma, and no single morphologic feature is diagnostic. For example, although prominent nucleoli are, on the average, helpful in indicating carcinoma, one study showed that about 10 percent of low-grade cancers did not have prominent nucleoli (166). The low-power pattern should be integrated with observations of nuclear, cytoplasmic, and luminal characteristics, and the presence of basal cells; carcinoma is usually separable from AAH by evaluating this constellation of features.

Clinical Significance. From a therapeutic perspective AAH is considered benign and patients should be followed conservatively (176). The term should not be used as a "wastebasket" for small acinar lesions that are difficult to classify, for those with a few suspicious glands considered below the threshold for carcinoma (see chapter 4), or if artifact precludes reliable histologic evaluation (144,176).

REFERENCES

Historical Perspective

1. Altenähr E, Kastendieck H, Siefert H. Coincidence of prostatic carcinoma and dysplasia in total prostatectomies and in autopsies. Verh Dtsch Ges Pathol 1979;63:415–8.
2. Amin MB, Ro JY, Ayala AG. Putative precursor lesions of prostatic adenocarcinoma: fact or fiction? Mod Pathol 1993;6:476–83.
3. Andrews CS. Latent carcinoma of the prostate. J Clin Pathol 1949;2:197–208.
3a. Anton RC, Kattan MW, Chakraborty S, Wheeler TM. Postatrophic hyperplasia of the prostate. Lack of association with prostate cancer. Am J Surg Pathol 1999;23:932–6.
4. Armenian NK, Lilienfeld AM, Diamond EL, Bross ID. Relation between benign prostatic hyperplasia and cancer of the prostate: a prospective and retrospective study. Lancet 1974;2:115–7.
5. Billis A. Latent carcinoma and atypical lesions of prostate. An autopsy study. Urology 1986;28:324–9.
6. Bostwick DG, Algaba F, Amin MB, et al. Consensus statement on terminology: recommendation to use atypical adenomatous hyperplasia in place of adenosis of the prostate. Am J Surg Pathol 1994;18:1069–70.
7. Bostwick DG, Brawer MK. Prostatic intra-epithelial neoplasia and early invasion in prostate cancer. Cancer 1987;59:788–94.
8. Bostwick DG, Cooner WH, Denis L, Jones GW, Scardino PT, Murphy GP. The association of benign prostatic hyperplasia and cancer of the prostate. Cancer 1992;70(Suppl):291–301.
9. Bostwick DG, Srigley J, Grignon D, et al. Atypical adenomatous hyperplasia of the prostate: morphologic criteria for its distinction from well-differentiated carcinoma. Hum Pathol 1993;24:819–32.
10. Bostwick DG, Srigley JR. Premalignant lesions. In: Bostwick DG, ed. Pathology of the prostate. New York: Churchill Livingstone, 1990:37–59.
11. Cheatle GL, Wale RS. A lesion common to breast and prostate glands. Br J Surg 1930;17:619–22.
12. Cheville JC, Bostwick DG. Postatrophic hyperplasia of the prostate. A histologic mimic of postatic adenocarcinoma. Am J Surg Pathol 1995;19:1068–76.
13. Dhom G. Early neoplastic changes in the prostate. Verh Dtsch Ges Pathol 1979;63:218–31.
14. Drago JR, Mostofi FK, Lee F. Introductory remarks and workshop summary. Urology, 1989;34(Suppl):2–3.
15. Epstein JI. Adenosis vs. atypical adenomatous hyperplasia of the prostate. Am J Surg Pathol 1994;18:1070–1.
16. Franks LM. Atrophy and hyperplasia in prostate proper. J Pathol Bacteriol 1954;68:617–21.
17. Franks LM. Latent carcinoma of prostate. J Pathol Bacteriol 1954;68:603–16.
18. Gaudin PB, Epstein JI. Adenosis of the prostate. Histologic features in transurethral resection specimens. Am J Surg Pathol 1994;18:863–70.
19. Greenwald P, Kirmss V, Polan AK, Dick VS. Cancer of the prostate among men with benign prostatic hyperplasia. JNCI 1974;53:35–40.
20. Helpap BG. The biological significance of atypical hyperplasia of the prostate. Virchows Arch (A) 1980;387:307–17.
21. Helpap BG, Bostwick DG, Montironi R. The significance of atypical adenomatous hyperplasia and prostatic intraepithelial neoplasia for the development of prostate carcinoma. Virchows Arch 1995;426:425–34.
22. Kastiendieck H, Altenähr E, Husselmann H, Bressel M. Carcinoma and dysplastic lesions of the prostate. A histomorphological analysis of 50 total prostatectomies by step–section technique. Z. Krebsforsch 1976;88:33–54.
23. Kastendieck H, Helpap B. Prostatic "dysplasia/atypical hyperplasia." Terminology, histopathology, pathobiology and significance. Urology 1989;34(Suppl 6):28–42.
24. Kovi J, Mostofi FK, Heshmat MY, et al. Large acinar atypical hyperplasia and carcinoma of the prostate. Cancer 1988; 61:555–61.
25. Liavag I. Atrophy and regeneration in the pathogenesis of prostatic carcinoma. Acta Pathol Microbiol Scand 1968;73:338–50.
26. McNeal JE. Age related changes in prostatic epithelium associated with carcinoma. In: Griffiths K, Pierrepoint CG, eds. Some aspects of the aetiology and biochemistry of prostatic cancer. Third Tenovus Workshop. Cardiff, Wales: Alpha Omega Alpha Publishing, 1970:23–32.
27. McNeal JE. Morphogenesis of prostatic carcinoma. Cancer 1965;18:1659–66.
28. McNeal JE, Bostwick DG. Intraductal dysplasia: a premalignant lesion of the prostate. Hum Pathol 1986;17:64–71.
29. Miller A, Seljelid R. Cellular atypia in the prostate. Scand J Urol Nephrol 1971;5:17–21.
30. Oertel H. Involutionary changes in prostate and female breast cancer in relation to cancer development. Can Med Assoc J 1926;16:237–41.
31. Parkinson MC. Pre-neoplastic lesions of the prostate. Histopathology 1995;27:301–11.
31a. Ruska KM, Sauvageot J, Epstein JI. Histology and cellular kinetics of prostatic atrophy. Am J Surg Pathol 1998;22:1073–7.
32. Tannenbaum M. Atypical epithelial hyperplasia or carcinoma of prostate gland. The surgical pathologist at an impasse? Urology 1974;4:758–60.

Prostatic Intraepithelial Neoplasia

33. Alexander EE, Qian J, Wollan PC, Myers RP, Bostwick DG. Prostatic intraepithelial neoplasia does not appear to raise serum prostate-specific antigen concentration. Urology 1996;47:693–8.
34. Allam CK, Bostwick DG, Hayes JA, et al. Interobserver variability in the diagnosis of high grade prostatic intraepithelial neoplasia and adenocarcinoma. Mod Pathol 1996;9:742–51.
35. Amin MB, Bostwick DG. Pigment in prostatic epithelium and adenocarcinoma: a potential source of diagnostic confusion with seminal vesicular epithelium. Mod Pathol 1996;9:791–5.
36. Amin MB, Ro JY, Ayala AG. Putative precursor lesions of prostatic adenocarcinoma: fact or fiction? Mod Pathol 1993;6:476–83.

37. Amin MB, Ro JY, Ayala AG. Prostatic intraepithelial neoplasia. Relationship to prostate adenocarcinoma. In: Rosen PP, Fechner RE, eds. Pathology annual (Part II). Norwalk CT: Appleton Lange, 1994:1–30.

38. Amin MB, Schultz DS, Zarbo RJ, Kubus J, Shaheen C. Computerized static DNA ploidy analysis of prostatic intraepithelial neoplasia. Arch Pathol Lab Med 1993;117:794–8.

39. Amin MB, Schultz DS, Zarbo RJ. Analysis of cribriform morphology in prostatic neoplasia using antibody to high-molecular-weight cytokeratins. Arch Pathol Lab Med 1994;118:260–4.

40. Anton R, Arakawa A, Wheeler TM. Survey of 5000+ prostatic needle biopsies over five–year period from a large urologic practice [Abstract]. Mod Pathol 1996;9:70A.

41. Ayala AG, Srigley JR, Ro JY, Abdul-Karim FW, Johnson DE. Clear cell cribriform hyperplasia of prostate. Report of 10 cases. Am J Surg Pathol 1986;10:665–71.

42. Baretton GB, Vogt T, Blasenbreu S, Lohrs U. Comparison of DNA ploidy in prostatic intraepithelial neoplasia and invasive carcinoma of the prostate: an image cytometric study. Hum Pathol 1994;25:506–13.

43. Bergerheim US, Kunimi K, Collins VP, Ekman P. Deletion of chromosomes 8,10 and 16 in human prostatic carcinoma. Genes Chromosom Cancer 1991;3:215–20.

44. Boag AH, Young ID. Immunohistochemical analysis of type IV collegenase expression in prostatic hyperplasia and adenocarcinoma. Mod Pathol 1993;6:65–8.

45. Bonkhoff H, Stein U, Remberger K. The proliferative function of basal cells in the normal and hyperplastic human prostate. Prostate 1994;24:114–8.

46. Bostwick DG. Evaluating prostate needle biopsy: therapeutic and prognostic significance. CA Cancer J Clin 1997;47:297–319.

47. Bostwick DG. High-grade prostatic intraepithelial neoplasia: the most likely precursor of prostate cancer. Cancer 1995;75:1823–36.

48. Bostwick DG. Premalignant lesions of the prostate. Semin Diagn Pathol 1988;5:240–53.

49. Bostwick DG. What is the clinical significance of high-grade PIN? Contemp Urol 1998:45–60.

50. Bostwick DG, Amin MB, Dundore P, Marsh W, Schultz DS. Architectural patterns of high-grade prostatic intraepithelial neoplasia. Hum Pathol 1993;24:298–310.

51. Bostwick DG, Brawer MK. Prostatic intra-epithelial neoplasia and early invasion in prostate cancer. Cancer 1987;59:788–94.

52. Bostwick DG, Dousa MK, Crawford BG, Wollan PC. Neuroendocrine differentiation in prostatic intraepithelial neoplasia and adenocarcinoma. Am J Surg Pathol 1994;18:1240–6.

53. Bostwick DG, Pacelli A, Lopez-Beltran A. Molecular biology of prostatic intraepithelial neoplasia. Prostate 1996;29:117–34.

54. Bostwick DG, Pacelli A, Lopez-Beltran A. Ultrastructure of prostatic intraepithelial neoplasia. Prostate 1997;33:32–7.

55. Bostwick DG, Qian J, Frankel K. The incidence of high–grade prostatic intraepithelial neoplasia in needle biopsies. J Urol 1995;154:1791–4.

56. Brawer MK. Prostatic intraepithelial neoplasia: a premalignant lesion. Hum Pathol 1992;23:242–8.

57. Brawer MK, Bigler SA, Sohlberg OE, Nagle RB, Lange PH. Significance of prostatic intraepithelial neoplasia on prostate needle biopsy. Urology 1991;38:103–7.

58. Brawer MK, Deering RE, Brown M, Preston SD, Bigler SA. Predictors of pathologic stage in prostatic carcinoma. The role of neovascularity. Cancer 1994;73:678–87.

59. Brawer MK, Lange PH. Prostate-specific antigen and premalignant change: implications for early detection. CA Cancer J Clin 1989;39:361–75.

60. Brawer MK, Rennels MA, Nagle RB, et al. Prostatic intraepithelial neoplasia: a lesion that may be confused with cancer on prostatic ultrasound. J Urol 1989;142:1510–2.

61. Colombel M, Symmans F, Gil S, et al. Detection of the apoptosis-suppressing oncoprotein bcl-2 in hormone-refractory human prostate cancers. Am J Pathol 1993;143:390–400.

62. Crissman JD, Sakr WA, Hussein ME, Pontes JE. DNA quantification of intraepithelial neoplasia and invasive carcinoma of the prostate. Prostate 1993;22:155–62.

63. Davidson D, Bostwick DG, Qian J, et al. Prostatic intraepithelial neoplasia is a risk factor for adenocarcinoma: predictive accuracy in needle biopsies. J Urol 1995;154:1295–9.

64. Deschenes J, Weidner N. Nucleolar organizer regions (NOR) in hyperplastic and neoplastic prostate disease. Am J Surg Pathol 1990;14:1148–55.

65. Devaraj LT, Bostwick DG. Atypical basal cell hyperplasia of the prostate. Immunophenotypic profile and proposed classification of basal cell proliferations. Am J Surg Pathol 1993;17:645–59.

66. Devonec M, Fendler JP, Monsallier M, et al. The significance of prostatic hypoechoic area: results in 226 ultrasonically guided prostatic biopsies. J Urol 1990;143:316–9.

67. Drago JR, Mostofi FK, Lee F. Introductory remarks and workshop summary. Urology, 1989;34(Suppl):2–3.

68. Emmert-Buck MR, Vocke CD, Pozzatt RO, et al. Allelic loss of chromosome 8p12-21 in microdissected prostatic intraepithelial neoplasia. Cancer Res 1995;55:2959–62.

69. Epstein JI, Cho KR, Quinn BD. Relationship of severe dysplasia to stage A (incidental) adenocarcinoma of the prostate. Cancer, 1990;65:2321–7.

70. Epstein JI, Grignon DJ, Humphrey PA, et al. Interobserver reproducibility in the diagnosis of prostatic intraepithelial neoplasia. Am J Surg Pathol 1995;19:873–86.

71. Garnett JE, Oyasu R. Urologic evaluation of atypical prostatic hyperplasia. Urology 1989;34(Suppl 6):66–9.

72. Gaudin PB, Sesterhenn IA, Wojno KJ, Mostofi FK, Epstein JI. Incidence and clinical significance of high-grade prostatic intraepithelial neoplasia in TURP specimens. Urology 1997;49:558–63.

73. Glannulis I, Montironi R, Galluzzi CM, deNictolis M, Diamanti L. Frequency and location of mitoses in prostatic intraepithelial neoplasia (PIN). Anticancer Res 1993;13:2447–51.

74. Gleason DF. Atypical hyperplasia, benign hyperplasia and well-differentiated adenocarcinoma of the prostate. Am J Surg Pathol 1985;9(Suppl):53–67.

75. Haggman MJ, Macoska JA, Wojno KJ, Oesterling JE. The relationship between prostatic intraepithelial neoplasia and prostate cancer: critical issues. J Urol 1997;158:12–22.

76. Hedrick L, Epstein JI. Use of keratin 903 as an adjunct in the diagnosis of prostate carcinoma. Am J Surg Pathol 1989;13:389–96.

77. Helpap B. Observations on the number, size and localization of nucleoli in hyperplastic and neoplastic prostatic disease. Histopathology 1988;13:203–11.

78. Helpap B. The biological significance of atypical hyperplasia of the prostate. Virchows Arch [A] 1980;387:307–17.

79. Humphrey PA. Mucin in severe dysplasia in the prostate. Surg Pathol 1991;4:237–43.

80. Ibrahim GK, Kerns BJ, MacDonald JA, et al. Differential immunoreactivity of epidermal growth factor receptor in benign, dysplastic and malignant prostatic tissues. J Urol 1993;149:170–3.

81. Jones EC, Young RH. The differential diagnosis of prostatic carcinoma. Its distinction from premalignant and pseudocarcinomatous lesions of the prostate gland. Am J Clin Pathol 1994;101:48–64.

82. Kappel TJ, Kuskowski M, Willmott L, Cherwitz DL. Prostatic intraepithelial neoplasia and atypical adenomatous hyperplasia (adenosis): a retrospective study with long-term follow-up. J Surg Pathol 1995;1:77–85.

83. Kastendieck H. Correlations between atypical primary hyperplasia and carcinoma of the prostate: a histologic study of 180 total prostatectomies. Pathol Res Pract 1980;169:366–87.

84. Kastendiek H, Helpap B. Prostatic "dysplasia/atypical hyperplasia." Terminology, histopathology, pathobiology and significance. Urology 1989;34(Suppl 6):28–42.

85. Keetch DW, Humphrey P, Stahl D, Smith DS, Catalona WJ. Morphometric analysis and clinical follow-up of isolated prostatic intraepithelial neoplasia in needle biopsy of the prostate. J Urol 1995;154:347–51.

86. Kovi J, Mostofi FK, Heshmat MY, et al. Large acinar atypical hyperplasia and carcinoma of the prostate. Cancer 1988;61:555–61.

87. Langer JE, Rovner ES, Coleman BG, et al. Strategy for repeat biopsy of patients with prostatic intraepithelial neoplasia detected by prostate needle biopsy. J Urol 1996:155:228–31.

88. Layfield LJ, Goldstein NS. Morphometric analysis of borderline atypia in prostatic aspiration biopsy specimen. Anal Quant Cytol Histol 1991;13:288–92.

89. Lee F, Torp-Pedersen ST, Carroll JT, Siders DB, Christensen-Day C, Mitchell AE. Use of transrectal ultrasound and prostate–specific antigen in diagnosis of prostatic intraepithelial neoplasia. Urology 1989;34(Suppl):4–8.

90. Macoska JA, Micale MA, Sakr WA, Benson PD, Wolman SR. Extensive genetic alterations in prostate cancer revealed by dual PCR and FISH analysis. Genes Chrom Cancer 1993;8:88–97.

91. Macoska JA, Trybus TM, Benson PD, et al. Evidence for three tumor suppressor gene loci on chromosome 8p in human prostate cancer. Cancer Res 1995;55:5390–5.

92. Markham CW. Prostatic intraepithelial neoplasia: detection and correlation with invasive cancer in fine–needle biopsy. Urology 1989;24(Suppl 6):57–61.

93. Maygarden SJ, Strom S, Ware JL. Localization of epidermal growth factor receptor by immunohistochemical methods in human prostatic carcinoma, prostatic intraepithelial neoplasia, and benign hyperplasia. Arch Pathol Lab Med 1992;116:269–73.

94. McNeal JE, Alroy J, Leav I, Redwine EA, Freiha FS, Stamey TA. Immunohistochemical evidence for impaired cell differentiation in the premalignant phase of prostate carcinogenesis. Am J Clin Pathol 1988;90:23–32.

95. McNeal JE, Bostwick DG. Intraductal dysplasia: a premalignant lesion of the prostate. Hum Pathol 1986;17:64–71.

96. McNeal JE, Leav I, Alroy J, Skutelsky E. Differential lectin staining of central and peripheral zones of the prostate and alterations in dysplasia. Am J Clin Pathol 1988;89:41–8.

97. McNeal JE, Reese JH, Redwine EA, Freiha FS, Stamey TA. Cribriform adenocarcinoma of the prostate. Cancer 1986;58:1714–9.

98. McNeal JE, Villers A, Redwine EA, Freiha FS, Stamey TA. Microcarcinoma in the prostate: its association with duct-acinar dysplasia. Hum Pathol 1991;22:644–52.

99. McNeal JE, Yemoto CE. Spread of adenocarcinoma within prostatic ducts and acini. Morphologic and clinical correlations. Am J Surg Pathol 1996;20:802–14.

100. Min KW, Jin JK, Blank J, Hemstreet G. AgNORs in the human prostatic gland. Am J Clin Pathol 1990;94:508.

101. Mirchandani D, Zheng J, Miller GJ, et al. Heterogeneity in intratumor distribution of p53 mutation in human prostate cancer. Am J Pathol 1995;147:92–101.

102. Montironi R, Braccischi A, Matera G, Scarpelli M, Pisani E. Quantitation of prostatic intraepithelial neoplasia. Analysis of the nuclear size, number and location. Pathol Res Pract 1991;187:307–14.

103. Montironi R, Magi Galluzzi CM, Diamanti L, Giannulis I, Pisani E, Scarpelli M. Prostatic intraepithelial neoplasia: expression and location of proliferating cell nuclear antigen in epithelial, endothelial and stromal nuclei. Virchows Arch [A] 1993;422:185–92.

104. Montironi R, Magi Galluzzi C, Diamanti L, Tabomor, Scarpelli M, Pisani E. Prostatic intra-epithelial neoplasia. Qualitative and quantitative analyses of the blood capillary architecture on thin tissue sections. Pathol Res Pract 1993;189:542–8.

105. Montironi R, Magi Galluzzi C, Scarpelli M, Giannulis I, Diamanti L. Occurrence of cell death (apoptosis) in prostatic intra-epithelial neoplasia. Virchows Arch [A] 1993;423:351–7.

106. Montironi R, Scarpelli M, Sisti S, et al. Quantitative analysis of prostatic intraepithelial neoplasia on tissue sections. Anal Quant Cytol Histol 1990;12:366–72.

107. Myers RB, Grizzle WE. Biomarker expression in prostatic intraepithelial neoplasia. Eur Urol 1996;30:153–66.

107a. Myers RB, Srivastava S, Oelschlager DK, Brown D, Grizzle WE. Expression of nm23-H1 in prostatic intra-epithelial neoplasia and adenocarcinoma. Hum Pathol 1996;27:1021–4.

108. Myers RB, Srivastava S, Oelschlager DK, Grizzle WE. Expression of p160erb-B3 and p185erb-B2 in prostatic intraepithelial neoplasia and prostatic adenocarcinoma. JNCI 1994;86:1140–5.

109. Nagle RB, Brawer MK, Kittelson J, Clark V. Phenotypic relationship of prostatic intraepithelial neoplasia to invasive prostatic carcinoma. Am J Pathol 1991;138:119–28.

110. Nagle RB, Petein M, Brawer M, Bowden GT, Cress AE. New relationships between prostatic intraepithelial neoplasia and prostatic carcinoma. J Cell Biochem 1992;16H(Suppl):26–9.

111. Oyasu R, Bahnson RR, Nowel SK, Garnett JE. Cytological atypia in the prostate gland: frequency, distribution and possible relevance to carcinoma. J Urol 1986;135:959–62.

112. Pacelli A, Bostwick DG. Clinical significance of high-grade prostatic intraepithelial neoplasia in transurethral resection specimens. Urology 1997;50:355–9.

113. Parkinson MC. Pre-neoplastic lesions of the prostate. Histopathology 1995;27:301–11.

114. Perlman EJ, Epstein JI. Blood group antigen expression in dysplasia and adenocarcinoma of the prostate. Am J Surg Pathol 1990;14:810–18.

115. Petein M, Michel P, Van Velthoven R, et al. Morpho-nuclear relationship between prostatic intraepithelial neoplasia and cancers as assessed by digital cell image analysis. Am J Clin Pathol 1991;96:628–34.

116. Qian J, Jenkins RB, Bostwick DG. Detection of chromosomal anomalies and c-myc gene amplification in the cribriform pattern of prostatic intraepithelial neoplasia and carcinoma by fluorescence in situ hybridization. Mod Pathol 1997;10:1113–9.

117. Qian J, Wollan P, Bostwick DG. The extent and multicentricity of high grade prostatic intraepithelial neoplasia in clinically localized prostatic adenocarcinomas. Hum Pathol 1997;28:143–8.

118. Quinn BD, Cho KR, Epstein JI. Relationship of severe dysplasia to stage B adenocarcinoma of prostate. Cancer 1990;65:2328–37.

119. Raviv G, Janssen T, Zlotta AR, Descamps F, Verhest A, Schulman CC. Prostatic intraepithelial neoplasia: influence of clinical and pathological data on the detection of prostate cancer. J Urol 1996;156:1050–5.

120. Reyes AO, Swanson PE, Carbone JM, Humphrey PA. Unusual histologic types of high–grade prostatic intraepithelial neoplasia. Am J Surg Pathol 1997;21:1215–22.

121. Ronnett BM, Carmichael MJ, Carter HB, Epstein JI. Does high-grade prostatic intraepithelial neoplasia result in elevated serum prostate specific antigen levels? J Urol 1993;150:386–9.

122. Sakr WA, Grignon DJ, Crissman JD, et al. High grade prostatic intraepithelial neoplasia (HGPIN). and prostatic adenocarcinoma between the ages of 20–69: an autopsy study of 249 cases. In Vivo 1994;8:439–44.

123. Sakr WA, Haas GP, Cassin BJ, Pontes JE, Crissman JD. The frequency of carcinoma and intraepithelial neoplasia of the prostate in young male patients. J Urol 1993;150:379–85.

124. Sakr WA, Macoska JA, Benson P, et al. Allelic loss in locally metastatic multisampled prostate carcinoma. Cancer Res 1994;54:3273–7.

125. Sakr WA, Sarkar FH, Sreepathi P, Drozdowicz S, Crissman JD. Measurement of cellular proliferation in human prostate by AgNOR, PCNA and SPF. Prostate 1993;22:147–54.

126. Schultz DS, Amin MB, Zarbo RJ. Type IV collagen basement membrane component of prostatic intraepithelial neoplasia and associated carcinoma. Appl Immunohist 1993;1:123–6.

127. Sentinelli S. Mucins in prostatic intraepithelial neoplasia and prostatic carcinoma. Histopathology 1993;22:271–4.

128. Sesterhenn IA, Becker RL, Avallone FA, et al. Image analysis of nucleoli and nucleolar organizer regions in prostatic hyperplasia, intraepithelial neoplasia and prostatic carcinoma. J Urogenit Pathol 1991;1:61–74.

129. Shah IA, Schlageter MO, Stinnett P, Lechago J. Cytokeratin immunohistochemistry as a diagnostic tool for distinguishing malignant from benign epithelial lesions of the prostate. Mod Pathol 1991;4:220–4.

130. Shepherd D, Keetch DW, Humphrey PA, Smith DS, Stahl D. Repeat biopsy strategy in men with isolated prostatic intraepithelial neoplasia on prostate needle biopsy. J Urol 1996;156:460–3.

131. Srigley J, King S, VanNostrand AW, Robinette M. The preneoplastic prostate: a giant section whole organ study of 72 radical prostatectomies [Abstract]. Lab Invest 1986;54:30A.

132. Srigley J, Toth P, Hartwick RW. Atypical histologic patterns in cases of benign prostatic hyperplasia [Abstract]. Lab Invest 1989;60:90A.

133. Tamboli P, Amin MB, Schultz DS, Linden MD, Kubus J. Comparative analysis of nuclear proliferative index (Ki-67) in benign prostate, prostatic intraepithelial neoplasia and prostatic carcinoma. Mod Pathol 1996;9:1015–9.

134. Tamboli P, Amin MB, Xu HJ, Linden MD. Immunohistochemical expression of retinoblastoma and p53 tumor suppressor genes in prostatic intraepithelial neoplasia: comparison with prostatic adenocarcinoma and benign prostate. Mod Pathol 1998;11:247–52.

135. Troncoso P, Babaian RJ, Ro JY, Grignon DJ, von Eschenbach AC, Ayala AG. Prostatic intraepithelial neoplasia and invasive prostatic adenocarcinoma in cystoprostatectomy specimens. Urology 1989;34(Suppl 6):52–6.

136. Turkeri LN, Sakr WA, Wykes SM, Grignon DJ, Pontes JE, Macoska JA. Comparative analysis of epidermal growth factor receptor gene expression and protein product in benign, premalignant, and malignant prostate tissue. Prostate 1994;25:199–205.

137. Varma M, Amin MB, Linden MD, Zarbo RJ. Discriminant staining patterns of small glandular and preneoplastic lesions of the prostate using high molecular weight cytokeratin (HMCK). A study of 301 consecutive needle biopsies [Abstract]. Mod Pathol 1997;10:93A.

138. Weaver MG, Abdul-Karim FW, Srigley J, Bostwick DG, Ro JY, Ayala AG. Paneth cell-like change of the prostate gland. A histologic, immunohistochemical and electron microscopic study. Am J Surg Pathol 1992;16:62–8.

139. Weinberg DS, Weidner N. Concordance of DNA content between prostatic intraepithelial neoplasia and concomitant invasive carcinoma. Evidence that prostatic intraepithelial neoplasia is a precursor of invasive prostatic carcinoma. Arch Pathol Lab Med 1993;117:1132–7.

140. Weinstein MH, Epstein JI. Significance of high-grade prostatic intraepithelial neoplasia on needle biopsy. Hum Pathol 1993;24:624–9.

141. Yantiss RK, Young RH. Transitional cell "metaplasia" in the prostate gland. A survey of its frequency and features based on 103 consecutive prostatic biopsy specimens. J Urol Pathol 1997;7:71–80.

Atypical Adenomatous Hyperplasia

142. Amin MB, Ro JY, Ayala AG. Putative precursor lesions of prostatic adenocarcinoma: fact or fiction? Mod Pathol 1993;6:476–83.

143. Bostwick DG, Algaba F, Amin MB, et al. Consensus statement on terminology: recommendation to use atypical adenomatous hyperplasia in place of adenosis of the prostate [Letter]. Am J Surg Pathol 1994;18:1069–70.

144. Bostwick DG, Iczkowski KA. Minimal criteria for the diagnosis of prostate cancer on needle biopsy. Ann Diagn Pathol 1997:1:104–29.

145. Bostwick DG, Qian J. Atypical adenomatous hyperplasia of the prostate. Relationship with carcinoma in 217 whole-mount radical prostatectomies. Am J Surg Pathol 1995;19:506–18.

146. Bostwick DG, Srigley J, Grignon D, et al. Atypical adenomatous hyperplasia of the prostate: morphologic criteria for its distinction from well-differentiated carcinoma. Hum Pathol 1993;24:819–32.

147. Brawn PN. Adenosis of the prostate: a dysplastic lesion that can be confused with prostate adenocarcinoma. Cancer 1982;49:826–33.

147a. Brawn PN, Speights VO, Contin JU, Bayardo RJ, Kuhl DH. Atypical hyperplasia in prostates of 20 to 40 year old men. J Clin Pathol 1989;42:383–6.

148. Cheng L, Shan A, Cheville JC, Qian J, Bostwick DG. Atypical adenomatous hyperplasia of the prostate: a premalignant lesion? Cancer Res 1998;58:389–91.

149. Epstein JI. Adenosis (atypical adenomatous hyperplasia): histopathology and relationship to carcinoma. Path Res Pract 1995;191:888–98.

150. Epstein JI. Adenosis vs. atypical adenomatous hyperplasia of the prostate [Letter]. Am J Surg Pathol 1994;18:1070–1.

151. Epstein JI, Fynheer J. Acidic mucin in the prostate: can it differentiate adenosis from adenocarcinoma? Hum Pathol 1992;23:1321–5.

152. Furman J, Zhu X, Kalcem Z, Torres C, Humphrey PA. Chromosome 8p22 allelic loss in atypical adenomatous hyperplasia (adenosis) and carcinoma of the prostate [Abstract]. Mod Pathol 1996;9:73A.

153. Gaudin PB, Epstein JI. Adenosis of the prostate. Histologic features in needle biopsy specimens. Am J Surg Pathol 1995;19:737–47.

154. Gaudin PB, Epstein JI. Adenosis of the prostate. Histologic features in transurethral resections specimens. Am J Surg Pathol 1994;18:863–70.

155. Ghazizadah M, Sasaki Y, Oguro T, Aihara K. Silver staining of nucleolar organizer regions in prostate lesions. Histopathology 1991;19:369–72.

156. Gleason DF. Atypical hyperplasia, benign hyperplasia, and well-differentiated adenocarcinoma of the prostate. Am J Surg Pathol 1985;9(Suppl):53–67.

157. Goldstein NS, Qian J, Bostwick DG. Mucin expression in atypical adenomatous hyperplasia of the prostate. Hum Pathol 1995;26:887–91.

157a. Grignon DJ, Sakr WA. Atypical adenomatous hyperplasia of the prostate: a critical review. Eur Urol 1996;30:2206–11.

158. Häussler O, Epstein JI, Amin MB, Heitz PU, Hailemariam S. Putative precursors of prostate cancer—adenosis (atypical adenomatous hyperplasia) and prostatic intraepithelial neoplasia—further investigation of cell kinetics, oncogene and tumor suppressor gene status and comparison with benign prostatic hyperplasia and cancer. Hum Pathol (in press).

159. Hedrick L, Epstein JI. Use of keratin 903 as an adjunct in the diagnosis of prostate carcinoma. Am J Surg Pathol 1989;13:389–96.

160. Helpap B. Cell kinetic studies on prostatic intraepithelial neoplasia (PIN) and atypical adenomatous hyperplasia (AAH) of the prostate. Pathol Res Pract 1995;191:904–7.

160a. Helpap B. Observations on the number, size, and localization of nucleoli in hyperplastic and neoplastic prostatic disease. Histopathology 1988;13:203–11.

161. Helpap B. The biological significance of atypical hyperplasia of the prostate. Virchows Arch [A] 1980;387:307–17.

161a. Humphrey PA, Zhu X, Crouch EC, Carbone JM, Keetch DW. Mass-formative atypical adenomatous hyperplasia of prostate. J Urol Pathol 1998;9:73–81.

162. Kappel TJ, Kuskowski M, Willmott L, Cherwitz DL. Prostatic intraepithelial neoplasia and atypical adenomatous hyperplasia (adenosis): a retrospective study with long-term follow up. J Surg Pathol 1995;1:77–85.

163. Kastendieck H, Helpap B. Prostatic "dysplasia/atypical hyperplasia." Terminology, histopathology, pathobiology, and significance. Urology 1989;34(Suppl 6):28–42.

164. Keane PF, Ilesley IC, O'Donoghue PN, Parkinson MC. Pathological classification and follow-up of prostatic lesions initially diagnosed as "suspicious of malignancy." Br J Urol 1990;66:306–11.

165. Kovi J, Mostofi FK. Atypical hyperplasia of prostate. Urology 1989;34(Suppl 6):23–7.

166. Kramer CE, Epstein JI. Nucleoli in low-grade prostate adenocarcinoma and adenosis. Hum Pathol 1993;24:618–23.

167. Lopez-Beltran A, Pacelli A, Rothenberg HJ, Sebo TJ, Qian J, Bostwick DG. Atypical adenomatous hyperplasia of the prostate: immunophenotype and DNA ploidy analysis. Mod Pathol (in press).

168. McNeal JE. Morphogenesis of prostatic carcinoma. Cancer 1965;18:1659–66.

169. McNeal JE, Redwine EA, Freiha FS, Stamey TA. Zonal distribution of prostatic adenocarcinoma. Correlation with histologic pattern and direction of spread. Am J Surg Pathol 1988;12:897–906.

170. Miller GJ. An atlas of prostatic biopsies: dilemmas of morphologic variance. In: Fenoglio-Preiser CM, Wolff M, Rilke F, eds. Progress in surgical pathology. Philadelphia: Field and Wood, 1988:81–112.

171. Mittal BV, Amin MB, Kinare SG. Spectrum of histologic lesions in 185 consecutive prostate specimens. J Postgrad Med 1989;35:157–61.

172. O'Malley FP, Grignon DJ, Shum DT. Usefulness of immunoperoxidase staining with high-molecular-weight cytokeratin in the differential diagnosis of small-acinar lesions of the prostate gland. Virchows Arch [A] 1990;417:191–6.

173. Parkinson MC. Pre-neoplastic lesions of the prostate. Histopathology 1995;27:301–11.

174. Shah IA, Schlageter MO, Stinnett P, Lechago J. Cytokeratin immunohistochemistry as a diagnostic tool for distinguishing malignant from benign epithelial lesions of the prostate. Mod Pathol 1991;4:220–4.

175. Srigley JR. Small acinar patterns in the prostate gland with emphasis on atypical adenomatous hyperplasia and small acinar carcinoma. Semin Diagn Pathol 1988;5:284–93.1

176. Srigley JR, Bullock M, Amin M. Small glandular patterns in the prostate gland: the differential diagnosis of small acinar carcinoma. In: Foster CS, Bostwick DG, eds. Pathology of the prostate. Philadelphia: WB Saunders, 1998:126–55.

177. Srigley JR, Toth P, Hartwick RW. Atypical histologic patterns in cases of benign prostatic hyperplasia [Abstract]. Lab Invest 1989;60:90A.

4

CARCINOMA OF THE PROSTATE GLAND
(EXCLUDING UNUSUAL VARIANTS AND SECONDARY CARCINOMAS)

GENERAL AND CLINICAL FEATURES

Establishing, or ruling out, the diagnosis of carcinoma of the prostate has been a well-known challenge for pathologists for many years (2,5,8, 9,12,13) and has become an even greater problem in recent times because of the increased number of biopsy specimens and the often limited amount of carcinoma, or questionable carcinoma, in such samples (1,3,4,6,7,10,11). In this chapter the various appearances of prostatic adenocarcinoma, except for the specific variants of prostatic carcinoma considered in chapter 5, are presented and the features important in the differential diagnosis emphasized.

General Features

Prostatic adenocarcinoma is the most common noncutaneous malignant neoplasm in humans, with an estimated prevalence, based on histologic studies, of over 30 percent in males older than 50 years. In the United States it represents the most common internal cancer, with an estimated 179,300 new cases in 1999 (60,101). Prostatic carcinoma is second only to lung cancer in mortality, accounting for an estimated 37,000 deaths in the United States in 1999 (60). Both incidence and mortality rates have increased over the last few decades (Table 4-1) (68,71,78,88). Between 1991 and 1995, however, the prostate cancer death rate decreased (49a). The changing incidence in successive decades until the 1990s is related, at least in part, to the advent of newer diagnostic tests such as serum prostate-specific antigen (PSA) and prostatic ultrasound, as well as increased public awareness of this disease (23,28,46,72).

There is a disparity in the frequency of carcinoma at autopsy compared to clinically manifest disease (90). The autopsy prevalence of prostatic adenocarcinoma ranges up to 80 percent in the ninth decade (21). Some authors have suggested that these "latent" carcinomas represent an intrinsically innocuous form of prostatic cancer, distinct from clinically manifest disease (14,17,

34,36,37,39,40,47,53,56,65,72,77,84). More recent studies indicate that carcinomas detected at autopsy or in radical cystoprostatectomy specimens for bladder cancer are not inherently different from clinically manifest prostatic carcinoma but are simply smaller and better differentiated and, therefore, less clinically significant (53,65).The lifetime risk for a 50-year-old man developing carcinoma discoverable at autopsy has been estimated at 42 percent, while the lifetime risk for developing clinical disease or dying from prostatic carcinoma is about 10 and 3 percent, respectively (86).

Clinically manifest prostatic cancer usually occurs in the sixth to eighth decades and is uncommon in patients under 50 years of age; cases diagnosed in the latter age group account for less than 1 percent of the total (56). Clinically recognizable prostatic carcinoma is rare in patients younger than 40 years but has been documented even in the first decade; many of the reported cases have been histologically aggressive neoplasms (32, 91). A recent autopsy study, however, has shown that prostatic intraepithelial neoplasia may be seen in males in their late twenties, and invasive carcinomas were detected in about one quarter of patients in their thirties (84). In the current era of PSA screening for prostate cancer many more

Table 4-1

**ANNUAL PROSTATE CANCER
INCIDENCE AND MORTALITY RATES
PER 100,000 POPULATION***

Year	Incidence	Mortality Rate
1994	144.0	26.7
1992	190.1	26.7
1990	132.0	26.5
1985	88.0	23.4
1976	73.5	22.1

*Adapted from: Ries LA, Kosary CL, Hankey BF, et al. (eds). SEER Cancer Statistics Review, 1973-1994 (NIH, Pub. No. 97-2789). Bethesda, MD, National Cancer Institute, 1997.

cases are detected in relatively young men between 40 and 55 years of age than in prior times.

There is considerable geographic variation in the incidence and mortality rates for prostatic cancer (18,35,56). Low rates are seen in the Far East and very high rates in Northern European and North American populations (fig. 4-1) (78). Men who move from low risk to high risk countries tend to acquire the risk profile of their destination (14,35). The marked difference between rates of clinical carcinoma among countries is not reflected by similar differing rates of prostatic carcinoma detected at autopsy (24,104). This suggests that in high risk populations there is a greater conversion rate of "latent" to clinical carcinomas.

From a racial perspective, the mortality rate among African-American men exceeds that of Caucasian males and greatly exceeds the rate among black men residing in Africa (56, 58,66,73,94). It is among the highest mortality rates in the world. American men of Asian origin have lower rates than Caucasian males (41,56). Lower mortality rates have been noted among Jewish men residing in New York compared to non-Jewish men (70,102). The differences in clinical behavior among racial groups are not reflected in different rates of carcinoma detected at autopsy (24,35). Socioeconomic status, marital status, and fertility status are not strongly linked to the development of prostatic carcinoma (87).

The etiology and pathogenesis of prostate cancer are poorly understood (37). Both genetic and epigenetic factors have been implicated. There is a well-documented familial association in a minority of cases (25–27,97,99,103). If a first-degree relative had prostatic cancer, a male has a twofold higher risk for this disease (99). If two or more first-degree relatives were affected the risk increases from five-fold to as much as eleven-fold (99). In pathologic studies of hereditary prostate cancer, the neoplasms were of lower grade than their sporadic counterpart, but no other substantial clinical or pathologic differences were noted (16,54). Currently, there is considerable ongoing research to detect molecular markers in families at high risk for the development of prostatic adenocarcinoma, and a putative prostate cancer susceptibility gene has been identified with genetic linkage to 1q24-25 in such families (96).

There is little current evidence to suggest an etiologic role for viruses; however, herpes sim-

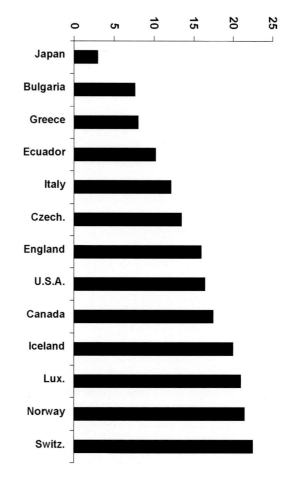

Age-adjusted death rates due to prostate cancer (per 100,000 population)

Figure 4-1
AGE-ADJUSTED DEATH RATES DUE TO PROSTATE CANCER PER 100,000 POPULATION IN VARIOUS COUNTRIES
(Data from Boring CC, Squires TS, Tong T. Cancer statistics 1992. CA Cancer J Clin 1992;42:19–39.)

plex virus type II, cytomegalovirus, and RNA viruses have been associated with prostatic carcinoma, and herpes-like viral particles have been detected by electron microscopy in some cancers (29,50,64,85). Cadmium exposure has been associated with higher risks of prostatic adenocarcinoma in some studies (55). Cadmium is known to be an inhibitor of zinc metabolism, and the prostate gland contains the highest levels of zinc of all body tissues. An increased risk of prostate cancer has been noted in workers exposed to chemicals in the rubber, textile, chemical, drug, fertilizer, and atomic energy industries (56). There have also been a number of studies linking a high fat diet to the development of prostatic carcinoma (74,76). The diet of Japanese men has considerably less fat content than that of American men, and, as the fat content has increased in recent years toward "Western" levels, there has been a rise in the incidence of prostate cancer in Japan (92). Both vitamin A deficiency and increased vitamin A intake have been linked with prostate cancer in some studies (57,67,75). Vitamin D deficiency has also been implicated in the development of prostate cancer. Prostate cancer is more common in northern countries than in those closer to the equator. Prostate cancer incidence and mortality rates have been inversely related to ultraviolet radiation exposure, a factor necessary for the synthesis of vitamin D (49,95).

Some studies have suggested men who underwent vasectomy have an increased risk of developing prostatic adenocarcinoma (43,44,80), but other studies have not supported this (93). Indeed, the validity of many of the published studies related to vasectomy has been questioned because of methodologic deficiencies (33,51). Both increased and reduced sexual activity levels have been associated with prostate cancer, but the role of sexual activity in prostatic carcinogenesis is uncertain (82,83,98).

The strongest risk factors for the development of prostate cancer are advancing age, race, heredity (as previously discussed), and hormonal activity. Testicular hormones are necessary for normal prostatic growth and maintenance (31). Prostatic adenocarcinoma apparently does not develop in males castrated before puberty or in male pseudohermaphrodites with 5-a-reductase deficiency (81). Furthermore, both primary and metastatic prostatic carcinoma commonly respond to surgical castration, exogenous estrogen therapy, and anti-androgen treatments. No consistent abnormalities in serum androgens have been detected in patients with prostatic carcinoma (37,42), but increased concentrations of testosterone, dihydrotestosterone, and androstenedione have been reported in prostate cancer tissues compared to normal tissues (48,59,63). Elevated urinary estrone/androsterone ratios have been detected in some studies (31). A reduced risk for prostate cancer has been documented in patients with cirrhosis (45,79); this may be related to the increased circu-

lating levels of estrogen and decreased levels of testosterone (56).

There are a number of studies of rodents and other experimental models in which prostate adenocarcinoma is induced by chemical carcinogens, radiation therapy, and hormone administration, details of which are beyond the scope of this work. The interested reader is referred to selected references (52,69,89,100).

Possible or probable precursor lesions of adenocarcinoma have already been discussed in chapter 3. There is little evidence that nodular hyperplasia or atrophy are directly related to the genesis of prostatic adenocarcinoma (30,38). Prostatic intraepithelial neoplasia, however, is strongly associated with invasive carcinomas, especially those arising in the peripheral zone. The role, if any, of atypical adenomatous hyperplasia is poorly understood (see page 95). There are limited data to suggest that some low-grade carcinomas of the transition zone may be related to it (15,19,20,22). The factors leading to the transformation of small, possibly clinically insignificant tumors to larger, potentially aggressive ones are unknown, although both hereditary and environmental factors may be involved.

Clinical Features

In several historical series encompassing a total of 5,291 patients and covering a span of years dating from prior to 1925 (112), from 1932 to 1956 (165), from 1966 to 1991 (171a), and from 1983 to 1993 (116), the average age of patients coming to medical attention for the treatment of prostate cancer was virtually the same, 64 to 65 years. The youngest patient was 31 years old (171a), and several additional patients were in their forties (112,116,165). In the largest series, 3,170 patients treated at the Mayo Clinic, there were no apparent age differences by stage or grade of the tumor (171a).

Patients with adenocarcinoma of the prostate gland are most often asymptomatic in this era, but locally extensive tumors may cause patients to present with pelvic pain, rectal obstruction, or bleeding as was seen more frequently in the past (128a,137a,138,151a,157,158). Symptoms of bladder outlet obstruction are common in patients who do not come to attention through PSA screening (118). In many of these cases these symptoms are related to coexistent nodular hyperplasia, but in some patients, especially those with large volume periurethral tumors, the adenocarcinoma itself may result in obstruction. Occasionally, the clinical presentation is that of a urethral neoplasm (see Secondary Tumors of Urethra, chapter 9). In most patients presenting with obstructive symptoms, the carcinoma is clinically unsuspected and detected in the material removed to relieve nodular hyperplasia. When both hyperplasia and carcinoma are present in large amounts, it is difficult to define the relative contributions of each process to the bladder outlet obstruction. In patients undergoing transurethral resection for clinical hyperplasia, carcinoma was detected in about 16 percent of cases derived from a composite series (125). The frequency of detection of carcinoma in these cases is directly dependent on the sampling strategy, with more cases detected with total submission of the tissue (148,153,167). Although many of these neoplasms are small volume, well-differentiated tumors, a sizable number are more extensive, and moderately to poorly differentiated.

Presenting symptoms of metastatic disease include bone pain and tenderness (112,118,138, 158). Involvement of the spinal column may lead to cord compression (141,154). Occasionally, enlarged lymph nodes, especially inguinal and sometimes cervical or axillary, lead to clinical detection (113,138). Symptoms related to ascites, pleural effusion, or visceral or bone metastases are uncommon presenting manifestations (107,121,133).

On rare occasions, prostatic carcinoma may manifest as a paraneoplastic syndrome. Ectopic hormone production (Cushing's syndrome due to adrenocorticotrophic hormone, inappropriate antidiuretic hormone secretion), hypercalcemia, and neuromuscular disorders have been reported, particularly with small cell carcinoma (105,130,142, 161,162,169). Disseminated intravascular coagulation and nonbacterial thrombotic endocarditis may be seen in some patients, particularly those with metastatic disease (114,153a), and dermatomyositis has also been reported as a presenting clinical manifestation (152).

In asymptomatic patients the tumor may be detected by an abnormal digital rectal examination (DRE). The detection rate of prostate carcinoma using DRE is about 0.8 to 2.7 percent in several large series (114,119,131,136,139a,140,

147,163,166). Many cancers detected by DRE are locally advanced. The predictive value of a positive DRE ranges from 21 to 39 percent (119,139a, 140,147,163,166). Abnormal findings include a discrete hard nodule, diffuse induration, and asymmetry in shape and texture. False positive observations are common and may result from spheroids of nodular hyperplasia and chronic prostatitis, especially of the granulomatous variety; calculi; infarct; and intraprostatic seminal vesicles. An important limitation of DRE is its lack of sensitivity (i.e., high false negative rate). Most carcinomas detected by transurethral resection and in PSA screening programs are not palpable.

In recent years, there has been increased interest in the early detection of prostatic adenocarcinoma. This stems from the fact that prostatic carcinoma is commonly silent and frequently has spread beyond the gland locally, or is metastatic at the time of presentation (128). Early detection is of paramount importance as therapy for localized disease increases cure rates. In addition to DRE, screening involves measurement of serum PSA, transrectal ultrasound (TRUS) (62), and biopsy in selected cases. The positive predictive value of a high PSA measurement (greater than 10 ng/ml) is about 66 percent (111,126,149); the positive predictive value of a low range abnormality (4 to 10 ng/ml) is from 22 to 35 percent. In a recent study, 22 percent of men with total serum PSA values of 2.6 to 4.0 ng/ml had prostatic carcinoma using a sextant biopsy approach (117). An elevation in the total serum PSA level, especially in the relatively low range (4 to 10 ng/ml), is sometimes unrelated to carcinoma but rather the result of benign processes, such as hyperplasia and prostatitis.

In order to improve the sensitivity and specificity of PSA for detecting carcinoma, a variety of other PSA indices have been developed, including age-specific PSA tables (see Table 2-2, page 34), PSA density which takes into account total serum PSA and prostatic volume, PSA velocity in which serum PSA values are measured over time, and the percentage of free (nonbound) serum PSA relative to the total serum PSA pool (108,115, 115a,150,164). These approaches can improve diagnostic sensitivity and specificity so that they exceed that of total PSA alone and, as a result, can eliminate many of the potentially negative prostate biopsies.

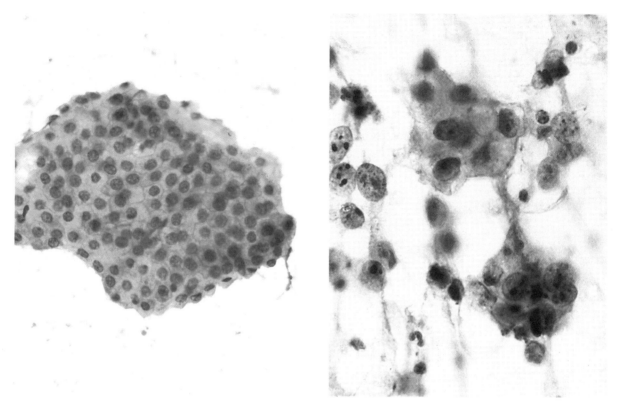

Figure 4-2
PROSTATIC CYTOLOGY SPECIMENS OBTAINED BY FRANZEN'S TECHNIQUE
Left: Benign glandular tissue. Note the uniform honeycomb appearance and regular round nuclei.
Right: Prostatic adenocarcinoma. Note the irregular clusters and individual cells showing nuclear membrane irregularity, parachromatin clearing, and prominent nucleoli. Occasional nuclei have multiple nucleoli.

In most patients with an abnormal PSA measurement there is no palpable tumor on DRE. On TRUS, areas of hypoechogenicity may be detected, but in some cases no abnormalities are seen (120,123,129,145). Directed biopsies of abnormal areas can be obtained, and, if no abnormalities are detected, multiple areas are systematically biopsied (134,135,160). Commonly, a sextant approach is undertaken: biopsies from the basal, mid, and apical portions of the gland, with or without the transition zone, are taken on both sides (132,160).

Whether investigating a clinically abnormal nodule or taking biopsies in the context of an elevated PSA measurement or hypoechogenic area on TRUS, a variety of biopsy methodologies may be used (124). Fine needle aspiration biopsy was popular in Europe and to some degree in North America until the advent of the spring-loaded thin core biopsy gun (139,143,159) and is still used

to some extent (171). Using a Franzen's needle guide, a needle is passed through the rectal wall into the prostate gland where numerous passes are needed to produce a cytology sample (fig. 4-2). The fine needle aspiration procedure has been largely replaced by the biopsy gun approach. The latter is a spring-loaded device, usually coupled with an 18-gauge needle, to obtain a biopsy core measuring 15 to 20 mm in length (124,139). The procedure can be done with or without ultrasound guidance and allows the urologist or radiologist to obtain a small sample, suitable for histology. There is minimal crushing of the tissues with resultant good histology. Also, the procedure is well tolerated by the patients, and complications are minimal to absent (122). The chief disadvantage is the lesser volume of tissue sampled which, to some extent, is overcome by obtaining multiple biopsies. Thin core needle biopsies can be performed in the office or

115

on an outpatient basis, and they do not require the anesthesia needed for larger core needle biopsies (122). Furthermore, the transperineal needle route can also be used, an approach associated with a very low rate of biopsy track-related soft tissue seeding of cancer (106). The biopsy gun procedure has largely supplanted large core needle biopsy devices such as Vim-Silverman, Tru-cut, and Hutchins (168). These latter devices often utilize 14-gauge needles and, although they yield more tissue, are associated with more complications including bleeding and infection (124).

CLINICAL STAGING

In order to deal with the diverse modes of presentation of prostate cancer and variations in the extent of local disease and prognosis, a number of staging systems have been devised. The system of Whitmore was one of the earliest and is the basis for the popular system still used in some institutions in North America (170). The Whitmore system separates prostate cancer into four groups: stage A, carcinoma is clinically unsuspected and disease is detected in tissue removed for the treatment of prostatic hyperplasia; stage B, clinically palpable tumor is judged to be confined to the gland; stage C, carcinoma is locally advanced with spread beyond the gland to involve the surrounding soft tissues, seminal vesicles, or rectal wall or bladder; stage D, tumor is metastatic to either lymph nodes or bone. This system was subsequently modified by Jewett to include subdivisions within each category as outlined in Table 4-2 (110,137).

The TNM system is also widely used for the stratification of prostatic carcinoma (156,159a) and is the recommended one, as consistent use of a standard system allows for easier scientific comparison of data across institutions throughout the world. The current revision of the TNM system (1997) is shown in Table 4-3 (159a), divided into clinical and pathologic stages. Each of the major clinical TNM categories will be briefly described. The corresponding Whitmore-Jewett stages, where applicable, are included in parenthesis.

Stage T1 (A). This category is for tumor that is an incidental histologic finding in tissue removed for other reasons, usually the treatment of prostatic hyperplasia and, strictly speaking, is not a

Table 4-2

MODIFIED WHITMORE-JEWETT STAGING SYSTEM FOR PROSTATE CANCER

A Clinically unsuspected (incidental)
A1 Focal microscopic tumor
A1 Diffuse microscopic tumor

B Confined to prostate
B1 Clinically palpable tumor involving one lobe
B2 Clinically palpable tumor involving more than one lobe

C Localized to periprostatic region
C1 No involvement of seminal vesicle; <70 g
C2 Involvement of seminal vesicle; >70 g

D Metastatic disease
D1 Regional lymph nodes
D2 Distant metastases

"clinical" stage. The T1a (A1) designation is used for tumors that occupy less than 5 percent of the surface area of the specimen, and the T1b (A2) designation applies to those tumors that occupy more than 5 percent of the surface area (fig. 4-3). (Prior methods of counting the number of involved chips are no longer recommended because of the problem caused by the representation of a single focus of tumor in multiple chips [125] and their lack of applicability to incidentally detected tumors in simple prostatectomy specimens.) Some authors have attempted to estimate tumor volume in transurethral resectates by measuring the diameter of carcinomatous foci. In this system, 1 cm^3 is used as a cut-off point to distinguish T1a and T1b disease (109,125,127).

Stage T1c is reserved for those cases identified on needle biopsies in the course of investigating an elevated PSA measurement, without a suspicious nodule by either DRE or TRUS.

Stage T2 (B). A stage T2 tumor is one that presents as a nodule on DRE or TRUS and appears to be organ confined. If the nodule involves only one side of the gland it is classified as T2a (fig. 4-4A). A T2b tumor involves both sides (fig. 4-4B,C).

Stage T3 (C). A stage T3 tumor involves adjacent structures such as periprostatic fat or seminal vesicles. A T3a designation is used when there is extraprostatic extension without seminal vesicle

Table 4-3

1997 TNM STAGING (CLINICAL AND PATHOLOGIC) OF PROSTATIC ADENOCARCINOMA*

Primary Tumor, Clinical (T)

TX   Primary tumor cannot be assessed
T0   No evidence of primary tumor
T1   Clinically inapparent tumor not palpable nor visible by imaging
    T1a   Tumor incidental histologic finding in 5% or less of tissue resected
    T1b   Tumor incidental histologic finding in more than 5% of tissue resected
    T1c   Tumor identified by needle biopsy (e.g., because of elevated PSA)
T2**   Tumor confined within prostate
    T2a   Tumor involves one lobe
    T2b   Tumor involves both lobes
T3   Tumor extends through the prostatic capsule
    T3a   Extracapsular extension (unilateral or bilateral)
    T3b   Tumor invades seminal vesicle(s)
T4   Tumor is fixed or invades adjacent structures other than seminal vesicles: bladder neck, external sphincter, rectum, levator muscles, and /or pelvic wall

Primary Tumor, Pathologic (pT)†

pT2‡   Organ confined
    pT2a One lobe involved
    pT2b Both lobes involved
pT3   Extraprostatic extension
    pT3a Extraprostatic extension¶
    pT3b Seminal vesicle invasion
pT4   Invasion of bladder, rectum

Regional Lymph Nodes (N)

NX   Regional lymph nodes cannot be assessed
N0   No regional lymph node metastasis
N1   Metastasis in regional lymph node or nodes

Distant Metastasis (M)§

MX   Distant metastasis cannot be assessed
M0   No distant metastasis
M1   Distant metastasis
    M1a   Nonregional lymph node(s)
    M1b   Bone(s)
    M1c   Other sites

Stage Grouping

Stage I	T1a	N0	M0 G1
Stage II	T1a	N0	M0 G2,3-4
	T1b	N0	M0 any G
	T1c	N0	M0 any G
	T1	N0	M0 any G
	T2	N0	M0 any G
Stage III	T3	N0	M0 any G
Stage IV	T4	N0	M0 any G
	any T	N1	M0 any G
	any T	any N	M1 any G

Grading

G1 - well differentiated; Gleason score 2-4
G2 - moderately differentiated; Gleason score 5-6
G3 - moderate to poorly differentiated; Gleason score 7
G4 - poorly differentiated; Gleason score 8-10

---

*From Sobin LH, Wittekind C, eds. TNM classification of malignant tumors. 5th ed. New York: Wiley-Liss, 1997:170–3.

**Tumor found in one or both lobes by needle biopsy, but not palpable or reliably visible by imaging is classified as T1c.

†No pT1 category exists because of insufficient tissue to permit a true pathologic staging of these cases.

‡Invasion into the prostatic apex or into (but not beyond) the prostatic capsule is classified as T2, not as T3.

§When more than one site of metastasis is present, the most advanced category is used. PM1c is most advanced.

¶Authors' footnote: extraprostatic extension (pT3a) generally refers to tumor beyond the capsule into periprostatic soft tissue (see page 179).

---

invasion, and T3b is used when at least one seminal vesicle is involved.

Stage T4 (C). Stage T4 applies to situations in which there is locally advanced tumor and corresponds to a subset of stage C2 in the Whitmore-Jewett system. Stage T4 is used when there is involvement of adjacent structures other than seminal vesicle. These include bladder neck, external sphincter, rectum, levator muscles, and pelvic wall.

Nodal Involvement (N). The N category is used to define the extent of regional lymph node involvement. NX is used when the regional nodes cannot be assessed; N0 indicates no involvement of the regional nodes; and N1 indicates involvement of a regional node or nodes.

Distant Metastasis (M). The M category refers to metastases beyond the regional lymph nodes. MX is used when the presence of distant metastases cannot be assessed; M0 indicates no

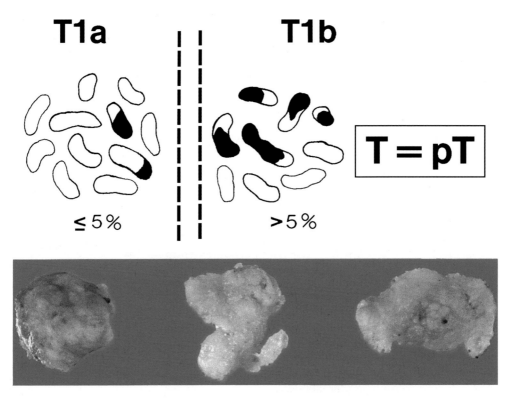

Figure 4-3
ADENOCARCINOMA IN PROSTATIC CHIPS
Top: This is a diagram of prostatic chips with T1a and T1b disease. In T1a cases, 5 percent or less of the tissue is involved. In T1b disease greater than 5 percent of the tissue is involved. (Fig. 348 from Hermanek P, Hutter RV, Sobin LH, Wagner G, Wittekind C. TNM atlas, 4th ed. Berlin: Springer-Verlag, 1997:274.)
Bottom: Carcinomatous areas are represented by irregular tan-yellow regions. (Fig. 1.23 from Ro JY, Grignon DJ, Amin MB, Ayala A. Atlas of surgical pathology of the male reproductive tract. Philadelphia: WB Saunders Co., 1997:11.)

distant metastases; M1a is nonregional lymph node involvement; M1b, bone; and M1c, other sites.

Stage Distribution at Presentation. The historical distribution of prostate cancer cases classified by stage is shown in Table 4-4 (155). Approximately 10 percent of patients had distant metastases (M+; D2) at the time of initial presentation. A further 50 percent had either locally advanced disease or regional lymph node involvement (T3,4 N0 M0 or T1-4 N1 M0; C,D1). Thirty percent of patients had clinically localized tumors that were amenable to therapy. The remaining 10 percent had incidental and microscopically focal disease (T1a).

In recent years, this stage distribution has changed (so-called stage migration) due, in part, to the advent of newer technologies for the early detection of prostate cancer including PSA assays, TRUS, and biopsy guns which obtain tissue samples with relative ease in the office practice setting. Early stage disease (T1-2) now represents a greater proportion of cases than previously (146, 151). In four large series of prostate cancer patients treated by radical prostatectomy from the early 1980s to the early 1990s, 37 to 64 percent of the tumors were organ confined, 25 to 48 percent extended extraprostatically, 7 to 17 percent involved the seminal vesicles, and 2 to 7 percent had metastasized to lymph nodes (116,150a,151,171a).

PATHOLOGIC FEATURES

The general pathologic aspects of prostatic adenocarcinoma including topographic, volumetric, gross, microscopic, and histologic grading are presented in this section. The specific guidelines for the handling and reporting of needle biopsies, transurethral resectates, and simple and radical

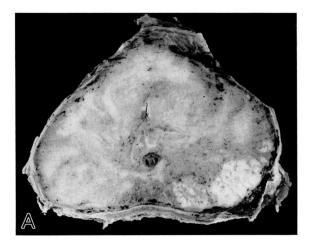

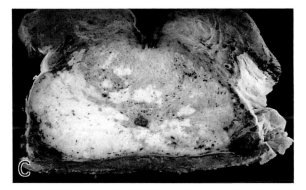

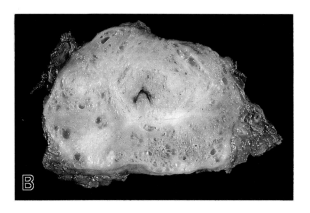

Figure 4-4
PROSTATE WITH ADENOCARCINOMA

A: Stage T2a adenocarcinoma. Note the poorly defined white area in the peripheral zone on the right side. (Fig. 3 from Fascicle 31B and 32, 1st Series.)

B: Stage T2b adenocarcinoma. The gland has been sectioned at the level of the verumontanum and shows three distinct foci of cancer, one in the transition zone and two in the peripheral zone. The dominant nodule (left posterior) abuts the capsule but does not involve it.

C: Stage T2b adenocarcinoma. The tumor is centered in the left peripheral zone but has spread to the right side and to the transition zone. There is "capsular invasion" on the left but there is no spread beyond the capsule (extraprostatic extension) and therefore this is still stage T2b. (Fig. 4 from Moore RA. A textbook of pathology. Philadelphia: W.B. Saunders Co., 1944:1157).

Table 4-4

PROSTATE CANCER: HISTORICAL STAGE DISTRIBUTION WITH PROGNOSIS, SURVIVAL RATE, AND CURE RATE*

Stage	Patients (%)	Prognosis	10-Year Cancer-Specific Survival Rate (%)	Estimated Cure Rate (%)
T1a (A1)	10	Treatment often "unnecessary"	95	85
T1b-T2 (A2-B2)	30	Often curable	80	65
T3-T4 (C1-2)	10	Occasionally curable	60	25
N+ (D1)	40	Rarely curable	40	<5
M+ (D2)	10	Incurable	10	<1
All stages	100		51	32
Excluding T1a			45	25

*Modified from reference 155.

prostatectomy specimens will not be reviewed in detail, although we do feel it is appropriate to discuss some issues regarding the handling of the radical prostatectomy specimen. Readers are referred to recent publications from the College of American Pathologists and the Association of Directors of Anatomic and Surgical Pathology for comprehensive recommendations (179,292,385a).

Several publications concerning the gross examination of radical prostatectomy specimens are available, and the interested reader should consult them for more detailed information

(203a,244,373,398a). The goal of the pathologic examination is to provide the necessary information to guide future therapy and assess the prognosis. Important features include the histologic type; Gleason score; the pathologic stage which includes assessment of extraprostatic extension, seminal vesicle status, and lymph node status; the status of the surgical margins and the amount (volume) of tumor in the gland; and status of vascular invasion.

Upon receipt in the laboratory, the prostate gland should be measured in three dimensions and weighed. The entire external surface should then be inked, and some may prefer to use different colors to assist with the orientation. The inked gland can then be briefly immersed in Bouin's solution which acts as a mordant to prevent the spread of the ink. We then prefer to immerse the inked gland in a generous volume of 10 percent formalin overnight, although some pathologists section the gland at this point. Following fixation, amputate the apex first, and section the rest of the prostate serially at 3 mm intervals in the anterior-posterior plane, perpendicular to the urethra. For those using the whole mount method, the sections are typically thicker, 4 to 5 mm, and the individual slices may require additional fixation.

The cut surfaces should then be closely inspected for the features of tumor as described on page 122. We recommend that the apical slice be sectioned in a radial fashion or in the sagittal/parasagittal plane and entirely submitted. Sagittal sections of the base are obtained to evaluate the bladder neck margin. Sections of the right and left seminal vesicles should be submitted at the point of insertion of the seminal vesicle into the prostate, to include a portion of the contiguous prostate.

It remains controversial how much of the prostate gland should be submitted for histologic examination (229a,303). Obviously, the more sections that are submitted, the more likely that microscopically positive margins or focal extraprostatic extension will be identified. Hall et al. (282) found that a high percentage of positive margins and extraprostatic extension could be detected by a method that submits less than all of the gland. For clinical stage T1 cases, all of any gross lesion should be submitted in addition to the apical and bladder neck margins, seminal vesicle sections, a slice adjacent to the apical margin, and alternate grossly normal complete cross

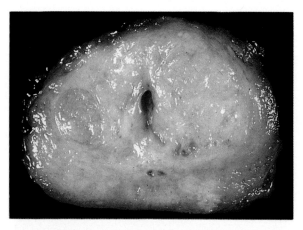

Figure 4-5
PROSTATE WITH ADENOCARCINOMA
A transverse section shows a small carcinoma with a yellow cut surface and ill-defined irregular border in the peripheral zone (lower right). Note the nodular hyperplasia of the transition zone surrounding the prostatic urethra.

sections. For clinical stage T2 lesions in which tumor is grossly apparent, all of the gross lesion should be submitted in addition to the routine margins, seminal vesicle sections, and a complete section adjacent to the apical margin; if no gross lesion is detected, alternate posterior slices should be submitted plus the other sections as detailed for gross lesions. With this approach, 95 percent of positive margins and 90 percent of the cases with extraprostatic extension are identified. The tumor volume can be given as a percentage of the examined prostate gland involved by tumor.

Tumor Location

Historically, it was thought that most prostatic adenocarcinomas arose in what is now referred to as the peripheral zone of the prostate gland, usually in the posterior and lateral regions (fig 4-5). Periurethral adenocarcinomas were restricted to the uncommon ductal variants or to tumors that represented central extension of neoplasms arising peripherally (fig. 4-6). The detailed anatomic studies of McNeal indicate that while most (70 to 75 percent) adenocarcinomas do arise in the peripheral zone, a significant minority (15 to 20 percent) originate in the transition zone (fig. 4-7) and about 10 percent are thought to arise in the central zone (329,330,334). In large tumors it is often difficult to establish the precise epicenter

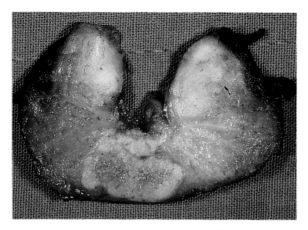

Figure 4-6
PROSTATE WITH ADENOCARCINOMA
A transverse section of a gland opened anteriorly along a prostatic urethra that had been widened by a previous transurethral curettage shows secondary involvement of the urethra by a large yellow carcinoma of peripheral zone origin. The remaining transition zone on each side is also involved by tumor.

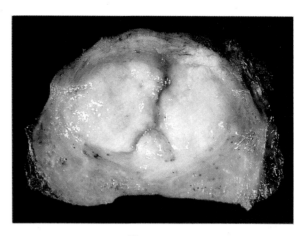

Figure 4-7
PROSTATE WITH ADENOCARCINOMA
The carcinoma is represented by the yellow tissue in the transition zone on the right side and has spread anteriorly. It contrasts with the tan-white tissue of the remaining transition zone involved by nodular hyperplasia. Note that the peripheral zone (bottom) is not involved by hyperplasia or carcinoma.

since several zones may be involved, and many cases display separate tumors in peripheral and transitional zones (fig. 4-8).

In general, tumors arising in the transition zone tend to be relatively low-volume and low-grade neoplasms while those occurring in the peripheral zone are usually of intermediate to high grade and display a wide range of tumor volumes (280,326). Duct adenocarcinomas (see chapter 5) often involve the verumontanum and large primary periurethral ducts (203,237). Extension into the deeper duct-acinar system is common, and these duct carcinomas are often associated with an acinar component in the peripheral zone (see chapter 5).

Tumor Focality

Multifocal adenocarcinoma is found in at least 50 percent of radical prostatectomy specimens (342,401,402). In most cases the additional tumors are small, many with a volume of less than 0.5 cm^3 (336), but some are easily appreciable and occasionally bulky on gross examination (figs. 4-4B, 4-6). Multiple carcinomas may be of either peripheral or transition zone origin, and sometimes both regions harbor carcinomas (fig. 4-8) (173,402). The apical region is a common location for second small carcinomas.

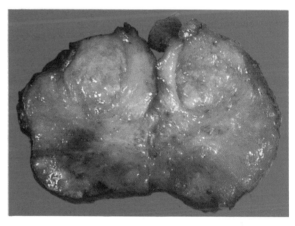

Figure 4-8
PROSTATE WITH ADENOCARCINOMA
There are multiple tan-yellow nodules of carcinoma in the peripheral and transition zones. (Courtesy of Dr. P. Troncoso, Houston, TX.)

Tumor Volume

Studies of McNeal and others have suggested that volume is an important predictor of outcome. The volume of a given tumor correlates with grade, extraprostatic extension, margin involvement, seminal vesicle invasion, regional lymph node status, recurrence rate, and survival (196,225,253, 308,326,332,333,338,387,389). Most prostatic adenocarcinomas discovered incidentally at autopsy are small lesions less than 1 cm^3 in volume (332). In one study of incidental carcinomas detected at cystoprostatectomy (thought to be likely similar to incidental tumors detected at autopsy), the median volume was 0.04 cm^3 (353). In contrast, most tumors that present clinically are greater than 0.5 cm^3 and some are larger than 5 cm^3. Tumors greater than 5 cm^3 have a high rate of seminal vesicle involvement and metastatic disease. In the PSA screening era, the mean volume of T1c (PSA detected) carcinomas is about 1.7 cm^3 (300). The importance of volume has led some investigators to propose a volume-based prognostic index (201).

Tumor volume cannot be prospectively measured with accuracy using current clinical or radiographic technology. At best, only rough estimates can be obtained in some cases. In pathologic material, tumor volume is measured by computer assisted image analysis of prostatectomy slices (332,333,389). The tumor areas in each slice are integrated and a total volume determined. These studies have indicated that the three-dimensional configuration of prostatic tumors is often quite irregular, with small tongues of tumor spreading along susceptible pathways such as perineural spaces and ejaculatory ducts (221). Detailed volumetric studies are quite time consuming and complex and not feasible for most laboratories. A grid-counting method has been developed by Humphrey (302) to measure intraglandular tumor extent, which is a surrogate for tumor volume. The number of grid squares containing tumor over the total number of squares containing prostatic tissue is expressed as a percentage which can be multiplied by the weight of the gland to estimate volume. Some authors have suggested that once the status of extraprostatic extension, grade, and margin involvement is known in radical prostatectomy specimens, the tumor volume is not additive in predicting prognosis and have questioned the need for including accurate tumor volume measurements (201a, 248). General estimates of percentage of surface area involved by tumor can easily be given by pathologists and thus is recommended in reporting results from needle biopsies, transurethral resectates, and prostatectomy specimens. These measures correlate well enough with more sophisticated methods to suffice for routine practice at this time (216,252,321,359).

Gross Findings

Tiny carcinomas are impossible to recognize grossly in transurethral resectates, but in cases with more abundant disease, the chips are often firmer and yellow or orange-yellow (fig. 4-3, bottom) compared to the tan-brown, more often spongy appearance of chips involved by nodular hyperplasia. In general, gross examination of chips has little practical role (303,343), particularly as benign processes such as granulomatous prostatitis may mimic carcinoma grossly (see page 310).

Adenocarcinoma can sometimes be identified grossly in radical prostatectomy specimens. In a consecutive prospective study, carcinoma was diagnosable accurately in 63 percent of cases, and no gross lesion was apparent in 22 percent of cases; the false positive rate for gross inspection was 19 percent (364). Those tumors that were grossly apparent were typically of higher stage, higher grade, and larger diameter than grossly subtle tumors. Ninety-two percent of T3 tumors, 81 percent of Gleason score 8 or higher tumors, and 72 percent of tumors with a diameter of 1 cm or more were grossly apparent (364). In another recent series carcinoma was correctly identified grossly in a similar number of cases to the above study, 65 percent (262a). In marked contrast, in a series from the older literature carcinoma was only suspected grossly in 1 of 23 occult carcinomas found at autopsy (185). In general, lesions under 5 mm in size are not grossly detectable (236a). Multifocal involvement is grossly apparent in 10 to 20 percent of the cases (236a).

On transverse sections the abnormal areas are usually posterior or posterolateral, frequently adjacent to the capsule, and are solid and smooth compared to the more often spongy or cystic appearance of adjacent benign tissue (figs. 4-4–4-9). Some may have a granular quality. An asymmetric appearance or displacement of the fibromuscular band separating the periurethral and peripheral prostate tissue are subtle signs of the cancer (282). The tumor is often firmer on palpation than the surrounding benign tissue, but subtle lesions even lack this feature. The color typically differs from the usual light tan appearance of adjacent benign tissue; many carcinomas are yellow or yellow-orange (due to intracytoplasmic lipid, see page 124), and others white to gray (figs. 4-4–4-9). Those that are white

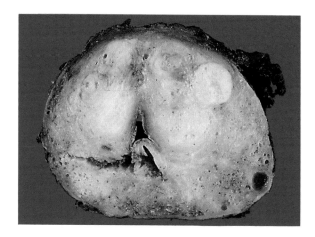 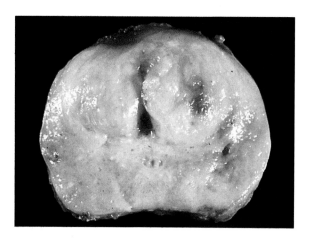

Figure 4-9
PROSTATE WITH ADENOCARCINOMA
Left: The tumor largely replaces the transition zone and is characterized by well-defined white nodules.
Right: The tumor is represented by a much more subtle, ill-defined, gray-tan area in the peripheral zone (right lower corner).
The transition zone shows typical benign nodular hyperplasia with compromise of the urethral lumen.

to gray may be mimicked by benign lesions such as healed infarcts, leiomyomatous hyperplasia, and atrophy, and yellow neoplasms may be mimicked by infectious processes including tuberculosis (310). In many cases, especially in clinical stage T1 disease, tumor is not identified grossly. The borders of the tumor are often indistinct, and microscopic examination nearly always reveals more tumor than suspected grossly.

Tumors located anteriorly are often difficult to see because of admixed stromal tissue. Large bilateral tumors may be overlooked because of their homogeneous appearance. Involvement of adjacent structures may be recognized, particularly when involvement is extensive; extraprostatic extension is grossly identifiable most commonly in the region of the junction of the seminal vesicles with the prostate (364). Positive margins and extraprostatic extension were evaluated successfully by gross examination in over 80 percent of the cases in one study (282) but were seen in only about 50 percent of the cases in another (364). The gross assessment of apical involvement, including the apical margins, is especially difficult (282). In contrast to many other types of carcinoma, hemorrhage and necrosis are rare both grossly and microscopically in prostatic carcinoma.

Microscopic Findings

Whole mount sections of the prostate gland are beneficial for academic interest and for re-

search purposes in showing the location of prostatic carcinoma in relation to the urethra and its zonal distribution (fig. 4-10), but they are not necessary in routine practice.

The accurate diagnosis of prostatic adenocarcinoma involves familiarity with its protean patterns and identification, in most cases, of features indicative of invasion and also abnormal cellular features, especially those related to the nucleus (Table 4-5). The diagnosis is usually made, or at least strongly suspected, at scanning magnification because of an abnormal arrangement of epithelial units (fig. 4-11), indicating infiltration, which is inconsistent with hyperplasia, atrophy, or the diverse other mimics of carcinoma (see chapter 7). However, judging whether a given process is truly infiltrative or "pseudoinfiltrative," as may be seen in atrophy, is not always easy and cytologic aspects are crucial in cases which are equivocal on architectural grounds.

Supportive cytoplasmic and luminal features also play a role (figs. 4-11C, 4-12A,B) and are also often noted on low-power magnification; however, they are never definitive on their own. Easily appreciable, to abundant, cytoplasm that is usually pale to clear or amphophilic is a feature of the majority of tumors, except some moderately differentiated tumors (see page 129) and many of those that are poorly differentiated, and may contrast with the staining properties of the cytoplasm of benign acini. Benign acini, particularly

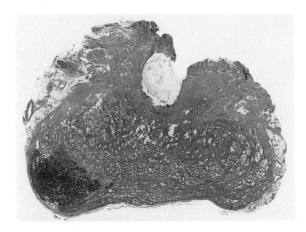

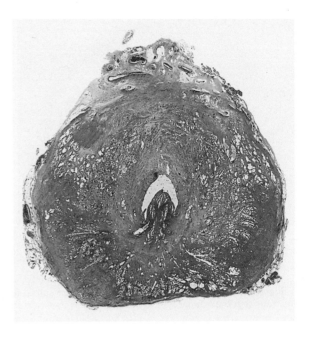

Figure 4-10
PROSTATE WITH ADENOCARCINOMA:
WHOLE MOUNT SECTIONS
Above: The peripheral zone on the left is involved by carcinoma in one discrete area.
Right: There is extensive multifocal carcinoma involving the peripheral zone.

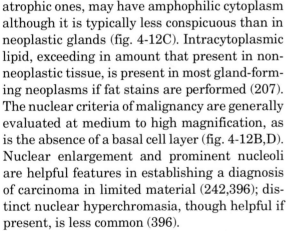

atrophic ones, may have amphophilic cytoplasm although it is typically less conspicuous than in neoplastic glands (fig. 4-12C). Intracytoplasmic lipid, exceeding in amount that present in non-neoplastic tissue, is present in most gland-forming neoplasms if fat stains are performed (207). The nuclear criteria of malignancy are generally evaluated at medium to high magnification, as is the absence of a basal cell layer (fig. 4-12B,D). Nuclear enlargement and prominent nucleoli are helpful features in establishing a diagnosis of carcinoma in limited material (242,396); distinct nuclear hyperchromasia, though helpful if present, is less common (396).

A variety of other microscopic features play varyingly important roles in the establishment of the diagnosis of cancer as detailed in subsequent sections, one of the most important being circumferential perineural invasion (fig. 4-13A). The absence of basal cells in cases of carcinoma can often be assessed in routine light microscopic sections but may be further evaluated by the use of an immunohistochemical stain for high molecular weight cytokeratin (fig. 4-13B). In general, stromal alterations play a minimal role in the diagnosis of carcinoma, particularly compared to certain other cancers. Desmoplasia is sometimes seen, particularly in prostatectomy specimens (fig. 4-13C), but the biopsy diagnosis is rarely

facilitated by this finding. Within the spectrum of conventional prostatic adenocarcinomas, there are a number of common patterns as well as several unusual ones. The various histologic patterns may be pure or mixed. The morphology of "latent" prostate cancers is usually that of well or moderately differentiated adenocarcinoma (Gleason grades 1, 2, and 3) of conventional type (188,212,239,260,261,296,365), and only exceptionally is a higher grade.

Histopathology of Adenocarcinoma According to the Gleason System of Pattern-Based Grading

The common patterns of prostatic adenocarcinoma are best described by referring to the now classic Gleason grading diagram (figs. 4-14, 4-15) (272, 273). The rarest pattern (Gleason grade 1) consists of a tightly packed collection of small to medium-sized acini, with relatively little variation in size and shape (fig. 4-15A, 4-16). It is generally agreed that it can only rarely, if ever, be diagnosed in thin core needle biopsy specimens, and we have not done so ourselves. This is because the caliber of the needle core does not generally enable all the edges of the nodule to be seen. The neoplastic focus has a smooth, rounded, "pushing" border; there is an abrupt transition between the abnormal focus and adjacent prostatic

Table 4-5

CHECKLIST OF FEATURES RELEVANT TO THE DIAGNOSIS OF PROSTATE CANCER

I. Architecture (usually assessed at low to intermediate power)
    Abnormal architecture
        Small closely packed glands
        Relatively uniform glands
        Glands differing in appearance from surrounding glands
        Glomeruloid structures
        Periglandular clefts
    Features indicative of invasion
        Small glands infiltrating between clearly benign glands
        Confluent glands, cords, single cells
        Splitting of muscle fibers
        Perineural (preferably circumferential) or intraneural invasion
        Extraprostatic spread, e.g., tumor in fat
        Glands unequivocally in vascular spaces

II. Absence of basal cell layer around problematic glands

III. Cytology (usually assessed at intermediate to high power)
    Nuclei (compare to benign glands in biopsy)
        Nucleomegaly
        Hyperchromasia
        Nuclear membrane irregularity
        Parachromatin clearing
        Mitotic figures
        Nucleoli
            Prominent (usually cherry red to purple)
            Multiple
            Eccentric

IV. Cytoplasm
        Tinctorially different from adjacent clearly benign glands
        Amphophilic cytoplasm
        Excessive clear or pale cytoplasm

V. Intraluminal contents
        Wispy blue mucin
        Flocculent pink granular material
        Crystalloids
        Necrosis

VI. Ancillary (or supportive) features
        Collagenous micronodules (may be luminal or juxtaluminal)
        High-grade prostatic intraepithelial neoplasia elsewhere in specimen
        Lack of high molecular weight cytokeratin around atypical glands

stroma. There is very little stroma separating individual glands in the acinar proliferation. The acini are of relatively uniform size, with "sharp" luminal edges. Some glands may contain geometric-shaped, eosinophilic crystalloids in the lumens (see page 146). The lining cells are usually cuboidal to columnar, uniform, and contain moderate amounts of clear to slightly granular pale cytoplasm. The basal cell layer is absent. The nuclei are slightly enlarged and show some degree of mild atypia, and at least a few nuclei usually contain nucleoli greater than 1.5 μm in diameter (288,312,314). Areas of clearing may be seen within the nuclear chromatin, so-called parachromatin clearing, but this and other cytologic abnormalities are sometimes inconspicuous

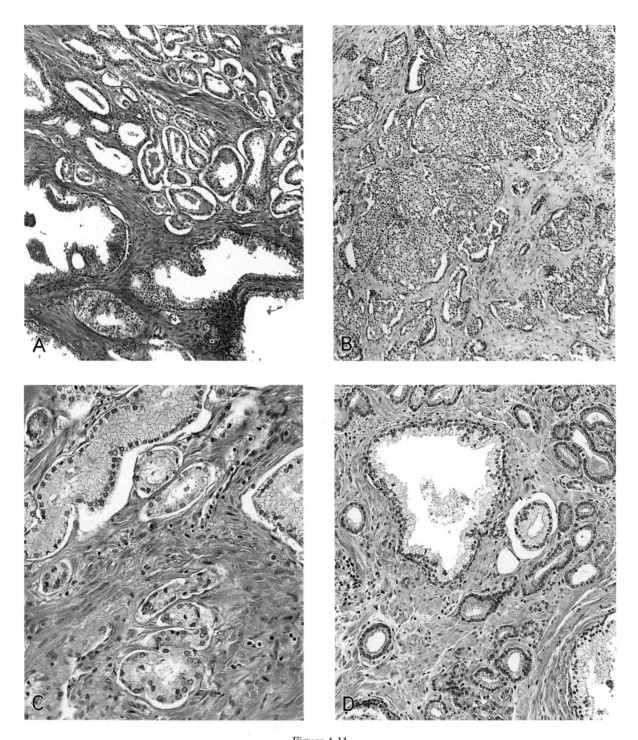

Figure 4-11
PROSTATIC ADENOCARCINOMA: TYPICAL MICROSCOPIC FEATURES (SEE ALSO FACING PAGE)
In A, small, closely packed, relatively uniform glands of invasive cancer (upper half) contrast with the larger noninvasive prostatic glands (bottom) which exhibit prostatic intraepithelial neoplasia. In B, there is prominent fusion of epithelial units corresponding to Gleason grade 4A adenocarcinoma. In C, several of the acini contain wispy, lightly basophilic mucin which is a clue to their neoplastic nature. In D, neoplastic glands with the typical size of many Gleason grade 3 adenocarcinomas encircle a non-neoplastic gland that retains a basal cell layer. Basal cells are not present in the neoplastic acini. Some of the neoplastic acini in A, C, and D are surrounded by clefts separating them from the adjacent stroma, a feature more typical of neoplastic than non-neoplastic acini.

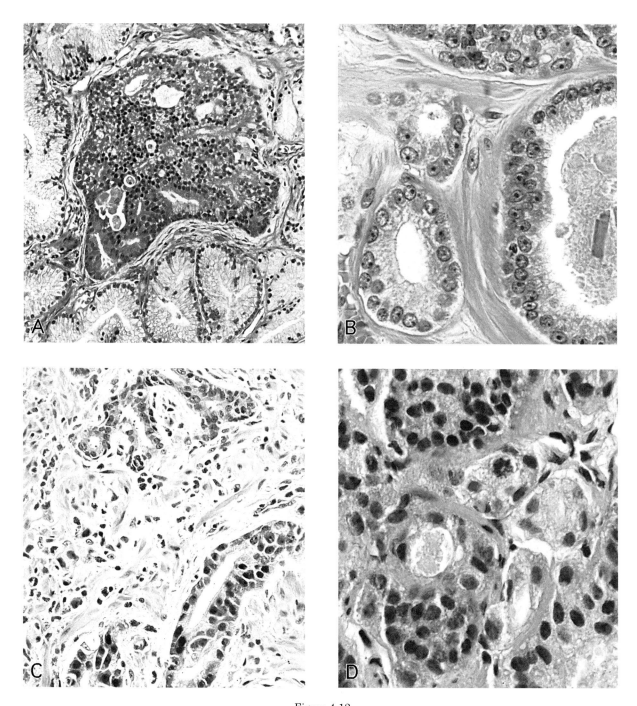

Figure 4-12
PROSTATIC ADENOCARCINOMA: TYPICAL MICROSCOPIC FEATURES (SEE ALSO FACING PAGE)

In A, some neoplastic acini have columnar cells with abundant clear cytoplasm whereas in other cells there is striking amphophilic cytoplasm. In B, the neoplastic acini show nuclear irregularity and, most importantly, strikingly enlarged nucleoli. Additionally, at the right there is a rod-shaped eosinophilic crystalloid which, although not diagnostic of carcinoma, is seen more often in neoplastic glands. In C, an important feature of many cases of prostatic carcinoma, namely the contrasting cytologic features of benign and neoplastic acini, is evident. A cluster of atrophic acini is seen at the top and a few neoplastic acini at the bottom. In the atrophic acini the cells have amphophilic cytoplasm, a finding that is overall more characteristic of neoplastic acini and is seen in the neoplastic acini in this case. Note that nucleoli are visible in the nuclei of some cells in the atrophic focus but are much less conspicuous than those in the neoplastic acini. Several of the nuclei in the neoplastic acini are hyperchromatic and somewhat "smudged," and there is also some degree of nuclear irregularity. In D, nucleoli are less prominent than in B and C, but there is unequivocal nuclear atypia and a mitotic figure.

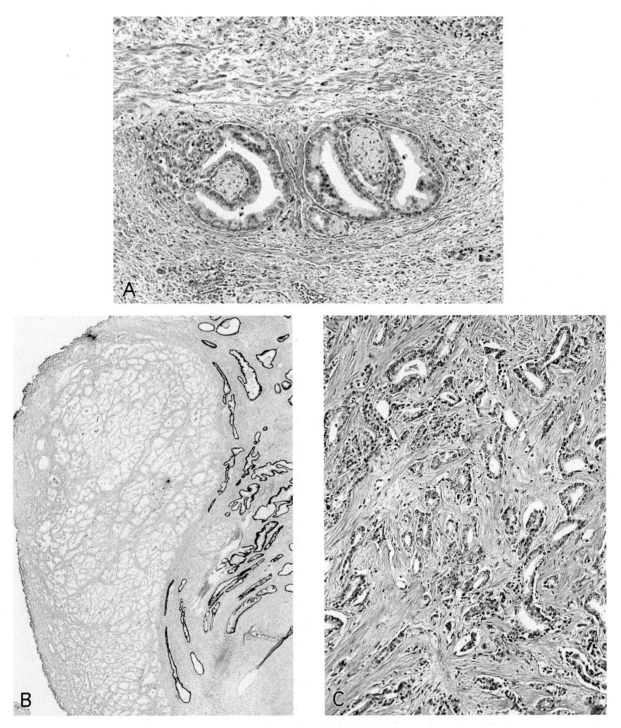

Figure 4-13
PROSTATIC ADENOCARCINOMA

A: Two nerves are completely surrounded by small acini, a finding diagnostic of carcinoma, an interpretation made particularly easy in this case because of the obvious cytologic features of carcinoma with prominent nucleoli visible even at this magnification.

B: A nodule of well-differentiated adenocarcinoma is completely devoid of basal cells in an immunostain for high molecular weight cytokeratin (clone 34βE12). This contrasts with the conspicuous investment of basal cells around the non-neoplastic glands on the right.

C: Stromal desmoplasia in a moderately differentiated (Gleason grade 3A) adenocarcinoma. Stromal changes play relatively little role in establishing the diagnosis of carcinoma.

PROSTATIC ADENOCARCINOMA
(Histologic Grades)

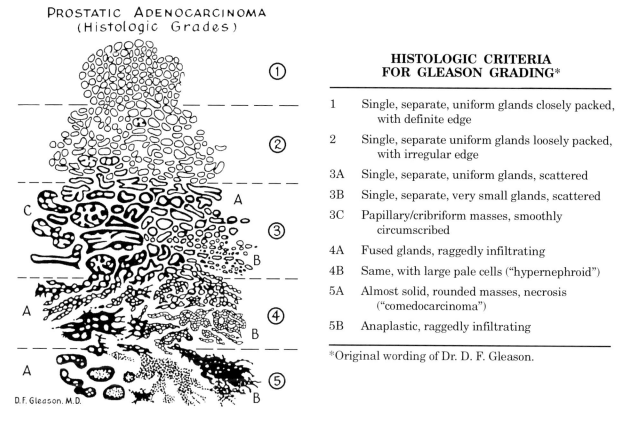

HISTOLOGIC CRITERIA
FOR GLEASON GRADING*

1	Single, separate, uniform glands closely packed, with definite edge
2	Single, separate uniform glands loosely packed, with irregular edge
3A	Single, separate, uniform glands, scattered
3B	Single, separate, very small glands, scattered
3C	Papillary/cribriform masses, smoothly circumscribed
4A	Fused glands, raggedly infiltrating
4B	Same, with large pale cells ("hypernephroid")
5A	Almost solid, rounded masses, necrosis ("comedocarcinoma")
5B	Anaplastic, raggedly infiltrating

*Original wording of Dr. D. F. Gleason.

Figure 4-14
GLEASON GRADING
Left: Histologic grades of prostatic adenocarcinoma as schematically depicted by Dr. D. F. Gleason.
Right: Description of Gleason grades.

in both Gleason grades 1 and 2 neoplasms. The grade 1 pattern of prostatic adenocarcinoma is virtually only seen in transition zone tumors. It is distinguished from atypical adenomatous hyperplasia (adenosis) (see chapter 3), which also occurs at this site, by an absent basal cell layer, more regular acini, and the presence of nuclear abnormalities, including significantly enlarged nucleoli.

There is greater separation of acini that are more variable in size and shape in a Gleason grade 2 carcinoma, which also shows limited infiltration of the adjacent prostatic tissue (figs. 4-15B, 4-17). Distinction between a Gleason grade 1 and 2 carcinoma is often difficult but of no practical significance. Most of these tumors also arise in the transition zone and are typically encountered in transurethral resectates or in prostatectomy specimens.

The carcinomas which constitute Gleason grades 3A (fig. 4-15C) and 3B (fig. 4-15D) show

a greater degree of gland separation than those of Gleason grades 1 and 2, and greater variation in the size and shape of the acini, especially in the 3A pattern (fig. 4-18). The glands are often irregular, angulated, and somewhat elongated or even branching (fig. 4-18C) in 3A cases. The glands may be medium to large and angulated (grade 3A) (see fig. 4-23) and somewhat dilated (fig. 4-19) or small and insidiously infiltrative (Gleason 3B) (fig. 4-20). The glands of 3B cases are smaller than those of Gleason grades 1 and 2 adenocarcinomas. Some 3B tumors have acini lined by cells with relatively scant cytoplasm, making the cells appear "dark." This pattern can be subtle and may simulate patterns of atrophy. These "atrophic" carcinomas (226,241,311), however, have a more infiltrative growth pattern than atrophy, sometimes show perineural invasion, and lack basal cells (see further discussion on page 168). Furthermore, on close inspection,

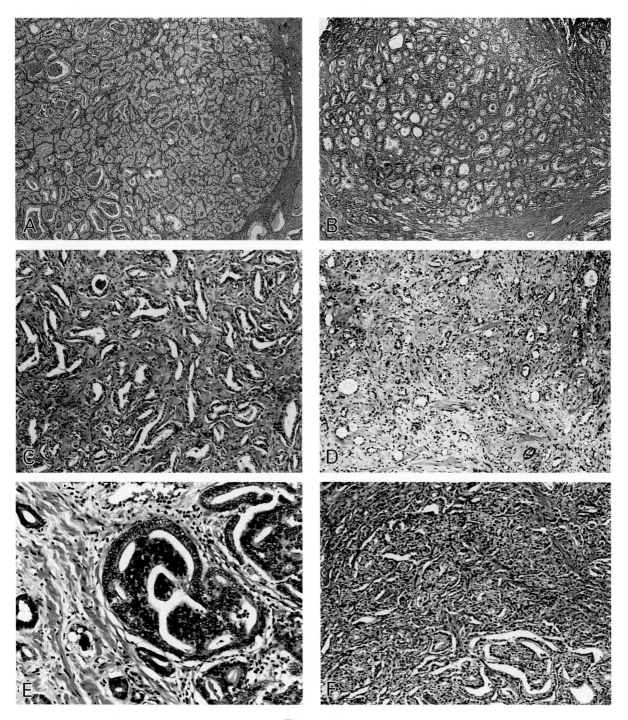

Figure 4-15
PROSTATIC ADENOCARCINOMA: GLEASON PATTERNS

A: Grade 1. Relatively uniform acini with a rounded pushing interface with the stroma.

B: Grade 2. Acini with some size and shape variation in a somewhat circumscribed arrangement. The interface between tumor and the surrounding stroma is more irregular than in grade 1 neoplasms.

C: Grade 3A. Angulated and elongated acini are haphazardly distributed in the stroma.

D: Grade 3B. Microacini have an irregular, infiltrative growth pattern.

E: Grade 3C. A rounded cribriform structure with a sieve-like pattern lacks necrosis. Small individual acini of grade 3B are also present.

F: Grade 4A. Note fused microacini and aggregates with an infiltrative growth pattern.

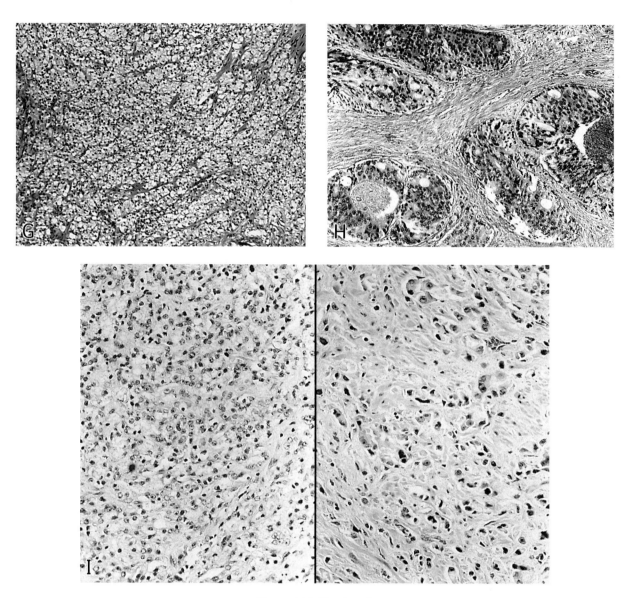

Figure 4-15 (Continued)

G: Grade 4B. Hypernephroid pattern. Note infiltrating nests of cells with abundant clear cytoplasm.

H: Grade 5A. Rounded duct-like structures showing central comedonecrosis.

I: Grade 5B. Solid (left) and cord-like and single cell patterns (right) of infiltrative growth. Glandular differentiation is inconspicuous.

nuclear features of adenocarcinoma are present. Small glands of Gleason grade 3B may be admixed with small nests of cells with inconspicuous lumens. Acinar fusion or the formation of elongated chains of glands or cords indicates a higher Gleason pattern.

An intermingling of neoplastic acini with non-neoplastic ones is an important feature of Gleason grade 3 tumors, in contrast to grades 1 and 2 (fig. 4-21). Occasional grade 3 adenocarcino-

mas are associated with prominent periacinar clefts, presumably due to retraction artifact (fig. 4-22), a feature that we, and others (283) who referred to the phenomenon as a "halo," have observed more often in association with neoplastic than non-neoplastic acini. Some grade 3A adenocarcinomas are associated with generally inconspicuous small papillae protruding into their lumens (fig. 4-23), papillae being more usual in grade 3C carcinomas (see below). Infiltration is

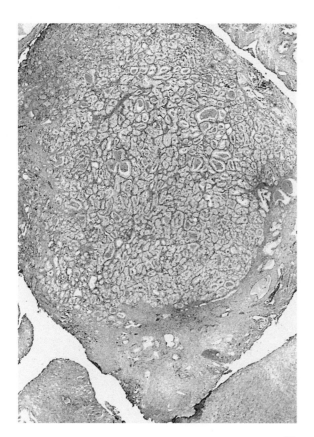 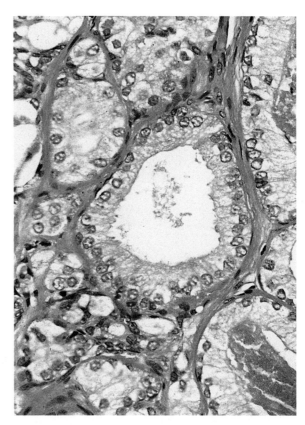

Figure 4-16
PROSTATIC ADENOCARCINOMA, GLEASON GRADE 1

Left: Note the proliferation of closely packed, small to medium-sized acini showing only mild size and shape variation. A smooth pushing interface with the adjacent stroma is noted where the edges of the lesion can be visualized.

Right: The cytologic features of carcinoma are confirmed on high-power microscopy.

usually readily evident in grade 3 carcinomas in transurethral resectates and prostatectomy specimens. Small acini, sometimes widely spaced from each other, are often seen dissecting between and "splitting" the otherwise normal fibromuscular stroma of the gland (fig. 4-24). Infiltration is generally more subtle in needle biopsy specimens but an important feature to look for (see page 168). Desmoplasia is sometimes seen, although uncommon overall in prostate carcinoma, as noted earlier, and is not a feature of Gleason grades 1 and 2 carcinomas.

There is usually a greater degree of cytologic atypia in Gleason grade 3 carcinomas than seen in grades 1 and 2. The individual cells show some variation in size and shape. The cytoplasm is often amphophilic, while in grades 1 and 2 the cytoplasm is usually clear. In some grade 3 tumors it is abundant and foamy (see page 148).

Nuclei also show greater atypia with more prominent enlargement and greater variation in size and shape; nucleoli and parachromatin clearing are usually quite conspicuous (figs. 4-18D, 4-25A,B,C). The nucleoli are often large and may be eccentric. Two, or rarely more, nucleoli may be seen (fig. 4-25D) (see page 168).

In the Gleason scheme, grade 3C (fig. 4-15E) consists of generally rounded, smooth, circumscribed masses of glands with a cribriform or papillary architecture (figs. 4-26, 4-27) (335); necrosis is not present in contrast to grade 5A tumors (see below). Although the "textbook description" is that of rounded, smoothly contoured aggregates with punched out, relatively uniform round glands imparting a sieve-like appearance, some deviation from this is allowable, in our opinion, with linkage of the epithelial aggregates, some of which may be elongated (fig. 4-26B). Although

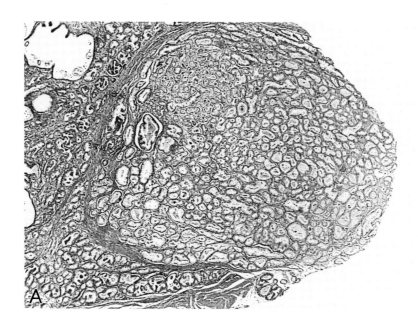

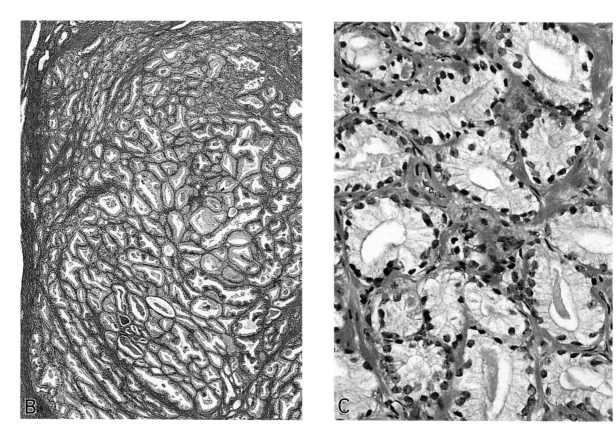

Figure 4-17
PROSTATIC ADENOCARCINOMA, GLEASON GRADE 2
Note the relatively well circumscribed proliferations of small to medium-sized acini with limited stromal invasion in two separate cases (A,B). There is more variation in size and shape of the acini than seen in Gleason grade 1 neoplasms. Cytologic features of carcinoma are seen on high power in another case (C).

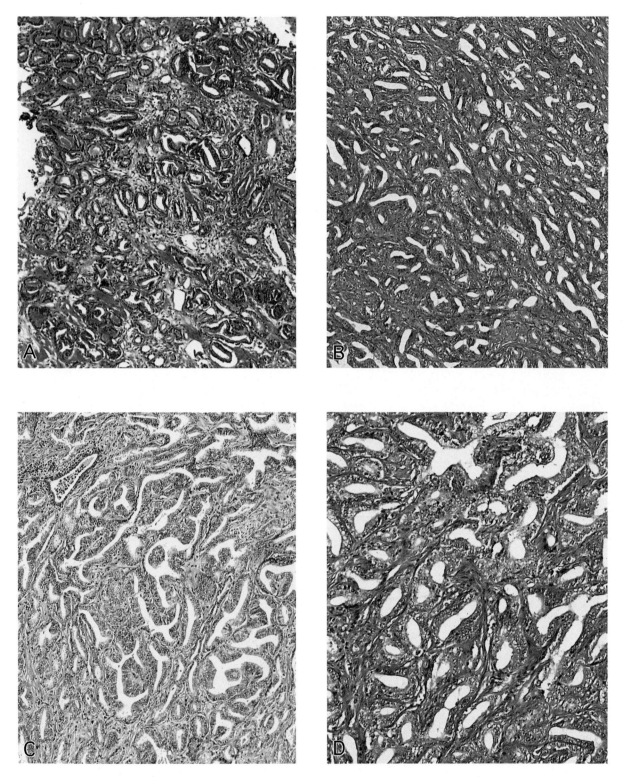

Figure 4-18
PROSTATIC ADENOCARCINOMA, GLEASON GRADE 3A
Four cases show the typical features. The luminal caliber is greater than in grade 3B carcinomas and the acini somewhat more irregular in size and shape, sometimes elongated or even branching (C). Typical cytologic features are easily visible in D, even at intermediate magnification.

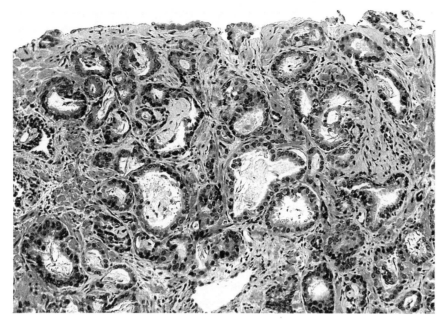

Figure 4-19
PROSTATIC
ADENOCARCINOMA,
GLEASON GRADE 3A
There is focally prominent dilatation of the gland lumens. Even at this magnification the absence of a basal cell layer and the nuclear features of carcinoma are evident, with many prominent nucleoli. The amphophilic cytoplasm typical of many grade 3 carcinomas is also seen.

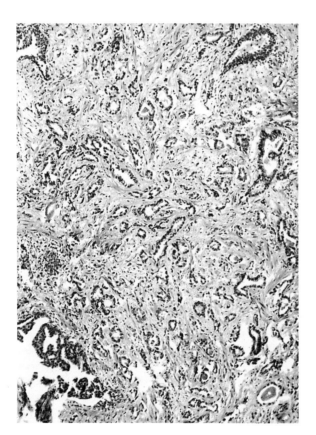

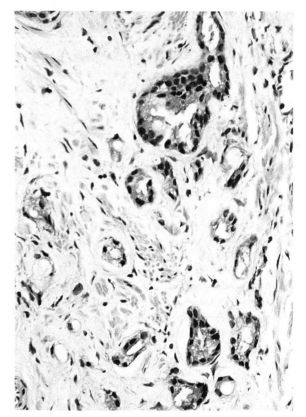

Figure 4-20
PROSTATE ADENOCARCINOMA, GLEASON GRADE 3B
Most of the acini are small and those with scant cytoplasm (left) have a superficial resemblance to atrophic non-neoplastic acini (so-called "atrophic" adenocarcinomas). The neoplastic acini in another case (right) have appreciable cytoplasm on high-power evaluation, a feature much more in keeping with grade 3 adenocarcinoma than atrophic acini. Prominent nucleoli are not evident in this field, indicating that this important feature of carcinoma is not always seen in neoplastic acini.

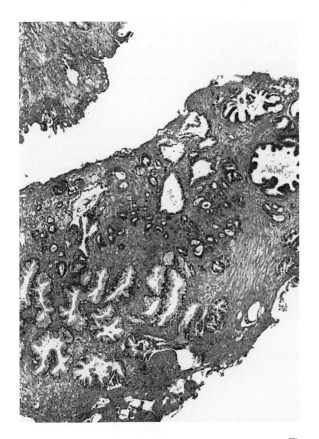
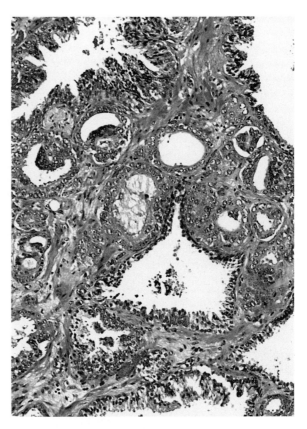

Figure 4-21
PROSTATIC ADENOCARCINOMA, GLEASON GRADE 3A
Low- (left) and high-power (right) views show the intermingling of neoplastic and non-neoplastic acini often seen with grade 3 carcinomas. Prostatic intraepithelial neoplasia is also evident.

Figure 4-22
PROSTATIC
ADENOCARCINOMA,
GLEASON GRADE 3A
Note the angulated acini surrounded by cleft-like spaces.

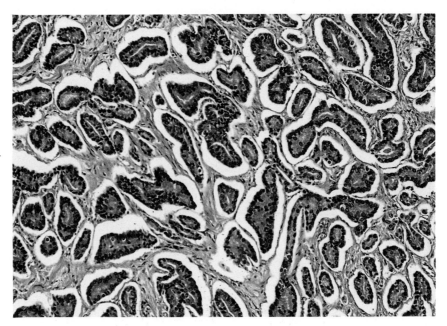

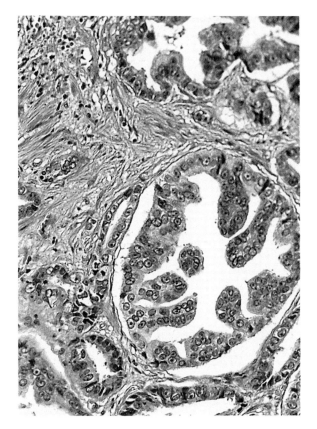

Figure 4-23
PROSTATIC ADENOCARCINOMA,
GLEASON GRADE 3A
There are a few intraluminal papillae.

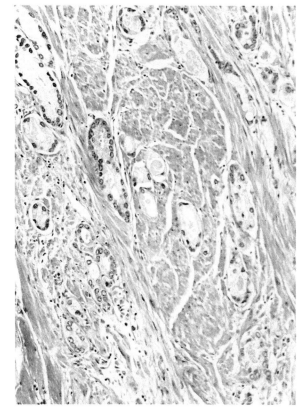

Figure 4-24
GLEASON GRADE 3 ADENOCARCINOMA
Small relatively uniform acini are dissecting within the fibromuscular stroma.

there may be cases in which the interpretation is difficult, in general, there is not the massive confluence seen in a Gleason grade 4 adenocarcinoma, and the majority of the glands in the grade 3C neoplasms are larger. Additionally, papillarity is not a feature of Gleason grade 4 adenocarcinomas. The neoplastic cells are often relatively uniform but display nuclear features of carcinoma with enlargement, prominent nucleoli, and parachromatin clearing. Rounded masses of tumor are seen infiltrating the stroma, and perineural invasion is sometimes present. The papillae of Gleason grade 3 lesions are typically thin with inconspicuous stromal cores (fig. 4-26C). In some instances, the Gleason grade 3C pattern may represent intraductal spread of adenocarcinoma; in such instances, residual basal cells should be apparent (339). Pure Gleason grade 3C tumors that are not in the category of duct carcinoma (see chapter 5) are rare, and a nonductal cribriform pattern is, in the great majority of cases, associated with carcinoma of another Gleason pattern, often another grade 3 pattern, or grade 4 or 5.

The distinction of high-grade prostatic intraepithelial neoplasia from a Gleason grade 3C carcinoma of either cribriform or papillary type may be difficult and depends on architectural and cytologic features. Basal cells are generally absent in cases that we interpret as grade 3C carcinoma of cribriform-papillary type (see page 91). For the diagnosis of prostatic intraepithelial neoplasia one needs to see a maintained normal relationship between glands and stroma whereas in cribriform-papillary carcinomas there is usually a complexity and irregularity of architecture indicative of invasion, in analogous fashion to the help these features provide in the distinction between cribriform carcinoma of the breast and intraductal carcinoma.

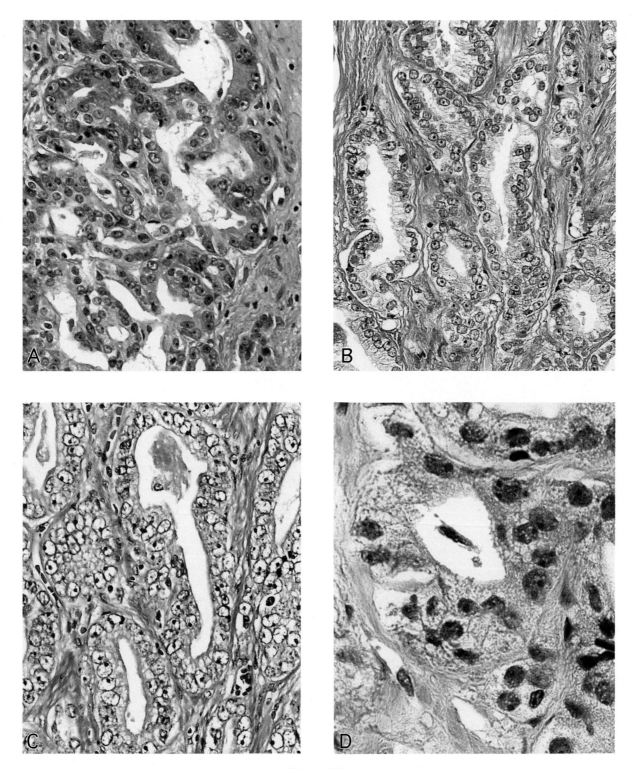

Figure 4-25
PROSTATIC ADENOCARCINOMA, GLEASON GRADE 3

The typical cytologic features are present. Note the nuclear atypia characterized by pleomorphism, parachromatin clearing, particularly in A, and enlarged strikingly prominent nucleoli. The cytoplasm is amphophilic in A and clear in B. Many nucleoli are eccentric in C and in D a few nuclei have two nucleoli. The glands are close together in A, suggesting the possibility of Gleason grade 4, but overall evaluation indicated this was due to artifactual crowding and not the true fusion of a Gleason grade 4 neoplasm.

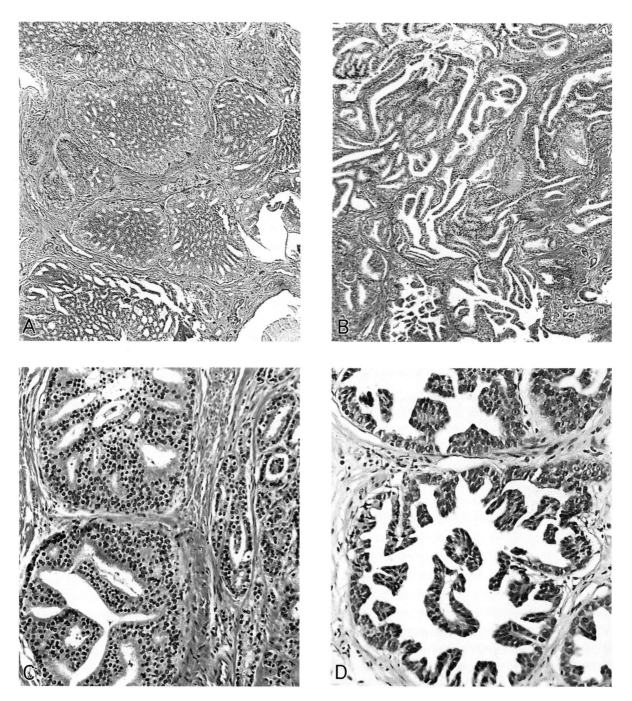

Figure 4-26
PROSTATIC ADENOCARCINOMA, GLEASON GRADE 3C

The low-power views (A,B) show a pure cribriform pattern in A and a mixed cribriform-papillary pattern in B. A shows the typical, sharply etched, smoothly contoured edges of the cribriform aggregates. There is focal grade 4 carcinoma due to fusion (top). B shows a more irregular pattern but the cribriform-papillary pattern of a grade 3C neoplasm is still striking. There is linkage of the epithelial units, which aids in distinction from prostatic intraepithelial neoplasia, and not the confluent gland fusion, nor the smaller caliber glands, characteristic of a Gleason grade 4 adenocarcinoma. A minor component of Gleason grade 3B is seen at the bottom right. The higher power views of cribriform (C) and papillary (D) patterns of Gleason grade 3C carcinoma show the typical cytologic features of carcinoma and a lack of basal cells. Taken in isolation it may be very difficult to distinguish individual foci of the type illustrated in C and D from high-grade prostatic intraepithelial neoplasia unless immunostains for basal cells are available but architectural features of the type illustrated in B, which were present in adjacent areas in both C and D, are helpful, and in many cases there is adjacent conventional small acinar (grade 3A or B) adenocarcinoma, as depicted in C (right) and present elsewhere in the tumor in D.

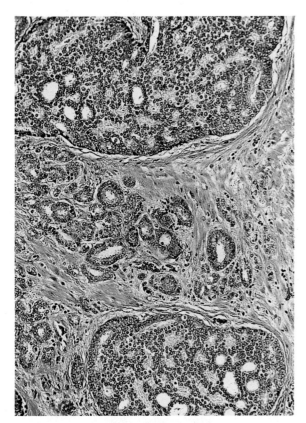

Figure 4-27
PROSTATIC ADENOCARCINOMA,
GLEASON GRADES 3C AND 3A
Note the rounded cribriform aggregates of grade 3C. There is no comedo-type necrosis. Small acini of noncribriform grade 3 carcinoma are also present.

Sometimes, relatively large glands, resembling those of normal or hyperplastic prostate tissue, constitute part of the neoplastic population in Gleason grade 3, or occasionally grade 2, tumors (fig. 4-28). They may be easily overlooked if the abnormal epithelial-stromal pattern is not recognized. This pattern must be suspected on low-power microscopy and confirmed on medium to high power by the absence of the basal cell layer and nuclear atypia, especially the presence of significantly enlarged nucleoli (fig. 4-28). This pattern, seen in about 10 percent of prostatectomy specimens, has been referred to as *pseudohyperplastic adenocarcinoma* (299).

Gleason grade 4 carcinoma is characterized by growth as fused glands or chains and cords of acini, with little or no stroma within the aggregates (fig. 4-29). It is very important that Gleason grade 4 tumors be recognized since they are associated with a significant deterioration in prognosis compared to tumors that are Gleason grade 3 or lower. Strict criteria should be applied in recognizing the gland fusion that is definitional for Gleason grade 4 neoplasms. Sometimes, artifactual aggregation of glands may erroneously suggest a grade 4 cancer. If a distinct uninterrupted line can be drawn around an acinus it is most likely not a component of a grade 4 neoplasm. A cribriform pattern is common in grade 4 neoplasms and should not lead to confusion with the cribriform pattern that represents grade 3C neoplasia. In the cribriform patterns of Gleason grade 4, the individual neoplastic aggregates are usually larger and more irregular in contour than those of Gleason 3C carcinomas. Also, the acini are generally smaller and not as evenly arranged as in 3C neoplasms and the spaces within the neoplastic aggregate often collapse and appear almost solid in appearance, contrasting with the neatly punched out, evenly spaced lumens of the cribriform glands of a Gleason 3C neoplasm. Most of these tumors are composed of cells with relatively scant (although distinctly appreciable) eosinophilic or amphophilic cytoplasm (grade 4A), but some have abundant clear cytoplasm (grade 4B) (fig. 4-30). The latter pattern has been referred to as hypernephroid because it has been likened to renal cell carcinoma, but the resemblance is only superficial, and metastatic renal cancer is rarely suspected. The degree of nuclear atypia is variable within Gleason grade 4. The nuclei in most cases are enlarged and irregular with prominent nucleoli, but in some the nuclei are relatively small and hyperchromatic with inapparent nucleoli (fig. 4-30). Gleason grade 4 tumors are often associated with a component of Gleason grade 3 carcinoma yielding a Gleason score of 7 out of 10.

The highest grade of prostatic adenocarcinoma is Gleason grade 5, and may be composed of rounded or irregular masses of cribriform tumor with central comedonecrosis (fig. 4-31). This picture is similar to that seen in intraductal comedocarcinoma of the breast. Sometimes, the rounded tumor masses are solid. Solid growth without specific features represents Gleason 5B. Sheets, cords, and irregular aggregates of tumor cells may show focal lumens or cytoplasmic vacuoles (fig. 4-32). These formations are more haphazardly arranged than in Gleason grade 4 carcinoma,

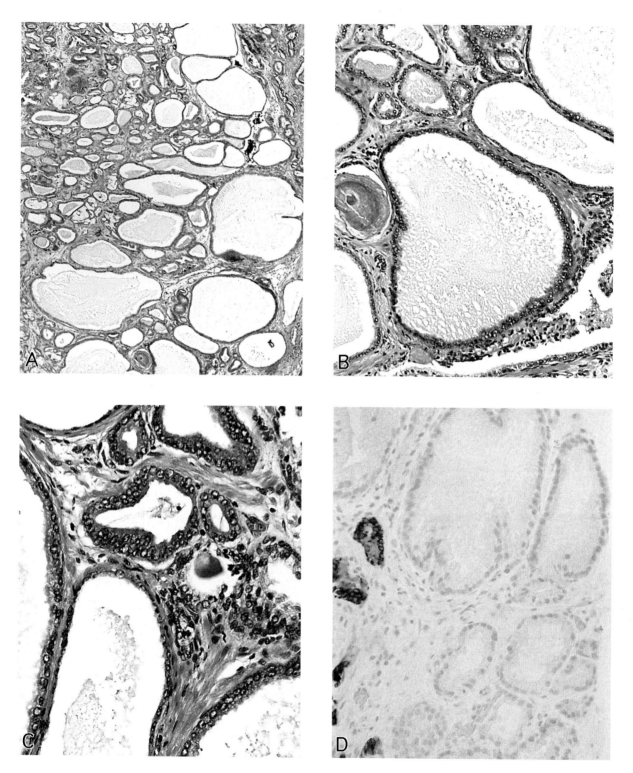

Figure 4-28
PROSTATIC ADENOCARCINOMA, GLEASON GRADE 3 (PSEUDOHYPERPLASTIC)
Note the striking variation in the size of the glands, many of them cystically dilated, imparting a pseudohyperplastic appearance. The cystic glands are more regular than in hyperplasia. Medium- and high-power views (B and C) show variably sized acini lined by a single cell layer; the nuclei have prominent nucleoli on careful scrutiny. A high molecular weight cytokeratin immunostain shows an absence of basal cells (D).

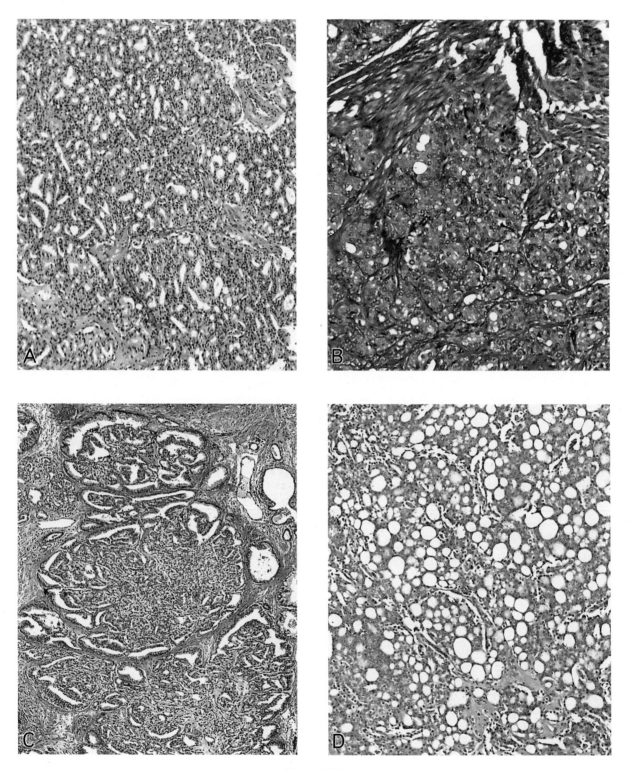

Figure 4-29
PROSTATIC ADENOCARCINOMA, GLEASON GRADE 4A

The microacini are fused, and the cytoplasm is eosinophilic to amphophilic in these four examples. The lumens may be relatively inconspicuous, as in B, but can be seen on close examination. In D, there is a cribriform (sieve-like) pattern indicating that a cribriform picture is not unique to Gleason grade 3C neoplasms; in contrast to the latter, however, this case has large, fused, expansile masses whereas the grade 3C examples are discrete with circumscribed borders.

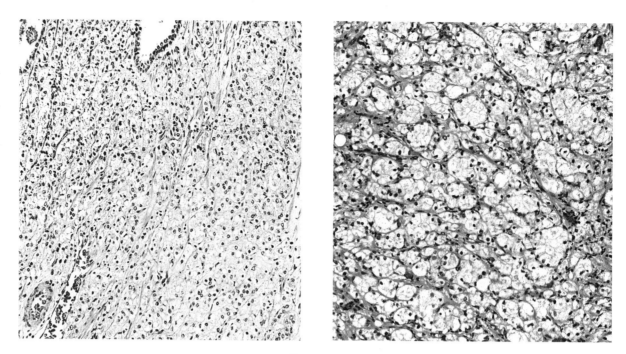

Figure 4-30
PROSTATIC ADENOCARCINOMA, GLEASON GRADE 4B

Left: Note the fused glands. Clear cytoplasm is conspicuous on low power.

Right: Tightly packed nests of cells have abundant clear cytoplasm and small dark nuclei. This pattern has been referred to as hypernephroid because of its superficial resemblance to clear cell renal carcinoma. Nucleoli may not be prominent, as in this case, but the diagnosis of carcinoma is generally not difficult because of the obvious architectural features indicative of invasion.

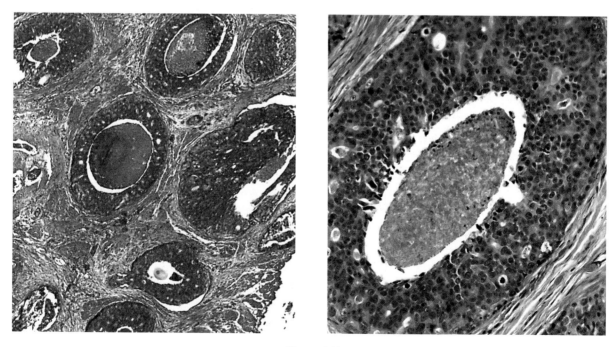

Figure 4-31
PROSTATIC ADENOCARCINOMA, GLEASON GRADE 5A

Note the large cribriform aggregates with comedonecrosis and overt cytologic atypia (right).

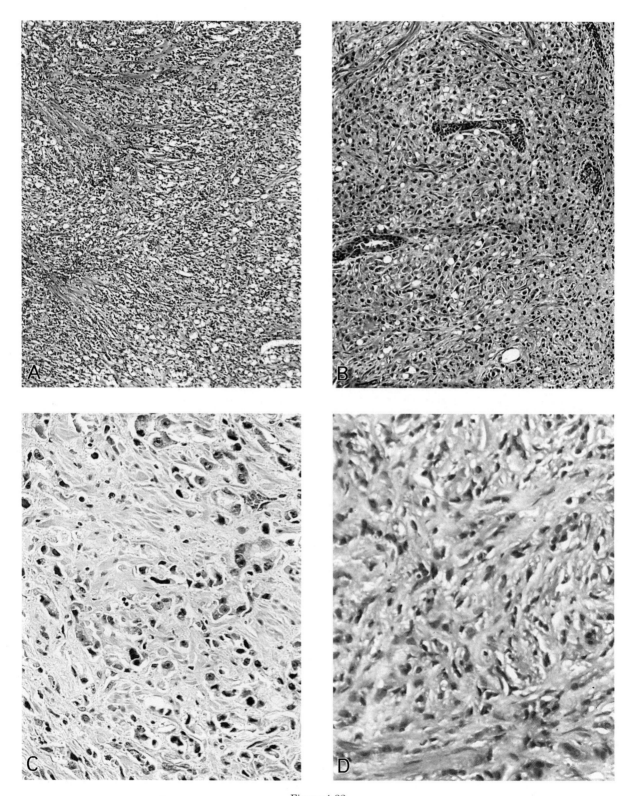

Figure 4-32
PROSTATIC ADENOCARCINOMA, GLEASON GRADE 5B
There is diffuse, featureless growth of poorly differentiated carcinoma cells (A). The tumor cells have abundant eosinophilic cytoplasm in B. Small nests and single cells are seen in C, and the tumor cells are focally spindled in D.

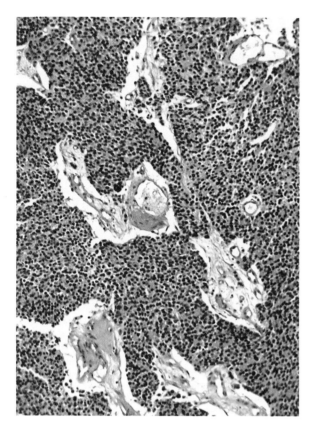

Figure 4-33
PROSTATIC ADENOCARCINOMA,
GLEASON GRADE 5B
  The pattern in this case, including growth as large trabeculae, suggested the possible diagnosis of transitional cell
carcinoma which was excluded by appropriate immunohistochemical stains. This photomicrograph shows the relative cellular uniformity that is a feature of many poorly differentiated
prostatic carcinomas in contrast, in general, to a greater degree
of pleomorphism in high-grade transitional cell carcinoma.

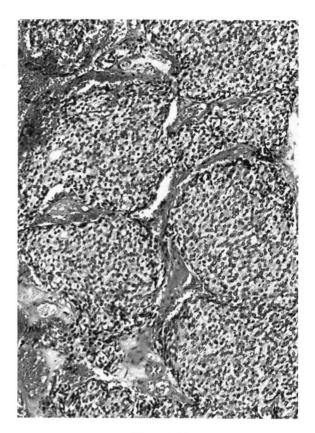

Figure 4-34
PROSTATIC ADENOCARCINOMA,
GLEASON GRADE 5B
There is growth in solid, irregularly rounded nests.

and individual infiltrating tumor cells, sometimes arranged in thin cords, are also common.
Occasional signet ring–like cells may be present
(see chapter 5). At times it is difficult to appreciate the tumor as adenocarcinoma except for focal
luminal differentiation or the accompanying
lower grade patterns that may be present. Some
grade 5 carcinomas grow in large trabeculae
which may be difficult to distinguish from transitional cell carcinoma (fig. 4-33) or as solid nests
(fig. 4-34) which rarely have rosette-like structures (fig. 4-35). In Gleason grade 5 tumors, the
nuclear morphology is highly variable (327).
Small dark and irregular nuclei with relatively
inconspicuous nucleoli may be seen, but in most

cases, atypical nuclei with enlarged nucleoli are
conspicuous. Tumor giant cells are occasionally
seen (fig. 4-36) but in general the nuclear pleomorphism of prostatic carcinoma is less striking
than in most other carcinomas.
  The various subcategories within Gleason
grades 3, 4, and 5 have been discussed because of
the morphologic differences between them,
but these subcategories within each grade have
no known prognostic significance, with the possible exception of 3C in the grade 3 category, and
are not necessary in routine reports.
  The various Gleason patterns of prostatic adenocarcinoma considered above have the characteristic cytologic features of this neoplasm, with the
exceptions noted. However, practically, their most
crucial role is in the consideration of needle
biopsy specimens, and cytologic features of prostate carcinoma are accordingly considered in
more detail in that section (see page 168).

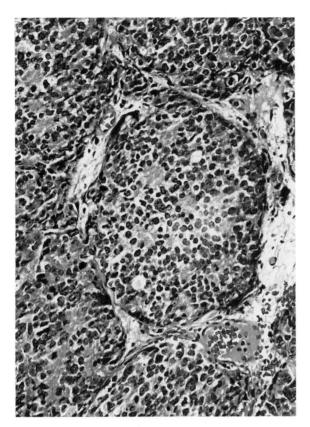

Figure 4-35
PROSTATIC ADENOCARCINOMA,
GLEASON GRADE 5B

In this case, otherwise solid nests are punctuated by small, rounded, rosette-like structures. There is a superficial resemblance to a carcinoid tumor.

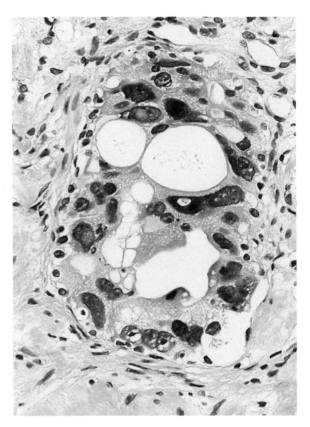

Figure 4-36
PROSTATIC ADENOCARCINOMA,
GLEASON GRADE 5B

A few acini are lined by cells with highly atypical nuclei, forming occasional giant cells. Nuclear pleomorphism of this degree is relatively uncommon even in high-grade prostatic adenocarcinoma. This case also illustrates that focal luminal differentiation may be seen in grade 5 carcinoma. Most other areas of this tumor had a featureless diffuse growth.

Luminal and Other Ancillary Histologic Features Relevant to the Diagnosis of Prostatic Adenocarcinoma

A great number of histologic features, in addition to those already presented, are useful in arriving at a diagnosis of prostatic adenocarcinoma (Table 4-5). The material present within gland lumens is frequently noteworthy. There is often an eosinophilic material which may be quite abundant and is pinker and more granular and flocculent than the redder more homogenous secretion seen in normal or hyperplastic glands (fig. 4-37). It is also less dense and not as hyaline in appearance as the eosinophilic luminal material in cases of the rare mesonephric remnant hyperplasia (see chapter 7) and lacks the lamellated appearance of corpora amylacea.

Eosinophilic crystalloids are relatively common, especially in low- and moderate-grade tumors (189,295,305), and are often present in the background of the flocculent material just referred to (fig. 4-37, right). They are needle-shaped, prismatic, rectangular, or rhomboid structures that are refractile, variable in length (fig. 4-38), and can usually be detected on scanning magnification. Special stains may enhance their detection; they are red with trichrome stain, blue with toluidine blue, and violet with phosphotungstic acid hematoxylin, but are negative with periodic acid–Schiff (PAS), alcian blue, prussian blue, and Congo red stains, as well as immunostains for PSA and PAP. Crystalloids were initially thought to be related to Bence-Jones protein (295), but more recent studies show little phenotypic

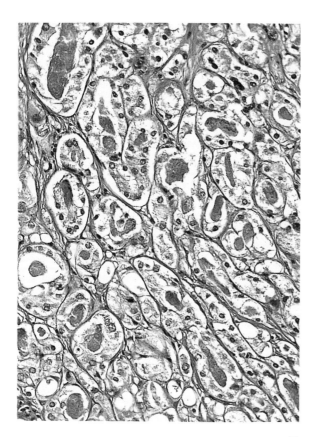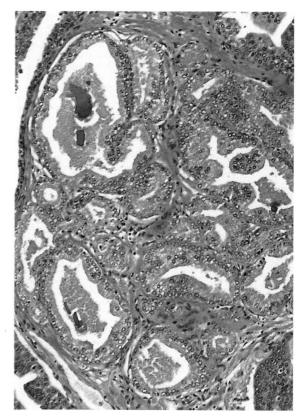

Figure 4-37
PROSTATIC ADENOCARCINOMA
Medium- (left) and high-power views (right) show granular, flocculent eosinophilic secretions. Needle-like crystalloids are also seen on the right.

similarity. They likely represent an altered secretory product of the neoplastic acinus and have been shown to contain sulfur, calcium, and phosphorous (234,366). Crystalloids may be found in atypical adenomatous hyperplasia, conventional hyperplasia, and benign glands, especially those adjacent to prostatic adenocarcinoma. When crystalloids are found unassociated with any other features that raise the suspicion of a precancerous or cancerous lesion, they have no significance; two studies have shown that this finding alone is not associated with an increased incidence of cancer on repeat biopsy (177,291). Nonetheless, when crystalloids are found in acini that are atypical they are one feature that should prompt the examination of multiple levels. We have personally seen cases in which this has disclosed foci diagnostic of carcinoma which were lacking in initial cuts.

Basophilic, "blue-tinged," mucinous secretions are commonly found in the acini of prostatic carcinoma (fig. 4-39). In some studies, they are present in about 60 percent of cases (319,367, 392). Mucin is recognized as a wispy, lightly basophilic luminal material (fig. 4-40D) and may be highlighted using acid mucin stains such as alcian blue or other stains (fig. 4-39B,C). The glands of normal prostate and nodular hyperplasia do not usually contain acid mucin, although they may harbor neutral mucosubstances (262,297). The presence of acid mucin is useful as a diagnostic adjunct in assessing small acinar lesions when the differential diagnosis includes atypical adenomatous hyperplasia and carcinoma (250,265, 385). This assessment is generally made by routine hematoxylin and eosin evaluation, special stains not being indicated. While not specific, the presence of luminal acidic mucin, especially if extensive, supports a diagnosis of carcinoma; focal acid mucin may be found rarely in atypical adenomatous hyperplasia, sclerosing adenosis, and postatrophic hyperplasia (250,278,331).

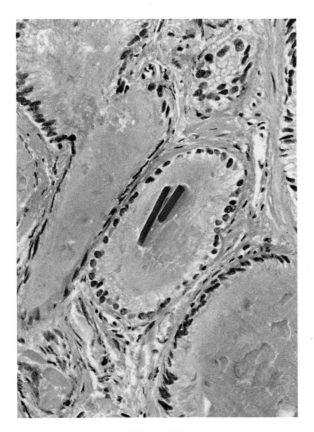

Figure 4-38
PROSTATIC ADENOCARCINOMA

Two typical, parallel, needle-like crystalloids are in an area that itself was not diagnostic of carcinoma but merged, on deeper cuts, with well-differentiated adenocarcinoma. Crystalloids may be seen in benign, atypical, and neoplastic acini.

Collagenous micronodules have been described in adenocarcinoma and are an important, albeit uncommon, feature (fig. 4-40) since they are considered pathognomonic of cancer (184a,206,331). They may cause a striking appearance on low-power microscopy when conspicuous (fig 4-40A) and appear to represent organization of mucin, being initially uncovered in an analysis of mucinous differentiation in prostatic carcinoma (331). This is supported by observations such as those in figure 4-40 C and D which show foci that are partly mucinous and partly collagenous. This has led some to refer to them as "mucinous fibroplasia" (245). The particular association with mucinous differentiation in prostatic carcinoma is highlighted by the findings in the initial study describing the entity. The process was found in 13 of 33 carcinomas with prominent mucin-secreting areas and none of 67 tumors without mucinous elements (331). In a subsequent investigation, the micronodules were found in 13 percent of a large series of carcinomas in prostatectomy specimens (206). In that series acid mucin was demonstrated in glands with the micronodules or in glands adjacent to them. In the same series, micronodules were identified in only 0.6 percent of needle biopsy specimens. The rarity of this finding in needle biopsies and its usual association with moderate- to high-grade carcinoma make it a relatively uncommon finding of crucial diagnostic significance. Two other findings have also been considered pathognomonic of carcinoma (184a) but are respectively relatively uncommon and rare in diagnostic biopsies: these are circumferential perineural invasion (see page 180) and glomeruloid structures (see page 154).

Other Features of Adenocarcinoma

Corpora amylacea are uncommon in areas of prostatic carcinoma (fig. 4-41), but they may be seen due to overgrowth of benign tissue by the infiltrating cancer (301). In a series investigating this topic, 11 of 100 cases of carcinoma contained corpora within neoplastic foci (301). In many instances, the corpora amylacea are present in benign glands and are literally entrapped by the advancing tumor which tends to be moderate to high grade (301). Less commonly, in our experience, corpora amylacea lie in neoplastic glands which may be relatively low grade (fig. 4-41, right). Rarely, cytoplasmic lipofuscin pigment is noted in prostatic adenocarcinoma (fig. 4-42, left). Occasionally, dystrophic calcification may be present in the lumens of malignant acini; rarely, they resemble psammoma bodies (fig. 4-42, right).

Some prostatic adenocarcinomas are composed of cells with abundant, foamy cytoplasm (fig. 4-43) (207,350). This "xanthomatous" or "foamy gland" variant may simulate xanthomatous prostatitis-xanthoma (see chapter 7), a differential that has been mentioned only rarely in the literature on prostatic carcinoma (340) until recently (350). The presence of well-defined nests and groups of foamy cells, often with intraluminal pink secretions, focal nuclear enlargement, and nucleolar prominence, are helpful diagnostic findings, although nuclear features are less helpful in these cases than in most other prostatic cancers.

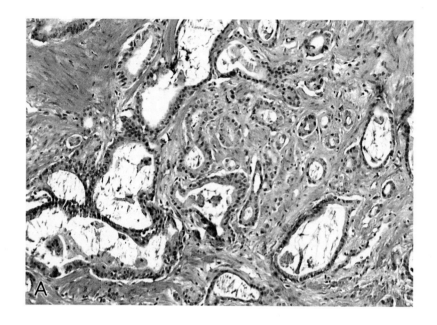

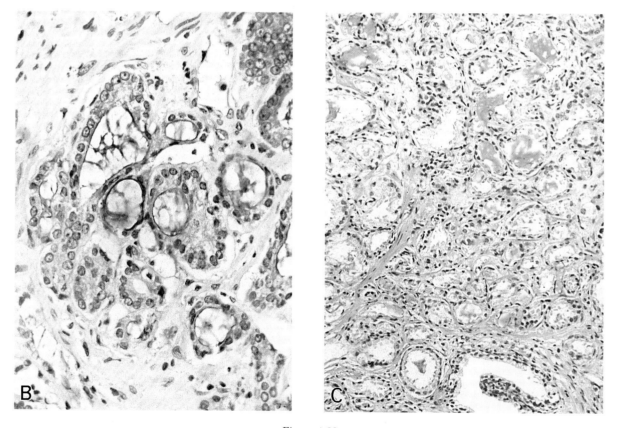

Figure 4-39
PROSTATIC ADENOCARCINOMA WITH LUMINAL MUCIN
A: There is wispy mucin within neoplastic acini.
B: The material in another case is stained with the mucicarmine technique.
C: The material in another case is positive with an alcian blue stain.

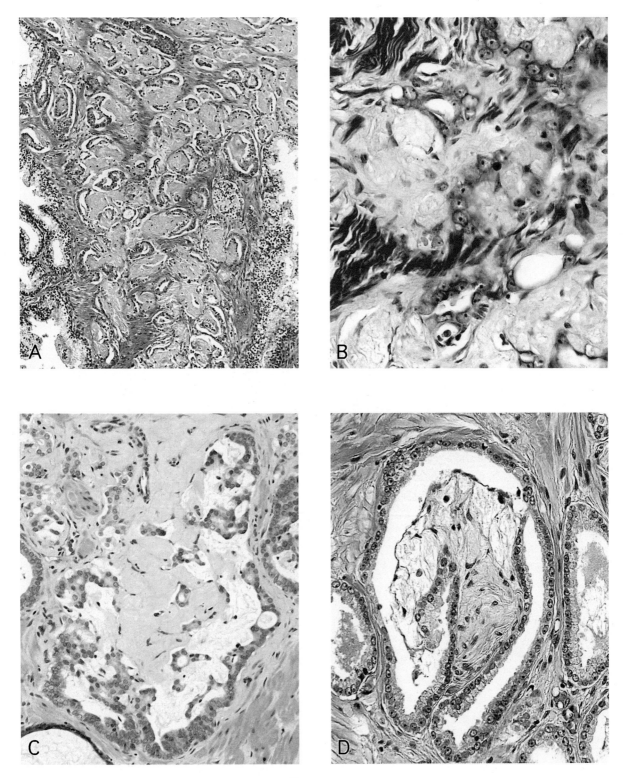

Figure 4-40
PROSTATIC ADENOCARCINOMA WITH COLLAGENOUS MICRONODULES
Collagenous micronodules occur as rounded, dense, hyaline-like material within and adjacent to neoplastic acini (A). A Masson trichrome stain (B) shows pale green-staining material consistent with collagen. An association with wispy basophilic mucin is seen in C and D; this has led some to use the term "mucinous fibroplasia" for this phenomenon.

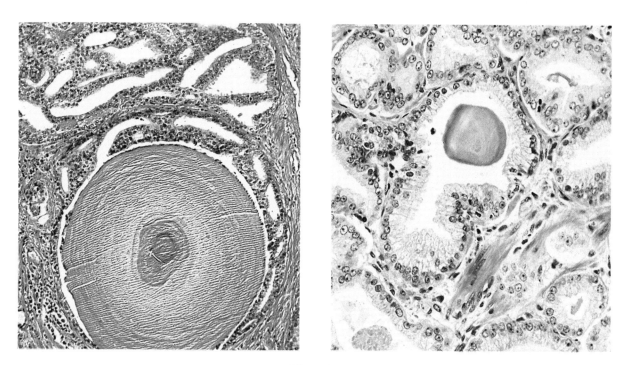

Figure 4-41
PROSTATIC ADENOCARCINOMA WITH CORPORA AMYLACEA
These are examples of one of several corpora amylacea present within two different carcinomas, one moderately differentiated (Gleason grade 3C; left) and the other well differentiated (Gleason grade 2; right).

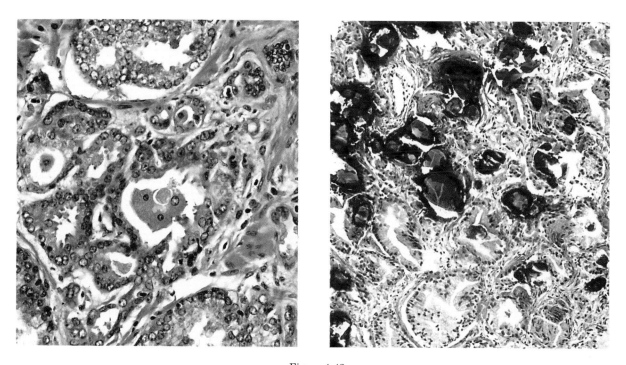

Figure 4-42
PROSTATIC ADENOCARCINOMA WITH LIPOFUSCIN OR CALCIFICATION
Left: There is focal cytoplasmic lipofuscin pigment within the cells of a small acinar carcinoma.
Right: Another case shows calcification with focal psammoma body features.

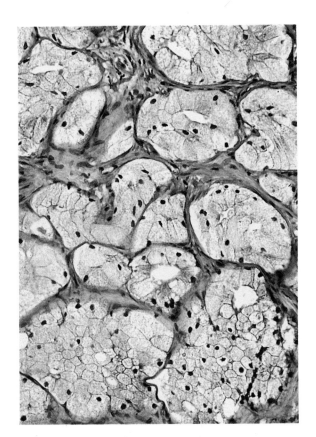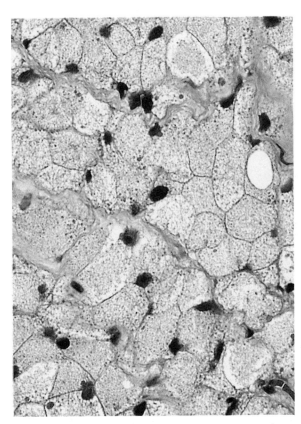

Figure 4-43
PROSTATIC ADENOCARCINOMA WITH FOAMY CYTOPLASM
Left: This is an example of the xanthomatous or "foamy gland" variant. Acini are lined by cells with voluminous foamy cytoplasm.
Right: In this typical example, most of the nuclei are small and dark lacking the usual cytologic hallmarks of carcinoma.

A similar foamy pattern of adenocarcinoma may be present in metastatic deposits within regional lymph nodes or bone (375a). The foamy nature of the cytoplasm in cases of "foamy gland" carcinoma serves to distinguish this variant from other prostatic carcinomas, particularly those of transition zone origin and the so-called hypernephroid variant of Gleason grade 4B, which are somewhat similar because of their abundant pale to clear cytoplasm. Distinction from the latter is not crucial as most foamy gland cancers are of intermediate to high grade, but it is important that they be distinguished from well-differentiated transition zone cancers. However, the distinctive foamy cytoplasm, architectural disposition of the glands that is usually indicative of at least a Gleason grade 3 neoplasm, and peripheral zone location of the foamy gland tumors should facilitate distinction (350). The foamy cytoplasm in

these cases is presumably due to lipid, although verification of this by appropriate staining of the reported cases is usually lacking.

Rare adenocarcinomas of the prostate are composed of cells with abundant, granular, eosinophilic cytoplasm resembling oncocytes (356,361). Ultrastructural studies of such cases have shown abundant mitochondria in these cells. Occasional other tumors may be partly composed of cells with granular, brightly eosinophilic cytoplasm resembling either intestinal Paneth cells (fig. 4-44, left) or, if the granules are subnuclear, argentaffin cells (172,285,408,409). Rare tumors are composed predominantly of these cells which stain for neuroendocrine markers such as neuron-specific enolase and chromogranin (fig. 4-44, right) (172,232,408,409). A wide range of neuroendocrine-type granules has been demonstrated by electron microscopy (fig.

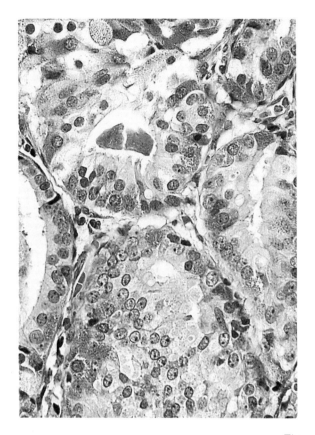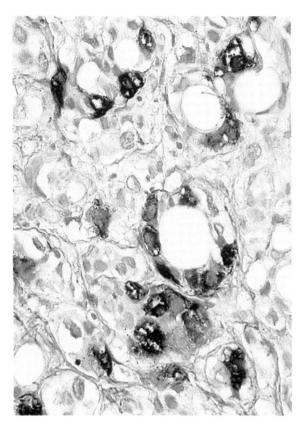

Figure 4-44
PROSTATIC ADENOCARCINOMA WITH PANETH CELL–LIKE CHANGE
Paneth cell–like change is manifest as many cells with granular eosinophilic cytoplasm (left). They stain for chromogranin (right). (Fig. 3 from Weaver MG, Abdul-Karim FW, Srigley JR. Paneth cell-like change and small cell carcinoma of the prostate. Two divergent forms of prostatic neuroendocrine differentiation. Am J Surg Pathol 1992;16:1013–6.)

4-45) (285,409). These findings indicate that the cells have a neuroendocrine nature, despite the fact that Paneth-like cells in the non-neoplastic prostate have been found to be due to lysosome accumulation in the cytoplasm (409).

Prostatic adenocarcinoma is occasionally composed of organoid nests and groups of relatively uniform cells, superficially resembling carcinoid tumor, a resemblance occasionally heightened by the presence of structures that simulate the acini of a carcinoid tumor (fig. 4-35) (175,181, 217,232,270,391,407). Argyrophilia and neuroendocrine immunoreactivity may further suggest carcinoid tumor (fig. 4-46). Such tumors usually have nuclear features similar to prostatic adenocarcinoma, with open chromatin and nucleolar prominence, rather than the granular chromatin and inconspicuous nucleoli of a carcinoid tumor. Strong immunoreactivity for PSA is usually de-

tected, and tumors with this carcinoid-like pattern are thought to represent an unusual variant of adenocarcinoma rather than true carcinoid tumor. Prostatic adenocarcinoma in metastatic sites may also have a carcinoid-like morphology; when such a pattern is encountered, a prostatic origin should be considered and investigated using immunohistochemistry (176).

Small acini of prostatic carcinoma are occasionally separated and encircled by fibroblast-like spindle cells, creating a picture that resembles sclerosing adenosis (fig. 4-47) (see chapter 7). This sclerosing pattern of carcinoma can be separated from sclerosing adenosis by its more infiltrative architecture, absence of basal cells, and nuclear abnormalities. Rarely, the stroma of prostatic carcinoma appears markedly atypical with, occasionally, multinucleate cells. The absence of mitotic activity and stromal overgrowth help separate this

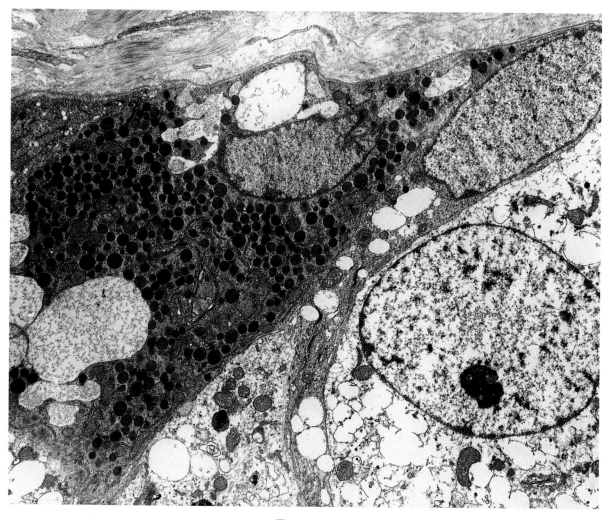

Figure 4-45

PROSTATIC ADENOCARCINOMA WITH NEUROENDOCRINE DIFFERENTIATION

Note the abundant cytoplasmic neurosecretory-type granules in this electron micrograph. (Courtesy of Dr. P.A. di Sant'Agnese, Rochester, NY.)

pseudosarcomatous stromal reaction from sarcomatoid carcinoma or sarcoma (222). The occasional multinucleation of the stromal cells is to be distinguished from neoplastic epithelial cells with a giant cell configuration (324).

Occasional adenocarcinomas display glomeruloid features with rounded or fused aggregates projecting into a space and surrounded by a crescentic space, resulting in the "glomeruloid" designation (fig. 4-48) (357). This unusual pattern is generally admixed with other typical areas of adenocarcinoma and, because of the fused acinar elements, is usually a variant pattern of a Gleason grade 4 neoplasm.

AN APPROACH TO THE DIAGNOSIS OF PROSTATIC CARCINOMA IN NEEDLE BIOPSY SPECIMENS

A systematic approach to the diagnosis of adenocarcinoma in needle biopsy specimens includes the following elements: 1) observation of architectural features; 2) analysis of cytology; 3) examination for ancillary features and other soft criteria supportive of carcinoma; 4) awareness of the spectrum of morphology of the various mimics of cancer (see chapters 2, 3, and 7); and 5) judicious application of immunohistochemical investigations. Representative examples of adenocarcinoma in

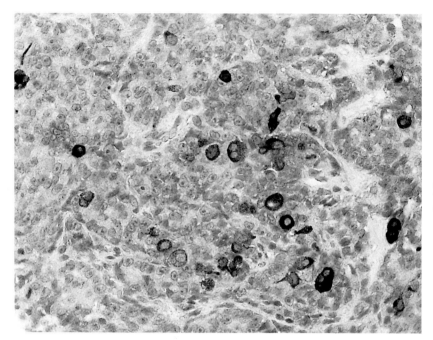

Figure 4-46
PROSTATIC
ADENOCARCINOMA
WITH NEUROENDOCRINE
DIFFERENTIATION
Scattered chromogranin-positive
cells are present in this tumor, which
was also positive for prostate-specific
antigen.

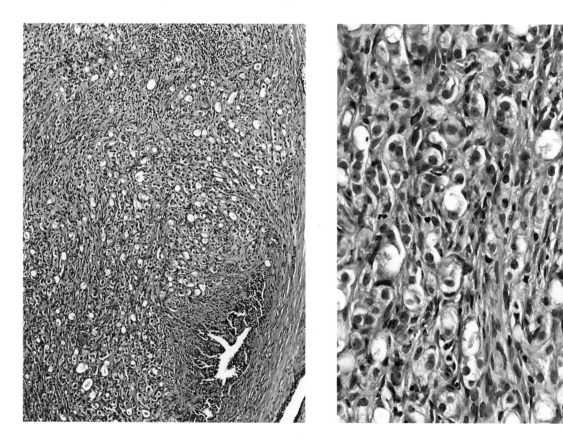

Figure 4-47
PROSTATIC ADENOCARCINOMA WITH SCLEROSIS
This tumor has a sclerosing pattern characterized by small acini and nests separated by a proliferative stroma. This pattern
of adenocarcinoma can simulate sclerosing adenosis (see chapter 7).

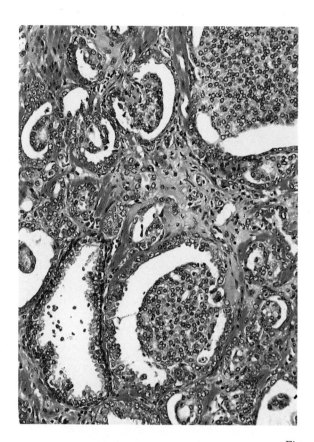
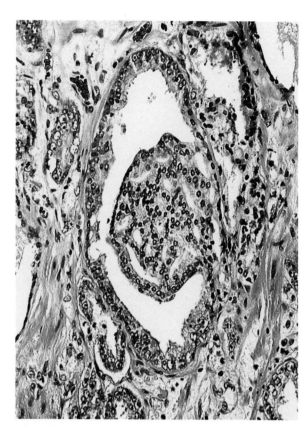

Figure 4-48
PROSTATIC ADENOCARCINOMA WITH GLOMERULOID FORMATIONS
Glomeruloid structures are created by rounded proliferations of neoplastic cells surrounded by often crescentic spaces resembling Bowman's space.

needle biopsy specimens are presented in figures 4-49–4-65. Those in figures 4-60–65 are progressively more difficult to diagnose as compared to earlier examples, and individual observers will vary in their degree of confidence in diagnosing cancer in cases of this type. The role of immunohistochemistry in aiding in the evaluation of difficult cases is discussed on page 192.

Many adenocarcinomas are easy to recognize based on architectural features in needle biopsy specimens. In the presence of fused glands, solid-cribriform patterns, with or without comedonecrosis, and sheets and cord-like patterns of growth, the diagnosis of cancer is usually obvious, unless the focus of questionable carcinoma is very small or the architecture, although florid, is still orderly (as in the case of cribriform hyperplasia), in which instance the cytologic criteria outlined below are applicable. For example, limited high-grade carcinoma and chronic prostatitis

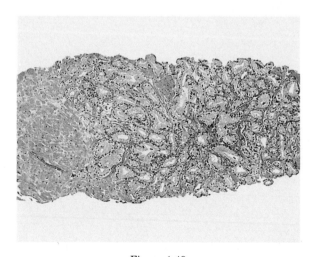

Figure 4-49
PROSTATIC ADENOCARCINOMA, NEEDLE BIOPSY
A needle biopsy specimen shows a proliferation of relatively uniform glands lined by columnar cells with abundant pale cytoplasm.

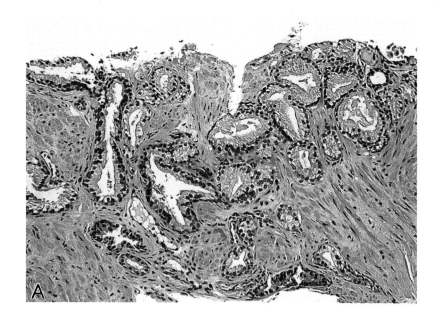

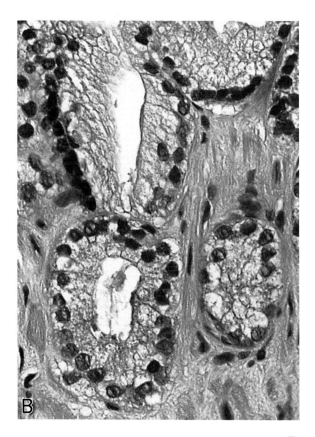

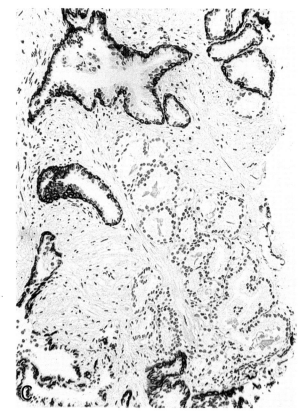

Figure 4-50
PROSTATIC ADENOCARCINOMA, NEEDLE BIOPSY

Three illustrations of the same needle core biopsy show on low power (A) an abnormal cluster of glands which, on high power (B), are lined by cells with the cytologic features of carcinoma, having irregular nuclei with focally prominent nucleoli. The abundant pale cytoplasm is also a feature of many relatively low-grade prostatic carcinomas. A diagnosis of carcinoma in this case was supported by negative cytokeratin immunoreactivity for basal cells within the problematic area (C).

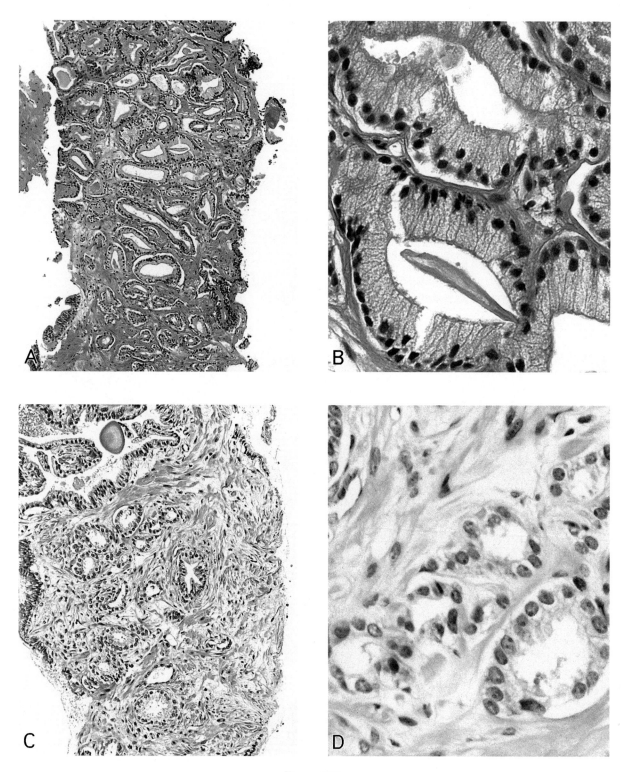

Figure 4-51
PROSTATIC ADENOCARCINOMA, NEEDLE BIOPSY

Figures A and B, and C and D represent low- and high-power views of needle biopsy specimens from two separate cases. Abnormal glandular patterns on low power with confirmatory abnormal cytologic findings on high power warrant the diagnosis of carcinoma. Cytologic features of carcinoma are more striking in D than in B, but the findings in B, in conjunction with the clearly neoplastic architecture, warrant the diagnosis of cancer.

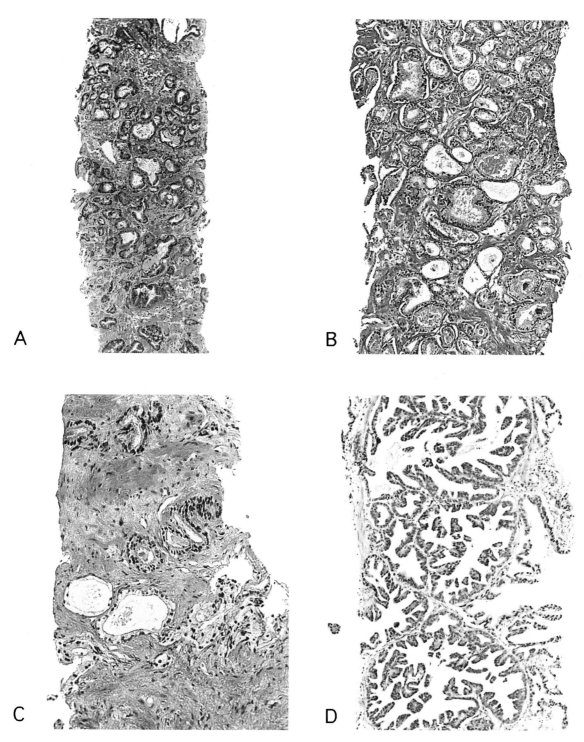

Figure 4-52
PROSTATIC ADENOCARCINOMA, NEEDLE BIOPSY

Representative needle biopsy examples of Gleason grade 3 adenocarcinoma. In A and B the architectural abnormalities are essentially diagnostic of adenocarcinoma. C is a good example of an appearance which mandates careful high-power scrutiny to confirm the diagnosis of carcinoma by appropriate cytologic findings which were present in this case. In D, the differential diagnosis is with high-grade prostatic intraepithelial neoplasia. In our opinion, the prominent papillary pattern and fusion of the abnormal epithelial units favor a diagnosis of carcinoma rather than intraepithelial neoplasia. An immediately adjacent area of this needle biopsy specimen showed conventional grade 3A adenocarcinoma.

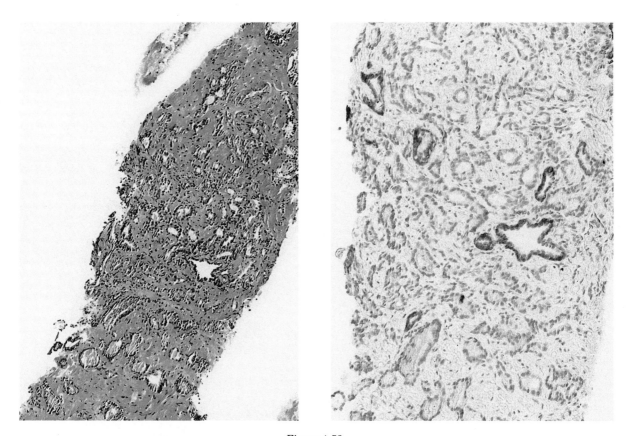

Figure 4-53
PROSTATIC ADENOCARCINOMA, NEEDLE BIOPSY
Left: This needle biopsy specimen shows predominantly Gleason grade 3B adenocarcinoma with, in areas, the appearance that has been referred to as "atrophic adenocarcinoma."
Right: An immunohistochemical stain for high molecular weight cytokeratin shows neoplastic acini without basal cells invading between residual non-neoplastic acini with basal cells.

Figure 4-54
PROSTATIC
ADENOCARCINOMA,
NEEDLE BIOPSY

A needle biopsy shows the Gleason grade 3C (cribriform) pattern at the bottom and a fused glandular pattern of grade 4 above it. Some might consider the latter area still in the 3C category, indicating one of the areas of variability and difficulty in Gleason grading.

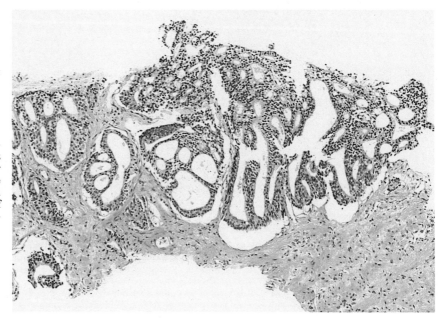

and in approximately 20 percent of grade 1 carcinomas (288). In the same investigation two nucleoli were present in some nuclei in approximately 12 percent of grade 3 carcinomas, 7 percent of grade 2 carcinomas, but in less than 1 percent of grade 1 carcinomas. More than two nucleoli are only exceptionally encountered, and then only in moderate- to high-grade neoplasms. It is our experience that eccentric nucleoli are a striking feature of some carcinomas, but we have seen this in benign cells also. While the nuclear features in carcinoma are often atypical, they are, paradoxically, commonly monomorphous and may at times be deceptively bland. As many as 25 percent of prostatic carcinomas in needle biopsy material lack conspicuous nucleoli, and in such instances the diagnosis of carcinoma is made by the identification of unequivocal infiltration and an absence of the basal cell layer (242). Cases lacking prominent nucleoli may have uniformly dense, hyperchromatic nuclei, but this is a relatively infrequent finding.

Mitoses are uncommon in most prostatic carcinomas of conventional type, especially those of low to moderate grade, but are occasionally present and cause concern for neoplasia if seen in an atypical acinus unassociated with inflammation or infarction. A high mitotic rate is often evident in the ductal variant of carcinoma (see chapter 5).

The luminal and other ancillary histologic features of cancer summarized on page 146 are also important in the diagnosis of carcinoma in needle biopsies. Intraluminal crystalloids are common but intraluminal wispy basophilic mucin is of more diagnostic value, being a stronger indicator of malignancy. Collagenous micronodules and glomeruloid structures ("glomerulations") have, to date, been associated only with malignant glands. They are exceptionally rarely the key diagnostic feature (184a). Collagenous micronodules should not be confused with the very rare hyaline spherules that have been seen in benign glands and have been likened to collagenous spherulosis of the breast (339a) (see page 334). Glands closely apposed to nerves suggest malignancy, but benign processes can also demonstrate this phenomenon, and only circumferential (fig. 4-13A) or near circumferential perineural involvement and intraneural invasion (see page 180) are diagnostic of carcinoma (184a). High-grade prostatic intraepithelial neoplasia (PIN) associated with an atypical small glandular focus provides supportive evidence for carcinoma, but this feature alone should not establish a diagnosis of cancer. Small acini with high-grade PIN may bud from larger ducts, and tangential sections may lack an apparent basal cell layer and lead to a misinterpretation as carcinoma (223,242). The diagnosis of carcinoma with an associated focus of high-grade PIN is usually more secure if the possible carcinoma is not directly adjacent to the PIN. Infiltration of periprostatic fat, and seminal vesicle or vascular invasion are essentially diagnostic of malignancy, although even with these criteria some caution is indicated with regard to reliance on one feature alone because mesonephric remnants and inflammatory processes may involve extraprostatic tissue, and tumor may be present within vessel lumens on an artifactual basis.

If small glands in a problematic focus appear to be emanating from a "parent" or central duct, one should be cautious since this usually occurs in atypical adenomatous hyperplasia, benign processes such as atrophy and postatrophic hyperplasia, or in normal anatomic structures such as seminal vesicle, ejaculatory duct, and Cowper's gland. When marked inflammation is present, there should be caution in the interpretation of cytologic features since regenerative nuclear atypia can simulate the nuclear changes of carcinoma. Nevertheless, carcinoma and prostatitis may coexist. If the atypical acini are crushed or poorly preserved, they should be interpreted cautiously.

Immunohistochemistry for high molecular weight cytokeratin (clone 34βE12) antibody can be used in selected situations to support a diagnosis of carcinoma by demonstrating a lack of basal cells (see page 192) (209,412,414). Low molecular weight keratins, pancytokeratins, and prostate-specific markers (PSA, PAP) can be used to establish the "epithelial" nature of a lesion in the setting of carcinoma versus xanthoma, or carcinoma versus granulomatous prostatitis, lymphoma, or sarcoma in crushed foci, and in treated cancers where neoplastic cells may be shrunken with vacuolated cytoplasm. Both prostate markers should be employed in these situations as one or the other may be negative in individual cases (257).

The frequency of various features that help establish a diagnosis of adenocarcinoma of the prostate in needle biopsy specimens, as determined in two studies, are shown in Table 4-6 (242,396). As these data indicate, no single feature is uniformly present, most cases show several features, and some of the most specific features are distinctly rare in the limited sampling provided by needle biopsy. Of particular note, prominent nucleoli are absent in one fourth to one third of the cases, although many pathologists consider them a necessary feature in establishing a diagnosis of carcinoma. It is often important, therefore, to evaluate many features before reaching a diagnostic conclusion.

In summary, we suggest the following algorithm be used for atypical small acinar processes, especially in needle biopsy material: 1) identify and characterize the small acinar process on low-power microscopy and compare its architecture with that of clearly benign tissue (if present); 2) confirm the absence of a basal cell layer on high power; 3) confirm the presence of significant nuclear abnormalities, especially enlarged nuclei, prominent nucleoli, or double nucleoli on high power; 4) look for other supportive evidence of neoplasia including cytoplasmic (usually amphophilia), luminal (wispy mucin or flocculent pink material), and miscellaneous other features such as perineural invasion; 5) unless the diagnosis of cancer is unequivocal consider the possibility that the appearance can be explained by one of the tumor-like lesions of the prostate (see chapter 7); and 6) use immunohistochemistry in selected instances. The gold standard for the diagnosis of prostatic carcinoma, however, still remains the hematoxylin and eosin–stained slide with the diagnosis usually being based on a constellation of histologic features that collectively indicate that malignant glands infiltrate the stroma (174,223, 242,281,304). In small foci, there is no set threshold for the minimum number of glands required for the diagnosis of cancer. While cancer may be diagnosable on the basis of one or two glands (provided, ideally, that two observers independently concur), at least three atypical glands fulfilling the criteria of carcinoma are usually required to make a confident diagnosis (174,236,281). In difficult cases a reasonable number of levels of each core should be examined, three levels per core being common in North America (206a)

Table 4-6

FEATURES HELPFUL IN ESTABLISHING A DIAGNOSIS OF LIMITED ADENOCARCINOMA OF THE PROSTATE IN NEEDLE BIOPSY SPECIMENS*

Features	Frequency
Nuclear enlargement	77–96%
Infiltrative pattern	88%
Prominent nucleoli	64–76%
Pink, amorphous secretions	53–72%
Amphophilic cytoplasm	36–39%
Blue-tinged mucinous secretions	18–34%
Associated high-grade prostatic intraepithelial neoplasia	13–40%
Nuclear hyperchromasia	30%
Intraluminal crystalloids	13–22%
Mitotic figures	2–11%
Perineural invasion	2–3%
Collagenous micronodules	2%

*Data from references 242 and 396.

When a diagnosis of carcinoma cannot be certain, descriptive designations such as "atypical small acinar proliferation" or "atypical glands suspicious for carcinoma" have been recommended (220,238,386). This is usually required when the number of atypical acini is such that the pathologist feels unable to make an unequivocal diagnosis of carcinoma, and factors such as suboptimal cytologic preservation may also be involved. The frequency with which such terminology is utilized will depend on the experience of the individual pathologist and the nature of the material being reviewed. It will be used much more often in needle biopsy material than in transurethral resection material. In a study of over 1,000 consecutive prostatic needle biopsy specimens from a community hospital practice, this interpretation accounted for almost 5 percent of the diagnoses (223). In another recent analysis of biopsy results from private practice settings, 2.9 percent of specimens had "suspicious" foci only (356a). In another large study of needle biopsies, an uncertain diagnosis was rendered in 7.1 percent of cases (351a). In our experience, the two dominant findings which result in an equivocal interpretation in these cases are the small number of atypical acini and the relative dearth of prominent nucleoli. Additionally, in some cases the presence of immediately adjacent high-grade PIN makes it difficult to rule out tangential sectioning of the latter as a cause for one or two atypical acini, although in general, coexistent PIN is good circumstantial support for a diagnosis of cancer. It should be borne in mind from the management viewpoint that in the current experience approximately 50 percent of cases diagnosed as "atypical small acinar proliferation" or essentially similar other terms are from patients subsequently proven to have prostatic adenocarcinoma (174a,220,396).

A PATTERN-BASED APPROACH TO THE DIFFERENTIAL DIAGNOSIS OF PROSTATIC CARCINOMA

The differential diagnosis of primary prostatic adenocarcinoma is complex (271,386,397). In many instances the differential is with normal prostatic tissue since the usual needle biopsy typically procures peripheral zone tissue, and this has been discussed in the preceding needle biopsy section. A wide variety of normal non-prostatic structures; benign pathologic processes such as inflammation, atrophy, metaplasia, hyperplasia, and treatment effects; and secondary tumors (see chapter 5) can simulate prostatic carcinoma to varying degrees. The various carcinomas, some of them discussed in chapter 5, and benign lesions they may be confused with are presented in Table 4-7. Most of the non-neoplastic lesions are presented in chapter 7, with comments on differential diagnosis, and the differential diagnosis of adenocarcinoma is restricted here to a consideration of each of the common patterns of prostatic adenocarcinoma, namely, small glandular, large glandular (including papillary and cribriform), fused glandular, clear cell, and solid. The various features that facilitate a diagnosis of carcinoma in general have already been discussed in the prior section and only aspects particular to these patterns are presented here.

A uniform theme, which is applicable to carcinoma of the prostate in its various guises as has already been emphasized, is that the diagnosis of cancer is made on the basis of a pattern or cytologic appearance that is different from that of hyperplasia in any of its forms or, of course, normal prostate. The importance of each of these two criteria is variable from case to case. For example, in cases of so-called pseudohyperplastic carcinoma cytologic evaluation is crucial even though there may be some subtle differences on low-power magnification compared to the appearance of hyperplasia. On the other hand, in many carcinomas, for example those in the grade 4 category, cursory evaluation of the architecture clearly mandates a diagnosis of carcinoma almost irrespective of cytologic features. The morphology must also be inconsistent with any of the specific mimics of carcinoma of diverse types (see chapter 7). Also, the morphology and pattern of involvement of the gland must be inconsistent with secondary involvement for the diagnosis of primary prostatic carcinoma to be rendered. Although architectural features often make the diagnosis of adenocarcinoma straightforward, confirmation of the diagnosis on cytologic grounds is often crucial, particularly in cases with limited diagnostic tissue, as emphasized above in the section on needle biopsies.

Small Glandular Pattern

Cases in this general category account for the majority of problematic interpretations since they exemplify the very common problem of distinguishing a Gleason grade 3B adenocarcinoma from atrophy, the most common mimic of so-called small acinar carcinoma, and miscellaneous other benign conditions. Key points in the differential diagnosis are presented in Table 4-8, and each individual benign lesion is considered on its own in chapter 7. Identification of true invasion is a crucial architectural aspect in the evaluation of these cases. In some cases atypical acini may be seen dissecting between benign glands and are therefore recognizable as clearly infiltrative, but this helpful growth feature is not always present. Nuclear features are critical for the confirmation of a diagnosis of small acinar carcinoma in the latter cases. The cytoplasmic features are varied: amphophilic (usually), eosinophilic, or basophilic cytoplasm may be seen. In a subset of Gleason grade 3 adenocarcinomas, the cytoplasm is relatively scant and causes particular difficulty in the distinction from atrophy if infiltration is not easily judged to be present and if the nuclear features of carcinoma are not striking.

Table 4-7

**TYPES OF PROSTATIC CARCINOMA
AND BENIGN CONDITIONS THEY MAY BE CONFUSED WITH**

Carcinoma	Benign Condition
Gleason 1, 2, and 3A,B adenocarcinoma	Atypical adenomatous hyperplasia (adenosis) Postatrophic hyperplasia Basal cell hyperplasia Nephrogenic adenoma Verumontanum mucosal gland hyperplasia Hyperplasia of mesonephric remnants
Gleason 3B carcinoma with "atrophic features"	Atrophy
Gleason 3C (cribriform) adenocarcinoma	Cribriform hyperplasia Normal central zone
Gleason 4B carcinoma	Granulomatous prostatitis Paraganglia
Gleason 5B carcinoma	Chronic prostatitis
Foamy gland adenocarcinoma	Xanthogranulomatous prostatitis/Xanthoma Cowper's gland
Pseudohyperplastic carcinoma	Benign nodular hyperplasia
Oxyphilic carcinoma	Malakoplakia
Carcinoma with prominent luminal eosinophilic material	Hyperplasia of mesonephric remnants
Carcinoma with sclerotic stroma	Sclerosing adenosis Sclerotic atrophy
Carcinoma, not otherwise specified	Reactive atypia including radiation change Seminal vesicle/ejaculatory duct
Carcinoma with hormonal therapy effect	Histiocytic infiltrate Atrophy
Carcinoma with radiation change	Atrophy
Duct adenocarcinoma	Prostatic-type polyp
Signet ring cell carcinoma	Artifactual change in benign smooth muscle cells and lymphocytes
Squamous cell carcinoma	Squamous metaplasia
Basaloid carcinoma	Basal cell hyperplasia
Transitional cell carcinoma	Transitional cell metaplasia
Small cell carcinoma	Chronic inflammation (especially if "squeeze" artifact)
Sarcomatoid carcinoma	Postoperative spindle cell nodule Inflammatory pseudotumor

In these cases, which have been descriptively referred to as "atrophic" adenocarcinomas, a combination of the growth pattern and nuclear appearance permits their recognition (fig. 4-53). Although recently re-emphasized (226,241,311), almost half a century ago Lewis (320) noted the similarities between atrophic acini and small neoplastic acini. Indeed, the similarity between many grade 3B adenocarcinomas and atrophic acini has been a major reason for emphasizing

cytologic features in the diagnosis of prostatic carcinoma, as pointed out by Totten et al. in their classic study (397) (see their figures 3A, 4, and 7). In one series, almost 16 percent of prostatic adenocarcinomas had cytoplasmic features that were similar to those of benign atrophic acini (311). The absence of a basal cell layer is helpful, and in difficult cases the judicious use of basal cell–specific cytokeratin immunostains (clone 34βE12) may be important (see page 192) (226,241).

Large Glandular Pattern

This category includes well-differentiated tumors (Gleason grades 1 and 2) that may be difficult to distinguish from atypical adenomatous hyperplasia or conventional nodular hyperplasia (204,268,269); the latter is included in the differential of so-called pseudohyperplastic carcinoma (see page 140). This category also includes tumors of Gleason grade 3C in which cribriform and papillary patterns are typically present, as well as some grade 5A neoplasms. Helpful features indicative of carcinoma include an abnormal architectural relationship with a haphazard distribution of large glandular elements in the stroma, a lack of luminal maturation of the cells, and packing of epithelial units together without intervening stroma such that stromal invasion can be inferred. Basal cells are generally absent around the periphery of the malignant foci. Moderate- to high-grade nuclear changes are usually present in grade 3C or 5A tumors, and in the latter comedonecrosis supports a malignant interpretation. The distinction between Gleason grade 3C carcinoma and high-grade PIN is discussed in chapter 3. In well-differentiated tumors with large glands cytologic features of carcinoma are also present on high-power evaluation although they are not as striking as with higher grade neoplasms. Another tumor with large glands that frequently contains necrotic luminal material, colorectal adenocarcinoma, rarely may be in the differential with grade 5A tumors, but a combination of the classic histologic features of colorectal carcinoma and the clinical findings make this an exceptionally rare realistic diagnostic challenge. In the rare situation in which it might be a consideration, immunostains for prostate markers should be definitive.

Fused Glandular Pattern

Fusion of glandular units is a useful criterion of prostatic adenocarcinoma and with occasional exceptions indicates a Gleason grade 4 tumor. The diagnosis is usually obvious: there are typically abnormal nuclear features including nucleolar prominence, and, in the occasional case in which there are not, architectural features such as confluent growth are diagnostic. On occasion, fused glandular elements of grade 4 carcinoma are difficult to distinguish from cribriform structures of Gleason grade 3C, but the individual fused glands are smaller and the masses of fused glands usually have more irregular or scalloped peripheral borders than the round, smooth borders of the cribriform structures of grade 3C.

Clear Cell Pattern

Two relatively common forms of adenocarcinoma have a clear cell morphology: the raggedly irregular pattern of Gleason 4B tumors and the clear cell pattern which is frequently seen in low-grade transition zone carcinomas. It is important that these two cancers be distinguished because of striking differences in prognosis. The 4B pattern, usually seen in peripheral zone carcinomas, is composed of individual acini, cells, and nests that typically fuse and infiltrate widely in the prostatic stroma. The cytoplasm is clear to bubbly and frequently the nuclei are small and dark, often with inconspicuous nucleoli. In contrast, the clear cell transition zone carcinoma is characterized by variably sized, usually separated acini, ranging from small through, more typically, medium to large and sometimes cystically dilated; they are often lined by cuboidal to columnar cells with abundant apical clear cytoplasm. The nuclei are enlarged and nucleoli generally at least focally prominent. As mentioned below (see page 189), cytoplasmic clearing is also a feature typical of antiandrogen effect. As has already been discussed (see page 148), a subset of prostatic carcinomas is characterized by cells with exceedingly abundant foamy cytoplasm (350). These tumors are most often Gleason grade 3 or 4, and the abundant pale cytoplasm in these cases should not lead to a mistaken diagnosis of a grade 4 carcinoma if the pattern is not the fused glandular one that is diagnostic of that tumor type. It should also not lead to their erroneous placement in the category of a better differentiated neoplasm such as one in the Gleason grade 1 or 2 grouping.

Solid Pattern

The solid pattern of poorly differentiated adenocarcinoma has a differential diagnosis which includes inflammatory processes and other poorly differentiated neoplasms. Both granulomatous inflammation and malakoplakia are discussed in chapter 7. The carcinomas that enter the differential diagnosis of solid high-grade

Table 4-8

SMALL ACINAR PATTERNS IN THE PROSTATE: DIFFERENTIAL DIAGNOSTIC FEATURES THAT ARE FREQUENTLY HELPFUL*

Entity	Architecture	Cytology	Other Features
Simple (lobular) atrophy	Lobular configuration Often larger central duct Two cell layers	Scant cytoplasm Shrunken, hyperchromatic, uniform, small nuclei	Peripheral zone (usually) May be treatment related HMCK positive**
Sclerotic atrophy	As for simple (lobular) atrophy Stromal sclerosis	As above	Lymphohistiocytic reaction HMCK positive
Postatrophic hyperplasia	Lobular arrangement, often vague Variability in shape and size of glands	Cytoplasmic blebs Nuclei hyperchromatic Occasional enlarged nucleoli	Inflammation + atrophy may be nearby HMCK positive
Small glandular variant of nodular hyperplasia	Well circumscribed Two cell layers Hyperplastic stroma between glands	Bland nuclei	Association with ordinary nodular hyperplasia and location in TZ
Atypical adenomatous hyperplasia	Well circumscribed, rarely infiltrative Variable-sized acini Often parent duct Two cell layers (discontinuous)	Mild cytologic atypia Occasional enlarged nuceoli	Often multifocal TZ lesion HMCK positive in discontinuous pattern Occasional cystalloids and mucin
Basal cell hyperplasia	Multiple layers of basal cells Hyperplastic stroma between nests	Scant, basophilic cytoplasm Basal cells may have "prominent" nucleoli Central secretory cells may be present	Occasional calcification Association with ordinary nodular hyperplasia HMCK positive
Sclerosing adenosis	Well circumscribed or pseudoinfiltrative Distorted acini Cellular fibrous or myxoid stroma	Mild cytologic atypia May have enlarged nucleoli Basal cells present	S-100-, smooth muscle actin-, and HMCK-positive basal cells
Nephrogenic adenoma	Haphazard arrangement Cystic dilatation of some tubules Suburothelial location	Combination of eosinophilic, cuboidal, and hobnail cells Usually lack prominent nucleoli	Clinical history of inciting agent (e.g., TUR) PSA and PAP negative
Verumontanum mucosal gland hyperplasia	Well circumscribed Back-to-back acini Two cell layers	Bland nuclei	Suburethral location Associated transitional epithelial-lined ducts Corpora amylacea Orange-brown concretions
Mucinous metaplasia	Usually peripheral zone Involves preexisting normal or atrophic glands Double layered	Mucinous cytoplasm Bland nuclei	Mucin positive HMCK positive

Table 4-8 (continued)

Entity	Architecture	Cytology	Other Features
Mesonephric duct remnants	Vaguely lobular Single cell layer Micropapillary infoldings May involve nerves or extend beyond prostate	Cuboidal cells Bland nuclei	Colloid-like luminal content PSA and PAP negative HMCK positive
Seminal vesicles/ ejaculatory duct	Noninfiltrative Sometimes cleft-like, or central branching duct Double-layered epithelium	Spotty nucleomegaly Hyperchromasia Lipofuscin pigment Intranuclear cytoplasmic inclusions	PSA and PAP negative HMCK-positive basal layer
Cowper's gland	Lobular, closely packed acini Single-layered epithelium Excretory duct Skeletal muscle at periphery	Voluminous, mucinous cytoplasm Small, basally located bland nuclei	Apical location Positive for acid and neutral mucins; HMCK positive PAS and PAP negative
Paraganglion	Organoid Lumina absent	Polygonal cells Oval, dark nuclei Amphophilic finely granular or clear cytoplasm	Associated with small nerves Chromogranin positive
Small acinar carcinoma	Small, usually separated Typically irregularly distributed May interdigitate between and around clearly benign glands	Variable cytologic atypia Nucleomegaly Parachromatin clearing Frequent prominent nucleoli	See Table 4-6

*Modified from reference 386.
**Abbreviations: HMCK = high molecular weight cytokeratin (34βE12); PSA = prostate-specific antigen; PAP = prostatic-specific acid phosphatase; TUR = transurethral resection; TZ = transition zone.

prostatic adenocarcinoma of conventional type are discussed in chapter 5, and the important role of immunohistochemistry in the differential with bladder cancer involving the prostate is discussed on page 196.

HISTOLOGIC GRADING

The earliest approaches to the grading of prostatic cancer were based on the four-grade Broders system (213). Since then, numerous systems have been developed (186,192,195,210,263,272,273, 289,343,346,348,376–378,399), the most common of which are contrasted in Table 4-9. They can be grouped into methods based solely on architectural criteria, those based on cytologic criteria, and those that take both into account. The most widely used system, and the one recommended by us, is the Gleason system (272,273,316). It has been used since the 1960s, has provided useful information for management and prognostication (275,341), and is practical (184). The system was originally based on a large Veterans Administration study of patients with prostatic adenocarcinoma (215,272,275,341). The basic Gleason patterns have been described above. The Gleason system can be applied using low- and intermediate-power objectives (273). The pattern which is most prevalent in terms of surface area of involvement is defined as the primary grade. The next most prevalent pattern is referred to as the secondary grade. The two grades are added together to arrive at a Gleason score which ranges from 2 (1+1) to 10 (5+5). If only one pattern is seen, the grade is doubled to yield a score on the 2 to 10 scale. The most common primary and

Table 4-9

GRADING SYSTEMS FOR PROSTATE ADENOCARCINOMA: SUMMARIES

Gleason	Broders and Mostofi (WHO)	M.D. Anderson	Böcking	Gaeta	Helpap
Pattern 1: Lobular aggregate of closely packed, single, separate, rounded, relatively uniform glands	Grade 1: Well differentiated, with slight nuclear anaplasia	Grade 1: 75–100% of tumor composed of glands	Grade 1: Uniform glands with or without nuclear and nucleolar variation	Grade 1: Single separate glands; small nuclei with inconspicuous nucleoli	Grade 1a: Well-differentiated glands
Pattern 2: Same as pattern 1, except for less uniformity of gland spacing and shape; limited infiltration	Grade 2: Moderately to poorly differentiated, with moderate nuclear anaplasia	Grade 2: 50–75% of tumor composed of glands	Grade 2: Cribriform, without nuclear anaplasia, or pleomorphic glands and small glands with variable nuclear and nucleolar size	Grade 2: Small or medium glands; pleomorphic nuclei with nucleolomegaly	Grade 1b: Moderately differentiated glands
Pattern 3: Separate, often irregular glands including cribriform and papillary patterns	Grade 3: Poorly differentiated, with marked nuclear anaplasia, or undifferentiated carcinoma	Grade 3: 25–50% of tumor composed of glands	Grade 3: Cribriform, with enlarged nuclei and nucleoli, or sheets of cells without glands and variable nuclear and nucleolar size	Grade 3: Small glands, including cribriform and scirrhous patterns; pleomorphic nuclei with nucleomegaly	Grade 2a:: Poorly differentiated, with moderate nuclear and nucleolar atypia or mixed pattern with minor cribriform component
Pattern 4: Fused glands and cords, solid and cribriform patterns; may be clear cells		Grade 4: 0–25% of tumor composed of glands		Grade 4: Sheets of cells without glands; nuclei and nucleoli of any size; mitotic figures >3 per high-power field	Grade 2b: Poorly differentiated with marked nuclear and nucleolar atypia, or mixed pattern with chiefly cribriform pattern
Pattern 5: Few or no glands; tumor in sheets or comedo pattern					Grade 3: Solid trabecular pattern with marked atypia, with or without cribriform pattern

*Modified from reference 423.

secondary grade is 3. Frequently, minor tertiary and quaternary patterns are also present, and these are usually ignored unless they are of a higher grade (272,341). Where three grades are present, and the second and third account for roughly the same amount of tumor, the higher grade is chosen for the purpose of Gleason scoring.

Gleason scoring of needle biopsy specimens has been criticized because of sampling issues. Indeed, about 30 to 45 percent of such specimens are undergraded when compared to the final prostatectomy grade (194,266,318,344). However, this is most often seen in low-grade tumors present in small amounts (194); for cases with intermediate to high-grade scores (6 and above) there is reasonably good correlation with the Gleason score in the prostatectomy specimen (266,318,344, 351,384). Recent studies using 18-gauge thin-core needles have shown similar results to those obtained with thicker core needles. There is a good correlation of the Gleason grade on needle biopsies even with minimal tumor (less than 1 mm) (396). Accordingly, when there is sufficient material to make a confident diagnosis of carcinoma, a Gleason grade should be assigned. This approach is in line with the recommendations of a consensus conference to provide Gleason grades if at all possible (174).

As mentioned earlier, Gleason grade 1 neoplasms are virtually never diagnosed in needle biopsy material since they are generally found in the transition zone, and a smooth pushing interface with the surrounding stroma cannot be clearly established because of the small caliber of the needle cores.

Gleason 2 neoplasms are also rare and difficult to diagnose in needle biopsy specimens. The acini have some variation in size and shape, and there is limited infiltration of the stroma. There should be no malignant acini between preexisting benign glands in a Gleason grade 2 tumor. When microacini are found between preexisting, clearly benign glands, the tumor is grade 3, and indeed this is the most common pattern seen in needle biopsy specimens.

Any degree of acinar fusion indicates Gleason grade 4. Even tiny areas of Gleason grade 4 tumor should be noted in a needle biopsy. Commonly, the primary Gleason grade is 3, and there are minor, often subtle areas of Gleason grade 4, yielding a score of 7/10. The lack of recognition of minor areas of grade 4 is a common explanation for "undergrading" of needle biopsy material. In radical prostatectomy cases, the most common Gleason score is 7. Another important problem is the undergrading of the hypernephroid (Gleason 4B) pattern. While glandular fusion may be inconspicuous, and some nests may contain lumens, the presence of solid, often closely packed nests of cells with abundant clear to foamy cytoplasm and small dark nuclei should point to the correct diagnosis.

The higher grade patterns such as comedo-cribriform, solid, cord-like, and miscellaneous other patterns of poorly differentiated carcinoma are usually readily identified as Gleason grade 5.

Numerous studies have confirmed the value of the Gleason scoring system (274,395) which has shown strong correlations with many parameters, including clinical stage, acid phosphatase levels, PSA levels, lymph node status, and survival. The fundamental conclusion of the Veterans Administration study was that the behavior of prostatic adenocarcinoma relates more to the average of the architectural patterns rather than to the worst area (273). This result differs from most other tumor systems in which cancers generally behave according to the most poorly differentiated foci. More recent data suggest, however, that any grade 4 tumor in a prostatic neoplasm is adverse, and patients with tumors with a primary grade of 4 and secondary grade of 3 do worse than those with tumors of primary grade 3 and secondary grade 4 (fig. 4-53) (293a). Moreover, some data suggest that in radical prostatectomy tissues the amount (percentage) of grade 4 and 5 carcinoma is an important prognostic factor (253b).

PATHOLOGIC STAGING AND PATTERNS OF SPREAD AND METASTASES

The pathologic staging of prostatic carcinoma is displayed, along with the clinical staging, in Table 4-3. There is no pT1 category because the amount of tissue available is insufficient to permit evaluation for a possible higher pT category. The criteria for the clinical stage T1 cases are discussed on page 116.

The pT2 category is used for those cancers that are treated by prostatectomy and found to be organ confined, with no evidence of extraprostatic extension. The term "extraprostatic extension" has been adopted to replace other terms including capsular penetration and capsular perforation (200,374). Those cases that involve only one lobe (side) of the gland are considered pT2a, whereas those that involve both sides are considered pT2b. Invasion into, but not beyond, the so-called capsule is very common in peripheral zone tumors, and is not considered prognostically important (fig. 4-66A) (180,225,249,326,328,332,333,337,358,369, 389). Currently, therefore, cases with capsular invasion without extraprostatic extension are still considered to be in the pT2 category. A recent study, however, found that in completely examined specimens capsular invasion without extraprostatic extension had some adverse prognostic impact and that all tumors that lacked any capsular invasion did not progress (411).

The pT3 category applies to those tumors treated by prostatectomy which are found to

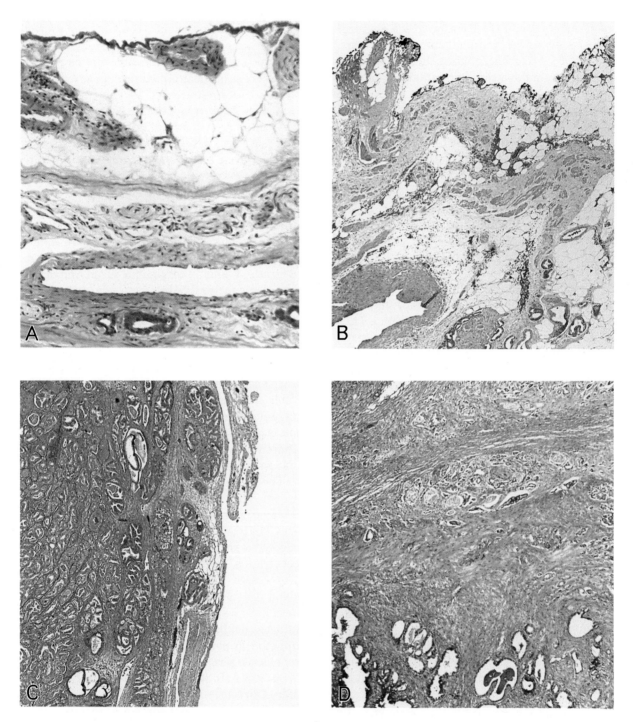

Figure 4-66
PROSTATIC ADENOCARCINOMA: LOCAL SPREAD

A: There is tumor within the capsule without extraprostatic extension. This is extremely common in peripheral zone carcinomas. Note the absence of tumor in periprostatic fat.

B: Focal extraprostatic extension shows obvious, but limited, involvement of periprostatic fat in one relatively small area. The inked surgical margin of the specimen is seen at the top and is free of involvement.

C: There is extensive spread through the capsule into the periprostatic fat, representing "established extraprostatic extension" because of the amount of tumor beyond the capsule.

D: Established extraprostatic extension is present because of obvious extensive spread beyond the gland boundary which is seen at the bottom. A fibrotic reaction to the invasive tumor has largely effaced the periprostatic fat.

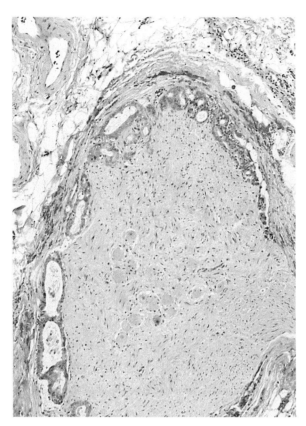

Figure 4-67
PROSTATIC ADENOCARCINOMA
WITH EXTRAPROSTATIC EXTENSION
The tumor encircles a neurovascular bundle in the periprostatic fat.

the involvement is more extensive. Extraprostatic extension is usually confirmed by finding neoplastic acini admixed with, or immediately juxtaposed to, adipocytes. Since fat is very rarely present in the substance of the prostate gland (229a), this almost always indicates extraprostatic spread. The most common site of extraprostatic extension is posterolateral along the neurovascular bundles. In this region there tends to be more adipose tissue attached to a radical prostatectomy specimen than elsewhere, and, additionally, tumor spreads along nerves and in soft tissue adjacent to nerves and vessels (180). The presence of neoplastic acini within extraprostatic neurovascular bundles, or spaces around them, is also a good indicator of extraprostatic spread, even if the neoplastic acini are not in direct contact with adipose tissue (fig. 4-67) (187). Occasionally, even in the absence of adipose tissue involvement (which may be effaced by invasive tumor and an associated connective tissue response), tumor can be easily judged to be clearly present beyond the normal contour of the prostatic edge and therefore to exhibit extraprostatic extension (fig. 4-66D). This situation is particularly likely to occur with large transition zone tumors that extend through the anterior fibromuscular stroma to involve adjacent connective tissue in a region deficient in adipose tissue. Desmoplasia in association with the invasive tumor can be particularly pronounced in cases in which neoadjuvant therapy has been given. The assessment of extraprostatic extension can be especially problematic at the anterolateral surface, apex, and base; the capsule is absent in these locations and there is a gradual merging of the anterior fibromuscular stroma with periprostatic smooth and skeletal muscle, and the prostate base blends imperceptibly with the smooth muscle of the bladder neck. Benign glands and skeletal muscle are normally admixed at the apex (see page 332) so involvement of skeletal muscle bundles by carcinoma in this location does not equate with extraprostatic extension.

When the tumor extensively invades local structures to involve the bladder, external sphincter, rectum, levator muscles, or pelvic wall, it is considered in the pT4 category.

Involvement of perineural spaces is extremely prevalent in prostatic adenocarcinoma; intraprostatic, capsular, or extraprostatic nerves may

extend outside the gland. Those cases that extend extraprostatically (unilateral or bilateral) but lack seminal vesicle involvement are considered pT3a, whereas tumors with seminal vesicle invasion (i.e., involving the muscular wall of the seminal vesicle) are considered pT3b. There are no data to suggest a worse outcome in patients with bilateral extraprostatic extension as opposed to those with unilateral extension. Quantifying the amount of tumor beyond the capsule in category pT3a cases into two subcategories, focal extraprostatic extension and established extraprostatic extension, has been shown to be of prognostic importance (253a,281a,411). The designation "focal extraprostatic extension" is used for cases in which there are only a few neoplastic glands outside the prostate in the periprostatic soft tissue and the term "established extraprostatic extension" is used when

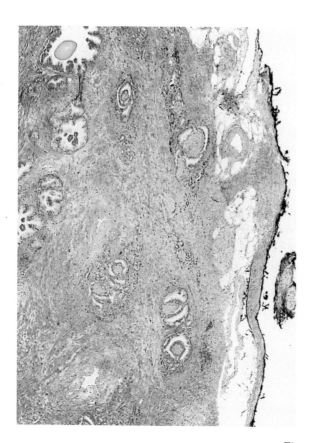 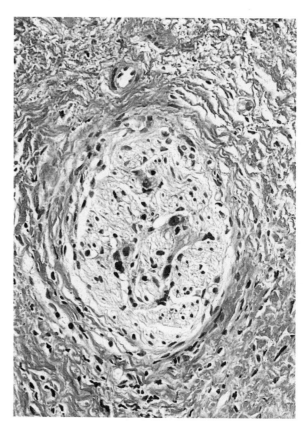

Figure 4-68
PROSTATIC ADENOCARCINOMA INVOLVING NERVES
There is circumferential perineural infiltration on the left and intraneural involvement on the right.

be involved (fig. 4-68, left) (240,244,368,404). Perineural involvement may represent a pathway of least resistance for the spread of neoplasm and appears to be a common mechanism for spread through the capsule to periprostatic fat (187,286,403). Sometimes, tumors located in the basal portion of the gland spread along the capsule and perineural spaces to reach extracapsular tissue. Occasionally, intraneural spread may also be seen (fig. 4-68, right). Ganglia and paraganglia may also be involved by tumor.

Most clinically significant carcinomas arise in the peripheral zone of the prostate, and those associated with local invasion usually have volumes greater than 1 to 2 cm^3 (255,300,326,332, 333,389). In some cases large peripheral zone carcinomas may extend anteriorly to involve the urethra (fig. 4-69), in which case they may clinically mimic a primary urethral tumor.

An important pathway of spread of prostatic adenocarcinoma, especially those arising in the peripheral zone, is to the seminal vesicle (fig. 4-70) (244,347,352,410). Tumor may reach the seminal vesicle by a number of routes (244,410). Commonly, there is extraprostatic extension in the posterolateral regions with secondary involvement of the muscular coat of the seminal vesicle. Seminal vesicle involvement requires invasion of the muscle coat, not just involvement of the connective tissue adjacent to the seminal vesicles (fig. 4-71). In some instances, there may be direct invasion of the seminal vesicle from a tumor located at the base of the prostate gland. Prostatic adenocarcinoma may also spread to the connective tissue around the ejaculatory duct to involve the substance of the seminal vesicle and rarely may involve the seminal vesicle epithelium in a pagetoid fashion. Occasionally, there may be metastatic involvement of the seminal vesicle due to lymphatic spread.

Lymphatic vessels have been identified in the substance of the prostate as well as within the

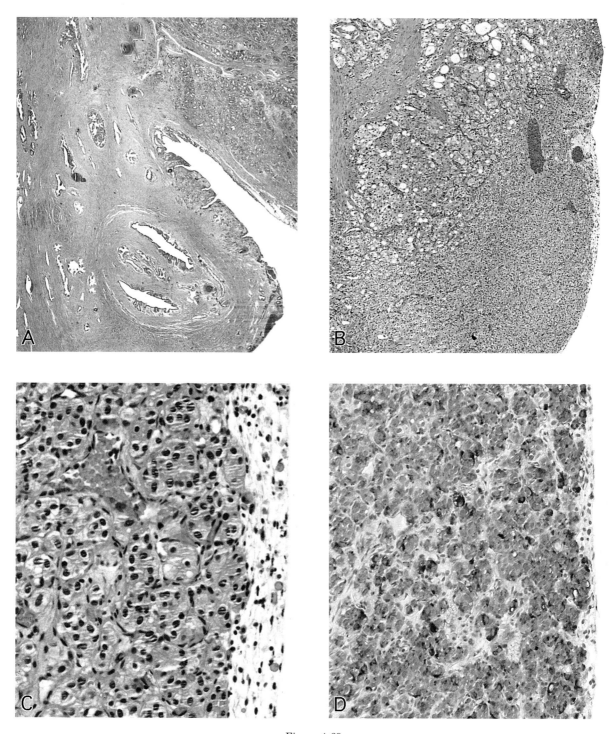

Figure 4-69
PROSTATIC ADENOCARCINOMA INVOLVING THE URETHRA

The submucosa of the urethra is involved in A (top). Note the dome-shaped verumontanum in the lower half of the illustration with its paired ejaculatory ducts surrounded by specialized stroma. Utricular glands are seen between the ejaculatory ducts. In another case there is submucosal involvement of the urethra (B and C) with the appearance in C closely resembling transitional cell carcinoma. The diagnosis of prostatic adenocarcinoma is indicated by an immunostain of the block represented in C which is positive for PSA (D). The small acinar features in B suggest the glandular differentiation of prostatic adenocarcinoma rather than that of transitional cell carcinoma; however, there is overlap in the morphology between these two neoplasms, and immunostains are indicated to aid in their distinction in cases of the type illustrated.

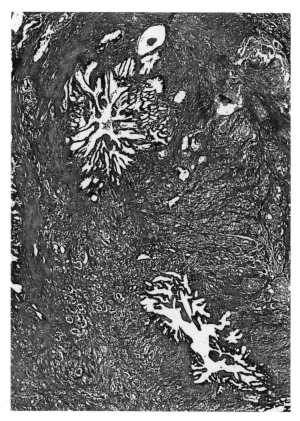

Figure 4-70
PROSTATIC ADENOCARCINOMA
A low-power photomicrograph shows extensive seminal vesicle involvement.

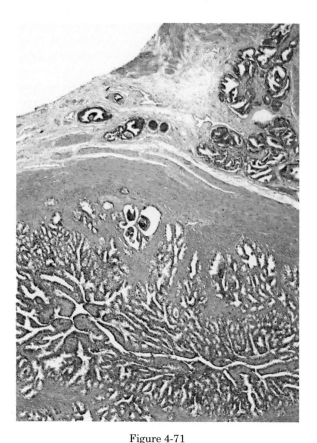

Figure 4-71
PROSTATIC ADENOCARCINOMA
This low-power view shows seminal vesicle with infiltrating carcinoma in the surrounding connective tissue. This does not constitute seminal vesicle invasion.

capsule and periprostatic tissue (382). Lymphatic invasion may be identified in tissues from radical prostatectomy specimens, and, on rare occasions, periurethral venous channels are also involved by tumor (183,375). Lymph-vascular involvement is more commonly seen in high-grade neoplasms (fig. 4-72) (375), but overall is still rare. The prognostic significance of vascular-lymphatic invasion in prostate cancer remains to be determined.

In radical prostatectomy specimens, prostatic carcinoma commonly extends close to, or to, the margins of resection (244,298,306,354,390,405). The apical, lateral, and posterior margins are most commonly affected; involvement of basal and anterior margins is much less frequent (244,337,405). The documentation of positive margins is very important since it correlates with other adverse pathologic factors and with

outcome (fig. 4-73) (191,201a,244,298,306,337, 390). The definition and biologic significance of tumor "closely" approaching the margin is uncertain (242), although a recent study suggests that close margins do not result in an increased risk of progression (254).

Prostatic carcinoma that has metastasized commonly involves regional lymph nodes, bone, and lung (198,393). The pelvic lymph nodes (obturator and iliac) are the first nodal sites of metastatic disease (211,293,315). Involvement may be macroscopic but is more commonly only identified on histologic examination. Early involvement consists of tiny subcapsular deposits of adenocarcinoma, usually with a fused glandular morphology. Involvement of perinodal soft tissue may be seen (fig. 4-74) (381). With more advanced disease, there is involvement of periaortic, intrathoracic, and cervical (especially

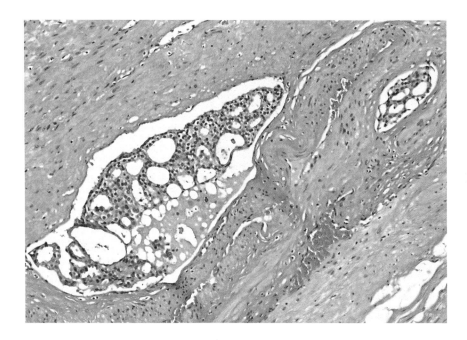

Figure 4-72
PROSTATIC
ADENOCARCINOMA
Lymphatic invasion is present.

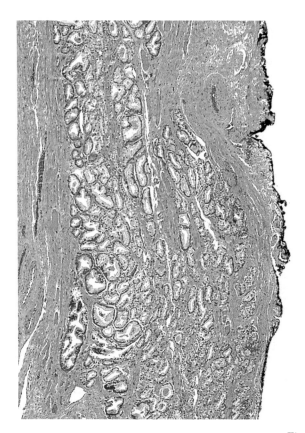 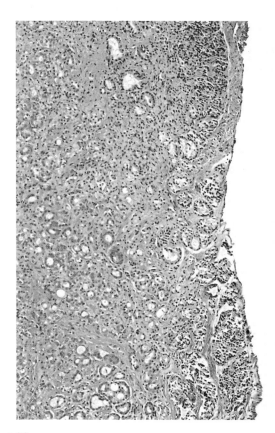

Figure 4-73
PROSTATIC ADENOCARCINOMA: MARGIN EVALUATION IN RADICAL PROSTATECTOMY SPECIMENS

On the left the tumor is close to, but not at, the margin. On the right the tumor reaches the inked margin of resection towards the bottom. A thin rim of uninvolved fibromuscular tissue is seen at the top. No extraprostatic tissue is present for evaluation of extraprostatic extension.

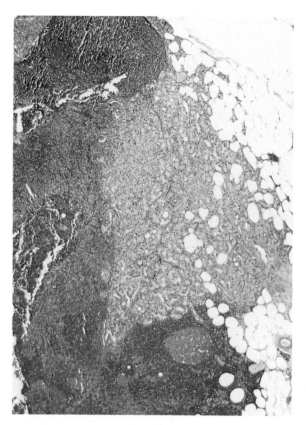

Figure 4-74
METASTATIC PROSTATIC ADENOCARCINOMA
A pelvic lymph node and the perinodal fat are involved.

left-sided supraclavicular) lymph nodes (211, 224,307,371,406,413), which may account for the clinical presentation.

In the PSA era, the rate of pelvic lymph node metastasis in radical prostatectomy series is low (246,276). The role of frozen section evaluation of pelvic lymph nodes prior to radical retropubic prostatectomy is somewhat controversial because of the relatively low rate of metastasis and the significant false negative rate, which may be related to surgical sampling, pathologic sampling, and technical difficulties in specimen processing. Frequently, the pelvic lymph nodes are quite fatty and difficult to analyze at frozen section (218,251). If an enlarged, clinically suspicious lymph node is encountered, frozen section should be obtained, and, if positive, the surgeon may elect not to proceed with the radical prostatectomy. In cases in which there are no clinically abnormal lymph nodes, the role of frozen section is not

entirely clear. If the urologist is committed to stop the operation based on the presence of even a single micrometastasis, then it may be justified to process all identifiable lymph node tissue, realizing that there will still be false negative results. When all factors are analyzed, including the low prevalence of nodal disease, the false negativity based on both surgical and pathologic sampling, and the additional time and expense required to carry out this procedure, it may be better to submit lymph node packets that are not clinically suspicious for permanent sections rather than for detailed frozen section analysis. Some urologists submit clinically negative lymph nodes for frozen section analysis based on information they consider places the patient at increased risk for occult metastases, including high Gleason grade and high PSA levels.

Hematogenous involvement usually manifests with osseous disease (233,372,388). The spinal column is most commonly involved, but the pelvis and appendicular skeleton may also be involved. The bony metastases are commonly osteoblastic (fig. 4-75). Spinal column involvement may lead to cord compression (370). Other sites of hematogenous spread include lungs, liver, and brain (388). Pulmonary involvement can be manifested as single or multiple nodules or, on occasion, an interstitial infiltrate secondary to extensive carcinomatosis (256). Central nervous system involvement is uncommon. Rarely, prostatic adenocarcinoma is associated with malignant ascites (219). The most common sites of metastatic disease at autopsy in two different series are presented in figure 4-76.

TREATMENT EFFECTS

Radiation Therapy

Radiation treatment is commonly used to treat locally advanced prostatic adenocarcinoma. Radiation can induce tumor necrosis and fibrosis, but in many instances, residual viable tumor is identified after completion of treatment (199,231,267, 290,294,322). When cribriform structures, fused glands, solid sheets, and cords are identified, the diagnosis can usually be made with confidence. In needle biopsies, distinguishing small acini with atypia induced by radiation (fig. 4-77) from microacinar carcinoma can be a difficult diagnostic

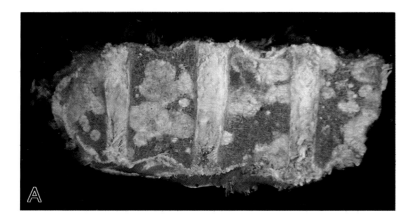

Figure 4-75
METASTATIC PROSTATIC
ADENOCARCINOMA TO BONE

There is extensive metastasis to the vertebral bodies (A). An osteoblastic metastasis (B) consists of a semi-circular area of increased bone formation with marrow fibrosis in the right two thirds of the illustration. A higher power view of an osteoblastic metastasis (C) shows numerous osteoblasts and almost nonexistent osteoclasts. The bony trabeculae show marked remodeling and the tumor fills the interosseous spaces. (B, C: Figs. 21 and 22 from Fascicles 31B and 32, 1st Series.)

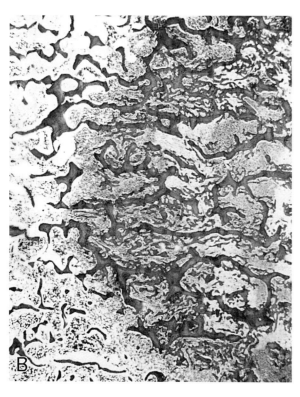

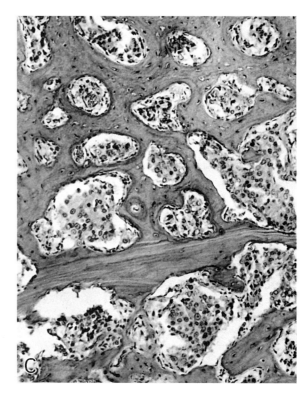

challenge (199,221a). An irregular distribution of acini in the stroma should increase the suspicion of cancer. The absence of basal cells is helpful, but at times the presence or absence of basal cells is difficult to judge because of acinar shrinkage and distortion. The application of a high molecular weight cytokeratin (clone 34βE12) stain may be useful to identify residual basal cells, thus excluding carcinoma (fig. 4-77) (208). The nuclear atypia associated with radiation can mimic that of carcinoma (267), although the spotty distribution of the atypia may be a clue in addition to the

history. Radiation may induce pleomorphism that often exceeds that of cancer. Immunostains for PSA help identify residual single or vacuolated tumor cells in the stroma that by routine light microscopy may mimic stromal cells with vacuolar change. It has been suggested that needle biopsy evaluation is of little value in the 12 months after radiation therapy because of the delayed manifestation of tumor cell death (231a,267). As yet, there is no valid method for assessing tumor viability after irradiation. In one study, strong immunoreactivity for PAP was

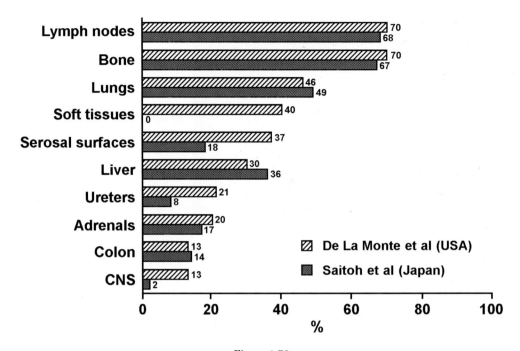

Figure 4-76
THE TEN MOST COMMON SITES OF PROSTATE CANCER METASTASES
AT AUTOPSY IN THE UNITED STATES AND JAPAN
(Fig. 4 from Bostwick DG, Eble JN. Prostatic adenocarcinoma metastatic to inguinal hernia sac. J Urol Pathol 1993;1:193–9).

identified in 23 of 27 irradiated adenocarcinomas, leading the authors to suggest that the tumor cells were capable of protein production and, by inference, may be able to divide and metastasize (323). In another study, the ultrastructural features of irradiated carcinoma were similar to untreated prostate carcinoma, suggesting that residual tumor was viable (313).

Estrogen and Androgen Deprivation Therapy

The morphologic effects induced by estrogen compounds such as diethylstilbestrol have been known for more that 50 years (309). There may be squamous metaplasia and individual tumor cells may display prominent cytoplasm, nuclear pyknosis, and loss of nucleoli (fig. 4-78, left) (236, 259,363,394). Irregular "empty" spaces representing remnants of shrunken neoplastic glands may be seen (fig. 4-78, right), similar to the changes seen with androgen deprivation therapy. Recent studies have analyzed the effects of anti-androgen neoadjuvant therapy, including total androgen blockade using drugs such as luteiniz-

ing hormone–releasing hormone agonists, flutamide, and cyproterone acetate (178,227,228, 258,276,287,317,345,349,380,383,398,400). The effects of finasteride, a 5-alpha-reductase inhibitor commonly used to treat hyperplastic and carcinomatous tissue, have recently been described (229). Finasteride produces less pronounced morphologic changes than other androgen deprivation strategies (414). In radical prostatectomy specimens, the neoadjuvant therapy leads to a reduction in tumor volume, reduced margin positivity, and an apparent down-staging effect, although the latter may be spurious.

Androgen deprivation has significant effects on both non-neoplastic and carcinomatous tissue. In non-neoplastic areas, there is pronounced glandular atrophy with shrinkage of the secretory cell compartment and basal cell prominence (fig. 4-79). Foci of basal cell hyperplasia are common, and squamous and transitional cell metaplasia may also be seen.

Carcinomatous glands exhibit shrinkage and cytoplasmic vacuolation (fig. 4-79). At times, there is a complete disappearance of the neoplastic acini leaving spaces, some of which may contain a

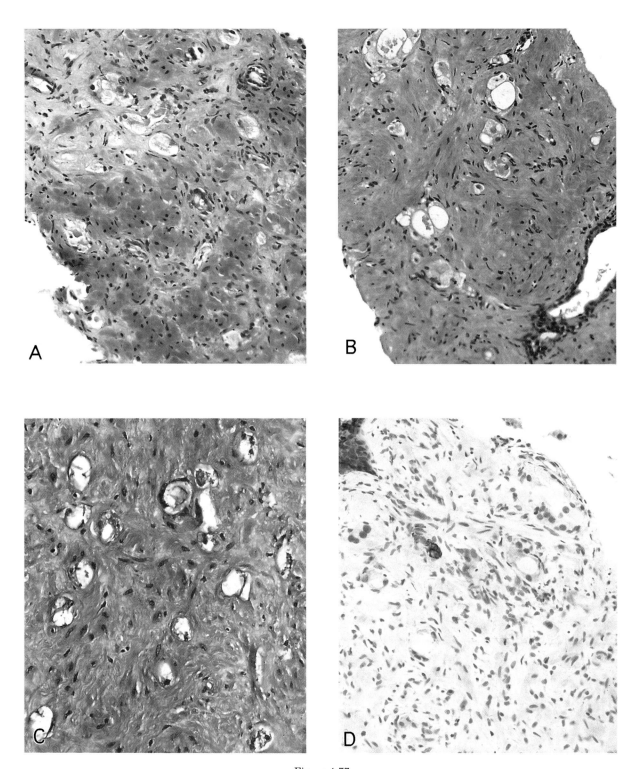

Figure 4-77
PROSTATIC ADENOCARCINOMA, POSTRADIATION TREATMENT

A,B: Needle biopsies show nests and acini composed of cells with abundant clear cytoplasm representing neoplastic glands. The non-neoplastic atrophic glands are lined by shrunken cells with a dark hyperchromatic appearance.

C: Some of the neoplastic glands contain blue-tinged luminal mucin.

D: An absence of high molecular weight cytokeratin (clone 34ßE12) staining is noted in the atypical glands. Occasional non-neoplastic glands showing cytokeratin-positive basal cells are noted. (Courtesy of Dr. D. Grignon, Detroit, MI.)

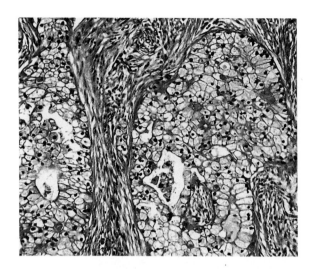 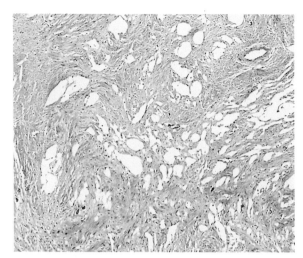

Figure 4-78
PROSTATIC ADENOCARCINOMA, POSTESTROGEN THERAPY
Left: Note the abundant clear cytoplasm.
Right: Shrunken glands have resulted in irregular "empty" spaces.

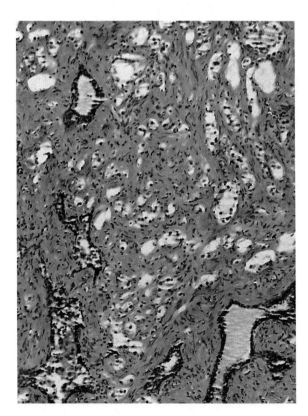 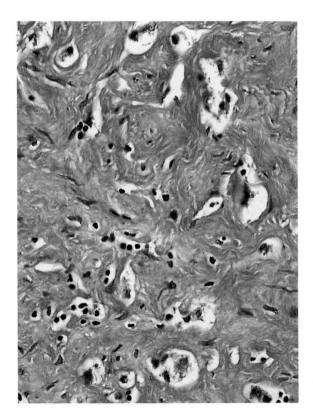

Figure 4-79
PROSTATIC ADENOCARCINOMA, POST-NEOADJUVANT ANDROGEN ABLATION THERAPY
Left: Note the atrophic non-neoplastic glands with a prominent basal cell layer. Numerous shrunken neoplastic acini with cytoplasmic clearing are seen in the stroma. In a few acini the epithelial cells are absent or barely perceptible, resulting in apparent empty spaces. Unless more obvious neoplastic acini are present, such spaces may be overlooked, and residual neoplasm not identified.
Right: Vacuolated cytoplasm and shrunken pyknotic nuclei are seen at high power.

mucosubstance which is highlighted with the alcian blue stain (fig. 4-80). This appearance has been likened to that of pseudomyxoma ovarii (398). Collagenous micronodules are often present and likely represent organization of extravasated mucin (fig. 4-81). Stromal proliferation resulting in a hemangiopericytoma-like appearance may be seen (fig. 4-80). Nuclear changes include nucleolysis, nuclear pyknosis, and fragmentation. Paneth cell–like change is sometimes prominent in treated carcinoma, and this correlates with increased numbers of neuroendocrine cells (fig. 4-81). The architectural changes associated with androgen deprivation therapy lead to an apparent worsening of the Gleason score when compared to the preoperative biopsy results (178,227,276,380,400). This change is likely spurious and related in great part to the cytoplasmic shrinkage and loss of lumens noted with the therapy. Studies utilizing DNA content and proliferating cell nuclear antigen (PCNA) have shown less proliferative activity in areas of apparently poor differentiation than in nontreated carcinomas with similar patterns, suggesting that the "upgrading" is artifactual (178). From a practical viewpoint, cases showing marked treatment effect should not be graded. In some situations, the neoadjuvant hormones have relatively little effect on tumor pattern, and in these situations a grade can be rendered, remembering not to overinterpret areas which superficially resemble Gleason grade 5 tumor. Some authors have advocated adjusting the Gleason score to compensate for the treatment effect, but this approach is not recommended since, in our opinion, some pseudo-grades 4 and 5 tumors in treated prostates cannot be reproducibly separated from de novo grades 4 and 5 (380). In some cases, residual carcinoma is very difficult to appreciate in the treated prostate tissue, and immunohistochemical stains for pancytokeratin and PSA are necessary to look for clandestine carcinoma cells (214). Stromal reactions, including a histiocytic infiltrate, may also mimic residual carcinoma cells, sometimes necessitating the use of macrophage and prostatic epithelial markers (see page 195). Antiandrogen therapy is one explanation for an apparent absence of carcinoma in a radical prostatectomy specimen, an event referred to as the "vanishing cancer phenomenon" (277).

Cryotherapy

In a number of centers, cryotherapy is being used to treat locally advanced tumors (182,230, 325,355). Postcryotherapy biopsies show a variety of histologic changes depending on the timing of the biopsy with respect to treatment (193,360, 379). Acute injury is manifested by necrosis, hemorrhage, and acute inflammation. Chronic changes include fibrosis, hyalinization, calcification, hemosiderin deposition, granulomatous inflammation, basal cell hyperplasia, and transitional and squamous metaplasia (fig. 4-82) (193, 284,379). Residual carcinoma is sometimes present, and it generally retains its original morphology and grade (193). Pathologic analysis of salvage prostatectomies performed after failed cryotherapy have revealed viable carcinoma in areas thought to be destroyed on intraoperative transrectal ultrasound (279).

SPECIAL STUDIES

A variety of special techniques have been used in cases of prostatic adenocarcinoma to facilitate diagnosis and to provide prognostic information. The diagnostic role of special studies, especially the morphologically based ones, is emphasized here. Newer phenotypic and especially genotypic studies show promise, especially in the area of prognosis (473).

Histochemistry

Mucin stains are not necessary in practice to assess the potential neoplastic nature of prostatic acini but will confirm the mucinous nature of the often blue-tinged luminal secretions frequently seen in neoplastic acini (419,495,510). While normal and hyperplastic prostatic glands may contain neutral mucosubstances, both neutral and acid mucopolysaccharides are found predominantly in neoplastic disease, including both prostatic intraepithelial neoplasia and adenocarcinoma (450,453,460,461). Usually, only small amounts of mucin are identified within lumens (fig. 4-39). The mucin can be highlighted using alcian blue and other stains for acid mucins according to individual preference. Other mimickers of adenocarcinoma such as atypical adenomatous hyperplasia (adenosis) may also contain acid mucin but less often than cancer (442).

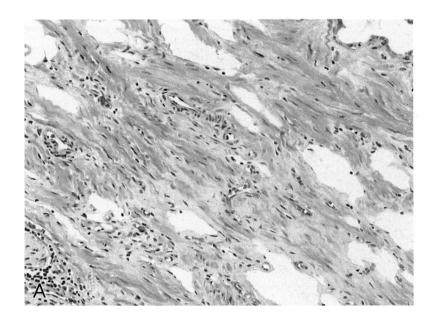

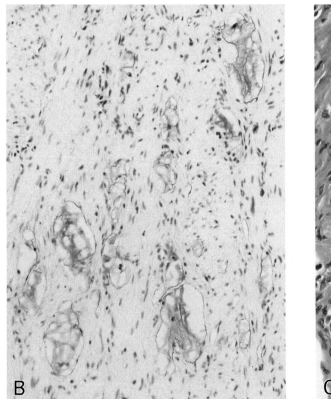

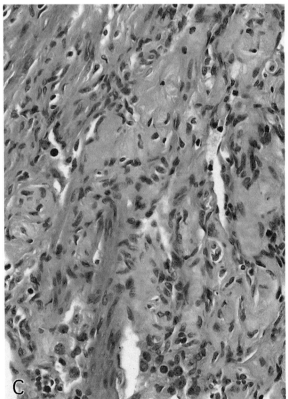

Figure 4-80
PROSTATIC ADENOCARCINOMA, POST-NEOADJUVANT ANDROGEN ABLATION THERAPY

A: Spaces within the fibromuscular stroma appear "empty" or contain faint, wispy, barely perceptible mucinous material.

B: Alcian blue stain shows abundant mucin within empty spaces.

C: Note the cellular stroma with a hemangiopericytoma-like vascular pattern. Occasional neoplastic cells, most with scant or virtually no cytoplasm and some appearing as "bare" nuclei, are seen.

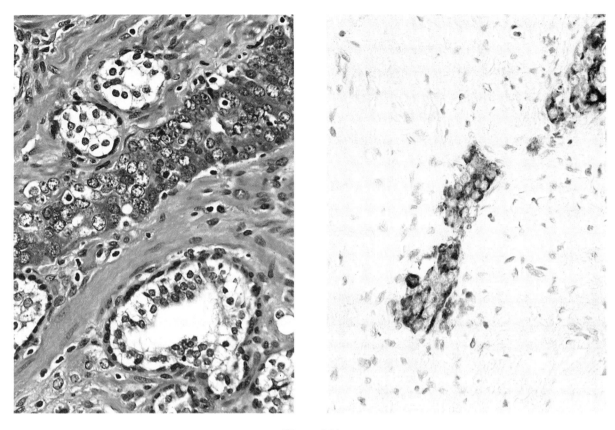

Figure 4-81
PROSTATIC ADENOCARCINOMA, POST-NEOADJUVANT ANDROGEN ABLATION THERAPY
Left: Note the neoplastic trabeculum with many cells that have eosinophilic granular cytoplasm resembling that of Paneth cells.
Right: A chromogranin stain is positive in the Paneth-like cells.

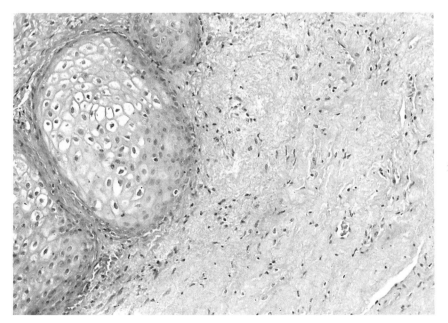

Figure 4-82
MORPHOLOGIC EFFECTS
OF CRYOTHERAPY
Late sequelae are represented by
fibrosis and squamous metaplasia.

Immunohistochemistry

Prostatic adenocarcinoma has been extensively studied with immunohistochemical markers. While the role of immunomarkers as providers of predictive or prognostic information remains to be established, a number of important diagnostic applications of immunohistochemistry have evolved (432,478,490); only these are discussed in this section.

High Molecular Weight Basal Cell–Specific Cytokeratin (34βE12). Broad spectrum keratins stain normal and hyperplastic secretory and basal cells along with cells of adenocarcinoma, but the high molecular weight (basal cell–specific) keratin, clone 34βE12, preferentially stains prostatic basal cells (428,493,514). Confirmation of the presence or absence of basal cells is helpful in the differential diagnosis of small acinar carcinoma (fig. 4-83) (432,457,459,489,490, 498,517). However, ductal spread of carcinoma may result in the presence of basal cells in cases of cancer (fig. 4-84, left) (339,359a). Also, overgrowth of benign glands by carcinoma represents another explanation for the presence of basal cells in carcinoma, analogous to the overgrowth of benign foci containing corpora amylacea by cancer in some cases (see fig. 4-41). In most cases of cancer in which basal cells are present the diagnosis of cancer is evident on other grounds and the application of pathologic "common sense" should preclude an erroneous diagnosis being made because one finding, admittedly one often helpful in pointing towards a different diagnosis, does not fit. It is also pertinent that several studies have shown that cancer cells themselves may be positive for high molecular weight cytokeratin in the prostate and at metastatic sites (fig. 4-84, right) (453a,475a). The frequency of this finding has ranged from relatively common to distinctly uncommon and is usually seen with high-grade tumors (453a,475a,512a,518a). The duration of fixation in formalin and type of antigen retrieval affect immunoreactivity (462a,512a) for high molecular weight cytokeratin and hence strict quality control is required. This may explain, at least in part, the differing rates of positivity for 34βE12 within carcinoma cells themselves just noted. The above comments not withstanding, use of high molecular weight cytokeratin immunostains remains a valuable tool in assessing prostate specimens for the presence of cancer (518a). Lesions such as lobular atrophy, postatrophic hyperplasia, sclerosing adenosis, and atypical adenomatous hyperplasia display at least focal 34βE12 positivity. When a minute, atypical, small acinar focus is encountered, especially in a needle biopsy, the absence of basal cells supported by immunohistochemistry may provide enough support to make a confident diagnosis of cancer (fig. 4-83). It is useful to save an unstained slide between two hematoxylin and eosin levels for this purpose (453b), and it is also important to have a positive internal control before concluding that a negative result in a suspicious focus is carcinoma. High molecular weight cytokeratin staining is also useful in irradiated or hormonally treated prostates to distinguish treatment effects from residual or recurrent adenocarcinoma (427). This stain is also used to help distinguish high-grade prostatic intraepithelial neoplasia and papillary-cribriform patterns of carcinoma: the presence of basal cells in a discontinuous fashion points to a diagnosis of the former, while a complete absence of basal cells suggests the latter (420). Unusual patterns of carcinoma, such as atrophic, may require confirmation by displaying a lack of high molecular weight cytokeratin–positive basal cells (430).

Prostatic-Specific Markers. Antibodies against prostate-specific antigen (PSA) and prostatic acid phosphatase (PAP) have been extensively studied in prostatic adenocarcinoma (423,424,429,432,469,475,483,490,518). One or both antibodies are usually positive in both primary and secondary lesions (432,441,446,484, 490,505). All Gleason patterns of prostatic adenocarcinoma are usually positive for PSA and PAP. The intensity of the immunoreactivity often varies from field to field, and it may be focal and weak or diffuse and strong. The lower grade tumors of acinar morphology generally show stronger reactivity than higher grade patterns, although wide variation in the staining intensity is commonplace. In a very small percentage of poorly differentiated prostatic adenocarcinomas, PSA and PAP are negative (424,440,468,507). In recent years prostate specific membrane (PSM) antigen, a membrane-bound antigen that is highly specific for benign and malignant prostate epithelial cells, has been shown to have maximal expression in high-grade (Gleason 4

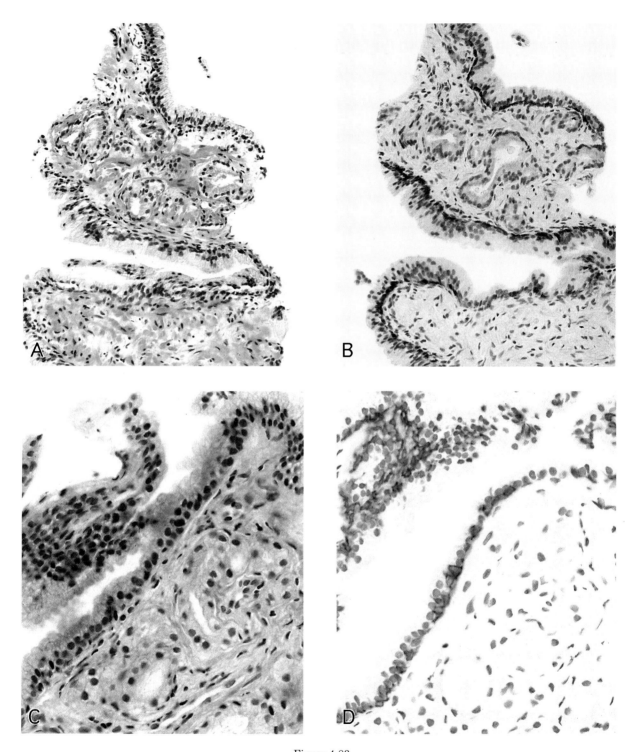

Figure 4-83
IMMUNOHISTOCHEMISTRY IN PROSTATIC PATHOLOGY

The use of high molecular weight basal cell–specific keratin (clone 34βE12) in supporting a diagnosis of prostatic adenocarcinoma.

A: An atypical small glandular focus suspicious for adenocarcinoma is seen in a needle biopsy specimen.

B: A negative 34βE12 keratin stain indicates the absence of basal cells and confirms the diagnosis of carcinoma. Note residual basal cells in non-neoplastic glands.

C,D: Similar findings in another case.

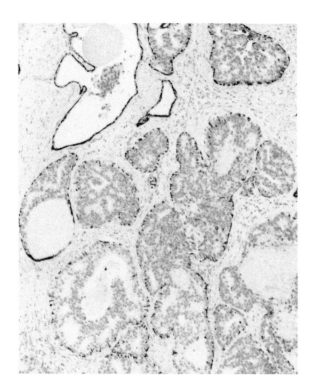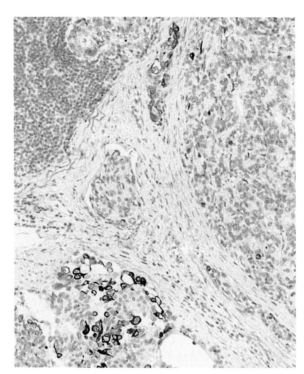

Figure 4-84
IMMUNOHISTOCHEMISTRY IN PROSTATIC PATHOLOGY

Left: This photomicrograph of prostatic adenocarcinoma within the gland shows prominent intraductal spread of carcinoma with the high molecular weight cytokeratin stain (clone 34βE12) displaying a liberal investment of basal cells in the periphery of the epithelial aggregates. Note a few non-neoplastic structures at the upper left. There is focal involvement of a non-neoplastic gland by carcinoma just above the 9 o'clock position. The expansive growth of carcinoma exhibited, in particular, by an elongated structure running vertically toward the right of the illustration argues strongly against a diagnosis of prostatic intraepithelial neoplasia as did the overall irregularity of the proliferation in this case.

Right: Metastatic carcinoma in a lymph node from the case illustrated on the left shows focal, striking cytoplasmic positivity with high molecular weight cytokeratin (clone 34βE12). A portion of the uninvolved nodal tissue is seen at the top left and tumor in a sinusoid is seen near the center of the illustration.

and 5 patterns) adenocarcinoma (425b). In contrast to PSA immunoreactivity which in general progressively decreases from benign prostate, to high-grade prostatic intraepithelial neoplasia, to cancer, PSM immunostaining shows an incremental immunoreactivity in the same spectrum of prostatic tissue.

Since normal, atrophic, hyperplastic, and carcinomatous glands are positive with these markers, PSA and PAP have a limited role in distinguishing prostatic adenocarcinoma from its mimics (432). Sometimes, florid granulomatous prostatitis may simulate high-grade carcinoma, necessitating the use of stains for PSA and PAP to confirm that the cells in the problematic focus are not prostatic epithelial cells (see chapter 7). Crushed inflammatory foci may also be a problem in the differential diagnosis with poorly dif-

ferentiated carcinoma, and the absence of PSA and PAP staining again helps support a benign interpretation. Xanthomatous inflammation may also mimic carcinoma, thus requiring immunohistochemistry to prove the identity of the cells (fig. 4-85) (497). PSA staining may be useful in separating small acinar carcinoma from adenotic seminal vesicle or ejaculatory duct, Cowper's gland, nephrogenic adenoma, and mesonephric duct remnants (465). PSA and PAP may also be used to identify the small tumor cells that are often difficult to visualize in cases of hormonally treated prostate cancer, although keratin stains are better in our experience (452).

The major role of prostatic-specific markers, however, is in the investigation of metastatic adenocarcinoma of unknown primary and poorly differentiated carcinomas involving the lower

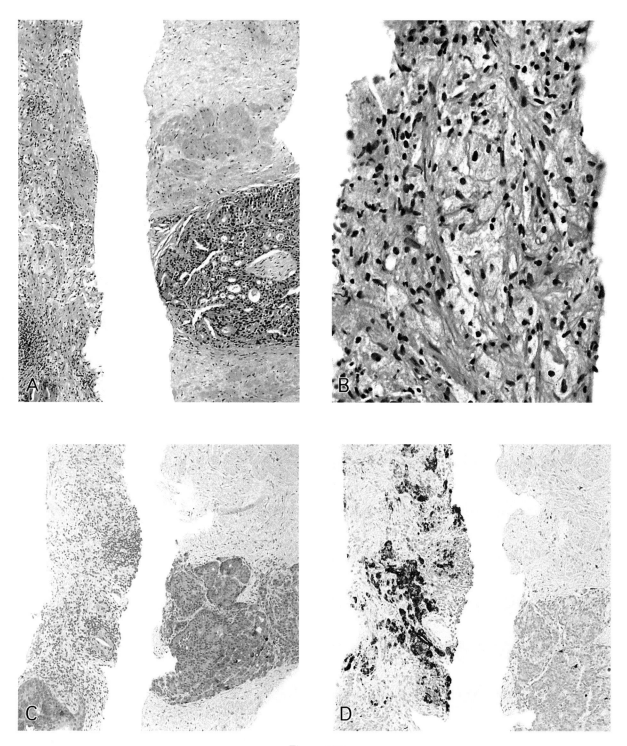

Figure 4-85
IMMUNOHISTOCHEMISTRY IN PROSTATIC PATHOLOGY

A: There are two prostatic cores, the one on the right containing grade 4 adenocarcinoma and the one on the left a foamy cell infiltrate. The differential diagnosis for the latter includes Gleason 4B adenocarcinoma and a histiocytic reaction.

B: High-power view of problematic foamy cells.

C: The foamy cells are negative for PSA, with positive staining in glandular areas.

D: CD68, a histiocytic marker, stains the foamy cells. This finding, and those in C, confirm that the foamy cells are non-neoplastic. (A–D courtesy of Dr. D.G. Bostwick, Rochester, MN.)

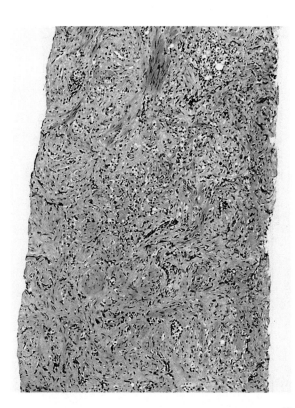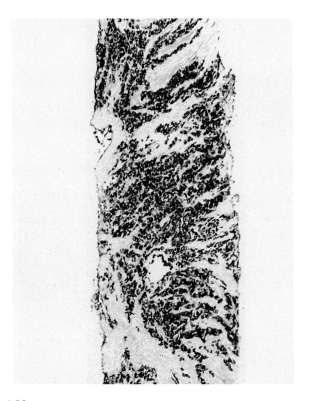

Figure 4-86
IMMUNOHISTOCHEMISTRY IN PROSTATIC PATHOLOGY
Left: Poorly differentiated carcinoma involves the bladder neck region.
Right: A positive stain for prostate-specific antigen indicates prostatic carcinoma rather than transitional cell carcinoma.

genitourinary tract (432,490). Not uncommonly, secondary adenocarcinomas are found in lymph nodes, lung, bone, liver, and other sites. The application of immunohistochemistry for PSA and PAP is of value in these situations, since if a prostatic origin is established, hormonal therapy can be instituted, often with some benefit.

When a poorly differentiated carcinoma involves bladder, bladder neck, or urethra and prostate gland, PSA and PAP are of value in establishing a prostatic origin (fig. 4-86). This is especially important when the pattern is that of a poorly differentiated solid carcinoma or a solid carcinoma containing occasional glands where transitional cell carcinoma with glandular differentiation enters the differential diagnosis. The latter tumors are generally negative for PSA and PAP although both markers have been identified in rare bladder adenocarcinomas (417,443,481). Rarely, colorectal adenocarcinoma or carcinomas of the "cloacogenic" type from the anorectal junction enter the differential diagnosis of a lower genitourinary mass, and

negative immunoreactivity for prostatic markers helps establish a diagnosis.

While PSA is a relatively specific marker of prostatic adenocarcinoma, it has been described in some extraprostatic tumors including mature teratoma, periurethral gland adenocarcinoma in females, villous adenoma and adenocarcinoma of the bladder, extramammary Paget's disease of the penis, and pleomorphic adenoma and carcinoma of the salivary gland in males. Likewise, PAP has been described in a number of extraprostatic tumors including adenocarcinoma of the urinary bladder, "cloacogenic" carcinoma of the anus, gastrointestinal carcinoid tumor, islet cell tumor of the pancreas, mature teratoma, and pleomorphic adenoma and carcinoma of the salivary gland in the male (see chapter 1). Caution must be exerted in situations where such lesions enter the differential diagnosis of prostatic adenocarcinoma. An immunohistochemical panel including PSA, PAP, and CD57 (see chapter 1) is useful in problem cases (477).

Prostatic-specific markers may also be of value in distinguishing transitional cell carcinoma of prostatic ducts from high-grade prostatic intraepithelial neoplasia and ductal patterns of prostatic adenocarcinoma (Gleason patterns 3C, 5A). The cells comprising transitional cell carcinoma of prostatic ducts are negative for the prostatic-specific markers (see chapter 5).

There are very few studies dealing with the prognostic value of immunoreactivity for PSA and PAP. Hammond et al. (458) reported that patients with advanced disease who had intense PAP staining were more likely to respond to hormonal therapy than those with weaker or absent reactions.

Neuroendocrine Markers. A large number of studies have looked at neuroendocrine markers in prostatic adenocarcinoma (435–437,485, 496). Neuroendocrine cells can be detected with antibodies directed against neuron-specific enolase, chromogranin, synaptophysin, and serotonin. When sensitive neuroendocrine markers are used in well-prepared tissue, most, if not all, prostatic adenocarcinomas display at least focal positivity. About 10 percent of cases show extensive positivity. In addition to the generic endocrine markers, other peptide markers such as somatostatin, calcitonin, calcitonin gene–related product, bombesin-like proteins, thyrotrophin-like peptide, and parathyroid hormone–related protein have been detected in prostatic adenocarcinoma (415, 434,438,439,463,496). The role of neuroendocrine cells in carcinoma is unknown, although a regulatory function has been proposed (435–437). The prognostic value of neuroendocrine differentiation in conventional adenocarcinoma is controversial (418,421,425,431,434–439,444,455,463,472, 485,496). A number of studies have challenged the original concept that increased numbers of neuroendocrine cells indicate a poor prognosis (418, 421, 425). There appears to be a progressive reduction in neuroendocrine differentiation with advancing tumor grade. The value of neuroendocrine staining in prostatic adenocarcinoma requires further study to assess its prognostic merit.

Ultrastructure

A number of studies have assessed the ultrastructural features of prostatic adenocarcinoma (426,445,467,504). In well-differentiated tumors

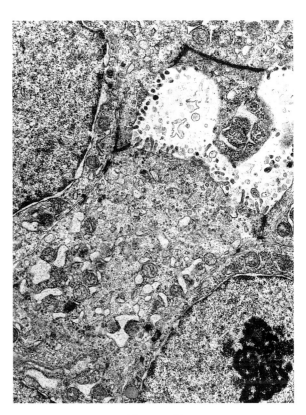

Figure 4-87
PROSTATIC ADENOCARCINOMA

An electron micrograph of a low-grade tumor with an acinar growth pattern shows an absence of basal cells, abundant cytoplasm, atypical nuclei, and a prominent nucleolus (lower right).

(Gleason 1, 2), the acini are lined by tall columnar cells which show only minimal deviation from normal secretory cells (fig. 4-87). In the tumors of Gleason patterns 3A and 3B, the acini are generally lined by cuboidal cells, and the ultrastructural nuclear findings, including prominent nucleoli, reflect those seen by light microscopy. The cytoplasm generally shows a reduction in organelles such as secretory vacuoles, endoplasmic reticulum, and mitochondria. With increasing grade, more heterogeneous and disorganized cell types develop. Intracellular lumens may be identified, and immature cells with scanty cytoplasmic organelles and highly atypical nuclear features may be apparent.

Electron microscopy has little or no practical role in the evaluation of prostatic adenocarcinoma, but may have value in some unusual epithelial and mesenchymal tumors discussed in chapters 5 and 6 (504).

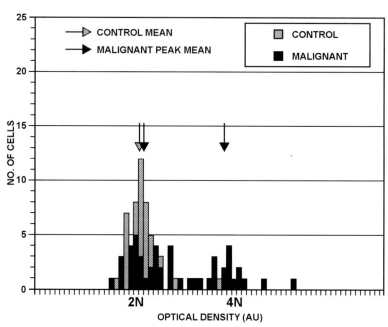

Figure 4-88
ANEUPLOID DNA
HISTOGRAM OF CARCINOMA
This image cytometry–generated histogram shows a distinct aneuploid peak. Tumor G0/G1 peak mean exceeds control G0/G1 peak by at least two standard deviations.

DNA Ploidy Analysis

The DNA content of prostatic adenocarcinoma has been extensively studied using a variety of techniques (416,422,433,447,448,454,462,464, 470,471,474,476,479,480,482,486,491,492,494, 499,500,502,506,509,511,512,516,519). It has been measured using fluorescence in situ hybridization (FISH), flow cytometry, and static image analysis (fig. 4-88) (447,474,492,508). However, the use of these techniques in routine practice is not widespread. Analysis of DNA ploidy has been shown to provide prognostic information in prostatic adenocarcinoma, independent of histologic grade and stage. Several studies using multiple regression analyses have shown DNA aneuploidy to correlate with poor survival and the potential for metastases (464,480,494,506,516,519). In general, patients with DNA diploid cancers survive longer and have better outcomes than those with aneuploid tumors. In addition, DNA diploid tumors are more responsive to hormone therapy (519).

The demonstrated value of DNA ploidy analysis lies in providing prognostic information after a radical prostatectomy. The utility of ploidy studies to predict extent of disease and assist with treatment decisions based on the analysis of needle biopsy specimens is questionable. Due to the heterogeneous nature of prostatic adenocarci-

noma, needle biopsy sampling may not be representative of areas of the tumor with the worst grade (454,488). However, some reports have shown a correlation between DNA ploidy analysis on needle biopsies and the subsequent radical prostatectomy specimen (474,509).

The limitations and advantages of DNA content analysis have been studied by an international DNA Cytometry Consensus Conference, and by the Prostate Cancer Working Group of the College of American Pathologists Conference XXVI on Clinical Relevance of Prognostic Markers in Solid Tumors (425a,456,500). Neither body recommends routine use of this technique for clinical practice as there are insufficient data available to justify it.

Genetic Alterations

The advent of molecular biologic techniques to detect abnormalities at the gene level has generated a plethora of papers on genetic alterations in prostate cancer (449,466,487,499). To date, a bewildering array of abnormalities has been reported, some of which seem to be consistently present while others appear to be random occurrences. Although a prostate cancer gene has been recently discovered, much work needs to be done to put these genetic findings in the context of other reported genetic abnormalities (473,501).

Genetic alterations in prostatic adenocarcinoma have been studied extensively using classic cytogenetic techniques, fluorescence in situ hybridization (FISH), loss of heterozygosity studies, nucleotide sequencing, and comparative genomic hybridization (466,513).

Cytogenetic analyses using metaphase spreads have been limited by sampling errors (as a majority of tumors are not evident on gross examination), poor growth of prostate cancer cells and their low mitotic rate, and overgrowth of stromal elements. Cytogenetics show frequent involvement of some chromosomes, particularly 2, 7, 8 10, and 16 (466,513). The use of FISH to detect chromosomal abnormalities in interphase nuclei has revealed such abnormalities in a greater number of cancers than detected by traditional cytogenetics, but FISH is limited by its ability to evaluate only a few regions at a time.

Loss of heterozygosity has most often been found at chromosomal regions 7q, 8p, 10q, 13q, 16q, 17q, and 18q (466). Using comparative genomic hybridization, deletions in these regions and in 6q and 9q have been reported (466). Although these deletions and loss of heterozygosity suggests the presence of tumor suppressor genes in these loci, to date very few specific genes have been identified as the ones responsible (449,466).

Among these myriad genetic alterations, there is the promise of finding a reliable prognostic marker which can be used prospectively for patient care. However, at this time, these discoveries are in a nascent phase, and much progress will have to be made before these can be used widely.

Other Studies

The list of other markers being studied is long and includes quantification of micro-vessel density, nuclear morphometry, proliferation markers (including S-phase fractions, Ki-67, MIB-1 [451,503], and PCNA [515]), apoptosis, PSA isoforms, cell adhesion molecules, androgen receptor status, reverse transcriptase polymerase chain reaction (RT-PCR) for PSA in serum, RT-PCR for prostate-specific membrane antigen, interphase cytogenetics, oncogenes, and tumor suppressor genes. Although there is voluminous literature on putative prognostic markers for prostate cancer, none of these studies have established their value in diagnosis or prognosis.

TREATMENT AND PROGNOSIS

Treatment can only commence after a certain diagnosis is established, which in many patients includes biopsies on more than one occasion if the initial material cannot be unequivocally considered malignant (525,543). In some instances repeat biopsies are performed to assess the extent of disease, which bears on the therapeutic decision (539). The management of patients with carcinoma of the prostate is complex (540,541, 553,568). The main treatment options include radical prostatectomy, external beam radiation therapy, radioactive seed implants, androgen deprivation therapy and, in selected situations, only surveillance with "watchful waiting" (541, 546,556,561,563,565,566). There is no established role for chemotherapy, although a number of promising agents such as estramustine are in the early phases of investigation. Other novel therapies such as laser ablation and cryosurgery are being actively studied. Many host and tumor factors impact on the choice of treatment: patient age, life expectancy, co-morbidity, clinical stage, tumor grade, and prostate-specific antigen levels (531,536,545). The natural history of many prostate cancers is lengthy, and long survival periods have been documented without treatment (522), justifying the watchful-waiting approach.

In general, treatment with intent to cure is used in clinically localized disease (T1b-T2) (524, 540,553,568). Such therapy includes radical prostatectomy and radiation therapy. Watchful waiting has been advocated by some in this situation. In the incidental, low-grade and low-volume tumors detected in prostatic curettings (T1a), watchful waiting is frequently employed, especially in older patients. However, it has been shown that 8 to 37 percent of stage T1a tumors progress when followed for more than 10 years (534,541,546,561). Some experts have, therefore, advocated aggressive therapy for these patients, especially those under the age of 60 years. The optimum treatment and prognosis for patients with T1c disease has not been established since this is a relatively recently described substage (532). In younger patients where tumor is detected by PSA screening and confirmed on needle biopsies, many surgeons recommend radical prostatectomy. The role of watchful waiting in these cases has not as yet been defined.

In more advanced stages (T3, T4), local radiotherapy is often employed (546,561,563). Androgen deprivation strategies have also been used in this situation and are the primary treatment of choice for patients with nodal (N+) or distant metastatic (M+) disease. More recently, neoadjuvant hormone therapies have been used in early stage disease, prior to radical prostatectomy or radiation therapy (542,547,562). The role of neoadjuvant hormone therapy looks particularly promising in the radiation setting (558a).

The prognosis for patients with prostatic adenocarcinoma is highly variable and dependent on a variety of host, tumor, and treatment parameters (520–524,526–538,544,546,548–552,554–559, 561,563,564,567). A recent consensus conference (520a) considered various prognostic parameters in three categories (Table 4-10) according to current knowledge of their importance: Category I includes factors which are well supported by the literature and recommended for widespread clinical use; Category II includes promising factors that may be recommended for use after large multicenter trials (investigational, promising); Category III includes factors with insufficient data for recommendation (investigational, unknown utility).

The historical 10-year cancer-specific survival rates are shown in Table 4-4 (560). Patients with T1a disease have a survival rate of 95 percent at 10 years, which is similar to the age-specific general survival. Patients with localized disease who are thought to be curable by surgery or radiation, have an 80 percent 10-year cause-specific survival rate, and those with more locally advanced disease (T3-T4) have a 60 percent 10-year survival. Estimated cure rates are considerably lower, indicating the long course of prostatic adenocarcinoma. Patients with nodal disease (N+) are thought to be rarely curable and have a 10-year cancer-specific survival rate of about 40

Table 4-10

PROGNOSTIC FACTORS FOR PROSTATE CANCER*

Category I	Serum PSA
	Gleason grade
	Pathologic stage
	Surgical margins
Category II	DNA ploidy
	Volume of cancer in radical prostatectomy
	Volume of cancer in needle biopsies
	Histologic subtypes
Category III	Perineural invasion
	Lymph node micrometastases
	Nuclear roundness
	Nuclear chromatin texture
	Mitotic figures
	MIB-1
	PCNA
	Apoptosis
	PSA derivatives (PSA velocity, PSA density, bound to free ratio, complexed PSA)
	Androgen receptors
	Neuroendocrine differentiation
	Human glandular kallikrein 2
	Prostate-specific membrane antigen
	Microvessel density
	Integrins
	TGF-Beta

*Data from reference 520a.

percent, and those with distant disease (M+) display a 10 percent 10-year survival rate. Overall, the death rate associated with prostatic adenocarcinoma appears to be falling, which may, in part, reflect diagnosis at earlier stages due to early detection strategies (524,528,538).

REFERENCES

General References

1. Algaba F, Epstein JI, Aldape HC, et al. Assessment of prostate carcinoma in core needle biopsy. Definition of minimal criteria for the diagnosis of cancer in biopsy material. Cancer 1996;78:376–81.
2. Andrews GS. Latent carcinoma of the prostate. J Clin Path 1949;2:197–208.
3. Bostwick DG, Iczkowski KA. Minimal criteria for the diagnosis of prostate cancer on needle biopsy. Ann Diagn Pathol 1997;1:104–29.
4. Epstein JI. The diagnosis and reporting of adenocarcinoma of the prostate in core needle biopsy specimens. Cancer 1996;78:350–6.
5. Kahler JE. Carcinoma of the prostate gland: a pathologic study. J Urol 1939;41:557–74.
6. Kastendieck H. Prostatic carcinoma: aspects of pathology, prognosis and therapy. J Cancer Res Clin Oncol 1980;96:131–56.

7. Kovi J. Microscopic differential diagnosis of small acinar adenocarcinoma of prostate. Pathol Annu 1985;20(part1):157–96.
8. Melicow MM. Cancer of the prostate: concepts and guidelines in histological diagnosis. J Urol 1966;95:791–800.
9. Moore RA. The morphology of small prostatic carcinoma. J Urol 1935;33:224–34.
10. Mostofi FK, Davis CJ Jr, Sesterhenn IA. Pathology of carcinoma of the prostate. Cancer 1992;70:235–53.
11. Mostofi FK, Sesterhenn IA, Davis CJ Jr. Prostatic carcinoma: problems in the interpretation of prostatic biopsies. Hum Pathol 1992;23:223–41.
12. Pugh RC. Pathology and natural history. Recent Results Cancer Res 1981;78:60–75.
13. Totten RS, Heinemann MW, Hudson PB, Sproul EE, Stout AP. Microscopic differential diagnosis of latent carcinoma of prostate. Arch Pathol 1953;55:131–41.

General Features

14. Akazaki K, Stemmermann GN. Comparative study of latent carcinoma of the prostate among Japanese in Japan and Hawaii. JNCI 1973;50:1137–44.
15. Amin MB, Ro JY, Ayala AG. Putative precursor lesions of prostatic adenocarcinoma: fact or fiction? Mod Pathol 1993;6:476–83.
16. Bastacky SI, Wojno KJ, Walsh PC, Carmichael MJ, Epstein JI. Pathological features of hereditary prostate cancer. J Urol 1995;153:887–92.
17. Bauer WC, McGavran MH, Carlin MR. Unsuspected carcinoma of the prostate in suprapubic prostatectomy specimens. A clinicopathological study of 55 consecutive cases. Cancer 1960;13:370–8.
18. Blair A, Fraumeni JF. Geographic patterns of prostate cancer in the United States. JNCI 1978;61:1379–84.
19. Bostwick DG. Grading of prostate cancer. Am J Clin Pathol 1994;102(Suppl):S38–56.
20. Bostwick DG. Prospective origins of prostate carcinoma. Prostatic intraepithelial neoplasia and atypical adenomatous hyperplasia. Cancer 1996;78:330–6.
21. Bostwick DG, Cooner WH, Denis L, Jones GW, Scardino PT, Murphy GP. The association of benign prostatic hyperplasia and cancer of the prostate. Cancer 1992;70:291–301.
22. Bostwick DG, Srigley JR. Premalignant lesions. In: Bostwick DG, ed. Pathology of the prostate. New York: Churchill Livingstone, 1990:37–59.
23. Brawer MK, Chetner MP, Beatie J, Buchner DM, Vessella RL, Lange PH. Screening for prostatic carcinoma with prostate-specific antigen. J Urol 1992;147:841–5.
24. Breslow N, Chan CW, Dhom G, et al. Latent carcinoma of prostate at autopsy in seven areas. Int J Cancer 1977;20:680–8.
25. Cannon L, Bishop DT, Skolnick M, et al. Genetic epidemiology of prostate cancer in the Utah Mormon genealogy. Cancer Surv 1982;1:47–69.
26. Carter BS, Beaty TH, Steinberg GD, Childs B, Walsh PC. Mendelian inheritance of familial prostate cancer. Proc Natl Acad Sci U S A 1992;89:3367–71.
27. Carter BS, Bova GS, Beaty TH, et al. Hereditary prostate cancer: epidemiologic and clinical features. J Urol 1993;150:797–802.
28. Catalona WJ, Smith DS, Ratcliff TL, et al. Measurement of prostate-specific antigen in serum as a screening test for prostate cancer. N Engl J Med 1991;324:1156–61.
29. Centifanto YM, Kaufman HE, Zam ZS, Drylie DM, Deardourff SL. Herpes virus particles in prostate carcinoma cells. J Virol 1973;12:1608–11.
30. Cheville JC, Bostwick DG. Postatrophic hyperplasia of the prostate. A histologic mimic of prostatic adenocarcinoma. Am J Surg Pathol 1995;19:1068–76.
31. Coffey DS. The molecular biology, endocrinology and physiology of the prostate and seminal vesicles. In: Walsh PC, Retik AB, Stamey TA, Vaughn ED Jr, eds. Campbell's urology, 6th ed. Philadelphia: WB Saunders, 1992:221–66.
32. Culkin DJ, Wheeler JS Jr, Castelli M, Fresco R, Canning JR. Carcinoma of the prostate in a 25-year-old man: a case report and review of the literature. J Urol 1986;136:684–5.
33. Der Simonian R, Clemens J, Spirtas R, et al. Vasectomy and prostate cancer risks: methodological review of the evidence. J Clin Epidemiol 1993;46:163–72.
34. Dhom G. Epidemiologic aspects of latent and clinically manifest carcinoma of the prostate. J Cancer Res Clin Oncol 1983:106:210–8.
35. Doll R. Geographic variation in cancer incidence: a clue to causation. World J Surg 1978;2:595–602.
36. Edwards CN, Steinthorsson E, Nicholson D. An autopsy study of latent prostatic cancer. Cancer 1953;6:531–4.
37. Flanders WD. Review: prostate cancer epidemiology. Prostate 1984;5:621–9.
38. Franks LM. Atrophy and hyperplasia in prostate proper. J Pathol Bacteriol 1954;68:617–21.
39. Franks LM. Latency and progression in tumors: the natural history of prostatic cancer. Lancet 1956;2:1037–9.
40. Franks LM. Latent carcinoma of the prostate. J Pathol Bacteriol 1954;68:603–16.
41. Fraumeni JF Jr, Mason TJ. Cancer mortality among Chinese-Americans, 1950–69. JNCI 1974;5:659–65.
42. Ghanadian R, Puah CM, O Donoghue EP. Serum testosterone and dihydrotestosterone in carcinoma of the prostate. Br J Cancer 1979;39:696–9.
43. Giovannucci E, Ascherio A, Rimm EB, Colditz GA, Stampfer MJ, Willett WC. A prospective cohort study of vasectomy and prostate cancer in U.S. men. JAMA 1993;269:873–7.
44. Giovanucci E, Tosteson TD, Speizer FE, Ascherio A, Vessey MP, Colditz GA. A retrospective cohort study of vasectomy and prostate cancer in U.S. men. JAMA 1993;269:878–82.
45. Glantz GM. Cirrhosis and carcinoma of the prostate gland. J Urol 1964;91:291–3.
46. Gohagan JK, Prorok PC, Kramer BS, Cornett JE. Prostate cancer screening in prostate, lung, colorectal and ovarian cancer screening trial of the National Cancer Institute. J Urol 1994;152:1905–9.
47. Greene LF, Simon HB. Occult carcinoma of the prostate. Clinical and therapeutic study of eighty-three cases. JAMA 1955;158:1494–8.
48. Habib FK. Studies on the in vitro binding and metabolism of testosterone in benign prostatic hypertrophy and carcinoma of the prostate: a correlation with endogenous androgen levels, In: Schroder FJ, de Voogt HJ, eds. Steroid receptors, metabolism and prostatic cancer. Amsterdam: Excerpta Medica, 1980:157.

49. Hanchette EL, Schwartz GG. Geographic patterns of prostate cancer: evidence for a protective effect of ultraviolet radiation. Cancer 1992;70:2861–9.

49a. Hankey BF, Feuer EJ, Clegg LX, et al. Cancer surveillance series: interpreting trends in prostate cancer—Part I: evidence of the effects of screening in recent prostate cancer incidence, mortality, and survival rates. JNCI 1999;91:1017–24.

50. Herbert JT, Birkhoff JD, Feorino PM, Caldwell GG. Herpes simplex virus type 2 and cancer of the prostate. J Urol 1976;116:611–2.

51. Howards SS, Peterson HB. Vasectomy and prostate cancer. Chance, bias, or a causal relationship? JAMA 1993;269:913–4.

52. Isaacs JT, Isaacs WB, Schalken J. Comparative aspects of multistep prostatic carcinogenesis in humans and rodents. Prog Clin Biol Res 1992;376:261–88.

53. Kabalin JN, McNeal JE, Price HM, Freiha FS, Stamey TA. Unsuspected adenocarcinoma of the prostate in patients undergoing cystoprostatectomy for other causes: incidences histology and morphometric observations. J Urol 1989;141:1091–4.

54. Keetch DW, Humphrey PA, Smith DS, Stahl D, Catalona WJ. Clinical and pathological features of hereditary prostate cancer. J Urol 1996;155:1841–3.

55. Kipling MD, Waterhouse JA. Cadmium and prostatic carcinoma. Lancet 1967;1:730.

56. Kirby RS, Christmas TJ, Brawer M. Prostate cancer. London: Mosby, 1996:23–31.

57. Kolonel LN, Hankin JH, Yoshizawa CN. Vitamin A and prostate cancer in elderly men: enhancement of risk. Cancer Res 1987;47:2982–5.

58. Kovi J, Heshmat MY. Incidence of cancer in negroes in Washington DC and selected African cities. Am J Epidemiol 1972;96:401–13.

59. Krieg M, Bartsch W, Janssen W, Voigt KD. A comparative study of binding, metabolism and endogenous levels of androgens in normal, hyperplastic and carcinomatous human prostate. J Steroid Biochem 1979;11:615–24.

60. Landis SH, Murray T, Bolden S, Wingo PA. Cancer statistics, 1999. CA Cancer J Clin 1999;49:8–31.

61. Latil A, Lidereau R. Genetic aspects of prostate cancer. Virchows Arch 1998;432:389–406.

62. Lee F, Littrup PJ, Torp-Pederson ST, et al. Prostate cancer: comparison of transrectal U.S. and digital rectal examination for screening. Radiology 1988;168:389–94.

63. Lieskovsky G, Bruchovsky N. Assay of nuclear androgen receptor in human prostate. J Urol 1979;121:54–8.

64. McCombs RM. Role of oncornaviruses in carcinoma of the prostate. Cancer Treat Rep 1977;61:131–2.

65. McNeal JE, Bostwick DG, Kindrachuk RA, Redwine EA, Freiha FS, Stanley TA. Patterns of progression in prostate cancer. Lancet 1986;1:60–3.

66. Miller BA, Ries LA, Hankey BF, et al. Cancer statistics review: 1973–1989. NIH publication 92–2789, Bethesda: National Cancer Institute, 1992.

67. Mills PK, Beeson WL, Phillips RL, Fraser GE. Cohort study of diet, life style, and prostate cancer in Adventist men. Cancer 1989;64:598–604.

68. Morra MN, Das S. Prostate cancer. Epidemiology and etiology. In Das S, Crawford ED, eds. Cancer of the prostate. New York: Marcel Dekker, 1993.

69. Muller WJ, Lee FS, Dickson C, Peters G, Pattengale P, Leder P. The int-2 gene product acts as an epithelial growth factor in transgenic mice. EMBO J 1990;9:907–13.

70. Newill VA. Distribution of cancer mortality among ethnic subgroups of the white population of New York City, 1953–58. JNCI 1961;26:405–17.

71. Nomura AM, Kolonel LN. Prostate cancer: a current perspective. Epidemiol Reviews 1991;13:200–27.

72. Oesterling JE, Chan DW, Epstein JL, et al. Prostate specific antigen in the preoperative and postoperative evaluation of localized prostatic cancer treated with radical prostatectomy. J Urol 1988;139:766–72.

73. Parker SL, Davis KJ, Wingo PA, Ries LA, Heath CW. Cancer statistics by race and ethnicity. CA Cancer J Clin 1998;48:31–48.

74. Pienta KJ, Esper PS. Is dietary fat a risk factor for prostate cancer? JNCI 1993;85:1538–40.

75. Pienta KJ, Nguyen NM, Lehr JE. Treatment of low volume prostate cancer in the rat with synthetic retinoid fenretinide. Cancer Res 1993;53:224–6.

76. Pollard M, Luckert PH. Promotional effects of testosterone and dietary fat on prostate carcinogenesis in genetically susceptible rats. Prostate 1985;6:1–5.

77. Rich AR. On the frequency of occurrence of occult carcinoma of the prostate. J Urol 1935;3:215–23.

78. Ries LA, Kosary CL, Hankey BF, et al, eds. SEER Cancer Statistics Review, 1973–1994 (NIH, Pub. No. 97–2789). Bethesda, MD: National Cancer Institute, 1997.

79. Robson MC. Cirrhosis and prostatic neoplasms. Geriatrics 1966;21:150–4.

80. Rosenberg L, Palmer JR, Zauber AG, et al. Vasectomy and the risk of prostate cancer. Am J Epidemiol 1990;132:1051–5.

81. Ross RK, Bernstein L, Lobo RA, et al. 5-alpha-reductase activity and risk of prostate cancer among Japanese and US white and black males. Lancet 1992;339:887–9.

82. Ross RK, Deapen DM, Casagrande JT, Paganini-Hill A, Henderson BE. A cohort study of mortality from cancer of the prostate in Catholic priests. Br J Cancer 1981;43:233–5.

83. Rotkin ID. Studies in the epidemiology of prostate cancer: expanded sampling. Cancer Treat Rep 1977;61:173–80.

84. Sakr WA, Haas GP, Cassin BF, Pontes JE, Crissman JD. The frequency of carcinoma and intraepithelial neoplasia of the prostate in young male patients. J Urol 1993;150:379–85.

85. Sanford EJ, Geder L, Laychock A, Rohner TJ Jr, Rapp F. Evidence for the association of cytomegalovirus with carcinoma of the prostate. J Urol 1977;118:789–92.

86. Scardino PT, Weaver R, Hudson MA. Early detection of prostate cancer. Hum Pathol 1992;23:211–22.

87. Schuman LM, Mandel J, Blackard C, Bauer H, Scarlett J, McHugh R. Epidemiologic study of prostatic cancer: preliminary report. Cancer Treat Rep 1977;61:181–6.

88. Seidman H, Mushinski MH, Gelb SK, Silverberg E. Probabilities of eventually developing or dying of cancer—United States, 1985. CA Cancer J Clin 1985;35:36–56.

89. Shain SA, Huot RI, Gorelic LS, Smith GC. Biochemical and morphological characterization of clonal AXC rat: prostate cancer cells. Cancer Res 1984;44:2033–42.

90. Sheldon CA, Williams RD, Fraley EE. Incidental carcinoma of the prostate: a review of the literature and critical reappraisal of classification. J Urol 1980;124:626–31.

91. Shimada H, Misugi K, Sasaki Y, Iizuka A, Nishihira H. Carcinoma of the prostate in childhood and adolescence: report of a case and review of the literature. Cancer 1980;46:2534–42.

92. Shimizu H, Ross RK, Bernstein L, et al. Cancer of the prostate and breast among Japanese and white immigrants in Los Angeles County. Br J Cancer 1981;63:963–6.

93. Sidney S. Vasectomy and the risk of prostatic cancer and benign prostatic hypertrophy. J Urol 1987;138:795–7.

94. Silverberg E. Statistical and epidemiologic data on urologic cancer. Cancer 1987;60:692–17.

95. Skowronski RJ, Peehl DM, Feldman D. Actions of vitamin D3 analogs on human prostate cancer cell lines: comparison with 1, 25-dihydroxyvitamin D3. Endocrinology 1995;136:20–6.

96. Smith JR, Freije D, Carpten JD, et al. Major susceptibility locus for prostate cancer on chromosome 1 suggested by a genome-wide search. Science 1996;274:1371–4.

97. Spitz MR, Currier RD, Fueger J, Childs B, Walsh PC. Familial patterns of prostate cancer: a case-control analysis. J Urol 1991;146:1305–7.

98. Steele R, Lees RE, Kraus AS, Roa C. Sexual factors in the epidemiology of cancer of the prostate. J Chronic Diseases 1971;24:29–37.

99. Steinberg GD, Carter BS, Beaty TH, Childs B, Walsh PC. Family history and the risk of prostate cancer. Prostate 1990;17:337–47.

100. Thompson TC, Southgate J, Kitchener GI, Land H. Multistage carcinogenesis induced by ras and myc oncogenes in a reconstituted organ. Cell 1989;56:917–30.

101. Wingo PA, Landis S, Ries LA. An adjustment to the 1997 estimate for new prostate cancer cases. CA Cancer J Clin 1997;47:239–42.

102. Winkelstein W Jr, Ernster VL. Epidemiology and etiology. In: Murphy GP, ed. Prostatic cancer. Littleton, MA: PSG Publishing, 1979.

103. Woolf CM. An investigation of the familial aspects of carcinoma of the prostate. Cancer 1960;13:739–44.

104. Yatani R, Chigusa L, Akazaki K, Stemmermann GN, Welsh RA, Correa P. Geographic pathology of latent prostatic carcinoma. Int J Cancer 1982;29:611–6.

Clinical Features and Clinical Staging

105. Barkin J, Crassweller PO, Roncari DA, Onrot J. Hypercalcemia associated with cancer of prostate without bony metastases. Urology 1984;24:368–71.

106. Bastacky SS, Walsh PC, Epstein JI. Needle biopsy associated tumor tracking of adenocarcinoma of the prostate. J Urol 1991;145:1003–7.

107. Baumann MA, Holoye PY, Choi H. Adenocarcinoma of prostate presenting as brain metastasis. Cancer 1984;54:1723–5.

108. Benson MC, Whang IS, Pantuck A, et al. Prostate-specific antigen density: a means of distinguishing benign prostatic hypertrophy and prostate cancer. J Urol 1992;147:815–6.

109. Blute ML, Zincke H, Farrow GM. Long-term follow-up of young patients with stage A adenocarcinoma of the prostate. J Urol 1996;36:840–3.

110. Bostwick DG, Myers RP, Oesterling JE. Staging of prostate cancer. Semin Surg Oncol 1994;10:60–72.

111. Brawer MK, Lange PH. Prostate specific antigen: its role in early detection, staging and monitoring of prostatic carcinoma. Endourology 1989;3(2):227–36.

112. Bumpus HC Jr. Carcinoma of the prostate. A clinical study of one thousand cases. Surg Gynecol Obstet 1926;43:150–5.

113. Butler JJ, Howe CD, Johnson DE. Enlargement of the supraclavicular lymph nodes as the initial sign of prostatic carcinoma. Cancer 1971;27:1055–63.

114. Carter HB, Partin AW. Diagnosis and staging of prostate cancer. In: Walsh PC, Retik AB, Vaughan ED Jr, eds. Campbell's urology, 7th ed. Philadelphia: WB Saunders, 1998:2509–17.

115. Carter HB, Pearson JD, Metter J, et al. Longitudinal evaluation of prostate-specific antigen levels in men with and without prostate disease. JAMA 1992;267:2215–20.

115a. Catalona WJ. Clinical utility of measurements of free and total prostate-specific antigen (PSA): a review. Prostate 1996;7(Suppl):64–9.

116. Catalona WJ, Smith DS. Five year tumor recurrence rates after anatomical radical prostatectomy for prostate cancer. J Urol 1994;152:1837–42.

117. Catalona WJ, Smith DS, Ornstein DK. Prostate cancer detection in men with serum PSA concentrations of 2.6–4.0 mg/ml and benign prostate examination. Enhancement of specificity with free PSA measurements. JAMA 1997;277:1452–5.

118. Caulk JR. Carcinoma of the prostate. J Urol 1937;37:832–9.

119. Chodak GW, Schoenberg HW. Progress and problems in screening for carcinoma of the prostate. World J Surg 1989;13:60–4.

120. Cooner WH, Mosley RB, Rutherford CL Jr, et al. Prostate cancer detection in a clinical urological practice by ultrasonography, digital rectal examination and prostate specific antigen. J Urol 1990;143:1146–52.

121. Davies AL. Prostatic carcinoma presenting as acute obstruction of large bowel. Cancer 1967;20:1035–7.

122. Desmond PM, Clark J, Thompson IM, Zeidman EJ, Mueller EJ. Morbidity with contemporary prostate biopsy. J Urol 1993;150:1425–6.

123. Devonec M, Chapelon JY, Cathignol D. Comparison of the diagnostic value of sonography and rectal examination in cancer of the prostate. Eur Urol 1988;14:189–95.

124. Eble JN, Angermeier PA. The roles of fine needle aspiration and needle core biopsies in the diagnosis of primary prostatic cancer. Hum Pathol 1992;23:249–57.

125. Eble JN, Epstein JI. Stage A carcinoma of the prostate. In: Bostwick DG, ed. Pathology of the prostate. New York: Churchill Livingstone, 1990:61–82.

126. Ellis WJ, Brawer MK. The role of tumor markers in the diagnosis and treatment of prostate cancer. In: Lepor H, Lawson RK, eds. Prostate diseases. Philadelphia: WB Saunders, 1993:276–92.

127. Epstein JI. The prostate and seminal vesicles. In: Sternberg SS, ed. Diagnostic surgical pathology, 2nd ed. New York: Raven Press, 1194:1807–53.

128. Epstein JI, Oesterling JE, Eggleston JC, Walsh PC. Frozen section detection of lymph node metastases in prostatic carcinoma: accuracy in grossly uninvolved pelvic lymphadenectomy specimens. J Urol 1986;136:1234–7.

128a. Foster MC, O'Reilly PH. Carcinoma of the prostate masquerading as rectal carcinoma. Report of 3 cases and review of the literature. Br J Urol 1990;66:193–5.

129. Fritzsche PJ, Axford PD, Ching VC, Rosenquist RW, Moore RJ. Correlation of transrectal sonographic findings in patients with suspected and unsuspected prostatic disease. J Urol 1983;130:272–4.

130. Ghandur-Mnaymneh L, Satterfield S, Block NL. Small cell carcinoma of the prostate gland with inappropriate antidiuretic hormone secretion: morphological, immunohistochemical, and clinical expressions. J Urol 1986;135:1263–6.

131. Gilbertsen VA. Cancer of the prostate gland: results of early diagnosis and therapy undertaken for cure of the disease. JAMA 1971;215:81–4.

132. Hammerer P, Huland H, Sparenberg A. Digital rectal examination, imaging and systematic-sextant biopsy in identifying operable lymph node-negative prostatic carcinoma. Eur Urol 1992;22:281–7.

133. Harper JM, Hunter WA. Unilateral exophthalmos secondary to metastatic carcinoma of the prostate: case report and review of the literature. J Urol 1963;89:75–7.

134. Hodge KK, McNeal SE, Terris MK, Stamey TA. Random systematic versus directed ultrasound–guided transrectal core biopsies of the prostate. J Urol 1989;142:71–5.

135. Hunter PT, Butler SA, Hodge GB, et al. Detection of prostatic cancer using transrectal ultrasound and sonographically guided biopsy in 1410 symptomatic patients. J Endourol 1989;3:167–75.

136. Jenson CB, Shahon DB, Wangensteen OH. Evaluation of annual examinations in the detection of cancer: special reference to cancer of the gastrointestinal tract, prostate, breast and female reproductive tract. JAMA 1960;174:1783–8.

137. Jewett HJ. The present status of radical prostatectomy for stages A and B prostatic cancer. Urol Clin N Am 1975;2:105–24.

137a. Kickham CJ. Diagnostic pitfalls in carcinoma of the prostate. J Urol 1941;45:92–101.

138. Kirby RS, Christmas TJ, Brawer M. Prostate cancer. London: Mosby, 1996:45–53.

139. Klotz, LH, Shaw PA, Srigley JR. Transrectal fine-needle aspiration and true cut needle biopsy of the prostate: a blinded comparison of accuracy. Can J Surg 1989;32:287–9.

139a. Lee F, Littrup PJ, Torp-Pederson ST, et al. Prostate cancer: comparison of transrectal U.S. and digital rectal examination for screening. Radiology 1988;168:389–94.

140. Lee F, Littrup PJ, Torp-Pedersen ST, et al. Prostate cancer: comparison of transrectal US and digital rectal examination for screening. Radiology 1988;168:389–4.

141. Liskow A, Chang CH, DeSanctis P, Benson M, Fetell M, Housepian E. Epidural cord compression in association with genitourinary neoplasms. Cancer 1986;58:949–54.

142. Mahedevia PS, Ramaswamy A, Greenwald ES, Wollner DI, Markham D. Hypercalcemia in prostatic carcinoma. Report of eight cases. Arch Intern Med 1983;143:1339–42.

143. Maksem JA, Galang CF, Johenning PW, et al. Aspiration biopsy cytology of the prostate. In: Bostwick DG, ed. Pathology of the prostate. New York: Churchill Livingstone, 1990.

144. McDowell PR, Fox WM, Epstein JI. Is submission of remaining tissue necessary when incidental carcinoma of the prostate is found on transurethral resection? Hum Pathol 1994;25:493–7.

145. Mettlin C, Lee F, Drago J, Murphy GP. The American Cancer Society National Prostate Cancer Detection Project. Findings on the detection of early prostate cancer in 2425 men. Cancer 1991;67:2949–58.

146. Mettlin CJ, Murphy GP, McGinnis LS, Menck HR. The national cancer data base report on prostate cancer. American College of Surgeons Commission on Cancer and the American Cancer Society. Cancer 1995;76:1104–12.

147. Mueller EJ, Crain TW, Thompson IM, Rodriguez FR. An evaluation of serial digital rectal examinations in screening for prostate cancer. J Urol 1988;140:1445–7.

148. Murphy WM, Dean PJ, Brasfield JA, Tatum L. Incidental carcinoma of the prostate. How much sampling is adequate? Am J Surg Pathol 1986;10:170–4.

149. Oesterling JE. Prostate specific antigen: a critical assessment of the most useful tumor marker for adenocarcinoma of the prostate. J Urol 1991;145:907–23.

150. Oesterling JE, Jacobsen SJ, Chute CG, et al. Serum prostate-specific antigen in a community-based population of healthy men: establishment of age-specific reference ranges. JAMA 1993;270:860–4.

150a. Ohori M, Goad JR, Wheeler TM, Eastham JA, Thompson TC, Scardino PT. Can radical prostatectomy alter the progression of poorly differentiated prostate cancer? J Urol 1994;152:1843–9.

151. Ohori M, Wheeler TM, Dunn JK, et al. Pathologic features and prognosis of prostate cancers detectable with current diagnostic tests. J Urol 1994;152:1714–20.

151a. Olsen BS, Carlisle RW. Adenocarcinoma of the prostate simulating primary rectal malignancy. Cancer 1970;25:219–22.

151b. Partin AW, Pound CR, Clemens JQ, Epstein JI, Walsh PC. Serum PSA after anatomic radical prostatectomy. The Johns Hopkins experience after 10 years. Urol Clin North Am 1993;20:713–25.

152. Rapoport AH, Omenn GS. Dermatomyositis and malignant effusions: rare manifestations of carcinoma of the prostate. J Urol 1968;109:183–7.

153. Rohr LR. Incidental adenocarcinoma in transurethral resections of the prostate. Partial versus complete microscopic examination. Am J Surg Pathol 1987;11:53–8.

153a. Rosen P, Armstrong D. Nonbacterial thrombotic endocarditis in patients with malignant neoplastic diseases. Am J Med 1973;54:23–9.

154. Rosenthal MA, Rosen D, Raghavan D, et al. Spinal cord compression in prostate cancer. A 10-year experience. Br J Urol 1992;69:530–3.

155. Scardino PT, Weaver R, Hudson MA. Early detection of prostate cancer. Hum Pathol 1992;23:211–22.

156. Schroder FH, Hermanek P, Denis L, Fair WR, Gospodarowicz MK, Pavore-Mocaluse M. The TNM classification of prostate cancer. Prostate 1992;4;129–38.

157. Scott R, Mutchnik DL, Laskowski TZ, Schmmhorst WR. Carcinoma of the prostate in elderly men: incidence, growth, characteristics and clinical significance. J Urol 1989;101;602–7.

158. See WA, Williams RD. Management of prostate cancer stage by stage. In: Das S, Crawford ED, eds. Cancer of the prostate. New York: Marcel Dekker, 1993.

159. Stilmant MM, Freelund MC, De Las Morenas A, Shepard RL, Oates RD, Siroky M. Expanded role for fine needle aspiration of the prostate. A study of 335 specimens. Cancer 1989;63:583–92.

159a. TNM classification of malignant tumors. Sobin LH, Witekind CH, eds. 5th ed. New York: Wiley-Liss, 1997.

160. Terris MK, McNeal JE, Stamey TA. Detection of clinically significant prostate cancer by transrectal ultrasound-guided systematic biopsies. J Urol 1992;148:829–32.

161. Tetu B, Ro JY, Ayala AG, Johnson DE, Logothetis CJ, Ordonez NG. Small cell carcinoma of the prostate. Part I. A clinicopathologic study of 20 cases. Cancer 1987;59:1803–9.

162. Tetu B, Ro JY, Ayala AG, Ordonez NG, Logothetis CJ, von Eschenbach AC. Small cell carcinoma of the prostate associated with myasthenia (Eaton-Lambert) syndrome. Urology 1989;33:148–52.

163. Thompson IM, Rounder JB, Teaque JL, Peek M, Spence CR. Impact of routine screening for adenocarcinoma of the prostate on stage distribution. J Urol 1987;137.424–6.

164. Vashi AR, Osterling JE. Present free prostate-specific antigen: entering a new year in the detection of prostate cancer. Mayo Clin Proc 1997;72:337–44.

165. Vickery AL Jr, Kerr WS Jr. Carcinoma of the prostate treated by radical prostatectomy. A clinicopathological survey of 187 cases followed for 5 years and 148 cases followed for 10 years. Cancer 1963;16:1598–608.

166. Vihko P, Kontturi M, Lukkarinen O, Ervasti I, Vihko R. Screening for carcinoma of the prostate. Rectal examination, and enzymatic and radioimmunologic measurements of serum acid phosphatase compared. Cancer 1985;56:173–7.

167. Vollmer RT. Prostate cancer and chip specimens: complete versus partial sampling, Hum Pathol 1986;17:285–90.

168. Von Eschenbach AC. Needle biopsy of the prostate. In: Johnson DE, Beileau MA, eds. Genitourinary tumors. Fundamental principles and surgical techniques. New York: Grune & Stratton, 1982:33–42.

169. Wenk RE, Bhagavan BS, Levy R, Miller D, Weisburger W. Ectopic ACTH, prostatic oat cell carcinoma, and marked hypernatremia. Cancer 1977;40:773–8.

170. Whitmore WF. Hormone therapy in prostatic cancer. Am J Med 1956;21:697–713.

171. Wojcik EM, Orozco R, O'Dowd GJ. The role of fine needle aspiration of the prostate in the era of an automated thin needle biopsy gun. J Urol Pathol 1997;7:89–97.

171a. Zincke H, Oesterling JE, Blute ML, Bergstrahl EJ, Myers RP, Barrett DM. Long-term (15 years) results after radical prostatectomy for clinically localized (stage T2c or lower) prostate cancer. J Urol 1994;152:1850–7.

Pathologic Features

172. Adlakha H, Bostwick DG. Paneth cell-like change in prostatic adenocarcinoma represents neuroendocrine differentiation: report of 30 cases. Hum Pathol 1994;25:135–9.

173. Aihara M, Wheeler TM, Ohori M, Scardino PT. Heterogeneity of prostate cancer in radical prostatectomy specimens. Urology 1994;43:60–6.

174. Algaba F, Epstein JI, Aldape HC, et al. Assessment of prostate carcinoma in core needle biopsy. Definition of minimal criteria for the diagnosis of cancer in biopsy material. Cancer 1996;78:376–81.

174a. Allen EA, Kahane H, Epstein JI. Repeat biopsy strategies for men with atypical diagnoses on initial prostate needle biopsy. Urology 1998;52:803–7.

175. Almagro UA, Tieu TM, Remeniuk E, Kueck B, Strumpf K. Argyrophilic carcinoid-like prostate carcinoma. Arch Pathol Lab Med 1986;110;916–9.

176. Ansari MA, Pintozzi RL, Choi YS, Ladove RF. Diagnosis of carcinoid-like metastatic prostatic carcinoma by an immunoperoxidase method. Am J Clin Pathol 1981;76:94–8.

177. Anton RC, Chakraborty S, Wheeler TM. The significance of intraluminal prostatic crystalloids in benign needle biopsies. Am J Surg Pathol 1998;22:446–9.

178. Armas OA, Aprikian AG, Melamed J, et al. Clinical and pathobiological effects of neoadjuvant total androgen ablation therapy on clinically localized prostatic adenocarcinoma. Am J Surg Pathol 1994;18:979–91.

179. Association of Directors of Anatomic and Surgical Pathology. Recommendations for the reporting of resected prostate carcinomas. Hum Pathol 1996;27:321–3.

180. Ayala AG, Jae JY, Babaian R, Troncoso P, Grignon DJ. The prostatic capsule: does it exist? Its importance in the staging and treatment of prostatic carcinoma. Am J Surg Pathol 1989;13:21–7.

181. Azumi N, Shibuya H, Ishikura M. Primary prostatic carcinoid tumor with intracytoplasmic prostatic acid phosphatase and prostate-specific antigen. Am J Surg Pathol 1984;8:545–51.

182. Bahn DK, Lee F, Solomon MH, Gontina H, Klionsky DL, Lee FT Jr. Prostate cancer: US-guided percutaneous cryoablation. Work in progress. Radiology 1995;194:551–6.

183. Bahnson RR, Dresner SM, Gooding W, Becich MJ. Incidence and prognostic significance of lymphatic and vascular invasion in radical prostatectomy specimens. Prostate 1989;15:149–55.

184. Bain G, Koch M, Hanson J. Feasibility of grading prostatic carcinomas. Arch Pathol Lab Med 1982;106:265–67.

184a. Blaire BL, Kahane H, Epstein JI. Perineural invasion, mucinous fibroplasia, and glomerulations. Diagnostic features of limited cancer on prostate needle biopsy. Am J Surg Pathol 1999;23:918–24.

185. Baron E, Angrist A. Incidence of occult adenocarcinoma of the prostate. After 50 years of age. Arch Pathol 1941;32.787–93.

186. Barzel W, Bean M, Hilaris B, et al. Prostatic adenocarcinoma: relationship of grade and local extent to pattern of metastases. J Urol 1977;118:278–82.

187. Bastacky ST, Walsh PC, Epstein JI. Relationship between perineural tumor invasion on needle biopsy and radical prostatectomy capsular penetration in stage B adenocarcinoma of the prostate. Am J Surg Pathol 1993;17:336–41.

188. Bauer WC, McGavran MH, Carlin MR. Unsuspected carcinoma of the prostate in suprapubic prostatectomy specimens. A clinicopathological study of 55 consecutive cases. Cancer 1960;13:370–8.

189. Bennett B, Gardner WA Jr. Crystalloids in prostatic hyperplasia. Prostate 1980;1:31–5.

190. Blom JH, Ten Kate FJ, Schroeder FH, van der Heul RO. Morphometrically estimated variation in nuclear size. A useful tool in grading prostatic cancer. Urol Res 1990;18:93–9.

191. Blute ML, Bostwick DG, Seay TM, et al. Pathologic classification of prostate carcinoma. The impact of margin status. Cancer 1998;82:902–8.

192. Bocking A, Kiehn J, Heinzel-Wach M. Combined histologic grading of prostatic carcinoma. Cancer 1982;50:288–94.

193. Borkowski P, Robinson MJ, Poppiti RJ Jr, Nash SC. Histologic findings in post cryosurgical prostatic biopsies. Mod Pathol 1996;9:807–11.

194. Bostwick DG. Gleason grading of prostatic needle biopsies. Correlation with grade in 316 matched prostatectomies. Am J Surg Pathol 1994;18:796–803.

195. Bostwick DG. Grading prostate cancer. Am J Clin Pathol 1994;102:S38–56.

196. Bostwick DG. The significance of tumor volume in prostate cancer. Urol Ann 1994;8:1–22.

197. Bostwick DG, Brawer MK. Prostatic intra-epithelial neoplasia and early invasion in prostate cancer. Cancer 1987;59:788–94.

198. Bostwick DG, Eble JN. Prostatic adenocarcinoma metastatic to inguinal hernia sac. J Urol Pathol 1993;1:193–9.

199. Bostwick DG, Egbert BM, Fajardo LF. Radiation injury of the normal and neoplastic prostate. Am J Surg Pathol 1982;6:541–51.

200. Bostwick DG, Foster CS. Examination of radical prostatectomy specimens: therapeutic and prognostic significance. In: Foster CS, Bostwick DG, eds. Pathology of the prostate. Philadelphia: WB Saunders, 1997:172–89.

201. Bostwick DG, Graham SD Jr, Napalkov P, et al. Staging of early prostate cancer: a proposed tumor volume-based prognostic index. Urology 1993;41:403–11.

201a. Bostwick DG, Grignon D, Amin MB, et al. Prognostic factors in prostate cancer: College of American Pathologists consensus statement 1999. Arch Pathol Lab Med 2000 (in press).

202. Bostwick DG, Iczkowski KA. Minimal criteria for the diagnosis of prostate cancer on needle biopsy. Ann Diagn Pathol 1997;1:104–29.

203. Bostwick DG, Kindrachuk RW, Rouse RV. Prostatic adenocarcinoma with endometrioid features. Am J Surg Pathol 1985;9:595–609.

203a. Bostwick DG, Montironi R. Evaluating radical prostatectomy specimens: therapeutic and prognostic importance. Virchows Arch 1997;430:1–16.

204. Bostwick DG, Srigley J, Grignon D, et al. Atypical adenomatous hyperplasia of the prostate: morphologic criteria for its distinction from well–differentiated carcinoma. Hum Pathol 1993;24:819–32.

205. Bostwick DG, Vonk J, Picado A. Pathologic changes in the prostate following contemporary 18-gauge needle biopsy. No apparent risk of local cancer seeding. J Urol Pathol 1994;2:203–12.

206. Bostwick DG, Wollan P, Adlakha K. Collagenous micronodules in prostate cancer. A specific but infrequent finding. Arch Pathol Lab Med 1995;119:444–7.

206a. Brat DJ, Wills ML, Lecksell KL, Epstein JI. How often are diagnostic features missed with less extensive histologic sampling of prostate needle biopsy specimens? Am J Surg Pathol 1999;23:257–62.

207. Braunstein H. Staining lipid in carcinoma of the prostate gland. Am J Clin Pathol 1964;41:44–8.

208. Brawer MK, Nagle RB, Pitts W, Freiha F, Gamble SL. Keratin immunoreactivity as an aid to the diagnosis of persistent adenocarcinoma in irradiated human prostates. Cancer 1989;63:454–60.

209. Brawer MK, Peebl DM, Stamey TA, et al. Keratin immunoreactivity in the benign and neoplastic human prostate. Cancer Res 1985;45:3663–7.

210. Brawn PN, Ayala AG, Von Eschenbach AC, Hussey DH, Johnson DE. Histologic grading study of prostate adenocarcinoma: the development of a new system and comparison with other methods—a preliminary study. Cancer 1982;49:525–32.

211. Brawn PN, Kuhl D, Johnson C III, Pandya P, McCord R. Stage D1 prostate carcinoma. The histologic appearance of nodal metastases and its relationship to survival. Cancer 1990;65:538–43.

212. Brawn PN, Kuhl D, Speights VO, Johnson III CF, Lind M. The incidence of unsuspected metastases from clinically benign prostate glands with latent prostate carcinoma. Arch Pathol Lab Med 1995;119:731–3.

213. Broders AC. Carcinoma grading and practical application. Arch Pathol Lab Med 1926;2:376–81.

214. Bullock MJ, Srigley JR, Klotz L, Chan J. Morphologic effects of cyproterone acetate (CPA) in normal, hyperplastic and neoplastic prostate specimens [Abstract]. Mod Pathol 1996;9:71A.

215. Byar D. The Veterans Administration Cooperative Urologic Group's studies of cancer of the prostate. Cancer 1973;32:1126–30.

216. Cantrell BB, DeKlerk DP, Eggleston JC, Boinett JK, Walsh PC. Pathological factors that influence prognosis in stage A prostatic cancer: the influence of extent versus grade. J Urol 1981;125:516–20.

217. Capella C, Usellini L, Buffa R, Frigerio B, Solcia E. The endocrine component of prostatic carcinomas, mixed adenocarcinoma-carcinoid tumours and non-tumour prostate. Histochemical and ultrastructural identification of the endocrine cells. Histopathology 1981;5:175–92.

218. Catalona WJ, Stein AJ. Accuracy of frozen section detection of lymph node metastases and prostatic carcinoma. J Urol 1982;127:460–1.

219. Catton PA, Hartwick RW, Srigley JR. Prostate cancer presenting with malignant ascites: signet-ring cell variant of prostatic adenocarcinoma. Urology 1992;39:495–7.

220. Chan TY, Epstein JI. Follow-up of atypical prostate needle biopsies. Urology 1999;53:351–5.

221. Chen ME, Troncoso P, Babaian R, Johnston D. Computer mapping of prostate cancer [Abstract]. Mod Pathol 1997;10:71A.

221a. Cheng L, Cheville JC, Bostwick DG. Diagnosis of prostate cancer in needle biopsies after radiation therapy. Am J Surg Pathol 1999;23:1173–83.

222. Chetty R, Gall JA. Prostatic adenocarcinoma with a bizarre stromal cell reaction. Histopathology 1993;22:193–5.

223. Cheville JC, Reznicek MJ, Clark JR, et al. The focus of atypical glands suspicious for malignancy in prostate needle biopsy specimens: incidence, histologic features, and clinical follow-up of cases diagnosed in a community practice. Am J Clin Pathol 1997;108:633–40.

224. Cho KR, Epstein JI. Metastatic prostatic carcinoma to supradiaphragmatic lymph nodes. A clinicopathologic and immunohistochemical study. Am J Surg Pathol 1987;11:457–63.

225. Christensen WN, Partin AW, Walsh PC, Epstein JI. Pathologic findings in clinical stage A2 prostate cancer. Relation of tumor volume, grade, and location to pathologic stage. Cancer 1990;65:1021–7.

226. Cina SJ, Epstein JI. Adenocarcinoma of the prostate with atrophic features. Am J Surg Pathol 1997;21:289–95.

227. Civantos F, Marcial MA, Banks ER, et al. Pathology of androgen ablation therapy in prostate carcinoma. A comparative study of 173 patients. Cancer 1995;75:1634–41.

228. Civantos F, Soloway MS. Prostate pathology after androgen blockade: effects of prostatic carcinoma and on non-tumor prostate. Adv Anat Pathol 1996;4:259–65.

229. Civantos F, Watson RB, Pinto JE, Korman HJ, Soloway MS. Finesteride effect of prostatic hyperplasia and prostate cancer: a comparative clinical pathology study of radical prostatectomies. J Urol Pathol 1997;6:1–13.

229a. Cohen MB, Soloway MS, Murphy WM. Sampling of radical prostatectomy specimens. How much is adequate? Am J Clin Pathol 1994;101:250–2.

229b. Cohen RJ, Stables S. Intraprostatic fat [Letter]. Hum Pathol 1998;29:424–5.

230. Coogan CL, McKiel CF. Percutaneous cryoablation of the prostate: preliminary results after 95 procedures. J Urol 1995;154:1813–7.

231. Cox JD, Stoffel TJ. The significance of needle biopsy after irradiation for stage C adenocarcinoma of the prostate. Cancer 1977;40:156–60.

231a. Crook J, Robertson S, Collin G, Zaleski V, Esche B. Clinical relevance of trans-rectal ultrasound, biopsy, and serum prostate-specific antigen following external beam radiotherapy for carcinoma of the prostate. Int J Rad Oncol Biol Phys 1993;27:31–7.

232. Dauge MC, Delmas V. APUD type endocrine tumour of the prostate: incidence and prognosis in association with adenocarcinoma. In: Murphy GP, Kuss R, Khoury S, et al., eds. Progress in clinical and biological medicine. Prostate cancer part A: research, endocrine treatment, and histopathology. New York: Alan R. Liss, 1987.

233. de la Monte SM, Moore GW, Hutchins GM. Metastatic behavior of prostate cancer. Cluster analysis of patterns with respect to estrogen treatment. Cancer 1986;58:985–93.

234. Del Rosario AD, Bui HX, Abdulla M, Ross JS. Sulfur-rich prostatic intraluminal crystalloids: a surgical pathologic and electron probe x-ray microanalytical study. Hum Pathol 1993;24:1159–67.

235. Dhom G. Unusual prostatic carcinomas. Path Res Pract 1990;186:28–36.

236. Dhom G, Degro S. Therapy of prostatic cancer and histopathologic follow-up. Prostate 1982;3:531–42.

236a. Dixon FJ, Moore RA. Tumors of the male sex organs. Atlas of Tumor Pathology, 1st series, Fascicles 31b & 32. Washington, D.C.: Armed Forces Institute of Pathology, 1952.

237. Dube VE, Farrow GM, Greene LF. Prostatic adenocarcinoma of ductal origin. Cancer 1973;32:402–9.

238. Dundore PA. Atypical small acinar proliferations (ASAP) suspicious for malignancy in prostate needle biopsies. J Urol Pathol 1998;8:21–9.

239. Edwards CN, Steinthorsson E, Nicholson D. An autopsy study of latent prostatic cancer. Cancer 1953;6:531–44.

240. Egan AJ, Bostwick DG. Prediction of extraprostatic extension of prostate cancer based on needle biopsy findings: perineural invasion lacks significance on multivariate analysis. Am J Surg Pathol 1997;21:1496–500.

241. Egan AJ, Lopez-Beltran A, Bostwick DG. Prostatic adenocarcinoma with atrophic features: malignancy mimicking a benign process. Am J Surg Pathol 1997;21:931–5.

242. Epstein JI. Diagnostic criteria of limited adenocarcinoma of the prostate on needle biopsy. Hum Pathol 1995;26:223–9.

243. Epstein JI. Evaluation of radical prostatectomy capsular margins of resection. The significance of margins designated as negative, closely approaching, and positive. Am J Surg Pathol 1990;14:626–32.

244. Epstein JI. The evaluation of radical prostatectomy specimens. Therapeutic and prognostic implications. Pathol Annu 1991;26;159–210.

245. Epstein JI. Interpretation of prostate biopsies. New York: Raven Press, 2nd Ed, 1995.

246. Epstein JI. Pathologic features that predict progression of disease following radical prostatectomy. In: Foster CS, Bostwick DG, eds. Pathology of the prostate. Philadelphia: WB Saunders, 1997:228–44.

247. Epstein JI, Berry SJ, Eggleston JC. Nuclear roundness factor. A predictor of progression in untreated stage A2 prostate cancer. Cancer 1984;54:1666–71.

248. Epstein JI, Carmichael M, Partin AW, Walsh PC. Is tumour volume an independent predictor of progression following radical prostatectomy? A multi-variable analysis of 185 clinical stage B adenocarcinomas of the prostate with five years of follow-up. J Urol 1993;149:1478–81.

249. Epstein JI, Carmichael MJ, Pizor G, Walsh PC. Influence of capsular penetration on progression following radical prostatectomy: a study of 196 cases with long-term follow-up. J Urol 1993;150:135–41.

250. Epstein JI, Fynheer J. Acidic mucin in the prostate: can it differentiate adenosis from adenocarcinoma? Hum Pathol 1992;23:1321–5.

251. Epstein JI, Oesterling JE, Eggleston JC, Walsh PC. Frozen section detection of lymph node metastases and prostatic carcinoma: accuracy in grossly uninvolved pelvic lymphadenectomy specimens. J Urol 1986;136:1234–7.

252. Epstein JI, Oesterling JE, Walsh PC. Tumor volume versus percentage of specimen involved by tumor correlated with progression in stage A prostatic cancer. J Urol 1988;139:980–4.

253. Epstein JI, Oesterling JE, Walsh PC. The volume and anatomical location of residual tumor in radical prostatectomy specimens removed for stage A1 prostate cancer. J Urol 1988;139:975–9.

253a. Epstein JI, Pizov G, Walsh PC. Correlation of pathologic findings with progression after radical retropubic prostatectomy. Cancer 1993;71:3582–93.

253b. Epstein JI, Pound CR, Partin AW, Walsh PC. Progression following radical prostatectomy in men with Gleason score 7 tumor. J Urol 1998;160:97–101.

254. Epstein JI, Sauvageot J. Do close but negative margins in radical prostatectomy specimens increase the risk of postoperative progression? J Urol 1997;157:241–3.

255. Epstein JI, Walsh PC, Carmichael M, Brendler CB. Pathologic and clinical findings to predict tumour extent of non-palpable (stage T1c) prostate cancer. JAMA 1994;271:368–74.

256. Fabozzi SJ, Schellhammer PF, el-Mahdi AM. Pulmonary metastases from prostate cancer. Cancer 1995;75:2706–9.

257. Feiner HD, Gonzales R. Carcinoma of the prostate with atypical immunohistological features. Clinical and histologic correlates. Am J Surg Pathol 1986;10:765–70.

258. Ferguson J, Zincke H, Ellison E, Bergstrahl E, Bostwick DG. Decrease of prostatic intraepithelial neoplasia following androgen deprivation therapy in patients with stage T3 carcinoma treated by radical prostatectomy. Urology 1994;44:91–5.

259. Franks LM. Estrogen-treated prostatic cancer. The variation in responsiveness of tumor cells. Cancer 1960;13:490–501.

260. Franks LM. Latency and progression in tumours. The natural history of prostatic cancer. Lancet 1956;2:1037–9.

261. Franks LM. Latent carcinoma of the prostate. J Path Bact 1954;68;603–16.

262. Franks LM, O'Shea JD, Thompson AE. Mucin in the prostate: a histochemical study in normal glands, latent, clinical, and colloid cancers. Cancer 1964;17:983–91.

262a. Furman J, Murphy WM, Rice L, Drew PA, Narayan P. Prostatectomy tissue for research. Balancing patient care and discovery. Am J Clin Pathol 1998;110:4–9.

263. Gaeta JF, Asirwatham JE, Miller G, Murphy GP. Histologic grading of primary prostatic cancer: a new approach to an old problem. J Urol 1980;123:689–93.

264. Gaffney EF, O'Sullivan SN, O'Brien A. A major solid undifferentiated carcinoma pattern correlates with tumour progression in locally advanced prostatic carcinoma. Histopathology 1992;21:249–55.

265. Gal R, Halpern M, Koren R, et al. Acid mucin and high molecular weight keratin in prostatic lesions: evaluation of a combined histochemical and immunohistochemical stain. Br J Urol 1995;76:57–60.

266. Garnett JE, Oyasu R, Grayhack JT. The accuracy of diagnostic biopsy specimens in predicting tumor grades by Gleason's classification of radical prostatectomy specimens. J Urol 1984;131:690–3.

267. Gaudin PB. Histopathologic effects of radiation and hormonal therapies on benign and malignant prostate tissues. J Urol Pathol 1998;8:55–67.

268. Gaudin PB, Epstein JI. Adenosis of the prostate. Histologic features in needle biopsy specimens. Am J Surg Pathol 1995;19:737–47.

269. Gaudin PB, Epstein JI. Adenosis of the prostate. Histologic features in transurethral resection specimens. Am J Surg Pathol 1994;18:863–70.

270. Ghali VS, Garcia RL. Prostatic adenocarcinoma with carcinoidal features producing adrenocorticotrophic syndrome. Immunohistochemical study and review of the literature. Cancer 1984;54:1042–8.

271. Gleason DF. Atypical hyperplasia, benign hyperplasia, and well–differentiated adenocarcinoma of the prostate. Am J Surg Pathol 1985;9(Suppl.):53–67.

272. Gleason DF. Classification of prostatic carcinomas. Cancer Chemother Rep 1966;50:125–8.

273. Gleason DF. Histologic grading and clinical staging of prostatic carcinoma. In: Tannenbaum M, ed. Urologic pathology: the prostate. Philadelphia: Lea & Febiger, 1977:171–97.

274. Gleason DF. Histologic grading of prostate cancer: a perspective. Hum Pathol 1992;23:273–9.

275. Gleason DF, Mellinger GT and the Veterans Administration Cooperative Urological Research Group. Prediction of prognosis for prostatic adenocarcinoma by combined histological grading and clinical staging. J Urol 1974;111:58–64.

276. Goldenberg SL, Klotz LH, Srigley J, et al. Radomized prospective controlled study comparing radical prostatectomy alone and neoadjuvant androgen in the management of localized prostate cancer. Canadian Urologic Oncology Group. J Urol 1996;156:873–7.

277. Goldstein NS, Begin LR, Grody WW, Novak JM, Quian J, Bostwick DG. Minimal or no cancer in all lower case radical prostatectomy specimens. Report of 13 cases of the "Vanishing Cancer Phenomenon." Am J Surg Pathol 1995;19:1002–9.

278. Goldstein NS, Qian J, Bostwick DG. Mucin expression in atypical adenomatous hyperplasia of the prostate. Hum Pathol 1995;26:887–91.

279. Grampsas SA, Miller GJ, Crawford ED. Salvage radical prostatectomy after failed transperineal cryotherapy. Histologic findings from prostate whole–mount specimens correlated with intraoperative transrectal ultrasound images. Urology 1995;45:936–41.

280. Greene DR, Wheeler TM, Egawa S, Dunn KJ, Scardino PT. A comparison of the morphological features of cancer arising in the transition zone and in the peripheral zone of the prostate. J Urol 1991;146:1069–76.

281. Grignon DJ. Minimal diagnostic criteria for adenocarcinoma of the prostate. J Urol Pathol 1998;8:31–43.

281a. Grignon DJ, Sakr WA. Pathologic staging of prostate carcinoma. What are the issues? Cancer 1996;78:337–40.

282. Hall GS, Kramer CE, Epstein JI. Evaluation of radical prostatectomy specimens. A comparative analysis of sampling methods. Am J Surg Pathol 1992;16:315–24.

283. Halpert B, Schmalhorst WR. Carcinoma of the prostate in patients 70 to 79 years old. Cancer 1966;19:695–8.

284. Hansen RI, Wanstrup J. Cryoprostatectomy. Histological changes elucidated by serial biopsies. Scand J Urol Nephrol 1973;7:100–4.

285. Haratake J, Horic A, Ho K. Argyrophilic adenocarcinoma of the prostate with Paneth cell-like granules. Acta Pathol Jpn 1987;37:831–6.

286. Hassan MO, Maksem J. The prostatic perineural space and its relation to tumor spread: an ultrastructural study. Am J Surg Pathol 1980;4:143–8.

287. Hellström M, Häggman M, Brändstedt S, et al. Histopathological changes in androgen-deprived localized prostatic cancer. A study in total prostatectomy specimens. Eur Urol 1993;24:461–5.

288. Helpap B. Observations on the number, size and location of nucleoli in hyperplastic and neoplastic prostatic disease. Histopathology 1988;13:203–11.

289. Helpap B. Review of the morphology of prostatic carcinoma with special emphasis on subgrading and prognosis. J Urol Pathol 1993;1:3–19.

290. Helpap B, Koch V. Histological and immunohistochemical findings of prostatic carcinoma after external or interstitial radiotherapy. J Cancer Res Clin Oncol 1991;117:608–14.

291. Henneberry JM, Kahane H, Humphrey PA, Keetch DW, Epstein JI. The significance of intraluminal crystalloids in benign prostatic glands on needle biopsy. Am J Surg Pathol 1997;21:725–8.

292. Henson DE, Hutter RV, Farrow GM. Practice protocol for the examination of specimens removed from patients with carcinoma of the prostate gland. A publication of the cancer committee, College of American Pathologists. Arch Pathol Lab Med 1994;118:779–83.

293. Hering F, Rist M, Roth J, Mihatsch M, Rutishauser G. Does microinvasion of the capsule and/or micrometastases in regional lymph nodes influence disease-free survival after radical prostatectomy? Br J Urol 1990;66;177–81.

293a. Herman CM, Kattan MW, Scardino PT, Wheeler TW. Predominant Gleason pattern is a significant predictor of disease progression in Gleason score 7 prostate cancer. Mod Pathol 1999;12:97A.

294. Herr HW, Whitmore WF Jr. Significance of prostatic biopsies after radiation therapy for carcinoma of the prostate. Prostate 1982;3:339–50.

295. Holmes EJ. Crystalloids of prostatic carcinoma: relationship to Bence-Jones crystals. Cancer 1977;39:2073–80.

296. Holund B. Latent prostatic cancer in a consecutive autopsy series. Scand J Urol Nephrol 1980;14:29–35.

297. Hukill PB, Vidone RA. Histochemistry of mucus and other polysaccharides in tumors. II. Carcinoma of the prostate. Lab Invest 1967;16:395–406.

298. Humphrey PA, Frazier HA, Vollmer RI, Paulson DF. Stratification of pathologic features in radical prostatectomy specimens that are predictive of elevated initial postoperative serum prostate-specific antigen levels. Cancer 1993;71:1821–7.

299. Humphrey PA, Kaleem Z, Swanson PE, Vollmer RT. Pseudohyperplastic prostatic adenocarcinoma. Am J Surg Pathol 1998;22:1239–46.

300. Humphrey PA, Keetch DW, Smith DS, Shepherd DL, Catalona WJ. Prospective characterization of pathological features of prostatic carcinomas detected via serum prostate-specific antigen based screening. J Urol 1996; 155:816–20.

301. Humphrey PA, Vollmer RT. Corpora amylacea in adenocarcinoma of the prostate: prevalence in 100 prostatectomies and clinicopathologic correlations. Surg Path 1990;3:133–41.

302. Humphrey PA, Vollmer RT. Intraglandular tumor extent and prognosis in prostatic carcinoma: application of a grid method to prostatectomy specimens. Hum Pathol 1990;21:799–804.

303. Humphrey PA, Walther PJ. Adenocarcinoma of the prostate. I. Tissue sampling considerations. Am J Clin Pathol 1993;99:746–59.

304. Iczkowski KA, MacLennan GT, Bostwick DG. Atypical small acinar proliferation suspicious for malignancy in prostate needle biopsies: clinical significance in 33 cases. Am J Surg Pathol 1997;21:1489–95.

305. Jensen PE, Gardner WA Jr, Piserchia PV. Prostatic crystalloids: association with adenocarcinoma. Prostate 1980;1:25–30.

306. Jones EC. Resection margin status in radical retropubic prostatectomy specimens: relationship to type of operation, tumor size, tumor grade and local tumor extension. J Urol 1990;144:89–93.

307. Jones H, Anthony PP. Metastatic prostatic carcinoma presenting as left-sided cervical lymphadenopathy: a series of 11 cases. Histopathology 1992;21:149–54.

308. Kabalin JN, McNeal JE, Price HM, Freiha FS, Stamey TA. Unsuspected adenocarcinoma of the prostate in patients undergoing cytoprostatectomy for other causes: incidence, histology and morphometric observations. J Urol 1989;141:1091–4.

309. Kahle PJ, Schencken JR, Burns EL. Clinical and pathologic effects of diethylstilbestrol and diethylstilbestrol dipropionate on carcinoma of the prostate gland: a continuing study. J Urol 1943;50:711–32.

310. Kahler JE. Carcinoma of the prostate gland: a pathologic study. J Urol 1939;41:557–574.

311. Kaleem Z, Swanson PE, Vollmer RT, Humphrey PA. Prostatic adenocarcinoma with atrophic features: a study of 202 consecutive completely embedded radical prostatectomy specimens. Am J Clin Pathol 1998;109:695–703.

312. Kelemen PR, Buschmann RJ, Weisz-Carrington P. Nucleolar prominence as a diagnostic variable in prostatic carcinoma. Cancer 1990;64:1017–20.

313. Kiesling VJ, Friedman HI, McAninch JW Nachtsheim DA, Nemeth TJ. The ultrastructural changes of prostate adenocarcinoma following external beam radiation therapy. J Urol 1979;122:633–6.

314. Kramer CE, Epstein JI. Nucleoli in low-grade prostate adenocarcinoma and adenosis. Hum Pathol 1993;24:618–23.

315. Kramer SA, Cline WA Jr, Farnham R, et al. Prognosis of patients with stage D1 prostatic adenocarcinoma. J Urol 1981;125:817–9.

316. Kramer SA, Spahr J, Brendler C, et al. Experience with Gleason's histopathologic grading in prostatic cancer. J Urol 1980;124:223–5.

317. Labrie F, Dupont A, Cussan L, et al. Downstaging of localized prostate cancer by neoadjuvant therapy with flutamide and lupron: the first controlled and radomized trial. Clin Invest Med 1993;16:499–509.

318. Lang PH, Narayan P. Understaging and undergrading of prostate cancer. Argument for postoperative radiation of adjuvant therapy. Urology 1983;21:113–8.

319. Levine AJ, Foster JD. The relation of mucicarmine staining properties of carcinomas of the prostate to differentiation, metastasis, and prognosis. Cancer 1964;17:21–5.

320. Lewis LG. Precancerous lesions of the prostate. Surg Clin N Am 1950;30:1777–82.

321. Lowe BA, Listrom MB. Incidental carcinoma of the prostate: an analysis of the predictors for progression. J Urol 1988;140:1340–4.

322. Lytton B, Collins JT, Weiss RM, Sahiff M Jr, McGuire EJ, Livolsi V. Results of biopsy after early stage prostatic cancer treatment by implantation of 125 I seeds. J Urol 1979;121:306–9.

323. Mahan DE, Bruce AW, Manley PN, Franchi L. Immunohistochemical evaluation of prostatic carcinoma before and after radiotherapy. J Urol 1980;124:488–91.

324. Mai KT, Burns BF, Morash C. Giant-cell carcinoma of the prostate. J Urol Pathol 1996;5:167–74.

325. Masson D, Bidair M, Shabaik A, Wilson S, Schmidt JD. Pathologic changes in prostate biopsies following cryoablation therapy [Abstract]. J Urol 1995;153:484A.

326. McNeal JE. Cancer volume and site of origin of adenocarcinoma in the prostate: relationship to local and distant spread. Hum Pathol 1992;23:258–66.

327. McNeal JE. Morphogenesis of prostatic carcinoma. Cancer 1965;18:1659–66.

328. McNeal JE. Normal histology of the prostate. Am J Surg Pathol 1988;12:619–33.

329. McNeal JE. Origin and development of carcinoma in the prostate. Cancer 1969;23:24–34.

330. McNeal JE. Regional morphology and pathology of the prostate. Am J Clin Pathol 1968;49:347–57.

331. McNeal JE, Alroy J, Villers A, Redwine EA, Freiha F, Stamey TA. Mucinous differentiation in prostatic adenocarcinoma. Hum Pathol 1991;22:979–88.

332. McNeal JE, Bostwick DG, Kindrachuk RA, Redwine EA, Freiha FS, Stamey TA. Patterns of progression in prostate cancer. Lancet 1986;1:60–3.

333. McNeal JE, Price HM, Redwine EA, Freiha FS, Stamey FS. Stage A versus stage B adenocarcinoma of the prostate: morphological comparison and biological significance. J Urol 1988;139:61–5.

334. McNeal JE, Redwine EA, Freiha FS, Stamey TA. Zonal distribution of prostatic adenocarcinoma. Correlation with histologic pattern and direction of spread. Am J Surg Pathol 1988;12:897–906.

335. McNeal JE, Reese JH, Redwine EA, Freiha FS, Stamey TA. Cribriform adenocarcinoma of the prostate. Cancer 1986;58:1714–9.

336. McNeal JE, Villers A, Redwine EA, Freiha FS, Stamey TA. Microcarcinoma in the prostate: its association with duct-acinar dysplasia. Hum Pathol 1991;22:644–52.

337. McNeal JE, Villers AA, Redwine EA, Freiha FS, Stamey TA. Capsular penetration in prostate cancer. Significance for natural history and treatment. Am J Surg Pathol 1990;14:240–7.

338. McNeal JE, Villers AA, Redwine EA, Freiha FS, Stamey TA. Histologic differentiation, cancer volume and pelvic lymph node metastasis in adenocarcinoma of the prostate. Cancer 1990;66:1225–33.

339. McNeal JE, Yemoto CE. Spread of adenocarcinoma within prostatic ducts and acini. Morphologic and clinical correlations. Am J Surg Pathol 1996;20:802–14.

339a. Melamed MR. Neoplastic lesions [letter]. Am J Surg Pathol 1998;22:903.

340. Melicow MM, Uson AC. A spectrum of malignant epithelial tumors of the prostate gland. J Urol 1976;115:696–700.

341. Mellinger GT, Gleason D, Bailar J III. The histology and prognosis of prostatic cancer. J Urol 1967;97:331–7.

342. Miller GJ, Cygan JM. Morphology of prostate cancer: the effects of multifocality on histological grade, tumor volume and capsule penetration. J Urol 1994;152:1709–13.

343. Mills SE, Bostwick DG, Murphy WM, Weiss MA. A symposium on the surgical pathology of the prostate. Pathol Annu 1990;25:109–58.

344. Mills SE, Fowler JE. Gleason histologic grading of prostatic carcinoma. Correlations between biopsy and prostatectomy specimens. Cancer 1986;57:346–9.

345. Montironi R, Magi-Galluzzi C, Muzzonigro G, Prete E, Polito M, Fabris G. Effects of combination endocrine treatment on normal prostate, prostatic intraepithelial neoplasia, and prostatic adenocarcinoma. J Clin Pathol 1994;47:906–13.

346. Mostofi FK. Grading of prostatic carcinoma. Cancer Chemother Rep 1975;59:111–7.

347. Mukamel E, deKernion JB, Hannah J, Smith RB, Skinner DG, Goodwin WE. The incidence and significance of seminal vesicle invasion in patients with adenocarcinoma of the prostate. Cancer 1987;59:1535–8.

348. Murphy GP, Whitmore WF Jr. A report of the workshops on the current status of the histologic grading of prostate cancer. Cancer 1979;44:1490–4.

349. Murphy WM, Soloway MS, Barrows GH. Pathologic changes associated with androgen deprivation therapy for prostate cancer. Cancer 1991;68:821–8.

350. Nelson RS, Epstein JI. Prostatic carcinoma with abundant xanthomatous cytoplasm. Foamy gland carcinoma. Am J Surg Pathol 1996;20:419–26.

351. Nemoto R, Uchida K, Harada M, et al. Experience with Gleason histopathologic grading of prostate cancer in Japan. Urology 1987;30:436–40.

351a. Novis DA, Zarbo RJ, Valenstein PA. Diagnostic uncertainty expressed in prostate needle biopsies. A College of American Pathologists Q-probes study of 15753 prostate needle biopsies in 332 institutions. Arch Pathol Lab Med 1999;123:687–92.

352. Ohori M, Scardino PT, Lapin SL, Seale-Hawkins C, Link J, Wheeler TM. The mechanisms and prognostic significance of seminal vesicle involvement by prostate cancer. Am J Surg Pathol 1993;17;1252–61.

353. Ohori M, Wheeler TM, Dunn JK, Stamey TA, Scardino PT. The pathological features and prognosis of prostate cancer detectable with current diagnostic tests. J Urol 1994;152:1714–20.

354. Ohori M, Wheeler TM, Kattan MW, Goto Y, Scardino PT. Prognostic significance of positive surgical margins in radical prostatectomy specimens. J Urol 1995; 154:1818–24.

355. Onik GM, Cohen JK, Reyes GD, Rubinsky B, Chang Z, Baust J. Transrectal ultrasound–guided percutaneous radical cryosurgical ablation of the prostate. Cancer 1993;72:1291–9.

356. Ordonez NG, Ro JY, Ayala AG. Metastatic prostatic carcinoma presenting as an oncocytic tumor. Am J Surg Pathol 1992;16:1007–12.

356a. Orozco R, O'Dowd G, Kunnel BM, Miller MC, Veltri RW. Observations on pathology trends in 62,537 prostate biopsies obtained from urology private practices in the United States. Urology 1998;51:186–95.

357. Pacelli A, Lopez-Beltran A, Egan AJ, Bostwick DG. Prostatic adenocarcinoma with glomeruloid features. Hum Pathol 1998;28:543–6.

358. Partin AW, Borland RN, Epstein JI, Brendler CB. Influence of wide excision of the neurovascular bundle(s) on prognosis in men with clinically localized prostate cancer with established capsular penetration. J Urol 1993;150:142–6.

359. Partin AW, Epstein JI, Cho KR, Gihelsohn AM, Walsh PC. Morphometric measurement of tumor volume and percent of gland involvement as predictors of pathological stage in clinical stage B prostate cancer. J Urol 1989;141:341–5.

359a. Pedersen J, Maruniak NA, Murphy WM. Can basal cells exist in carcinomatous prostatic glands? J Urol Pathol 1999;10:1–8.

360. Peterson DS, Milleman LA, Rose EF, et al. Biopsy and clinical course after cryosurgery for prostatic cancer. J Urol 1978;120:308–11.

361. Pinto JA, Gonzalez JE, Granadillo MA. Primary carcinoma of the prostate with diffuse oncocytic changes. Histopathology 1994;25:286–8.

362. Prout GR Jr, Heaney JA, Griffin PP, Daly JJ, Shipley WU. Nodal involvement as a prognostic indicator in patients with prostatic carcinoma. J Urol 1980;124:226–31.

363. Prout GR Jr, Kliman B, Daly JJ, MacLaughlin RA, Griffin PP, Young HH. Endocrine changes after diethylstilbestrol therapy. Effects on prostatic neoplasm and pituitary-gonadal axis. Urology 1976;7:148–55.

364. Renshaw AA. Correlation of gross morphologic features with histologic features in radical prostatectomy specimens. Am J Clin Pathol 1998;110:38–42.

365. Rich AR. On the frequency of occurrence of occult carcinoma of the prostate. J Urol 1935;33:215–23.

366. Ro JY, Ayala AG, Ordonez NG, Cartwright J Jr, Mackay B. Intraluminal crystalloids in prostatic adenocarcinoma. Immunohistochemical, electron microscopic, and x-ray microanalytic studies. Cancer 1986;57:2397–407.

367. Ro JY, Grignon DJ, Troncoso P, Ayala AG. Mucin in prostatic adenocarcinoma. Semin Diagn Pathol 1988;5:273–83.

368. Rodin AE, Larson DL, Roberts DK. Nature of the perineural space invaded by prostatic carcinoma. Cancer 1967;20:1772–9.

369. Rosen MA, Golstone L, Lapin S, Wheeler T, Scardino PT. Frequency and location of extracapsular extension and positive surgical margins in radical prostatectomy specimens. J Urol 1992;148:331–7.

370. Rosenthal MA, Rosen D, Raghavan D, et al. Spinal cord compression in prostate cancer. A 10-year experience. Br J Urol 1992;69:530–3.

371. Saeter G, Fossa SD, Ous S, Blom GP, Kaalhus O. Carcinoma of the prostate with soft tissue or non-regional lymphatic metastases at the time of diagnosis: a review of 47 cases. Br J Urol 1984;56:385–90.

372. Saitoh H, Hida M, Shimbo T, Nakamura K, Yamagata J, Satoh T. Metastatic patterns of prostatic cancer. Correlation between sites and number of organs involved. Cancer 1984;54:3078–84.

373. Sakr WA, Grignon DJ, Visscher DW, Wolman SR, Crissman JD. Evaluating the radical prostatectomy specimen. A protocol for establishing parameters and harvesting fresh tissue samples. J Urol Pathol 1995;3:355–64.

374. Sakr W, Wheeler T, Blute M, et al. Staging and reporting of prostate cancer—sampling of the radical prostatectomy specimen. Cancer 1996;78:366–8.

375. Salomao, DR, Graham, SD, Bostwick DG. Microvascular invasion in prostate cancer correlates with pathologic stage. Arch Pathol Lab Med 1995;119:1050–4.

375a. Samaratunga H, Williamson R. Metastatic foamy gland carcinoma of the prostate. A potential diagnostic pitfall. J Urol Pathol 1998;9:155–61.

376. Schroeder FH, Blom JH, Hop WC, Mostofi FK. Grading of prostatic cancer: I. An analysis of the prognostic significance of single characteristics. Prostate 1985;6:81–100.

377. Schroeder FH, Blom JM, Hop WC, Mostofi FK. Grading of prostatic cancer: II. The prognostic significance of the presence of multiple architectural patterns. Prostate 1985;6:403–15.

378. Schroeder FH, Hop WC, Blom JH, Mostofi FK. Grading of prostate cancer: III. Multivariate analysis of prognostic parameters. Prostate 1985;7:13–20.

379. Shabaik A, Wilson S, Bidair M, Masson D, Schmidt J, Parsons CL. Pathologic changes in prostate biopsies following cryoablation therapy of prostate carcinoma. J Urol Pathol 1995;3:183–93.

380. Smith DM, Murphy WM. Histologic changes in prostatic carcinomas treated with leuprolide (luteinizing hormone-releasing hormone effect). Distinction from poor tumor differentiation. Cancer 1994;73;1472–7.

381. Smith JA Jr, Middleton RG. Implications of volume of nodal metastasis in patients with adenocarcinoma of the prostate. J Urol 1985;133:617–9.

382. Smith MJ. The lymphatics of the prostate. Invest Urol 1966;3:439–44.

383. Soloway MS, Hachiya T, Civantos F, Murphy WM, Gomez CC, Ruiz HE. Androgen deprivation prior to radical prostatectomy for T2b and T3 prostate cancer. Urology 1994;43:52–6.

384. Spires SE, Cibull ML, Wood DP Jr, Miller S, Spires SM, Banks ER. Gleason histologic grading in prostatic carcinoma: correlation of 18-gauge core biopsy with prostatectomy. Arch Pathol Lab Med 1994;118:705–8.

385. Srigley JR. Small-acinar patterns in the prostate gland with emphasis on atypical adenomatous hyperplasia and small acinar carcinoma. Semin Diagn Pathol 1988;5:254–72.

385a. Srigley JR, Amin MB, Bostwick D, Grignon D, Hammond E. Practice protocol for the examination of specimens removed from patients with carcinoma of the prostate. A publication of the Cancer Committee, College of American Pathologists. Arch Pathol Lab Med 2000;124:1034–9.

386. Srigley JR, Bullock M, Amin MB. Small glandular patterns in the prostate gland: the differential diagnosis of small acinar carcinoma. In: Pathology of the prostate. Foster CS, Bostwick DG, eds. Philadelphia: WB Saunders, 1997:127–56.

387. Stamey TA, Freiha FS, McNeal JE, Redwine EA, Whittemore AS, Schumid HP. Localized prostate cancer. Relationship of tumor volume to clinical significance for treatment of prostate cancer. Cancer 1993;71:933–8.

388. Stamey TA, McNeal JE. Adenocarcinoma of the prostate. In: Walsh PC, Retik AB, Stamey TA, Darracott Vaughan E Jr, eds. Campbell's urology, 6th ed., Philadelphia: WB Saunders 1992:1159–221.

389. Stamey TA, McNeal JE, Freiha FS, Redwine E. Morphometric and clinical studies on 68 consecutive radical prostatectomies. J Urol 1988;139:1235–41.

390. Stamey TA, Villers AA, McNeal JE, Link PC, Freiha FS. Positive surgical margins at radical prostatectomy: importance of the apical dissection. J Urol 1990;143:1166–73.

391. Stratton M, Evans DJ, Lampert IA. Prostatic adenocarcinoma evolving into carcinoid: selective effect of hormonal treatment? J Clin Pathol 1986;39:750–6.

392. Taylor NS. Histochemistry in the diagnosis of early prostatic carcinoma. Hum Pathol 1979;10:513–20.

393. Tell DT, Khoury JM, Taylor HG, Veasey SP. Atypical metastasis from prostatic cancer. Clinical utility of the immunoperoxidase technique for prostate-specific antigen. JAMA 1985;253:3574–5.

394. Tetu B, Srigley JR, Boivin JC, et al. Effect of combination endocrine therapy (LHRH agonist and flutamide) on normal prostate and prostatic adenocarcinoma. A histopathologic and immunohistochemical study. Am J Surg Pathol 1991;15:111–20.

395. Thomas R, Lewis R, Sarma D, et al. Aid to accurate clinical staging—histopathologic grading in prostatic cancer. J Urol 1982;128:726–8.

396. Thorson P, Vollmer RT, Arcangeli C, Keetch DW, Humphrey PA. Minimal carcinoma in prostate needle biopsy specimens: diagnostic features and radical prostatectomy follow-up. Mod Pathol 1998;11:543–51.

397. Totten RS, Heinemann MW, Hudson PB, Sproul EE, Stout AP. Microscopic differential diagnosis of latent carcinoma of prostate. Arch Pathol 1953;55:131–41.

398. Tran TA, Jennings TA, Ross JS, Nazeer T. Pseudomyxoma ovarii-like posttherapeutic alteration in prostatic adenocarcinoma. A distinctive pattern in patients receiving neoadjuvant androgen ablation therapy. Am J Surg Pathol 1998;22:347–54.

398a. True LD. Surgical pathology examination of the prostate gland. Practice survey by American Society of Clinical Pathologists. Am J Clin Pathol 1996;102:572–9.

399. Utz DC, Farrow GM. Pathologic differentiation and prognosis of prostatic carcinoma. JAMA 1969;209:1701–3.

400. Vailancourt L, Tetu B, Fradet Y, et al. Effect of neoadjuvant endocrine therapy (combined androgen blockade) on normal prostate and prostatic carcinoma. A randomized study. Am J Surg Pathol 1996;20:86–93.

401. Villers A, McNeal JE, Freiha FS, Boccon-Gibod L, Stamey TA. Invasion of Denonvilliers' fascia in radical prostatectomy specimen. Urology 1993;149:793–8.

402. Villers A, McNeal JE, Freiha FS, Stamey TA. Multiple cancers in the prostate. Morphologic features of clinically recognized versus incidental tumors. Cancer 1992;70:2313–8.

403. Villers A, McNeal JE, Redwine EA, Freiha FS, Stamey TA. Pathogenesis and biological significance of seminal vesicle invasion in prostatic adenocarcinoma. J Urol 1990;143:1183–7.

404. Villers A, McNeal JE, Redwine EA, Freiha FS, Stamey TA. The role of perineural space invasion in the local spread of prostatic adenocarcinoma. J Urol 1989;142:763–8.

405. Voges GE, McNeal JE, Redwine EA, Freiha FS, Stamey TA. Morphologic analysis of surgical margins with positive findings in prostatectomy for adenocarcinoma of the prostate. Cancer 1992;69:520–6.

406. Warren MM, Furlow WL. Carcinoma of the prostate presenting as a mass in the neck. JAMA 1970;213:620–1.

407. Wasserstein PW, Goldman RL. Primary carcinoid of prostate. Urology 1979;13:318–20.

408. Weaver MG, Abdul-Karim FW, Srigley J. Paneth cell-like change and small cell carcinoma of the prostate. Two divergent forms of prostatic neuroendocrine differentiation. Am J Surg Pathol 1992;16:1013–6.

409. Weaver MG, Abdul-Karim FW, Srigley J, Bostwick DG, Ro JY Ayala AG. Paneth cell-like change of the prostate gland. A histological, immunohistochemical and electron microscopic study. Am J Surg Pathol 1992;16:62–8.

410. Wheeler TM. Anatomic considerations in carcinoma of the prostate. Urol Clin North Am 1989;16:623–34.

411. Wheeler TM, Dillioglugil O, Kattan MW, et al. Clinical and pathological significance of the level and extent of capsular invasion in clinical stage T1-2 prostate cancer. Hum Pathol 1998;29:856–62.

412. Wojno KJ, Epstein JI. The utility of basal cell-specific anti-cytokeratin antibody (34 beta E12) in the diagnosis of prostatic cancer. A review 228 cases. Am J Surg Pathol 1995;19:251–60.

413. Yam LT, Winkler CF, Janckila AJ, Li CY, Lam KW. Prostatic cancer presenting as metastatic adenocarcinoma of undetermined origin. Immunodiagnosis by prostatic acid phosphatase. Cancer 1983;51:283–7.

414. Yang XJ, Lecksell K, Short K, et al. Does long-term finasteride therapy affect the histologic features of benign prostatic tissue and prostate cancer on needle biopsy? Urology 1999;53:696–700.

Special Studies

415. Abrahamsson PA, Lilja H. Partial characterization of a thyroid-stimulating hormone-like peptide in neuroendocrine cells of the human prostate gland. Prostate 1989;14:71–81.

416. Adolfsson J. Prognostic value of deoxyribonucleic acid content in prostate cancer: a review of current results. Int J Cancer 1994;58:211–6.

417. Al Adnani MS. Origin of carcinomas causing bladder neck obstruction demonstrated by immunoperoxidase localisation of specific antigens. Br J Urol 1986;58:283–6.

418. Allen FJ, Van Velden DJ, Heyns CF. Are neuroendocrine cells of practical value as an independent prognostic parameter in prostate cancer? Br J Urol 1995;75:751–4.

419. Allsbrook WC, Simms WW. Histochemistry of the prostate. Hum Pathol 1992;23:297–305.

420. Amin MB, Schultz DS, Zarbo RJ. Analysis of cribriform morphology in prostatic neoplasia using antibody to high-molecular-weight cytokeratins. Arch Pathol Lab Med 1994;118:260–4.

421. Aprikian AG, Cordon-Cardo C, Fan WR, Reuter VE. Characterization of neuroendocrine differentiation in human benign prostate and prostatic adenocarcinoma. Cancer 1993;71:3952–65.

422. Bocking A, Chatelain R, Orthen U, et al. DNA-grading of prostatic carcinoma: prognostic validity and reproducibility. Anticancer Res 1988;8:129–35.

423. Bostwick DG. Neoplasms of the prostate. In: Urologic surgical pathology. Bostwick DG, Eble JN, eds. Mosby-Yearbook, St. Louis, 1996:343–422.

424. Bostwick DG. Prostate-specific antigen. Current role in diagnostic pathology of prostate cancer. Am J Clin Pathol 1994;102:S31–7.

425. Bostwick DG, Dousa MK, Crawford BG, Wolan PC. Neuroendocrine differentiation in prostatic intraepithelial neoplasia and adenocarcinoma. Am J Surg Pathol 1994;18:1240–6.

425a. Bostwick DG, Grignon D, Amin MB, et al. Prognostic factors in prostate cancer: College of American Pathologists consensus statement 1999. Arch Pathol Lab Med 2000;124:995–1000.

425b. Bostwick DG, Pacelli A, Blute M, Roche P, Murphy GP. Prostate specific membrane antigen expression in prostatic intraepithelial neoplasia and adenocarcinoma: a study of 184 cases. Cancer 1998;82:2256–61.

426. Brandes D, Kircheim D, Scott WW. Ultrastructure of human prostate: normal and neoplastic. Lab Invest 1964;13:1541–60.

427. Brawer MK, Nagle RB, Pitts W, Freiha F, Gamble SL. Keratin immunoreactivity as an aid to the diagnosis of persistent adenocarcinoma in irradiated human prostates. Cancer 1989;63:454–60.

428. Brawer MK, Peehl DM, Stamey TA, Bostwick DG. Keratin immunoreactivity in the benign and neoplastic human prostate. Cancer Res 1985;45:3663–7.

429. Cho KR, Epstein JI. Metastatic prostatic carcinoma to supradiaphragmatic lymph nodes. A clinicopathologic and immunohistochemical study. Am J Surg Pathol 1987;11:457–63.

430. Cina SJ, Epstein JI. Adenocarcinoma of the prostate with atrophic features. Am J Surg Pathol 1997;21:289–95.

431. Cohen RJ, Glezerson G, Haffejee Z. Neuro-endocrine cells—a new prognostic parameter in prostate cancer. Br J Urol 1991;68:258–62.

432. Cote RJ, Taylor CR. Prostate, bladder and kidney. In: Taylor CR, Cote RJ, eds. Immunomicroscopy: a diagnostic tool for the surgical pathologist. 2nd ed. Philadelphia: WB Saunders, 1994:256–76.

433. Dejter SW Jr, Cunningham RE, Noguchi PD, et al. Prognostic significance of DNA ploidy in carcinoma of prostate. Urology 1989;33:361–6.

434. di Sant'Agnese PA. Calcitonin-like immunoreactive and bombesin-like immunoreactive endocrine-paracrine cells of the human prostate gland. Arch Pathol Lab Med 1986;110:412–5.

435. di Sant'Agnese PA. Neuroendocrine differentiation in carcinoma of the prostate. Diagnostic, prognostic, and therapeutic implications. Cancer 1992;70:254–68.

436. di Sant'Agnese PA. Neuroendocrine differentiation in prostatic carcinoma. Recent findings and new concepts. Cancer 1995;75:1850–9.

437. di Sant'Agnese PA, Crockett AT. Neuroendocrine differentiation in prostatic malignancy. Cancer 1996;78:357–61.

438. di Sant'Agnese PA, de Mesy Jensen KL. Calcitonin, katacalcin and calcitonin gene-related peptide in the human prostate. An immunocytochemical and immunoelectron microscopic study. Arch Pathol Lab Med 1989;113:790–6.

439. di Sant'Agnese PA, de Mesy Jensen KL. Somatostatin and/or somatostatin-like immunoreactive endocrine-paracrine cells in the human prostate gland. Arch Pathol Lab Med 1984;108:693–6.

440. Ellis DW, Leffers S, Davies JS, Ng AB. Multiple immunoperoxidase markers in benign hyperplasia and adenocarcinoma of the prostate. Am J Clin Pathol 1984;81:279–84.

441. Epstein JI, Eggleston JC. Immunohistochemical localization of prostate-specific acid phosphatase and prostate-specific antigen in stage A2 adenocarcinoma of the prostate: prognostic implications. Hum Pathol 1984;15:853–9.

442. Epstein JI, Fynheer J. Acidic mucin in the prostate: can it differentiate adenosis from adenocarcinoma. Hum Pathol 1992;23:1321–5.

443. Epstein JI, Kuhajda FP, Lieberman PH. Prostate-specific acid phosphatase immunoreactivity in adenocarcinomas of the urinary bladder. Hum Pathol 1986;17:939–42.

444. Epstein JI, Partin AW, Veltri RW. Neuroendocrine (NE) differentiation in prostate cancer; enhanced prediction of progression following radical prostatectomy. Lab Invest 1995;72:72–5A.

445. Fisher ER, Sieracki JC. Ultrastructure of human, normal and neoplastic prostate. Pathol Annu 1970;5:1–26.

446. Fishleder A, Tubbs RR, Levin HS. An immunoperoxidase technique to aid in differential diagnosis of prostatic carcinoma. Cleve Clin Q 1981;48:331–5.

447. Fordham MV, Burdge AH, Matthew J, Cooke T, Williams G. Prostatic carcinoma cell DNA content measured by flow cytometry and its relation to clinical outcome. Br J Surg 1986;73:400–3.

448. Forsslund G, Zetterberg A. Ploidy level determinations in high-grade and low-grade malignant variants of prostatic carcinoma. Cancer Res 1990;50:4281–5.

449. Foster CS, Abel PD. Clinical and molecular techniques for diagnosis and monitoring of prostatic cancer. Hum Pathol 1992;23:395–401.

450. Franks LM, O Shea JD, Thompson AE. Mucin in the prostate: a histochemical study in normal glands, latent, clinical and colloid cancers. Cancer 1964;17:983–91.

451. Goel A, Abou-Ellela A, DeRose PB, Cohen C. The prognostic significance of proliferation in prostate cancer. Image cytometric quantitation of MIB–1. J Urol Pathol 1996;4:213–23.

452. Goldenberg SL, Klotz LH, Srigley J, et al. Randomized, prospective, controlled study comparing radical prostatectomy alone and neoadjuvant androgen withdrawal in the treatment of localized prostate cancer. Canadian Urologic Oncology Group. J Urol 1996;156:873–7.

453. Goldstein N, Qian J, Bostwick DG. Mucin expression in atypical adenomatous hyperplasia of the prostate. Hum Pathol 1995;26:887–91.

453a. Googe PB, McGinley KM, Fitzgibbon JF. Anti-cytokeratin antibody 34βE12 staining in prostate carcinoma. Am J Clin Pathol 1997;107:219–23.

453b. Green R, Epstein JI. Use of intervening unstained slides for immunohistochemical stains for high molecular weight on prostate needle biopsies. Am J Surg Pathol 1999;23:567–70.

454. Greene DR, Taylor SR, Wheeler TM, Scardino PT. DNA ploidy by image analysis of individual foci of prostate cancer: a preliminary report. Cancer Res 1991;51:4084–9.

455. Grignon D, Caplan R, Sakr W, et al. Neuroendocrine (NE) differentiation as a prognostic indicator in locally advanced prostate cancer (PCa) [Abstract]. Lab Invest 1995;72:76A.

456. Grignon DJ, Hammond EH. College of American Pathologists Conference XXVI on clinical relevance of prognostic markers in solid tumors. Report of the prostate cancer working group. Arch Pathol Lab Med 1995;119;1122–6.

457. Guinan P, Shaw M, Targonski P, Ray V, Rubenstein M. Evaluation of cytokeratin markers to differentiate between benign and malignant prostatic tissue. J Surg Oncol 1989;42:175–80.

458. Hammond ME, Sause WT, Martz KL, et al. Correlation of prostate-specific antigen acid phosphatase and prostate-specific immunocytochemistry with survival in prostate carcinoma. Cancer 1989;63:461–6.

459. Hedrick L, Epstein JI. Use of keratin 903 as an adjunct in the diagnosis of prostate cancer. Am J Surg Pathol 1989;13:389–96.

460. Hukill PB, Vidone RA. Histochemistry of mucus and other polysaccharides in tumors. II. Carcinoma of the prostate. Lab Invest 1967;16:395–405.

461. Humphrey PA. Mucin in severe dysplasia in the prostate. Surg Pathol 1991;4:137–43.

462. Humphrey PA, Walther PJ. Adenocarcinoma of the prostate. Part II. Tissue prognosticators. Am J Clin Pathol 1991;100:256–69.

462a. Iczkowski KA, Cheng L, Crawford BA, Bostwick DG. Steam heat with EDTA buffer and protease digestion optimizes immunohistochemical expression of basal cell-specific antikeratin 34βE12 to discriminate cancer in prostatic epithelium. Mod Pathol 1999;12:1–4.

463. Iwamura M, Wu G, Abrahamsson PA, di Sant Agnese PA, Crockett AT, Deftos LJ. Parathyroid hormone-related protein is expressed by prostatic neuroendocrine cells. Urology 1994;43:667–74.

464. Jones EC, McNeal J, Bruchovsky N, de Jong G. DNA content in prostatic adenocarcinoma. A flow cytometry study of the predictive value of aneuploidy for tumor volume, percentage Gleason grade 4 and 5, and lymph node metastases. Cancer 1990;66:752–7.

465. Jones EC, Young RH. The differential diagnosis of prostatic carcinoma. Its distinction from premalignant and pseudocarcinomatous lesions of the prostate gland. Am J Clin Pathol 1994;101:48–64.

466. Kallioniemi OP, Visakorpi T. Genetic basis and clonal evolution of human prostate cancer. Adv Cancer Res 1996;68:225–55.

467. Kastendieck H. Ultrastructural pathology of the human prostate gland. Cyto- and histomorphogenesis of atrophy, hyperplasia, metaplasia, dysplasia, and carcinoma. Prog Pathol 1977;106:1–63.

468. Keillor JS, Aterman K. The response of poorly differentiated prostatic tumors to staining for prostate specific antigen and prostatic acid phosphatase: a comparative study. J Urol 1987;137:894–6.

469. Kirby RS, Christmas TJ, Brawer MK. Prostate cancer. London: Mosby, 1996:155–66.

470. Kleer E, Larson-Keller JJ, Zincke H, Oesterling JE. Ability of preoperative serum prostate-specific antigen value to predict pathologic stage and DNA ploidy. Urology 1993;41:207–16.

471. Konchuba AM, Schellhammer PF, Kolm P, Clements MA, Wright GL Jr. Deoxyribonucleic acid cytometric analysis of prostate core biopsy specimens: relationship to serum prostate specific antigen and prostatic acid phosphatase, clinical stage and histopathology. J Urol 1993;150:115–9.

472. Labrie F, Dupont A, Cusan L, et al. Downstaging of localized prostate cancer by neoadjuvant therapy with flutamide and lupron: the first controlled and randomized trial. Clin Invest Med 1993;16:499–509.

473. Latil A, Lidereau R. Genetic aspects of prostate cancer. Virchows Arch 1998;432:389–406.

474. Leung CS, Zbieranowski I, Demers J, Murray D. DNA image cytometry of prostatic carcinoma: a comparison of needle core biopsy specimens and subsequent prostatectomy specimens. Mod Pathol 1994;7:195–9.

475. Li CY, Lam WK, Yam LT. Immunohistochemical diagnosis of prostatic cancer with metastasis. Cancer 1980;46:706–12.

475a. Lindemann N, Weidner N. Immunohistochemical profile of prostatic and urothelial carcinoma: impact of heat-induced epitope retrieval and presentation of tumors with intermediate features. Appl Immunohistochem 1996;4:264–75.

476. Lundberg S, Carstensen J, Rundquist I. DNA flow cytometry and histopathological grading of paraffin-embedded prostate biopsy specimens in a survival study. Cancer Res 1987;47:1973–7.

477. May EE, Perentes E. Anti-Leu 7 immunoreactivity with human tumours: its value in the diagnosis of prostatic adenocarcinoma. Histopathology 1987;11:295–304.

478. Maygarden SJ. Applications of immunohistochemistry to the diagnosis and prognostication of prostate cancer and prostatic intraepithelial neoplasia. Pathol Annu 1994;29(pt1):303–20.

479. McIntire TL, Murphy WM, Coon JS, et al. The prognostic value of DNA ploidy combined with histologic substaging for incidental carcinoma of the prostate. Am J Clin Pathol 1988;89:370–3.

480. Miller J, Horsfall DJ, Marshall VR, Rao DM, Leong SY. The prognostic value of deoxyribonucleic acid flow cytometric analysis in stage D2 prostatic carcinoma. J Urol 1991;145:1192–6.

481. Minkowitz G, Peterson P, Godwin TA. A histochemical and immunohistochemical study of adenocarcinomas involving urinary bladder [Abstract]. Mod Pathol 1990;3:68A.

482. Montgomery BT, Nativ O, Blute ML, et al. Stage B prostate adenocarcinoma. Flow cytometric nuclear DNA ploidy analysis. Arch Surg 1990;125:327–31.

483. Nadji M, Tabei SZ, Castro A, Chu TM, Morales AR. Prostatic origin of tumors. An immunohistochemical study. Am J Clin Pathol 1980;73:735–9.

484. Nadji M, Tabei SZ, Castro A, et al. Prostatic–specific antigen: an immunohistologic marker for prostatic neoplasms. Cancer 1981;48:1229–32.

485. Nakopoulou L, Stefanaki K, Deliveliotis C, Lazaris AC, Kondothanasis D, Dimopoulos CA. Neuroendocrine differentiation and proliferation state estimation in the hyperplastic and neoplastic human prostate. J Urol Pathol 1996;4:239–51.

486. Nativ O, Winkler HZ, Raz Y, et al. Stage C prostatic adenocarcinoma: flow cytometric nuclear DNA ploidy analysis. May Clin Proc 1989;64:911–9.

487. Netto GJ, Humphrey PA. Molecular biologic aspects of human prostatic carcinoma. Am J Clin Pathol 1994;102:S57–64.

488. O'Malley FP, Grignon DJ, Keeney M, Kerkvleit N, McLean C. DNA heterogeneity in prostatic adenocarcinoma. A DNA flow cytometric mapping study with whole organ sections of prostate. Cancer 1993;71:2797–802.

489. O'Malley FP, Grignon DJ, Shum DT. Usefulness of immunoperoxidase staining with high-molecular-weight cytokeratin in the differential diagnosis of small-acinar lesions of the prostate gland. Virchows Arch [A] 1990;417:191–6.

490. Ordonez NG, Ro JY, Ayala AG. Application of immunohistochemistry in the pathology of the prostate. In: Pathology of the prostate. Bostwick DG, ed. New York: Churchill Livingstone, 1990:137–60.

491. Palazzo JP, Ellison D, Petersen RO. DNA content in prostate adenocarcinoma. Correlation with Gleason score, nuclear grade and histologic subtypes. J Urol Pathol 1993;1:283–92.

492. Persons DL, Gibney DJ, Katzmann JA, Lieber MM, Farrow GM, Jenkins RB. Use of fluorescent in situ hybridization for deoxyribonucleic acid ploidy analysis of prostatic adenocarcinoma. J Urol 1993;150:120–5.

493. Purnell DM, Heatfield BM, Anthony RL, Trump BF. Immunohistochemistry of the cytoskeleton of human prostatic epithelium. Evidence for disturbed organization in neoplasia. Am J Pathol 1987;126:384–95.

494. Ritchie AW, Dorey F, Layfield LJ, Hannah J, Lovrekovich H, deKernion JB. Relationship of DNA content to conventional prognostic factors in clinically localised carcinoma of prostate. Br J Urol 1988;62:245–60.

495. Ro JY, Grignon DJ, Troncoso P, Ayala AG. Mucin in prostatic adenocarcinoma. Semin Diagn Pathol 1988;5:273–83.

496. Schmid KW, Helpap B, Totsch M, et al. Immunohistochemical localization of chromogranins A and B and secretogranin II in normal hyperplastic and neoplastic prostate. Histopathology 1994;24:233–9.

497. Sebo TJ, Bostwick DG, Farrow GM, Eble JN. Prostatic xanthoma: a mimic of prostatic adenocarcinoma. Hum Pathol 1994;25:386–9.

498. Shah IA, Schlageter MO, Stinnett P, Lechago J. Cytokeratin immunohistochemistry as a diagnostic tool for distinguishing malignant from benign epithelial lesions of the prostate. Mod Pathol 1991;4:220–4.

499. Shankey TV, Jin JK, Dougherty S, Flanigan RC, Graham S. DNA ploidy and proliferation heterogeneity in human prostate cancers. Cytometry 1995;21:30–9.

500. Shankey TV, Kallioniemi OP, Koslowski JM, et al. Consensus review of the clinical utility of DNA content cytometry in prostate cancer. Cytometry 1993;14:497–500.

501. Smith JR, Freije D, Carpten JD, et al. Major susceptibility locus for prostate cancer on chromosome 1 suggested by a genome-wide search. Science 1996;274:1371–4.

502. Song J, Chen WS, Cupps RE, Earle JD, Farrow CM, Lieber MM. Nuclear deoxyribonucleic acid content measured by static cytometry: important prognostic association for patients with clinically localized prostate carcinoma treated by external beam radiotherapy. J Urol 1992;147:794–7.

503. Speights Jr. VO, Arber DA, Riggs MW, Arber J, Chen PY. Proliferative index of organ-confined prostatic adenocarcinoma determined by MIB-1. J Urol Pathol 1996;4:25–30.

504. Srigley JR, Hartwick WJ, Edwards V, de Harven E. Selected ultrastructural aspects of urothelial and prostatic tumors. Ultrastruct Pathol 1988;12:49–65.

505. Stein BS, Vangore S, Peterson RO, Kendal AR. Immunoperoxidase localization of prostate-specific antigen. Am J Surg Pathol 1982;6:553–7.

506. Stephenson RA, James BC, Gay H, Fair WR, Whitmore WF, Melamed MR. Flow cytometry of prostate cancer: relationship of DNA content to survival. Cancer Res 1987;47:2504–7.

507. Svanholm H. Evaluation of commercial immuno-peroxidase kits for prostate specific antigen and prostatic specific acid phosphatase. APMIS 1986;94:7–12.

508. Takahashi S, Quian J, Brown JA, et al. Potential markers of prostate cancer aggressiveness detected by fluorescence in situ hybridization in needle biopsies. Cancer Res 1994;54:3574–9.

509. Takai K, Goellner JR, Katzmann JA, Myers RP, Lieber MM. Static image and flow DNA cytometry of prostatic adenocarcinoma. Studies of needle biopsy and radical prostatectomy specimens. J Urol Pathol 1994;2:39–47.

510. Taylor NH. Histochemistry in the diagnosis of early prostatic carcinoma. Hum Pathol 1979;10:513–20.

511. Tinari N, Naroli C, Angelucci D, et al. DNA and S-phase fraction analysis by flow cytometry in prostate cancer. Clinicopathologic implications. Cancer 1993;71:1289–96.

512. van den Ouden D, Tribukait B, Blom JH, et al. Deoxyribonucleic acid ploidy of core biopsies and metastatic lymph nodes of prostate cancer patients: impact on time to progression. The European Organization for Research and Treatment of Cancer Genitourinary Group. J Urol 1993;150:400–6.

512a.Varma M, Linden MD, Amin MB. Effect of formalin fixation and epitope retrieval techniques on antibody 34βE12 immunostaining of prostatic tissues. Mod Pathol 1999;12:472–8.

513. von Eschenbach AC, Brawer MK, di Sant Agnese PA, et al. Exploration of new pathologic factors in terms of potential for prognostic significance and future applications. Cancer 1996;78:372–5.

514. Wernert N, Seitz G, Achtstatter T. Immunohistochemical investigation of different cytokeratins and vimentin in the prostate from the fetal period up to adulthood and in prostate carcinoma. Path Res Pract 1987;182:617–26.

515. Wiatrowska BA, Robertson S, Crook JM. Measures of proliferative activity in prostatic adenocarcinoma. J Urol Pathol 1997;6:131–8.

516. Winkler HZ, Rainwater LM, Myers RP, et al. Stage D1 prostatic adenocarcinoma: significance of nuclear DNA ploidy patterns studied by flow cytometry. May Clin Pro 1988;63:103–12.

517. Wojno KJ, Epstein JI. The utility of basal cell-specific anti-cytokeratin antibody (34 beta E12) in the diagnosis of prostatic cancer. A review 228 cases. Am J Surg Pathol 1995;19:251–60.

518. Yam LT, Winkler CF, Janckila AJ, Li CY, Lam KW. Prostatic cancer presenting as metastatic adenocarcinoma of undetermined origin. Cancer 1983;51:283–7.

518a.Yang XJ, Lecksell K, Gaudin P, Epstein JI. Rare expression of high molecular weight cytokeratin in adenocarcinoma of the prostate. A study of 110 cases of metastatic and locally advanced prostate cancer. Am J Surg Pathol 1999;23:147–52.

519. Zincke H, Bergstralh EJ, Larson-Keller JJ, et al. Stage D1 prostate cancer treated by radical prostatectomy and adjuvant hormonal treatment. Evidence for favorable survival in patients with DNA diploid tumors. Cancer 1992;70:311–23.

Treatment and Prognosis

520. Bastacky SI, Walsh PC, Epstein JI. Relationship between perineural tumor invasion on needle biopsy and radical prostatectomy capsular penetration in clinical stage B adenocarcinoma of the prostate. Am J Surg Pathol 1993;17:336–41.

520a.Bostwick DG, Grignon D, Amin MB, et al. Prognostic factors in prostate cancer: College of American Pathologists consensus statement 1999. Arch Pathol Lab Med 2000;124:995–1000.

521. Bruce RG, Rankin WR, Cibull ML, Rayens MK, Banks ER, Wood DP Jr. Single focus of adenocarcinoma in the prostate biopsy specimen is not predictive of pathologic stage of disease. Urology 1996;48:75–9.

522. Byar DP and The Veterans Administration Cooperative Urological Research Group. Survival of patients with incidentally found microscopic cancer of the prostate: results of a clinical trial of conservative treatment. J Urol 1972;108:908–13.

523. Byar DP, Mostofi FK and The Veterans Administration Cooperative Urological Research Group. Carcinoma of the prostate: prognostic evaluation of certain pathologic features in 208 radical prostatectomies. Examined by the step–section technique. Cancer 1972;30:5–13.

524. Carter HB, Sauvageot J, Walsh PC, Epstein JI. Prospective evaluation of men with stage T1C adenocarcinoma of the prostate. J Urol 1997;157:2206–9.

525. Chan TY, Epstein JI. Follow up of atypical needle biopsies suspicious for cancer. Urology 1999;53:351–5.

526. Christensen WN, Partin AW, Walsh PC, Epstein JI. Pathologic findings in clinical stage A2 prostate cancer. Relation of tumor volume, grade, and location to pathologic stage. Cancer 1990;65:1021–7.

527. Cupp MR, Bostwick DG, Myers RP, Oesterling JE. The volume of prostate cancer in the biopsy specimen cannot reliably predict the quantity of cancer in the radical prostatectomy specimen on an individual basis. J Urol 1995;153:1543–8.

528. DiGiuseppe JA, Sauvegeot J, Epstein JI. Increasing incidence of minimal residual cancer in radical prostatectomy specimens. Am J Surg Pathol 1997;21:174–8.

529. Egan AJ, Bostwick DG. Prediction of extraprostatic extension of prostate cancer based on needle biopsy findings: perineural invasion lacks significance on multivariate analysis. Am J Surg Pathol 1997;21:1496–500.

530. Epstein JI. Evaluation of radical prostatectomy capsular margins of resection. The significance of margins designated as negative, closely approaching, and positive. Am J Surg Pathol 1990;14:626–32.

531. Epstein JI. The evaluation of radical prostatectomy specimens. Therapeutic and prognostic implications. Path Annu 1991;26(pt.1):159–210.

532. Epstein JI. Pathologic features that predict progression of disease following radical prostatectomy. In: Pathology of the prostate. Foster CS, Bostwick DG, eds. Philadelphia: WB Saunders, 1997:228–44.

533. Epstein JI, Carmichael MJ, Partin AW, Walsh PC. Small high grade adenocarcinoma of the prostate in radical prostatectomy specimens performed for neopalpable disease: pathogenetic and clinical implications. J Urol 1994;151:1587–92.

534. Epstein JI, Paull G, Eggleston JC, Walsh PC. Prognosis of untreated stage A1 prostatic carcinoma: a study of 94 cases with extended follow up. J Urol 1986;136:837–9.

535. Epstein JI, Pizov G, Walsh PC. Correlation of pathologic findings with progression after radical retropubic prostatectomy. Cancer 1993;71:3582–93.

536. Epstein JI, Pound CR, Partin AW, Walsh PC. Progression following radical prostatectomy in men with Gleason score 7 tumor. J Urol 1998;160:97–100.

537. Epstein JI, Steinberg GD. The significance of low-grade prostate cancer on needle biopsy. A radical prostatectomy study of tumor grade, volume, and stage of the biopsied and multifocal tumor. Cancer 1990;66:1927–32.

538. Epstein JI, Walsh PC, Carmichael M, Brendler CB. Pathologic and clinical findings to predict tumor extent of nonpalpable (stage T1c) prostate cancer. JAMA 1994;271:368–74.

539. Epstein JI, Walsh PC, Sauvageot J, Carter HB. Utility of repeat sextant and transition zone biopsies for assessing extent of prostate cancer. J Urol 1997;158:1886–90.

540. Fleming C, Wasson JH, Albertsen PC, Barry MJ, Wennberg JE. A decision analysis of alternative treatment strategies for clinically localized prostate cancer. JAMA 1993;269:2650–8.

541. Gittes RF. Carcinoma of the prostate. N Engl J Med 1991;324:236–45.

542. Goldenberg SL, Klotz LH, Srigley JR, et al. Randomized prospective controlled study comparing radical prostatectomy alone and neoadjuvant reversible androgen withdrawal therapy with cyproterone acetate in the management of localized prostate cancer. J Urol 1996;156:873–7.

543. Grignon DJ. Minimal diagnostic criteria for adenocarcinoma of the prostate. J Urol Pathol 1998;8:31–43.

544. Grignon DJ, Sakr WA. Pathologic staging of prostate carcinoma. What are the issues? Cancer 1996;78:337–40.

545. Helpap B. Review of the morphology of prostatic carcinoma with special emphasis on subgrading and prognosis. J Urol Pathol 1993;1:3–19.

546. Kirby RS, Christmas TJ, Brawer M. Prostate cancer. London: Mosby, 1996:93–166.

547. Labrie F, Dupont A, Cusan L, et al. Downstaging of localized prostate cancer by neoadjuvant therapy with flutamide and lupron: the first controlled and randomized trial. Clin Invest Med 1993;16:511–2.

548. McNeal JE. Cancer volume and site of origin of adenocarcinoma in the prostate: relationship to local and distant spread. Hum Pathol 1992;23:258–66.

549. McNeal JE, Bostwick DG, Kindrachuk RA, Redwine EA, Freiha FS, Stamey TA. Patterns of progression in prostate cancer. Lancet 1986;1:60–3.

550. McNeal JE, Villers AA, Redwine EA, Freiha FS, Stamey TA. Histologic differentiation, cancer volume, and pelvic lymph node metastasis in adenocarcinoma of the prostate. Cancer 1990;66:1225–33.

551. McNeal JE, Villers AA, Redwine EA, Freiha FS, Stamey TA. Capsular penetration in prostate cancer. Significance for natural history and treatment. Am J Surg Pathol 1990;14:240–7.

552. Mettlin CJ, Murphy GP, McGinnis LS, Menck HR. The National Cancer Data Base report on prostate cancer. Cancer 1995;76:1104–12.

553. Middleton RG. The management of clinically localized prostate cancer: guidelines from the American Urological Association. CA Cancer J Clin 1996;46:249–53.

554. Ohori M, Scardino PT, Lapin SL, Seale Hawkins C, Link J, Wheeler TM. The mechanisms and prognostic significance of seminal vesicle involvement by prostate cancer. Am J Surg Pathol 1993;17:1252–61.

555. Oesterling JE, Brendler CB, Epstein JI, Kimball AW Jr, Walsh PC. Correlation of clinical stage, serum prostatic acid phosphatase and preoperative Gleason grade with final pathological stage in 275 patients with clinically localized adenocarcinoma of the prostate. J Urol 1987;138:92–8.

556. Partin AW, Lee BR, Carmichael M, Walsh PC, Epstein JI. Radical prostatectomy for high grade disease: a reevaluation 1994. J Urol 1994;151:1583–6.

557. Partin AW, Steinberg GD, Pitcock RV, et al. Use of nuclear morphometry, Gleason histologic scoring, clinical stage, and age to predict disease-free survival among patients with prostate cancer. Cancer 1992;70:161–168.

558. Pfister S, Kleinschmidt-DeMasters BK. Dural metastases from prostatic adenocarcinoma. Report of five cases and review of the literature. J Urol Pathol 1995;3:119–27.

558a. Pilepich MV, Krall JM, Al-Sarraf M, et al. Androgen deprivation with radiation therapy compared with radiation therapy alone for locally advanced prostatic carcinoma: a randomized comparative trial of the radiation therapy oncology group. Urology 1995;45:616–23.

559. Pontes JE, Wajsman Z, Huben RP, et al. Prognostic factors in localized prostatic carcinoma. J Urol 1985;134:1137–9.

560. Scardino PT, Weaver R, Hudson ML. Early detection of prostate cancer. Hum Pathol 1992;23:211–22.

561. See WA, Williams RD. Management of prostate cancer stage by stage. In: Das S, Crawford ED, eds. Cancer of the prostate. New York: Marcel Dekker, 1993.

562. Soloway MS, Hachiya T, Civantos F, Murphy WM, Comez CC, Ruiz HE. Androgen deprivation therapy prior to radical prostatectomy for T2b and T3 prostate cancer. Urology 1994;43:52–6.

563. Stamey TA, McNeal JE. Adenocarcinoma of prostate. In: Campbell's urology. Walsh PC, Retik AB, Stamey Ta, Vaughan, eds. Philadelphia: WB Saunders, 1992:1159–221.

564. Steinberg DM, Sauvageot J, Piantadosi S, Epstein JI. Correlation of prostate needle biopsy and radical prostatectomy Gleason grade in academic and community settings. Am J Surg Pathol 1997;21:566–76.

565. Thompson IM. Observation alone in the management of localized prostate cancer: the natural history of untreated disease. Urology 1994;43(Suppl):41–6.

566. Vickery Jr AL, Kerr Jr WS. Carcinoma of the prostate treated by radical prostatectomy. A clinicopathological survey of 187 cases followed for 5 years and 148 cases followed for 10 years. Cancer 1963;16:1598–608.

567. Voges GE, McNeal JE, Redwine EA, Freiha FS, Stamey TA. Morphologic analysis of surgical margins with positive findings in prostatectomy for adenocarcinoma of the prostate. Cancer 1992;69:520–6.

568. Whitmore WF Jr. Management of clinically localized prostatic cancer. An unresolved problem [Editorial]. JAMA 1993;269:2676–7.

5

VARIANTS OF PROSTATIC ADENOCARCINOMA, OTHER PRIMARY CARCINOMAS OF PROSTATE, AND SECONDARY CARCINOMAS

The primary carcinomas considered here (Table 5-1), which account for 5 to 10 percent of prostatic carcinomas, include all those that differ from the various forms of "conventional" adenocarcinoma discussed in chapter 4. Their recognition is important since many have a poor prognosis, and their differential diagnosis often differs from that of conventional prostatic carcinoma. Several of them raise the possibility of an origin from an extraprostatic local or distant site, and for that reason secondary carcinomas are also considered in this chapter. The primary neoplasms discussed here exhibit a diverse histologic spectrum and rarely occur in pure form, usually being associated with conventional neoplasia. The Gleason grading scheme, although designed for conventional adenocarcinoma, can often be applied to these variants, which almost always are grade 3 or higher.

Table 5-1

PRIMARY CARCINOMAS OF THE PROSTATE (OTHER THAN CONVENTIONAL ADENOCARCINOMA) AND SECONDARY CARCINOMAS OF THE PROSTATE*

Primary carcinomas other than conventional
    adenocarcinoma
  Prostatic duct adenocarcinoma
  Mucinous (colloid) adenocarcinoma
  Signet ring cell carcinoma
  Adenosquamous and squamous carcinomas
  Basaloid and adenoid cystic carcinomas
  Transitional cell carcinoma
  Small cell carcinoma
  Sarcomatoid carcinoma
  Lymphoepithelioma-like carcinoma
  Undifferentiated carcinoma, not otherwise
    specified

Secondary carcinomas
  Transitional cell carcinoma
  Other tumors extending from adjacent viscera
  Metastatic solid tumors from more distant sites

* Carcinosarcoma is discussed in this chapter with sarcomatoid carcinoma, as explained in the text.

PROSTATIC DUCT ADENOCARCINOMA

General and Clinical Features. This variant was described by Melicow and Pachter in 1967 (20) as "endometrioid adenocarcinoma" because it histologically often resembles adenocarcinoma of the endometrium. It was initially thought to be of müllerian origin and was postulated to arise from the müllerian-derived prostatic utricle. Multiple studies based on routine light microscopy, immunohistochemistry, and ultrastructural analysis have shown, however, that this tumor is of prostatic epithelial cell origin (5,8,13,18,24,26,31,34). Additionally, it has recently been suggested that a male müllerian regression factor promotes involution of müllerian structures, and prostatic epithelium supervenes as the lining of the utricle (14).

These tumors account for about 1 percent of prostatic adenocarcinomas; Dube et al. (11) identified 55 in a review of 4,286 prostatic adenocarcinomas from the Mayo Clinic. Up to 50 percent of the tumors are associated with a component of conventional carcinoma that is usually minor (23a). Whether ductal adenocarcinoma is a unique variant of prostatic carcinoma and inherently distinct from the cribriform and comedo forms of conventional carcinoma is an issue that remains unresolved (4a,19). We consider it sufficiently distinctive pathologically, especially when seen in pure form, to merit separate consideration here.

The mean patient age is 65 years and, unlike conventional adenocarcinoma, hematuria and urinary obstruction are the two most frequent presenting symptoms (2–18,21–25,28–34). Cystoscopy may show a papillary growth at the verumontanum; as a result, these tumors are frequently discovered in transurethral resectates (2,11,25). Serum prostatic acid phosphatase (PAP) and prostate-specific antigen (PSA) levels may be normal or elevated, being more often normal in cases of organ-confined duct carcinoma than in cases of conventional non-duct carcinoma. In cases of peripheral tumors or those extensively involving the prostate, the gland

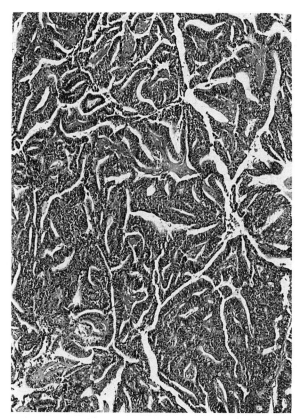

Figure 5-1
PROSTATIC DUCT CARCINOMA, TYPE A
This low-power view shows the complex tubulopapillary architecture.

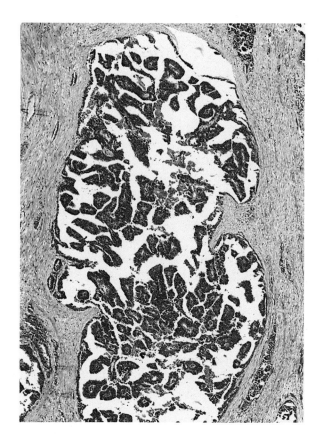

Figure 5-2
PROSTATIC DUCT CARCINOMA, TYPE A
There is cystic dilatation of a duct with a complex intraluminal papillary proliferation.

may be abnormal on digital examination. The tumors may be clinically unsuspected (stage T1; A) but more commonly present as locally advanced (stage T3; C) or metastatic disease. The pattern of spread is similar to typical prostatic carcinoma. Pelvic lymph nodes may be involved, and bone metastasis is common; the latter may be lytic but is more frequently blastic (5,22).

Gross Findings. Centrally occurring tumors may appear as friable, papillary, grayish white masses growing within a sometimes dilated prostatic urethra. Prostatic parenchymal involvement may or may not be apparent, and is not distinct from that of other carcinomas.

Microscopic Findings. The tumors grow in one of two ways: as papillary or polypoid masses within the prostatic urethra and periurethral ducts where there is more space for growth than within the prostatic parenchyma, or diffusely with extensive involvement of the gland, includ-

ing the transition and peripheral zones. Histologically, two basic patterns, arbitrarily designated types A (figs. 5-1–5-5) and B (figs. 5-6–5-8), have been described (2,26). Eight of the 55 cases in the series of Dube et al. (11) involved large central periurethral prostatic ducts and were called "adenocarcinoma of primary prostate ducts," and 47 were multicentric involving intermediate and small ducts, "adenocarcinoma of the secondary prostate ducts." These two categories roughly correspond to the above type A and B patterns, respectively. Subdivision into these categories is not required in routine practice. Type A shows an exuberant papillary and tubulo-papillary growth, with the tubules and papillae lined by cells ranging from a single layer to stratified, tall columnar epithelium (figs. 5-4, 5-5). The cells have appreciable eosinophilic cytoplasm; basally located or stratified, elongated nuclei; prominent nucleoli; irregular chromatin; and

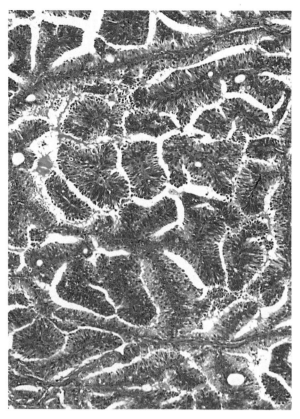

Figure 5-3
PROSTATIC DUCT CARCINOMA, TYPE A
Papillae are lined by high-grade tumor cells ranging from a single layer to pseudostratified columnar.

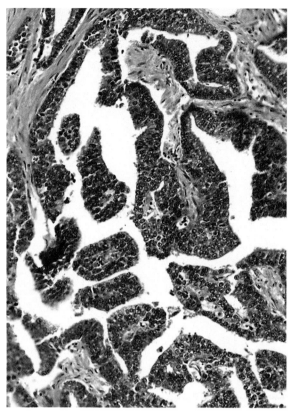

Figure 5-4
PROSTATIC DUCT CARCINOMA, TYPE A
Note the cellular stratification.

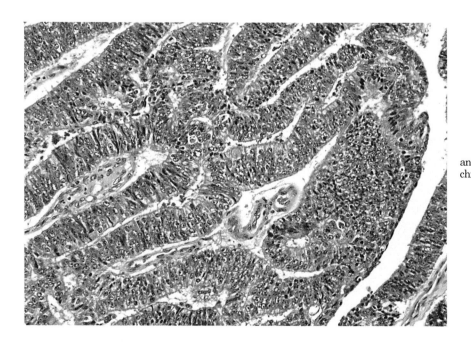

Figure 5-5
PROSTATIC DUCT
CARCINOMA, TYPE A
The tumor cells are elongated and pseudostratified, with irregular chromatin and prominent nucleoli.

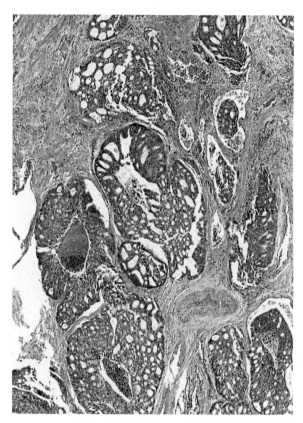

Figure 5-6
PROSTATIC DUCT CARCINOMA, TYPE B
There is a complex cribriform growth with comedonecrosis.

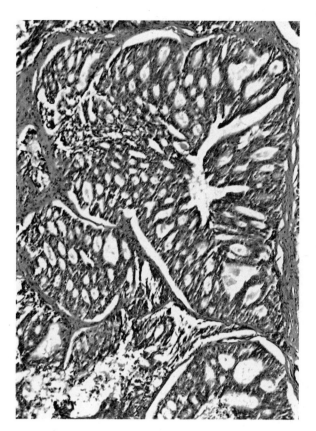

Figure 5-7
PROSTATIC DUCT CARCINOMA, TYPE B
Higher power view of the cribriform pattern.

frequent mitoses (fig. 5-8). Type B is more heterogeneous and characterized by intraductal papillary, solid, or complex glandular (cribriform) growth, with or without comedonecrosis (figs. 5-6, 5-7). This form is frequently associated with tumors located deeper within the prostatic parenchyma. The two patterns often coexist and may merge (2,26).

Except for some type A cancers which may have more banal nuclear features, most ductal carcinomas show high-grade cytologic atypia and more frequent mitotic activity than conventional acinar carcinomas (25). They are most frequently of Gleason pattern 4 (tumor masses containing anastomosing, irregular, cribriform glands) or Gleason pattern 5 (presence of comedonecrosis); infrequently the intraductal papillary-cribriform pattern has smooth rounded edges (Gleason 3C).

The tumor is positive on immunohistochemical staining for PSA (fig. 5-9) and PAP (fig. 5-10) and may be weakly and focally positive for carcinoembryonic antigen (CEA) (5,13,17,18,26,29). The stain for basal cell–specific high molecular weight cytokeratin (clone 34βE12) is negative in most areas. However, this stain often shows basal cells in some foci, chiefly at the periphery of neoplastic aggregates, consistent with growth within preexistent ducts (27). Ultrastructural examination shows well-developed glands with distinct basal lamina, luminal microvilli, abundant rough endoplasmic reticulum, lysosomes, and desmosomes; ciliated cells are not present in most reports, and putative examples may represent artifactual disruption of the cell membrane (5,7,13, 26). Two cell types, light and dark, are seen: the latter are basally located and have large nucleoli, and the former contain lipid, lysosomes, rough endoplasmic reticulum, and mitochondria (34).

Differential Diagnosis. Establishing a diagnosis of carcinoma in these cases is rarely, if ever, a problem, particularly when compared to the

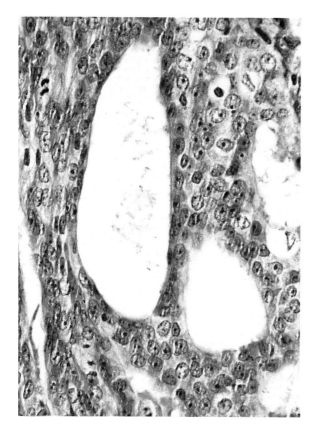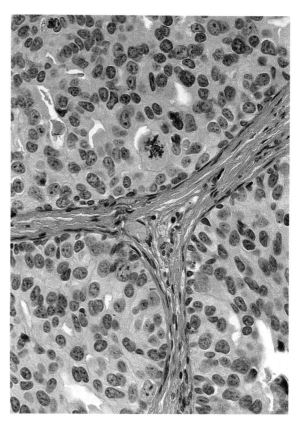

Figure 5-8
PROSTATIC DUCT CARCINOMA, TYPE B
These high-power views depict the high-grade nuclear features that are characteristically present. Note the brisk mitotic activity and the frequently irregular chromatin distribution.

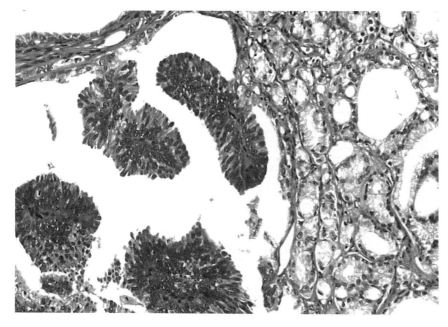

Figure 5-9
PROSTATIC DUCT
CARCINOMA WITH
ASSOCIATED
CONVENTIONAL
ADENOCARCINOMA
COMPONENT

The high-grade nuclear features of the ductal carcinoma (left) contrast with the monotonous nuclei of the conventional carcinoma (right). (Fig. 4-65 from Ro JY, Grignon DJ, Amin MB, Ayala AG. Atlas of surgical pathology of the male reproductive tract. Philadelphia: W.B. Saunders, 1997:65.)

221

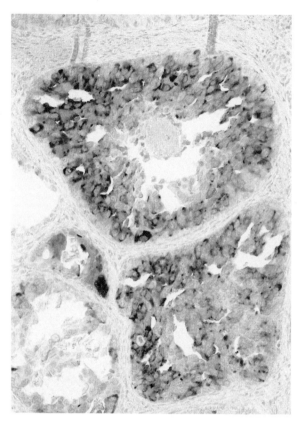

Figure 5-10
PROSTATIC DUCT CARCINOMA
There is positivity for prostatic acid phosphatase.

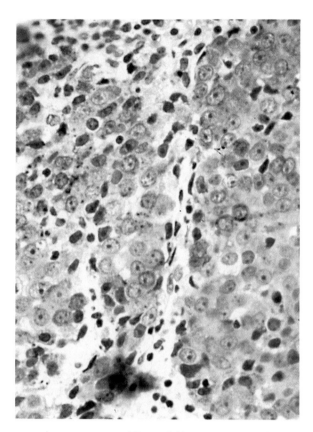

Figure 5-11
PROSTATIC DUCT CARCINOMA
There is diffusely positive immunostaining for prostate-specific antigen.

frequent problems making a definitive diagnosis in cases of conventional carcinoma. As noted earlier, distinction from conventional adenocarcinoma with similar patterns may be extremely difficult but is not of major consequence with regard to therapeutic decisions. If the majority of the tumor shows ductal patterns, and has high-grade nuclear features, the diagnosis of ductal carcinoma is appropriately rendered in parenthesis after the primary diagnosis and grading, e.g., prostatic adenocarcinoma, Gleason grade 4 + 4 = score 8 (ductal variant). Such a subcategorization should generally not be made on needle biopsy findings alone, as it is not possible to reliably distinguish ductal carcinoma and conventional carcinoma with a cribriform-papillary pattern in limited material. If a high nuclear grade and brisk mitotic activity is evident, a ductal tumor is suggested (fig. 5-11) (3,25). High-grade prostatic intraepithelial neoplasia and transitional cell carcinoma involving prostatic

ducts and acini may enter the differential. The former does not show the same degree of crowding, back to back arrangement, gland fusion, growth along true fibrovascular cores, and nuclear atypia as ductal carcinoma, and it consistently retains a basal cell layer to a greater extent (fig. 5-12) (1). Transitional cell carcinoma may also show considerable nuclear atypia but usually lacks gland differentiation (see discussion of primary and secondary transitional cell carcinoma) and lacks immunoreactivity for PSA and PAP. When presenting as a urethral mass ductal carcinoma may mimic a urethral primary (see chapter 8).

Prognosis. When this tumor was first recognized, it was characterized as low grade because of its early presentation, frequent localization within the prostate, and relatively favorable short-term prognosis (5,21,22,29,34). Recent studies (5,8, 13,26), however, indicate that most prostatic duct adenocarcinomas present at advanced stage and

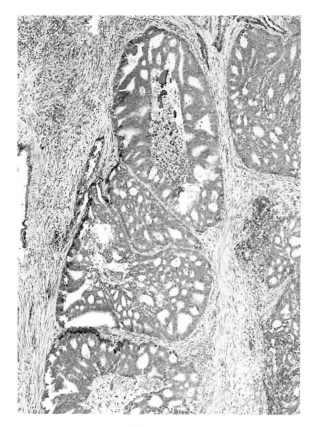

Figure 5-12
PROSTATIC DUCT CARCINOMA
Immunostains for basal cell-specific cytokeratin (clone 34βE12) are negative around the cribriform nests of prostatic duct carcinoma. Note the circumferential staining of adjacent benign glands.

pursue an aggressive course. Dube et al. (11) found a 5-year survival rate of 42.8 percent (similar to usual carcinoma) for carcinomas of primary ducts but only 24.2 percent for tumors of the secondary ducts which accounted for the majority of their cases. In one series of 10 cases, 50 percent of the patients had metastatic disease (13). The 5-year survival rates in two other series were 15 and 30 percent, with median survival times of 37 and 46.3 months, respectively (5,26). Finally, in an analysis of prostatectomies, Christensen et al. (8) reported that these tumors were at a more advanced pathologic stage than clinically suspected and had a higher recurrence rate than conventional carcinomas of similar clinical stage. Ninety-three percent of the tumors penetrated the capsule, 47 percent involved the surgical margin; 40 percent invaded the seminal vesicle, and 27 percent spread to pelvic lymph nodes.

MUCINOUS (COLLOID) ADENOCARCINOMA

Intraluminal mucin, apparent as blue wispy material under light microscopy, is seen in up to 34 percent of needle biopsy specimens and 60 percent of transurethral resection and prostatectomy specimens of conventional adenocarcinomas (38). Using mucin stains, such as alcian blue at pH 2.5, it can be found in 60 to 90 percent of carcinomas (41,43–45,55). The term "mucinous carcinoma," however, is reserved for tumors meeting the following criteria: 1) at least 25 percent of the resected neoplasm must be composed of tumor cells floating in lakes of extracellular mucin; 2) glands containing intraluminal mucin (commonly seen in conventional adenocarcinoma) do not qualify as mucinous carcinoma; and 3) an extraprostatic origin must be excluded (42,53,54).

General and Clinical Features. Applying the above criteria, two groups found that mucinous adenocarcinoma represents approximately 0.4 percent of all prostatic carcinomas (42,54). A portion of the tumor is almost invariably typical adenocarcinoma if entirely examined. Some early reports that did not use standardized criteria suggested that mucinous carcinoma is histogenetically, and perhaps clinically, different from conventional adenocarcinoma, with a more favorable outcome (35,39,40,46–48,50,56). Using strict diagnostic criteria, more recent reports show that the patient age, clinical symptoms, disease stage, metastatic patterns, and hormone responsiveness are similar to those of conventional carcinoma of similar grade (42,49,54,57). These tumors may present problems in diagnosis and staging by magnetic resonance imaging (MRI) due to an atypical signal intensity on the T2-weighted images which approximates or exceeds that of the uninvolved peripheral zone (51). In one series, 7 of 12 patients died of disease (mean follow-up, 56 months), and 5 were alive with disease (mean follow-up, 32.2 months) (54).

Gross Findings. A mucoid appearance may be appreciable on gross examination (fig. 5-13), but many tumors are not grossly distinctive.

Microscopic Findings. Lakes of extracellular mucin contain cribriform and anastomosing masses or nests of cells, with occasional well-formed acini (figs. 5-14–5-16) (42,53,54). Signet ring cells or goblet cells are uncommon. Cytologic features vary

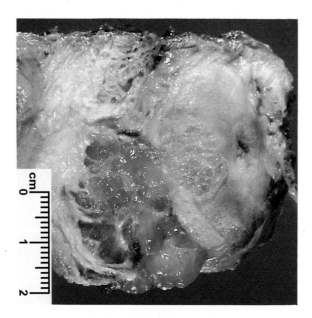

Figure 5-13
MUCINOUS ADENOCARCINOMA
Large globules of glistening mucinous material are evident. (Fig. 4-56 from Ro JY, Grignon DJ, Amin MB, Ayala AG. Atlas of surgical pathology of the male reproductive tract. Philadelphia: W.B. Saunders, 1997:62.)

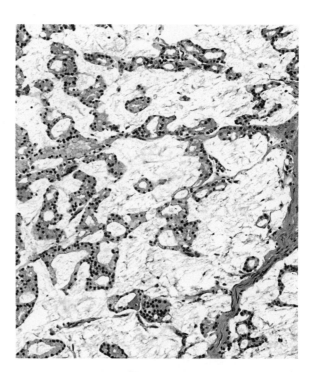

Figure 5-14
MUCINOUS ADENOCARCINOMA
Abundant extracellular mucin contains anastomosing neoplastic acini.

from relatively bland to atypical with prominent nucleoli. The grade of the accompanying typical carcinoma is usually high and, based on the fused glands of most cases, the Gleason grade of the mucinous component is typically 4 (37).

The extracellular mucin may be highlighted by a variety of histochemical stains including periodic acid–Schiff (PAS), mucicarmine, and alcian blue at pH 2.5 (fig. 5-17). The staining is markedly diminished at pH 0.9 indicating that the acid mucin is of the nonsulfated variety. The intraluminal mucin found in a high proportion of typical carcinomas has a similar staining profile. The tumor cells are positive for PSA (fig. 5-18) and PAP, but do not usually stain for CEA; mucin stains may show luminal rimming and apical membrane staining, but intracytoplasmic staining is generally absent (42,54).

Differential Diagnosis. Extraprostatic primary mucinous carcinomas from the colon, bladder, prostatic urethra, and Cowper's gland should be ruled out, although the component of typical prostatic adenocarcinoma readily permits this distinction in most cases (36,52); in addition the arrangement of the epithelial aggregates in the mucin as small acini is more typical

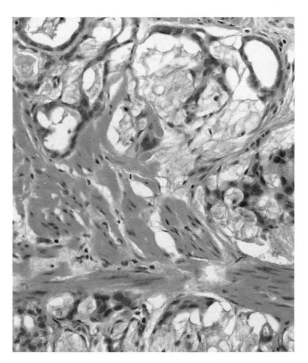

Figure 5-15
MUCINOUS ADENOCARCINOMA
Pools of mucin separate neoplastic acini.

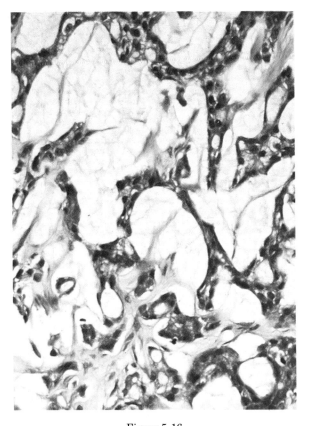

Figure 5-16
MUCINOUS ADENOCARCINOMA
The cytologic features are relatively bland with only occasional prominent nucleoli.

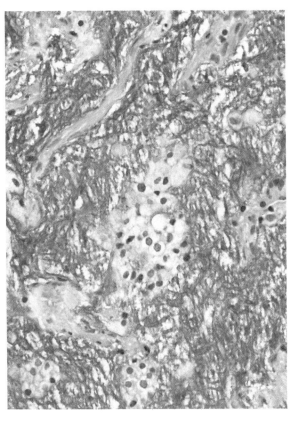

Figure 5-17
MUCINOUS ADENOCARCINOMA
Alcian blue at pH 2.5 highlights the abundant extracellular mucin.

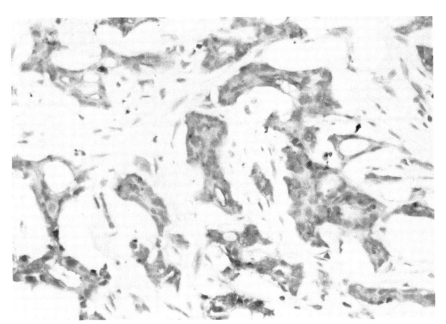

Figure 5-18
MUCINOUS
ADENOCARCINOMA
There is cytoplasmic immuno-staining for PSA in the neoplastic cells.

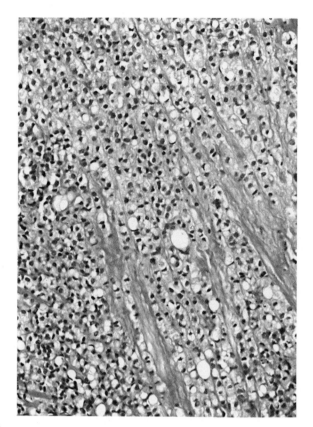

Figure 5-19
SIGNET RING CELL CARCINOMA
Signet ring cells extensively infiltrate the prostatic parenchyma.

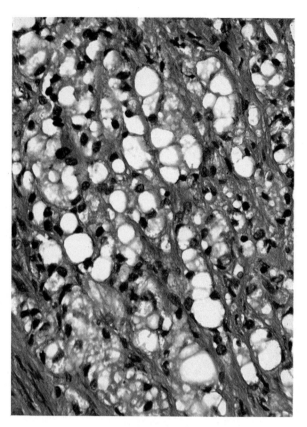

Figure 5-20
SIGNET RING CELL CARCINOMA
A high-power field shows the typical morphology.

of prostatic neoplasia than the other tumor types. Immunostains for PSA and PAP will be definitive in a problematic case.

SIGNET RING CELL CARCINOMA

General and Clinical Features. Signet ring cells may be seen focally within otherwise typical adenocarcinoma, and we require that they compose 25 percent of the tumor before using the designation, signet ring cell carcinoma. This cutoff is arbitrary but is recommended, since most of the reported tumors appear to fulfill this criterion.

This tumor is rare, with less than 25 cases reported (58–60,62,64–66,68–70). The age range (sixth to ninth decade), symptoms, and signs are similar to those of conventional prostatic carcinoma. The serum PSA level is frequently elevated. Some patients have presented with enlarged supraclavicular lymph nodes, and one presented with malignant ascites (61,63,66). In one series of eight patients, five had stage C disease and three stage D; five died 32 to 60 months after diagnosis (66).

Pathologic Findings. No specific gross features have been described. The neoplastic signet ring cells usually grow in clusters and singly and are widely infiltrative (fig. 5-19). They are associated with conventional high-grade prostatic carcinoma in a variety of patterns. A Gleason grade of 4 or 5 is usual. The tumors often demonstrate extracapsular extension, and blood vascular-lymphatic and perineural invasion. The signet ring cells have optically clear vacuoles which displace the nucleus (fig. 5-20). High-grade prostatic intraepithelial neoplasia with signet ring cell features may be identified in the invasive cancer or at its periphery (see chapter 3) (65). There is usually no associated mucinous carcinoma component. In the majority of the cases stains for cytokeratin, PSA (fig. 5-21), and PAP are positive, and 20

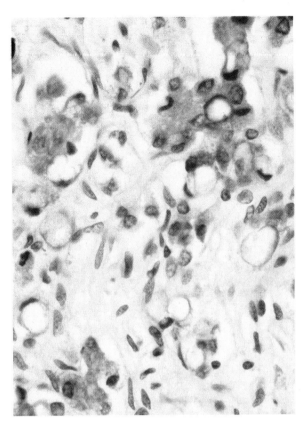

Figure 5-21
SIGNET RING CELL CARCINOMA
Immunostains for PSA are positive.

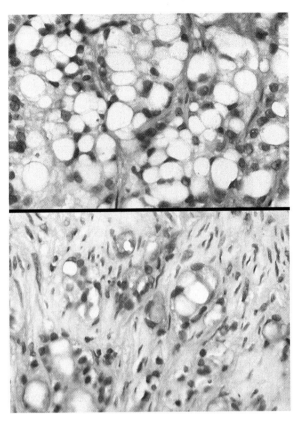

Figure 5-22
SIGNET RING CELL CARCINOMA
In most cases the cytoplasmic vacuoles do not stain for mucin (top), but occasionally they are positive (bottom). (Alcian blue at pH 2.5.) (Fig. 4-61 from Ro JY, Grignon DJ, Amin MB, Ayala AG. Atlas of surgical pathology of the male reproductive tract. Philadelphia: W.B. Saunders, 1997:64.)

percent are positive for CEA (63,66). Most tumors are negative for intracytoplasmic mucin (PAS, mucicarmine, alcian blue). Occasional positivity for mucin is seen but is usually focal and relatively unimpressive (69a), only rarely approaching in amount the staining seen with conventional signet ring cell carcinoma of other organs (fig. 5-22) (68). One tumor stained with Sudan black, indicating fat as the cause of the signet ring cell appearance (67). Ultrastructural examination of 10 cases (59,62,66) revealed intracytoplasmic lumens, occasional microvilli, and cytoplasmic vacuoles, without mucin or fat. This variability in immunohistochemical and ultrastructural findings suggests that the origin of the signet ring cell morphology may be varied, including the accumulation of excess PSA and PAP, mucin, or fat, or the formation of empty intracytoplasmic lumens.

Differential Diagnosis. In biopsy specimens lacking evidence of conventional acinar carcinoma, metastatic signet ring cell carcinoma must be ruled out. Clinical findings often help. Additionally, in contrast to signet ring cell carcinomas of other origins, those derived from the prostate are usually mucin negative. Their staining for PSA and PAP is further discriminatory. If a metastatic signet ring cell carcinoma in a male patient is negative for mucin, a prostatic origin should be considered. Other possible pitfalls include signet ring cell change in lymphocytes, and occasionally in smooth muscle cells with cautery artefact (see chapter 7). However, the cells in these cases lack cytologic atypia, and most signet ring tumors have other patterns that facilitate the diagnosis. If the diagnosis of carcinoma versus an artifactual change is a serious question, PSA, PAP, or leukocyte common antigen (LCA) immunostaining is often helpful.

227

ADENOSQUAMOUS AND SQUAMOUS CELL CARCINOMA

General and Clinical Features. These constitute less than 0.5 percent of all malignant tumors of the prostate (71,74-76,78,80,81,83,84, 87–94). Most adenosquamous carcinomas develop several years after a diagnosis of conventional adenocarcinoma that has been treated by radiation or hormonal therapy (78,82). One tumor arose in a patient treated with leuprolide and flutamide for stage D1 cancer (76). However, occasional cases may lack any association with prior adenocarcinoma (79). Pure squamous cell carcinoma usually occurs de novo and must meet the following criteria: 1) demonstrate unequivocal features of malignancy, i.e., nuclear anaplasia and stromal invasion; 2) have definitive squamous differentiation, i.e., intracytoplasmic keratin, pearl formation, or intercellular bridges; 3) lack a conventional carcinoma component; 4) lack prior treatment with radiation or hormones; and 5) lack squamous carcinoma elsewhere (73).

The age of the patient and the clinical presentation of these carcinomas are similar to those of prostatic carcinoma in general. Some squamous tumors have been associated with bone pain due to metastases (87) that are usually osteolytic rather than osteoblastic (77,88,93). PSA and PAP levels are not elevated, even in patients with metastatic squamous cell carcinoma. Both tumors are aggressive, with a mean survival period of 15 months for pure squamous cell carcinoma (84,88,89,91,92,94).

The origin of the pure squamous cell tumors is unclear. Occurrence in a patient with *Schistosoma hematobium* has been reported (72), suggesting a similar metaplastic to neoplastic sequence as seen in the bladder. Schistosomiasis has also been described in association with prostatic adenocarcinoma without squamous elements (85). One tumor occurred as a single nodule in the transition zone (86). Three cases of squamous cell carcinoma have reportedly stained for PSA, supporting a prostatic origin (72,90). In some cases mixtures of neoplastic transitional and squamous cells suggest that squamous cell carcinoma may be of urothelial derivation (75).

Gross Findings. Squamous cell tumors may be firm and gray-white to yellow (87).

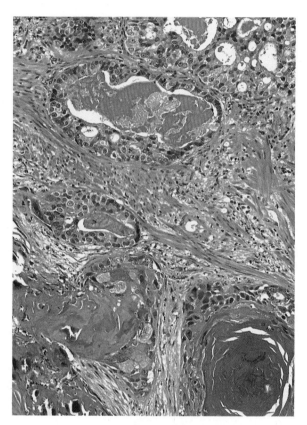

Figure 5-23
ADENOSQUAMOUS CARCINOMA
Adenocarcinoma (top) is juxtaposed with squamous carcinoma (bottom).

Microscopic Findings. Adenosquamous carcinoma exhibits a glandular pattern with unequivocal squamous differentiation (figs. 5-23, 5-24). The adenocarcinoma is usually high grade. Immunohistochemical stains may demonstrate positivity for PSA and PAP in the adenocarcinoma, but generally not in the squamous component (fig. 5-25) (78,82). There is frequently extraprostatic spread.

Squamous cell carcinomas are similar to those observed at other sites. They are usually moderately differentiated, with nests and sheets of cells with abundant eosinophilic cytoplasm displaying keratin pearls, intracellular keratin, and intercellular bridges; an intraductal component may be focally evident (fig. 5-26).

Differential Diagnosis. In both squamous and adenosquamous carcinomas it is crucial that secondary spread from a bladder or urethral

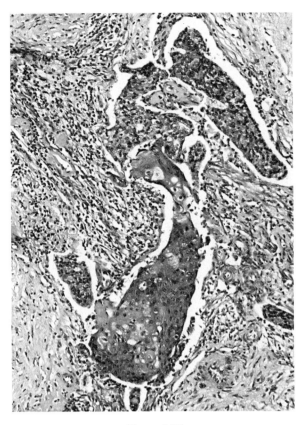

Figure 5-24
ADENOSQUAMOUS CARCINOMA
This neoplasm shows less conspicuous gland differentiation than the tumor in figure 5-23.

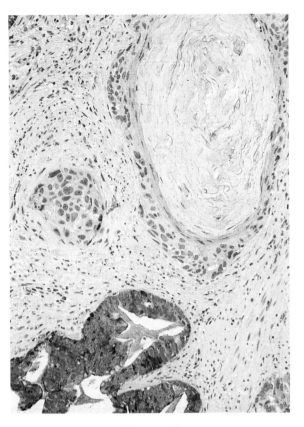

Figure 5-25
ADENOSQUAMOUS CARCINOMA
The glandular component is intensely positive for PSA while the squamous component is negative.

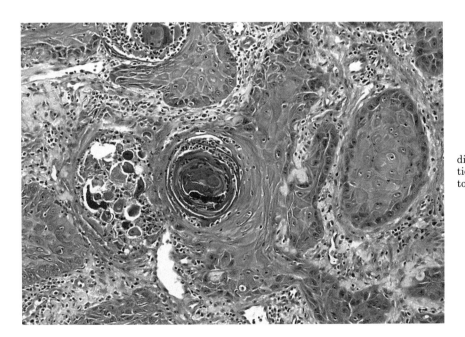

Figure 5-26
SQUAMOUS CELL CARCINOMA
There is unequivocal squamous differentiation with keratin production. (Courtesy of Dr. J.Y. Ro, Houston, TX.)

cancer (squamous cell carcinoma or transitional cell carcinoma with extensive squamous differentiation) be ruled out by an appropriate clinical work-up. Metastatic spread from more distant sites such as lung should similarly be excluded. When these are ruled out realistic problems in differential diagnosis are rare. Distinction of a pure squamous cell tumor from squamous metaplasia is considered in chapter 7.

BASALOID AND ADENOID CYSTIC CARCINOMAS

Malignant basal cell tumors of the prostate include neoplasms with little or no luminal differentiation (basaloid carcinomas) and those with extensive luminal differentiation that often show the regular cribriform pattern typical of adenoid cystic carcinomas of the salivary gland. Because of their rarity diagnostic histologic criteria are not clearly defined, and some reported "adenoid cystic carcinomas" are almost certainly hyperplastic (101,102,105,107,108,111). We have designated such cases "adenoid cystic-like hyperplasia" (see chapter 7), because they are expansive, noninfiltrative, nodular proliferations that often contain foci of typical basal cell hyperplasia. The following discussion includes information distilled from lesions we consider malignant, and combines basaloid and adenoid cystic carcinoma because of their overlapping features.

Clinical Features. The patient age range is wide, from 28 to 72 years (mean, 50 years) (95,97, 98). The patients present with symptoms such as nocturia, urgency, hesitancy, dysuria, and progressive or acute urinary retention (95,98-100, 103,104,106,109,110). One patient presented with a history of perianal pain and tenderness which clinically correlated with a firm and fixed mass on rectal examination; histologically, this tumor demonstrated extensive extraprostatic extension (104). The serum PSA and PAP are usually normal. Follow-up information is limited and available in only three cases (97,98,106): two patients died due to disease, one with pulmonary metastasis (106) and the other with local recurrence (Dr. R. Cohen, personal communication, 1995).

Gross Findings. The tumors form a mass with ill-defined infiltrative edges. The cut section does not have distinctive features (95,106).

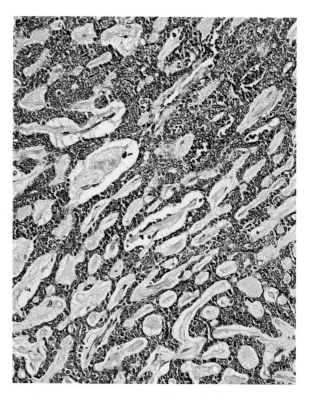

Figure 5-27
BASALOID CARCINOMA
Basaloid cells grow in cords.

Microscopic Findings. Basaloid tumors grow in infiltrating nests, cords, trabeculae, and sheets and may exhibit peripheral palisading (figs. 5-27, 5-28) (106). Adenoid cystic tumors are focally punctuated by cribriform spaces lined by a double layer of cells that surround eosinophilic, hyaline, basement membrane–like material or basophilic mucinous secretion that is positive for PAS and mucicarmine (figs. 5-29–5-31). Sebaceous differentiation and squamous metaplasia may be present within the tumor; the latter may rarely form keratinaceous cysts (106). There may be coexistent adenocarcinoma which is usually spatially distinct.

Necrosis, perineural invasion, angiolymphatic invasion, and extraprostatic extension may be seen (figs. 5-32, 5-33). The neoplastic cells have scant, pale or acidophilic cytoplasm, and round or angulated nuclei with finely stippled chromatin. Cells in apposition to the cystic spaces of adenoid cystic tumors may be larger, with more appreciable acidophilic cytoplasm. Mitotic activity is often not striking.

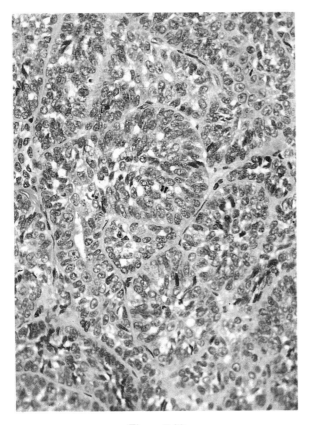

Figure 5-28
BASALOID CARCINOMA
Nests of basaloid cells show some peripheral palisading.
Note the overtly malignant features.

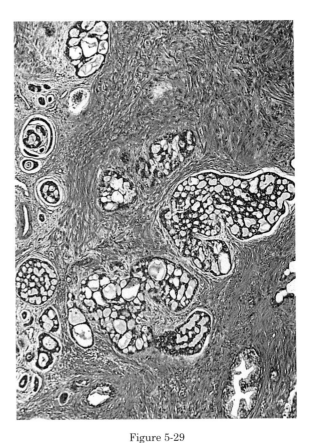

Figure 5-29
ADENOID CYSTIC CARCINOMA
The prostatic parenchyma is diffusely infiltrated by a
tumor with striking cribriform spaces.

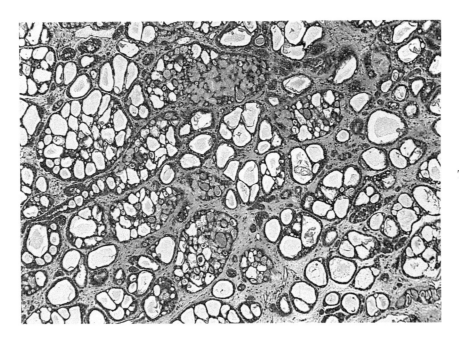

Figure 5-30
ADENOID CYSTIC
CARCINOMA
There is cystic dilatation of acini.

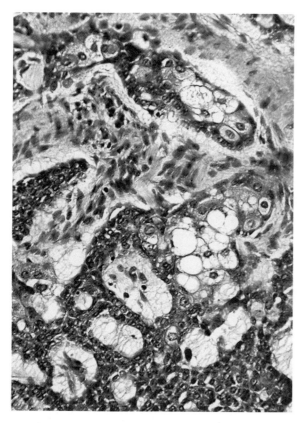

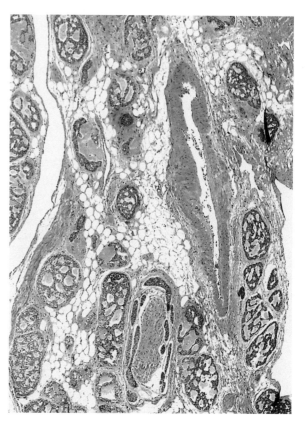

Figure 5-31
ADENOID CYSTIC CARCINOMA
There are basaloid tumor cells, basophilic luminal mucin, and focal sebaceous differentiation.

Figure 5-32
ADENOID CYSTIC CARCINOMA
The tumor shows extensive perineural invasion and extension into periprostatic fat.

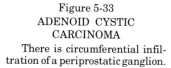

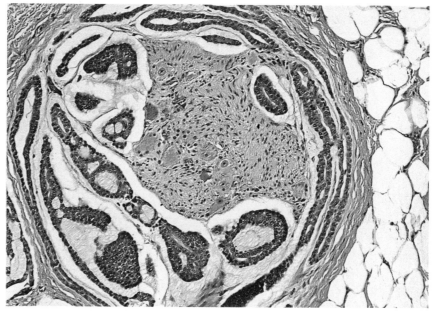

Figure 5-33
ADENOID CYSTIC
CARCINOMA
There is circumferential infiltration of a periprostatic ganglion.

The tumor cells are usually negative for PSA and PAP, although some cases have been reported to be focally positive. High molecular weight cytokeratin (clone 34βE12) and S-100 protein are frequently positive, but the staining is weak (99,103). CEA positivity has also been reported (97). Smooth muscle actin immunostaining is negative.

Ultrastructural studies of the adenoid cystic tumors have shown occasional true lumens with microvilli and tight junctions; convincing myoepithelial differentiation has not been demonstrated (97). The prostatic adenoid cystic tumors differ from salivary gland adenoid cystic carcinomas by the occasional presence of squamous metaplasia and rare acinar differentiation, and the absence of cytoplasmic myofilaments.

Differential Diagnosis. Distinguishing basaloid carcinomas from basal cell hyperplasia, including atypical variants, depends on identifying unequivocal stromal invasion, which may include extracapsular, angiolymphatic or perineural invasion. Necrosis may also be helpful in indicating the neoplastic nature of the process. The tumors usually have more atypia and mitotic activity than hyperplasia. The differential diagnosis of the adenoid cystic cases depends on similar criteria and is summarized in Table 7-2. The differential diagnosis also includes a cloacogenic carcinoma from the anus or adenoid cystic carcinoma of Cowper's gland infiltrating the prostate (96). Clinical features and determination of the epicenter of the mass may be crucial in ascertaining the primary site.

TRANSITIONAL CELL CARCINOMA

General and Clinical Features. Transitional cell carcinoma in the prostate may be primary or represent extension from the bladder (113,123). In a retrospective study of 3600 cases of carcinoma of the prostate from the Mayo Clinic, Greene et al. (116) identified 83 transitional cell carcinomas (2.3 percent); 26 were judged primary and 57 secondary from the bladder. The frequency of primary tumors in an expanded series of 5700 prostate carcinomas from the same institution was 2.8 percent (117). Others have suggested that the frequency of "primary tumors" may be lower because multiple bladder biopsies in patients with such tumors may dis-

close occult in situ bladder carcinoma (122,128). Secondary transitional cell carcinomas involving the prostate are discussed separately below (see page 242). Primary transitional cell carcinomas may arise from the transitional epithelium of the periurethral glands or conceivably on a background of transitional cell metaplasia of ducts and acini (see chapter 7), with a continuum from dysplasia to carcinoma in situ to invasive cancer (115,120,129,131,133).

Patients with primary transitional cell carcinoma have a clinical presentation similar to that of patients with prostatic duct adenocarcinoma; urinary obstructive symptoms and hematuria are most common (116,126). The mean patient age is in the 60s, (range, 45 to 90 years) (116,118). Patients may present with symptoms of metastatic disease such as bone pain due to osteolytic metastases.

Microscopic Findings. The histologic appearance is usually that of a moderately to poorly differentiated invasive carcinoma, with malignant cells infiltrating the stroma as nests, cords, and individually (figs. 5-34, 5-35) (112,125,130–132). The "transitional" nature of the tumors is variably conspicuous, as is the case with grade 2 or 3 transitional cell carcinoma of the bladder; nuclear grooves may be seen, at least focally, in some cases. Foci of squamous or glandular differentiation may be present. In some cases, the neoplastic cells may be confined to the duct-acinar system, consistent with an origin there (fig. 5-36) (117,118). In situ disease may involve the larger periurethral ducts alone or in combination with smaller ducts and acini of the transition and peripheral zones. The diagnosis of stromal invasion should be restricted to cases in which there is irregular stromal infiltration (fig. 5-34) as expansion of ducts and acini without stromal invasion sometimes produces a striking picture analogous to the appearance that may be seen in the endocervix when neoplastic cells expand cervical glands. The presence of focal subtle stromal invasion may be highlighted by high molecular weight cytokeratin immunostains which will demonstrate loss of the basal cell layer in the foci of early invasion (113a). Involvement of the prostatic urethra is rare (118); adenocarcinoma of the usual type may be incidentally discovered and is usually spatially distinct from the transitional cell carcinoma (119,124).

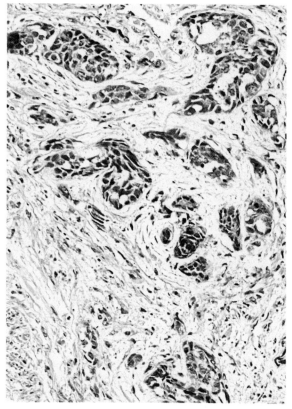

Figure 5-34
PRIMARY TRANSITIONAL CELL CARCINOMA,
POORLY DIFFERENTIATED,
WITH STROMAL INVASION

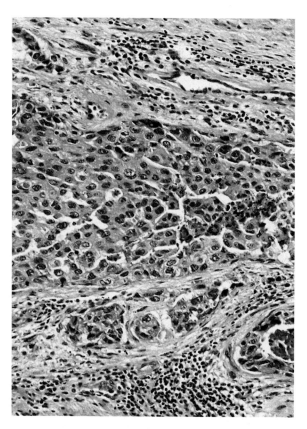

Figure 5-35
PRIMARY TRANSITIONAL CELL CARCINOMA

Figure 5-36
PRIMARY
TRANSITIONAL CELL
CARCINOMA
The tumor has high-grade cytologic features and provokes an inflammatory response.

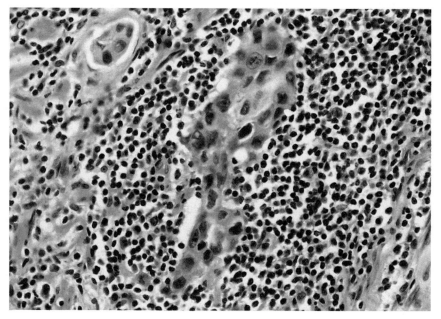

Differential Diagnosis. Diagnosing tumors that spread from the urinary bladder or urethra depends on careful clinical evaluation. Transitional cell carcinoma is distinguished from poorly differentiated adenocarcinoma or adenosquamous carcinoma of the prostate by usual positivity of the latter two neoplasms with immunohistochemical stains for PSA and PAP (127). Evidence of a histologic transition from a moderately differentiated conventional prostatic adenocarcinoma to poorly differentiated carcinoma may also be helpful. High-grade prostatic adenocarcinomas frequently have more monotonous round nuclei in contrast to transitional cell carcinoma which usually shows more pleomorphism. Patients with adenosquamous carcinomas often have a history of prior therapy for prostate cancer.

Prognosis. For patients with transitional cell carcinoma with prostatic stromal invasion, the prognosis is poor (survival, 1 month to 5 years; average, 18 months) (113,117,121). Cheville et al. reported a 45 percent 5-year disease-specific survival rate in 19 cases (114). On the other hand, there is a 100 percent survival rate for patients with primary transitional cell carcinoma in situ of the prostatic urethra, ducts, and acini when treated by cystoprostatectomy (114). The tumors are refractory to hormonal therapy.

SMALL CELL CARCINOMA

General and Clinical Features. This tumor occurs at a median age of 67 years (135–137,139–141,144,149,151). Most patients present with advanced stage disease: large primary masses, extraprostatic involvement, and distant metastases to lung, liver, brain, or other sites (139). Bone metastases are rare and are osteolytic instead of the typical osteoblastic type of most prostatic adenocarcinomas (150). There may be no significant elevation of serum PSA, although some have reported elevated levels, varying according to the stage (142,144,151). Elevated levels of serum carcinoembryonic antigen and calcium have also been reported in a few cases (136,148). Rarely, there are associated paraneoplastic syndromes including Cushing's syndrome (most commonly), the Eaton-Lambert syndrome, hyperglucagonemia, inappropriate antidiuretic hormone secretion, hypercalcemia, and thyrotoxicosis (137,141–144,147,150,151). Advanced

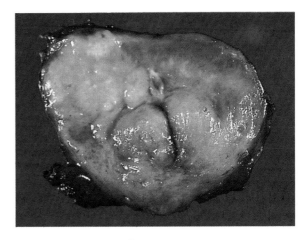

Figure 5-37
SMALL CELL CARCINOMA
In this radical prostatectomy specimen the small cell carcinoma component corresponds to the tan-white, poorly circumscribed area at the upper left.

clinical stage at presentation, metastasis to unusual sites, and sudden, rapid growth of a previously indolent adenocarcinoma should raise the suspicion of a small cell carcinoma component. Small cell carcinoma apparently arises de novo in close to half of the patients (147,149) but is preceded by adenocarcinoma (reported interval, 7 months to 8 years) in the other half.

Gross Findings. The gross features are not distinctive, but since the neoplasm is usually large and has a diffuse growth pattern, it is often grossly more obvious than most adenocarcinomas and may obliterate the prostatic parenchyma (fig. 5-37).

Microscopic Findings. The tumor grows predominantly in diffuse sheets (fig. 5-38) but clusters, cords (fig. 5-39), and single cell patterns may be seen. The cells are of the oat or intermediate cell types. They have minimal cytoplasm, salt and pepper–type chromatin, nuclear molding, and inconspicuous nucleoli (fig. 5-40). A brisk mitotic rate is usual, and necrosis is frequent. The frequently associated component of conventional adenocarcinoma is usually juxtaposed to the small cell carcinoma component which typically predominates (figs. 5-39, 5-41) (135,145,149).

Immunohistochemical and electron microscopic studies often demonstrate neuroendocrine differentiation with positive staining for neuron-specific enolase or serotonin in greater than 50 percent of cases (135,140,144,145,147) and dense core neurosecretory granules in 20 to

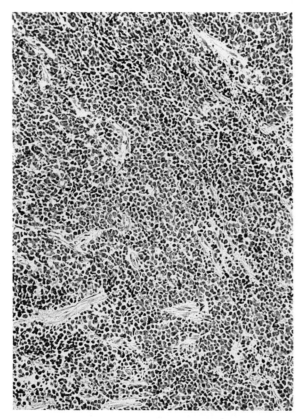

Figure 5-38
SMALL CELL CARCINOMA
Typical diffuse growth.

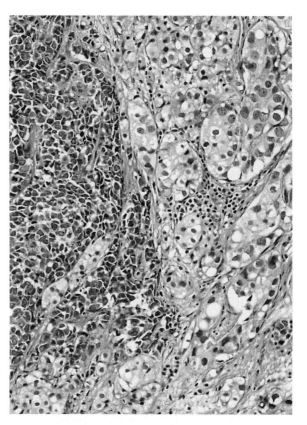

Figure 5-39
SMALL CELL CARCINOMA WITH
ADJACENT CONVENTIONAL
POORLY DIFFERENTIATED CARCINOMA

Figure 5-40
SMALL CELL CARCINOMA
Note the characteristic cyto-
logic features.

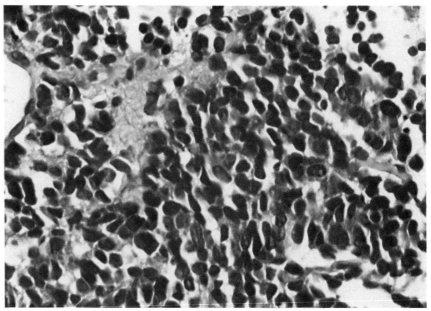

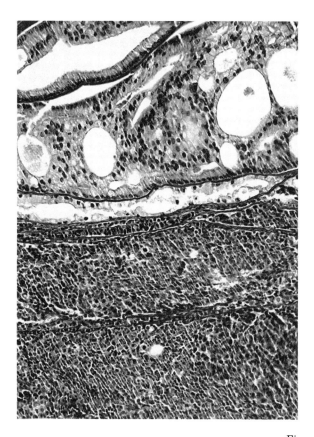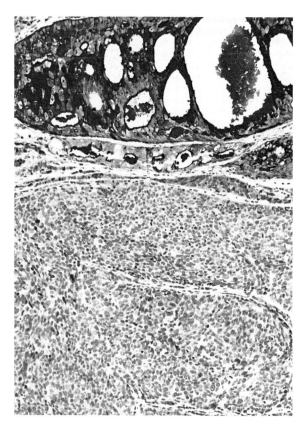

Figure 5-41
SMALL CELL CARCINOMA
Left: Small cell carcinoma (bottom) with cribriform carcinoma (top).
Right: There is negative immunoreactivity for PSA in the small cell component but intense positivity in the cribriform adenocarcinoma.

25 percent (136,140,145). Epithelial membrane antigen, carcinoembryonic antigen, and pancytokeratin cocktail (AE1/AE3 and CAM5.2) have shown variable but often strong immunoreactivity in the neoplastic cells; the cytokeratin cocktail stain may exhibit a paranuclear dot-like immunoreactivity. PSA and PAP are positive within the small cell component in less than 10 percent of cases (fig. 5-41, right), and are usually weak (140,145). A wide range of other immunohistochemical products have been expressed, including bombesin, inhibin, calcitonin, calcitonin gene-related peptide, human chorionic gonadotropin, and adrenocorticotrophic hormone (138,144). Because of the association with adenocarcinoma and the heterogeneous immunohistochemical and ultrastructural profile, small cell carcinoma probably does not arise from a specific prostatic neuroendocrine cell (145,146).

Differential Diagnosis. The differential diagnosis primarily includes metastatic small cell carcinoma, poorly differentiated prostatic adenocarcinoma, transitional cell carcinoma, and malignant lymphoma. Clinical findings are paramount in excluding metastasis. In our experience, the presence of PSA or PAP immunoreactivity, especially with strong intensity, is substantial evidence against a diagnosis of small cell carcinoma of the prostate and favors poorly differentiated prostatic adenocarcinoma. The latter may be composed of "small cells" but they do not have the distinctive architectural and cytologic features of small cell carcinoma as characteristically seen in the lung. A cytokeratin stain may also be helpful: paranuclear immunoreactivity favors small cell carcinoma, while diffuse cytoplasmic positivity is typical of conventional high-grade adenocarcinoma. This is an important differential since nonsmall cell

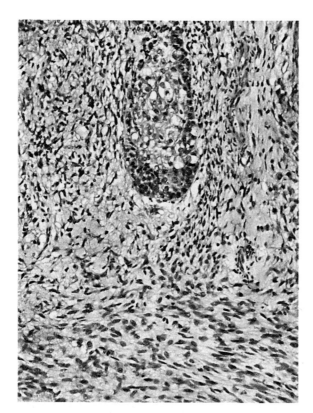

Figure 5-42
CARCINOSARCOMA
A nest of carcinoma with squamous features is present within a neoplastic spindle cell proliferation.

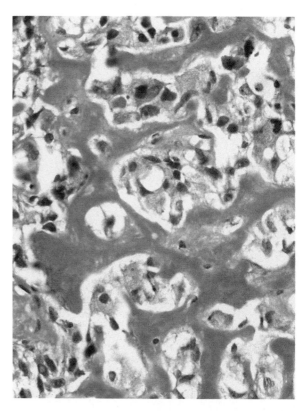

Figure 5-43
CARCINOSARCOMA
This tumor has an osteosarcomatous component. (Fig. 4-73 from Ro JY, Grignon DJ, Amin MB, Ayala AG. Atlas of surgical pathology of the male reproductive tract. Philadelphia: W.B. Saunders, 1997:68.)

carcinomas of the prostate are more likely to respond to hormonal management. Use of neuroendocrine markers such as chromogranin, neuron-specific enolase, or synaptophysin alone is not sufficient to make a diagnosis of small cell carcinoma since these may be expressed in many prostatic adenocarcinomas (134). Some transitional cell carcinomas have small cells and, particularly when there is "squeeze" artifact, they may resemble, on low-power microscopy, small cell carcinoma, but the typical cytologic features of the latter are lacking. Distinction from malignant lymphoma is also based on the differing cytologic features of the cells in the two tumors. A simple panel of immunostains including LCA and cytokeratin will be helpful in a difficult case. Immunostains also help in the very rare situation in which a metastatic melanoma composed of small cells is in the differential.

Prognosis. The prognosis is poor, with an average median survival following diagnosis of

7.7 to 17.1 months (135,144,149). Traditional hormonal therapy is characteristically ineffective. Chemotherapy regimens used for small cell carcinoma of the lung have prolonged survival, particularly in patients with only regional lymph node spread (135,142,149).

SARCOMATOID CARCINOMA AND CARCINOSARCOMA

General and Clinical Features. This topic is clouded by the differing criteria for sarcomatoid carcinoma, some equating the lesion with the tumor we separately designate carcinosarcoma. By our criteria, carcinosarcoma has a haphazard admixture of obvious epithelial and spindle cell foci, with the latter being truly sarcomatous, often with heterologous tissues such as cartilage or skeletal muscle (figs. 5-42–5-45) (157,166). In sarcomatoid carcinoma there is, by definition, no

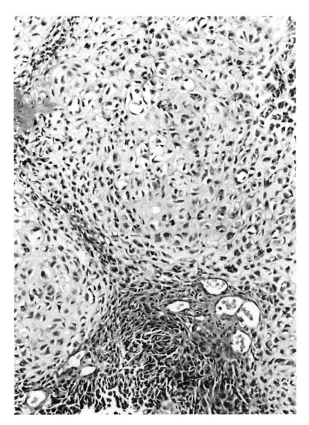

Figure 5-44
CARCINOSARCOMA
A chondrosarcomatous component dominates the field.

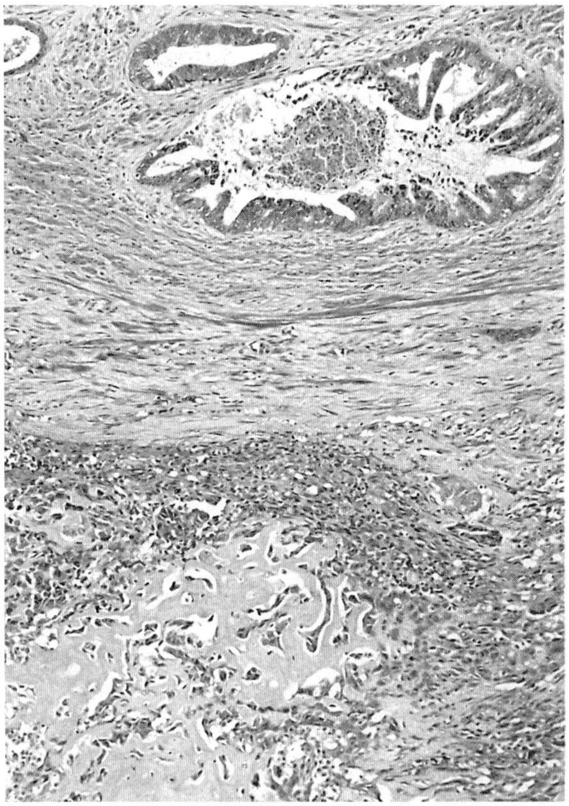

Figure 5-45
CARCINOSARCOMA
The epithelial component (top) shows a ductal histology.
There is osseous differentiation (bottom).

heterologous differentiation, and there are overtly epithelial and spindle cell elements that are typically spatially separated, although they may merge in areas (figs. 5-46, 5-47). If carcinosarcomas are excluded, only a few sarcomatoid carcinomas have been described in the usual age range and with the usual presentation of prostatic carcinoma (164). The following review groups both tumors together as the total number of reported cases is few, and some series include both categories as "sarcomatoid carcinoma," making separate analysis of the two groups impractical. The histologic distinction between them would be critical if their biologic potential differed, but it appears that sarcomatoid carcinoma and carcinosarcoma have relatively similar, poor outcomes.

The mean patient age in three large series was 67 to 71 years (152,156,162,164). Most patients present with obstructive symptoms and hence the tumors are usually first diagnosed in transurethral resection specimens. The majority have metastatic disease at the time of diagnosis, and approximately 50 percent have a previous history of adenocarcinoma of the prostate treated by radiation or hormonal therapy (159,161,164). The serum PSA and PAP are normal in approximately half of the patients (156). The most common sites of metastases are lung and bone; less frequent sites include liver, brain, peritoneum, skin, and lymph nodes (156,159,164,166).

Gross Findings. The gross appearance is characteristically "sarcoma-like," dull gray with infiltrative margins (fig. 5-46).

Microscopic Findings. The sarcomatoid or sarcomatous areas are usually composed of markedly atypical spindle cells with large, pleomorphic, hyperchromatic nuclei, typically with brisk mitotic activity, including atypical forms (fig. 5-47, right). The cytoplasm is variable but is often abundant

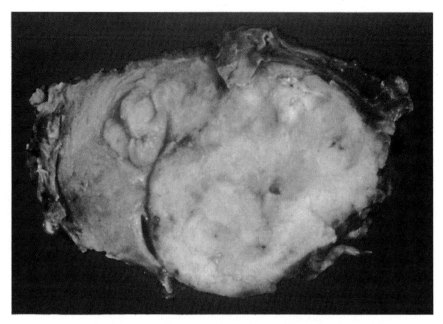

Figure 5-46
SARCOMATOID CARCINOMA
There are gray-white and tan-yellow areas of tumor. (Fig. 4-71 from Ro JY, Grignon DJ, Amin MB, Ayala AG. Atlas of surgical pathology of the male reproductive tract. Philadelphia: W.B. Saunders, 1997:68.)

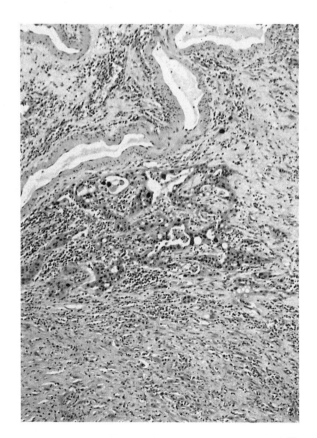
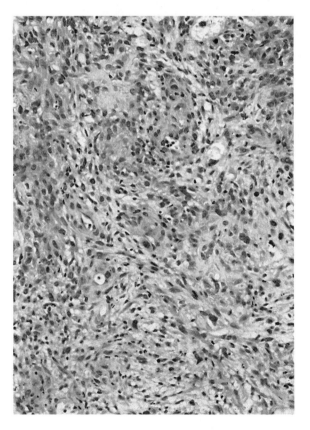

Figure 5-47
SARCOMATOID CARCINOMA
Left: Neoplastic glands (center) are associated with spindled cells (bottom).
Right: Epithelial-like and spindled components merge.

and eosinophilic. The pattern in most cases resembles that of an undifferentiated high-grade sarcoma, malignant fibrous histiocytoma, or, occasionally, fibrosarcoma. The most frequent heterologous components are osteosarcoma (57 percent), chondrosarcoma (34 percent), and rhabdomyosarcoma (14 percent); in approximately one third of the cases multiple types of heterologous differentiation are present (156,158–162,164–167).

The concurrent adenocarcinoma, which is usually present but may be difficult to identify, is typically poorly differentiated (fig. 5-47, left), however, it occasionally may be of lower grade (159). The morphologically recognizable epithelial component stains for keratin (fig. 5-48), PSA, and PAP, and the spindle cell component may do likewise, particularly with cytokeratin but to a more limited degree (156,159,160,163,164,166). Rhabdomyosarcomatous differentiation may be confirmed by appropriate stains but is usually obvious by light microscopy. Ultrastructural analysis may show desmosomes and tonofilaments, although in two cases no electron microscopic evidence of epithelial differentiation was found (160,164).

Differential Diagnosis. The cytologic atypia of sarcomatoid carcinomas excludes non-neoplastic lesions such as the postoperative spindle cell nodule and inflammatory pseudotumor (pseudosarcomatous fibromyxoid tumor; see chapter 7). The lack of atypical mitoses in both non-neoplastic lesions and the typical myxoid background with granulation tissue type vascularity of the inflammatory pseudotumor are helpful features, although rare sarcomatoid carcinomas are somewhat myxoid. Associated epithelial components are, of course, helpful in excluding the two rare non-neoplastic spindle cell lesions. True carcinosarcomas should be distinguished from the rare carcinoma with metaplastic, benign-appearing bone or cartilage in the stroma, in contrast to the malignant osseous and cartilaginous components in carcinosarcomas (153–155).

Prognosis. The median survival period of the nine patients in the M.D. Anderson Cancer Center series was only 12 months (164). In the series of carcinosarcomas of the prostate from the Mayo Clinic, Dundore et al. (156) reported a 41 percent 5-year and a 14 percent 7-year cancer-specific survival rate. Eighteen of 21 patients died of disease (median, 9.5 months).

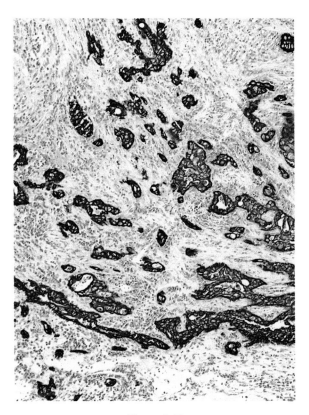

Figure 5-48
SARCOMATOID CARCINOMA
A cytokeratin immunostain highlights the overt epithelial component.

LYMPHOEPITHELIOMA-LIKE CARCINOMA

Lymphoepithelioma-like carcinoma of the prostate is an undifferentiated malignant epithelial tumor, histologically similar to nasopharyngeal lymphoepithelioma, and distinguished by its syncytial growth pattern and prominent lymphoid infiltrate. Only one tumor has been reported. It had areas of acinar carcinoma, but the two patterns were not intermingled (169). In situ hybridization was negative for Epstein-Barr virus (169). Immunohistochemistry showed a predominantly T-cell type lymphoid population. The possibility of extension from the bladder must be excluded before a diagnosis of a prostatic primary is established (168). It is important to be aware of this pattern and not to misinterpret it as malignant lymphoma or chronic inflammation, especially in crushed transurethral resectates or needle biopsy material. Immunostains to document the epithelial cell component are helpful.

UNDIFFERENTIATED CARCINOMA, NOT OTHERWISE SPECIFIED

These are high-grade tumors that lack differentiation by routine microscopy. The tumor cells may be small (but if they have the particular features of small cell carcinoma they should be classified as such), intermediate, or large. A single case of giant cell carcinoma that merged with acinar adenocarcinoma has been described (170). The giant cell carcinoma showed focal weak positivity for PSA and PAP while the adenocarcinoma showed diffuse moderate immunoreactivity. The differential diagnosis of undifferentiated carcinomas includes spread from the bladder or urethra and metastasis from distant sites. Focal immunoreactivity for PSA and PAP may be crucial in indicating the prostatic nature of an undifferentiated carcinoma.

SECONDARY CARCINOMAS

The most common secondary tumors of the prostate gland are hematopoietic malignancies (see chapter 6) and tumors directly extending from adjacent viscera (e.g., bladder, rectum, and anus). Hematogenous spread to the prostate is extremely rare.

Transitional Cell Carcinoma

Clinical Features. As noted earlier (see page 233), in one large series, 57 of 83 transitional cell carcinomas involving the prostate gland were secondary (180). The frequency of secondary involvement of the prostate by transitional cell carcinoma may be rising (190). One possible reason for this trend is the better conservative management of superficial bladder cancer by a combination of cystoscopic ablation and intravesical topical therapy. These methods, however, do not treat adequately the prostatic urethra and underlying prostatic ducts which remain, therefore, susceptible to direct spread or implantation of carcinoma (190,201). An additional consideration is a possible artifactual increase in secondary involvement because of closer surveillance of the prostate in patients with known bladder cancer.

The frequency of prostatic involvement in patients with bladder neoplasia varies from 10 to 50 percent (178,186,195). It is highest when the prostate gland is serially sectioned and entirely submitted for histologic analysis (186,189,197, 198,203). Patients with carcinoma in situ of the bladder are most likely to have prostatic involvement (68 to 80 percent) (176,194) which is particularly common in those with multifocal disease, disease refractory to intravesical therapy, or if the trigone is involved (177,181,188,203).

Secondary transitional cell carcinomas involving the prostate are usually restricted to the duct-acinar system, without stromal invasion, and consequently, obstructive symptoms are infrequent and, when present, suggest stromal invasion; there may be symptoms related to the bladder disease such as hematuria and bladder irritability. Less commonly, prostatic involvement results from direct invasion of the prostate from a bladder carcinoma that has extended through the muscularis propria (178). The frequency of detection of prostatic involvement is directly related to the tissue sampling technique, being 20 percent, 40 percent, and 90 percent for transrectal needle biopsy, fine needle aspiration, and transurethral resection, respectively, in two studies (195,203).

There is an apparently increased frequency of concurrent prostatic acinar carcinoma (up to 45 percent) in cystoprostatectomy specimens performed for transitional cell carcinoma of the bladder (184,189).

Microscopic Findings. Transitional cell carcinoma secondarily involving the prostate gland has no distinctive gross features and has two major microscopic forms (171,178). The carcinoma may spread directly along mucosal surfaces or may result from direct transmural spread of a transitional cell carcinoma of the bladder or prostatic urethra, usually from tumors that are high grade and known to be locally advanced clinically. The secondary spread is usually obvious pathologically and readily correlated with the clinical findings. Nonetheless, careful evaluation of morphology is imperative since some patients may have an incidentally discovered high-grade prostatic carcinoma as well as the secondary neoplasm, and the tumors may merge almost imperceptibly. The collision of the two tumors may cause diagnostic confusion (fig. 5-49) in which case immunostains may help delineate the two components. In other cases the prostatic adenocarcinoma is topographically distinct from the transitional cell carcinoma. In cases of mucosal spread, the prostatic involvement

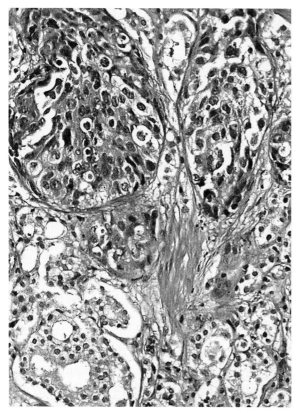

Figure 5-49
COLLISION OF PROSTATIC CARCINOMA
WITH TRANSITIONAL CELL CARCINOMA
SECONDARILY INVOLVING THE PROSTATE
Focal basal cells are preserved in the transitional cell carcinoma component, indicating its restriction to the duct-acinar system.

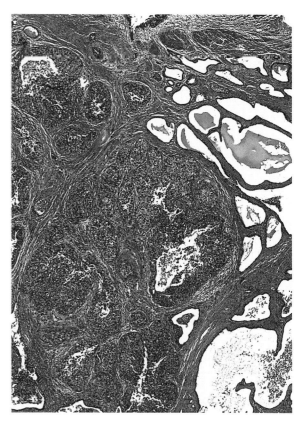

Figure 5-50
TRANSITIONAL CELL CARCINOMA SECONDARILY
INVOLVING PROSTATIC DUCTS AND ACINI
The tumor is limited to the more central region of the gland (the urethral mucosa is barely visible at the top center).

may be confined entirely to ducts and acini without stromal invasion, or there may be varying degrees of penetration into the stroma, the latter being of significant adverse prognostic significance (178). The involvement of ducts and acini is frequently limited to the more central region of the gland and thus is seen commonly in transurethral resection specimens (fig. 5-50), but occasionally the involvement may be widespread such that peripheral disease is sampled by needle biopsy. Confinement to ducts and acini is seen commonly in patients on surveillance for carcinoma in situ of the bladder. In most cases, there is expansion of the duct-acinar apparatus by neoplastic cells which usually are moderately or markedly atypical (figs. 5-51, 5-52); comedonecrosis may be present in the center of the ducts. Uncommonly, the cytologic features

may be relatively low grade (fig. 5-53). The secretory cells of the duct-acinar structures are usually entirely replaced by neoplastic transitional cells, although occasionally, a pagetoid form of growth may be seen. The least common pattern of transitional cell carcinoma involving ducts and acini is one in which there is an intraluminal papillary proliferation (fig. 5-54).

Invasion of the prostatic stroma may be focal or prominent. Detection of early invasion may be difficult but has prognostic implications and must be ruled out diligently. In cases in which invasion is equivocal by light microscopy, staining for high molecular weight cytokeratin (clone 34βE12) may be useful (fig. 5-55) (174a). Although the tumor cells may also be positive, this immunostain consistently highlights the circumferential basal cells of the ducts and acini whose basement

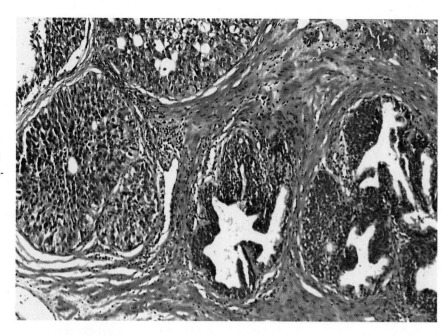

Figure 5-51
TRANSITIONAL CELL
CARCINOMA SECONDARILY
INVOLVING THE PROSTATE
There is expansion of the pros-
tatic ducts by tumor cells.

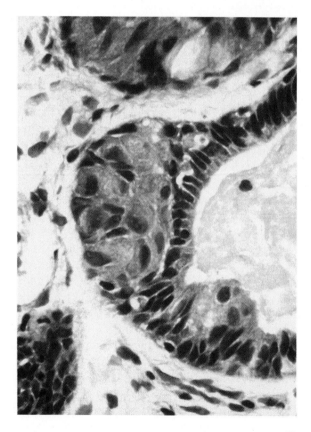 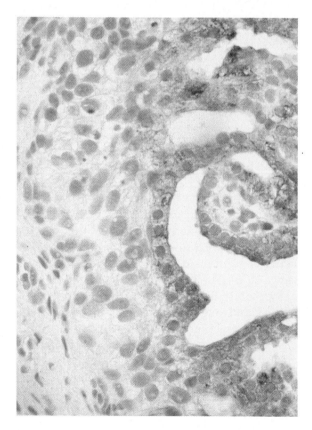

Figure 5-52
TRANSITIONAL CELL CARCINOMA SECONDARILY INVOLVING THE PROSTATE
Left: The tumor cells grow in a pagetoid fashion beneath the residual secretory cells.
Right: The secretory cells stain positively for PSA, but the transitional cells are negative. (Fig. 4-98 from Ro JY, Grignon DJ, Amin MB, Ayala AG. Atlas of surgical pathology of the male reproductive tract. Philadelphia: W.B. Saunders, 1997:78.)

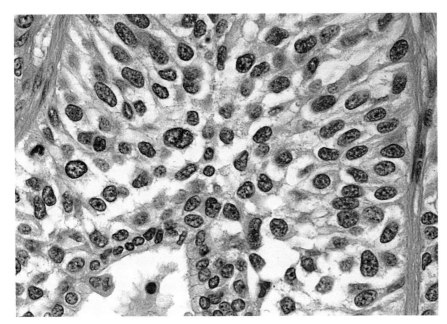

Figure 5-53
TRANSITIONAL CELL
CARCINOMA SECONDARILY
INVOLVING THE PROSTATE
In this example the cytologic
features are relatively low grade.
The neoplastic cells are somewhat
fusiform, with rare nuclear
grooves. Note the preservation of
the prostatic secretory cell layer
(bottom left).

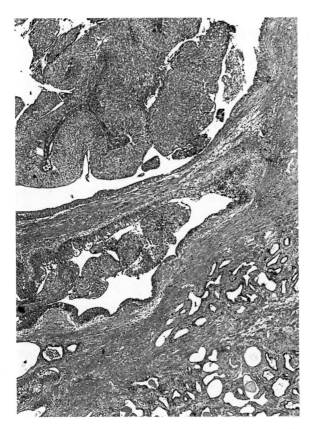

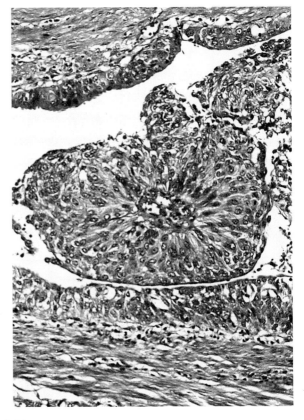

Figure 5-54
TRANSITIONAL CELL CARCINOMA SECONDARILY INVOLVING PROSTATIC DUCTS AND ACINI
A papillary pattern is retained. Note the absence of stromal invasion. (Courtesy of Dr. J. Grignon, Detroit, MI.)

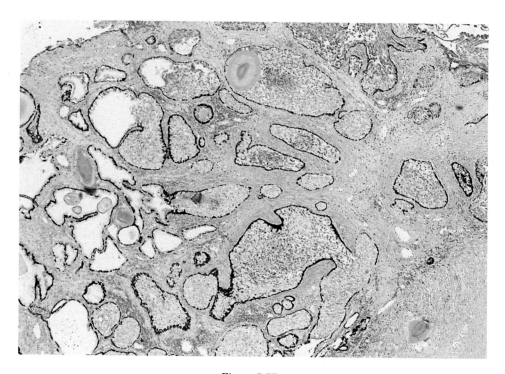

Figure 5-55
TRANSITIONAL CELL CARCINOMA SECONDARILY INVOLVING THE PROSTATE
A high molecular weight cytokeratin immunostain (clone 34βE12) shows circumferential investment of expanded ducts and acini containing intraluminal tumor, indicating a lack of invasion in this area.

membrane has not been breached and, conversely, is negative around nests of invasive carcinoma. In obvious cases of stromal invasion irregular sheets, nests, and cords of cells are haphazardly distributed in a desmoplastic stroma.

Differential Diagnosis. The differential diagnosis of transitional cell carcinoma involving ducts and acini without invasion includes ductal carcinoma and high-grade prostatic intraepithelial neoplasia; for invasive cases poorly differentiated prostatic adenocarcinoma of conventional type and basaloid carcinoma must be considered.

Prostatic duct carcinoma shares with transitional cell carcinoma a high nuclear grade and comedonecrosis, however, the tubulopapillary and complex cribriform growth of anastomosing large ductal structures of the former is not a feature of the latter. PSA and PAP immunostains, being positive in prostatic duct carcinoma, are useful in difficult cases or limited samples (171). These stains are also important in the differential with poorly differentiated adenocarcinoma of nonductal type. An overt basaloid pattern should be seen before basaloid carcinoma is entertained.

Prostatic intraepithelial neoplasia enters the differential diagnosis because of its intraductal growth of cytologically atypical cells. The degree of nuclear pleomorphism is less than that of transitional cell carcinoma involving prostatic ducts and acini; mitoses, comedonecrosis, and solid intraductal growth are also uncommon to rare in prostatic intraepithelial neoplasia (172).

Prognosis. The prognosis is dramatically worse in patients with carcinoma invasive into the prostatic stroma and in whom the carcinoma invades directly through the bladder wall (175, 177,178,190–192). The 5-year disease-specific survival rate is 52 percent. It is 100 percent for patients with carcinoma in situ involving the prostatic urethra, ducts, and acini; 45 percent in cases with stromal invasion; 30 percent for those with lymph node metastases; and 0 percent with extra-prostatic extension and seminal vesicle invasion (175). One study showed that only 11 percent of patients with transitional cell carcinoma limited to ducts and acini had metastatic disease compared to 100 percent of those with stromal invasion (202). In a study of 143 cases, there was a 71 percent 5-year survival rate for patients with secondary involvement of the prostate limited to the ducts and acini, but only a 36 percent 5-year survival rate in the presence of prostatic stromal invasion (178), a result comparable to the 20 percent rate reported in another series in spite of aggressive neoadjuvant radiotherapy and radical surgery (198). In the former study, the 5-year overall survival was 21 percent for patients in whom tumors directly invaded the prostate from the bladder (178). Transitional cell carcinoma limited to ducts and acini only did not alter the prognosis of the primary bladder tumor (178). Involvement of the prostatic urethra is associated with an increased risk for penile urethral recurrence (191). Another important pathologic parameter with therapeutic and possibly prognostic implications is the extent and location of involvement of the prostatic ducts and acini: central, noninvasive tumors may be amenable to conservative therapy while peripheral tumors usually require radical surgery or radiation (174,179,182).

Tumors Extending from Adjacent Viscera

In one series of 6000 male autopsies, 143 tumors (2.3 percent) had spread to the prostate from adjacent organs or involved the prostate as part of widespread pelvic dissemination (204). The primary tumors included bladder or urethral cancers (41.2 percent), colonic and rectal carcinomas (27.2 percent) (fig. 5-56), genitourinary malignant lymphomas (17.6 percent) (see chapter 6), and miscellaneous tumors (14 percent).

If a good clinical history is available, the differential diagnosis with primary prostatic tumors is relatively straightforward. The morphology of many secondary tumors is sufficiently unusual for the prostate such that secondary spread is suggested when they are encountered. A selective panel of immunohistochemical stains including PSA, PAP, and villin (a 93-kD, acidic, actin-binding protein found in epithelial cells with a brush border and which is positive in most colonic adenocarcinomas) (fig. 5-56C,D), may be helpful in problematic cases (196).

Metastatic Solid Tumors from More Distant Sites

The frequency of metastatic tumors in two large series of 6000 and 1474 male autopsies was 3.1 and 0.5 percent, respectively (183,196). The types included lung carcinoma (41 percent) (fig. 5-57), malignant melanoma (28 percent), pancreatic carcinoma (5 percent) (fig. 5-58), gastric carcinoma (5 percent), germ cell tumor (4 percent), and renal cell carcinoma (3 percent) (fig. 5-59) (173,185,187,193,199,200). Other tumors reported to spread to the prostate include cancers of the thyroid, esophagus, penis, and larynx, and a goblet cell carcinoid of the appendix. If the clear cells predominate in metastatic renal cell carcinoma, it may be difficult to distinguish from a primary prostatic adenocarcinoma with clear cells. The distinctive arborizing, delicate vascular pattern of clear cell renal cell carcinoma (fig. 5-59) and negative immunoreactivity for PSA and PAP are helpful, as are the clinical findings in many cases (187).

Only 3 of 18 patients in one series of metastatic cases (17 percent) were diagnosed on the basis of clinical findings; in each case the presentation was due to obstructive symptoms. Two patients survived 4 months and one, 18 months. All other patients had widespread disease at autopsy. As with local secondary spread, the morphology of these metastatic tumors is typically incompatible with or unusual for prostate cancer, and this facilitates the diagnosis (183).

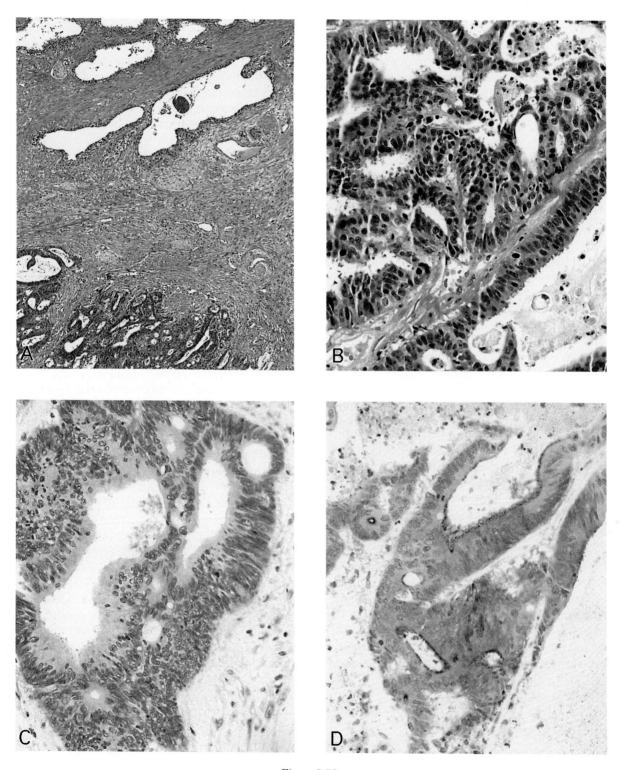

Figure 5-56
ADENOCARCINOMA OF RECTUM WITH DIRECT EXTENSION INTO PROSTATIC PARENCHYMA
A: Typical histology.
B: Anastomosing glands and cribriform architecture with focal dirty necrosis may mimic prostatic ductal carcinoma.
C: Negative PSA stain.
D: Luminal and cytoplasmic staining for villin.

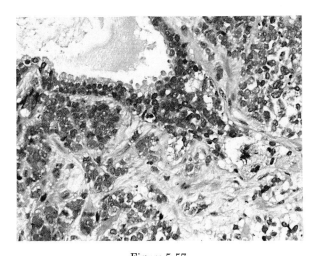

Figure 5-57
PULMONARY SMALL CELL CARCINOMA
METASTATIC TO THE PROSTATE
Transurethral resection specimen obtained for hyperplasia shows focal aggregates of small cell carcinoma.

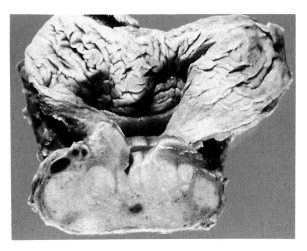

Figure 5-58
PANCREATIC ADENOCARCINOMA
METASTATIC TO THE PROSTATE
Note the multiple nodules throughout the peripheral and transition zone of the gland. (Fig. 5-21 from Ro JY, Grignon DJ, Amin MB, Ayala AG. Atlas of surgical pathology of the male reproductive tract. Philadelphia: W.B. Saunders, 1997:92.)

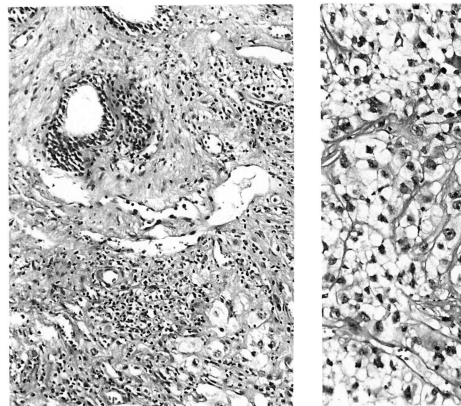

Figure 5-59
RENAL CELL CARCINOMA METASTATIC TO THE PROSTATE
Left: A low-power view shows infiltration of the prostatic stroma.
Right: A high-power view demonstrates the typical histologic features of renal cell carcinoma, clear cell type.

REFERENCES

Prostatic Duct Adenocarcinoma

1. Amin M, Schultz D, Zarbo R. Analysis of cribriform morphology in prostate neoplasia using antibody to high-molecular-weight cytokeratins. Arch Pathol Lab Med 1994;118:260–4.

2. Amin MB, Ro JY, Ayala AG. Clinical relevance of histologic variants of prostate cancer. Cancer Bull 1993; 45:403–10.

3. Amin MB, Ro JY, Ayala AG. Putative precursor lesions of prostatic adenocarcinoma: fact or fiction? Mod Pathol 1993;6:476–83.

4. Aydin F. Endometrioid adenocarcinoma of prostatic urethra presenting with anterior urethral implantation. Urology 1993;41:91–5.

4a.Bock BJ, Bostwick DG. Does prostatic ductal adenocarcinoma exist? Am J Surg Pathol 1999;23:781–5.

5. Bostwick DG, Kindrachuk RW, Rouse RV. Prostatic adenocarcinoma with endometrioid features. Clinical, pathologic, and ultrastructural findings. Am J Surg Pathol 1985;9:595–609.

6. Cantrell BB, Leifer G, DeKlerk DP, Eggleston JC. Papillary adenocarcinoma of the prostatic urethra with clear-cell appearance. Cancer 1981;48:2661–7.

7. Carney JA, Kelalis PP. Endometrial carcinoma of the prostatic utricle. Am J Clin Pathol 1973;60:565–9.

8. Christensen WN, Steinberg C, Walsh PC. Prostatic duct adenocarcinoma. Findings at radical prostatectomy. Cancer 1991;67:2118–24.

9. Cueva C, Urdiales M, Nogales F, Varela-Duran J. Papillary endometrioid carcinoma of the prostate. Br J Urol 1988;61:98–9.

10. Dictor M. Priapism in patient with endometrioid prostatic carcinoma. A case report. Urology 1988;43:245–7.

11. Dube VE, Farrow GM, Greene LF. Prostatic adenocarcinoma of ductal origin. Cancer 1973;32:402–9.

12. Elgamal AA, Van de Voorde W, Van Poppel H, Vandeursen H, Baert L, Lauweryns J. Exophytic papillary prostatic duct adenocarcinoma with endometrioid features, occurring in prostatic urethra after TURP. Urology 1994;43:737–42.

13. Epstein JI, Woodruff JM. Adenocarcinoma of the prostate with endometrioid features. A light microscopic and immunohistochemical study of ten cases. Cancer 1986;57:111–9.

14. Gilbert RF, Ibarra J, Tansey LA, Shanberg AM. Adenocarcinoma in a mullerian duct cyst. J Urol 1992;148:1262–4.

15. Greene LF, Farrow GM, Ravits JM, Tomera FM. Prostatic adenocarcinoma of ductal origin. J Urol 1979;121:303–5.

16. Kopelson G, Harisiadis L, Romas NA, Veenema RJ, Tannenbaum M. Periurethral prostatic duct carcinoma: clinical features and treatment results. Cancer 1978;42:2894–902.

17. Kuhajda FP, Gipson T, Mendelsohn G. Papillary adenocarcinomas of the prostate. An immunohistochemical study. Cancer 1984;54:1328–32.

18. Lee SS. Endometrioid adenocarcinoma of the prostate: a clinicopathologic and immunohistochemical study. J Surg Oncol 1994;55:235–8.

19. McNeal J, Yemoto C. Spread of adenocarcinoma within prostatic ducts and acini: morphologic and clinical correlations. Am J Surg Pathol 1996;20:802–14.

20. Melicow MM, Pachter MR. Endometrial carcinoma of prostate utricle (uterus masculinus). Cancer 1967;20:1715–22.

21. Melicow MM, Tannenbaum M. Endometrial carcinoma of uterus masculinus (prostatic utricle). Report of 6 cases. J Urol 1971;106:892–902.

22. Merchant RF, Graham AR, Bucher WC Jr, Parker DA. Endometrial carcinoma of prostatic utricle with osseous metastases. Urology 1976;8:169–73.

23. Odom DG, Westphal KW, Hawksley VC, Deshon GE. Endometrioid carcinoma of prostate. Urology 1988;31:217–9.

23a.Oxley JD, Abbott CD, Gillatt DA, MacIver AG. Ductal carcinomas of the prostate: a clinicopathological and immunohistochemical study. Br J Urol 1998;81:109–15.

24. Perrapato SD, Shah PC, Huben RP, Gaeta JF. Locally recurrent endometrioid adenocarcinoma of the prostate after radical prostatectomy. J Urol 1991;145:373–5.

25. Randolph T, Amin MB, Ro JY. Histologic variants of the prostatic adenocarcinoma and other carcinomas of the prostate. Mod Pathol 1997;10:612–29.

26. Ro J, Ayala A, Wishnow K, Ordóñez NG. Prostatic duct adenocarcinoma with endometrioid features: immunohistochemical and electron microscopic study. Semin Diagn Pathol 1988;5:301–11.

27. Samaratunga H, Singh M. Distribution pattern of basal cells detected by cytokeratin 34 beta E12 in primary prostatic duct adenocarcinoma. Am J Surg Pathol 1997;21:435–40.

28. Sufrin G, Gaeta J, Staubitz WJ, Ajrawat HS, Murphy GP. Endometrial carcinoma of prostate. Urology 1986;27:18–23.

29. Vale JA, Patel A, Ball AJ, Hendry WF, Chappell ME, Fisher C. Endometrioid carcinoma of the prostate: a misnomer? J Royal Soc Med 1992;85:394–6.

30. Walker AN, Mills SE, Fechner RE, Perry JM. Endometrial adenocarcinoma of the prostatic urethra arising in a villous polyp. A light microscopic and immunoperoxidase study. Arch Pathol Lab Med 1982;106:624–7.

31. Walther MM, Nassar V, Harruff RC, Mann BB Jr, Finnerty DP, Hewen-Lowe KO. Endometrial carcinoma of the prostatic utricle: a tumor of prostatic origin. J Urol 1985;134:769–73.

32. Wernert N, Luchtrath H, Seeliger H, Schäfer M, Roeggels R, Dhom G. Papillary carcinoma of the prostate, location, morphology and immunohistochemistry: the histogenesis and entity of so-called endometrioid carcinoma. Prostate 1987;10:123–31.

33. Young BW, Lagios MD. Endometrial (papillary) carcinoma of the prostatic utricle: response to orchiectomy. A case report. Cancer 1973;32:1293–300.

34. Zaloudek C, Williams JW, Kempson RL. Endometrial adenocarcinoma of the prostate: a distinctive tumor of prostatic duct origin. Cancer 1976;37:2255–62.

Mucinous (Colloid) Adenocarcinoma

35. Alfthan O, Koivuniemi A. Mucinous carcinoma of the prostate: case report. Scand J Urol Nephrol 1977;4:78–80.

36. Amin MB, Young RH. Primary carcinoma of urethra. Sem Diag Pathol 1997;14:147–60.

37. Bostwick DG. Neoplasms of the prostate. In: Bostwick DG, Eble JN, eds. Urologic surgical pathology. St. Louis: Mosby, 1997:343–421.

38. Bostwick DG, Iczkowski KA. Minimal criteria for the diagnosis of prostate cancer on needle biopsy. Ann Diagn Pathol 1997;1:104–29.

39. Chica G, Johnson DE, Ayala AG. Mucinous adenocarcinoma of the prostate. J Urol 1977;118:124–5.

40. Elbadawi A, Craig W, Linke CA, Cooper RA Jr. Prostate mucinous carcinoma. Urology 1979;13:658–66.

41. Epstein JI, Fynheer J. Acidic mucin in the prostate: can it differentiate adenosis from adenocarcinoma? Hum Pathol 1992;23:1321–5.

42. Epstein JI, Lieberman PH. Mucinous adenocarcinoma of the prostate gland. Am J Surg Pathol 1985;9:299–308.

43. Franks IM, O'Shea JD, Thomson AE. Mucin in the prostate: a histochemical study in normal glands, latent, clinical and colloid cancers. Cancer 1964;17:983–91.

44. Goldstein NS, Quian J, Bostwick DG. Mucin expression in atypical adenomatous hyperplasia of the prostate. Hum Pathol 1995;26:887–91.

45. Hukill PB, Vidone RA. Histochemistry of mucus and other polysaccharides in tumors. Lab Invest 1967;16:395–406.

46. Lee DW, Ro JY, Sahin AA, Lee JS, Ayala AG. Mucinous adenocarcinoma of the prostate with endobronchial metastasis. Am J Clin Pathol 1990;94:641–6.

47. Lightbourn GA, Abrams M, Seymour L. Primary mucoid adenocarcinoma of the prostate gland with bladder invasion. J Urol 1969;101:78–80.

48. Manne RK, Haddad FS. Mucinous adenocarcinoma of prostate. Urology 1989;33:247–9.

49. McNeal JE, Alroy J, Villers A, Redwine EA, Freiha FS, Stamey TA. Mucinous differentiation in prostatic adenocarcinoma. Hum Pathol 1991;22:979–88.

50. Odom DG, Donatucci CF, Deshon GE. Mucinous adenocarcinoma of the prostate. Hum Pathol 1986;17:863–5.

51. Outwater E, Schrieber ML, Tomaszewski JE, Schnall MD, Kressel HY. Mucinous carcinomas involving the prostate: atypical findings at MR imaging. J Mag Res Imaging 1992;2:597–600.

52. Proia AD, McCarty KS, Woodard BH. Prostatic mucinous adenocarcinoma. A Cowper gland carcinoma mimicker. Am J Surg Pathol 1981;5:701–6.

53. Randolph TL, Amin MB, Ro JY. Histologic variants of the prostatic adenocarcinoma and other carcinomas of the prostate. Mod Pathol 1997;10:612–29.

54. Ro JY, Grignon DJ, Ayala AG, Fernandez PL, Ordonez NG, Wishnow KI. Mucinous adenocarcinoma of the prostate: histochemical and immunohistochemical studies. Hum Pathol 1990;21:593–600.

55. Ro JY, Grignon DJ, Troncoso P, Ayala AG. Mucin in prostatic adenocarcinoma. Sem Diag Pathol 1988; 5:273–83.

56. Sika JV, Buckley JJ. Mucus-forming adenocarcinoma of prostate. J Urol 1977;118:124–5.

57. Teichman JM, Shabaik A, Demby AM. Mucinous adenocarcinoma of the prostate and hormone sensitivity. J Urol 1994;151:701–2.

Signet Ring Cell Carcinoma

58. Alline KM, Cohen MB. Signet-ring cell carcinoma of the prostate. Arch Pathol Lab Med 1992;116:99–102.

59. Catton PA, Hartwick RW, Srigley JR. Prostate cancer presenting with malignant ascites: signet-ring cell variant of prostatic adenocarcinoma. Urology 1992;39:495–7.

60. Das S, Brewer L, Bell S. Signet-ring cell carcinoma of the prostate. J Urol Pathol 1996;5:149–55.

61. Guerin D, Hasan N, Keen CE. Signet ring cell differentiation in adenocarcinoma of the prostate: a study of five cases. Histopathology 1993;22:367–71.

62. Hejka A, England D. Signet ring cell carcinoma of prostate: immunohistochemical and ultrastructural study of a case. Urology 1989;34:155–8.

63. Leong FJ, Leong AS, Swift J. Signet-ring cell carcinoma of the prostate. Path Res Pract 1996;192:1232–8.

64. Remmele W, Weber A, Harding P. Primary signet ring cell carcinoma of the prostate. Hum Pathol 1988;19:478–80.

65. Reyes AO, Swanson PE, Carbone JM, Humphrey PA. Unusual histologic types of high grade prostatic intraepithelial neoplasia. Am J Surg Path 1997;21:1215–22.

66. Ro JY, El-Naggar A, Ayala AG, Mody DR, Ordonez NG. Signet-ring-cell carcinoma of the prostate. Electron-microscopic and immunohistochemical studies of eight cases. Am J Surg Pathol 1988;12:453–60.

67. Segawa T, Kakehi Y. Primary signet ring cell adenocarcinoma of the prostate: a case report and literature review. Acta Urol Jpn 1993;39:565–8.

68. Skodras G, Wang J, Kragel PJ. Primary prostatic signet-ring cell carcinoma. Urology 1993;42:338–42.

69. Smith C, Feddersen RM, Dressler L, McConnell T, Milroy M, Smith AY. Signet ring cell adenocarcinoma of prostate. Urology 1994;43:397–400.

69a. Torbenson M, Dhir R, Nangia A, Becich MJ, Kapadia SB. Prostatic carcinoma with signet ring cells: a clinicopathologic and immunohistochemical analysis of 12 cases, with review of the literature. Mod Pathol 1998;11:552–9.

70. Uchijima Y, Ito H, Takahashi M, Yamashina M. Prostate mucinous adenocarcinoma with signet ring cells. Urology 1990;36:267–8.

Squamous and Adenosquamous Carcinoma

71. Accetta PA, Gardner WA Jr. Adenosquamous carcinoma of prostate. Urology 1983;22:73–5.

72. Al Adani MS. Schistosomiasis, metaplasia and squamous cell carcinoma of the prostate: histogenesis of the squamous cells determined by localization of specific markers. Neoplasia 1985;32:613–22.

73. Amin MB, Ro JY, Ayala AG. Clinical relevance of histologic variants of prostate cancer. Cancer Bull 1993;45:403–10.

74. Arnheim FK. Carcinoma of the prostate: a study of post-mortem findings in 176 cases. J Urol 1948;60:599–603.

75. Bennett RS, Edgerton EO. Mixed prostatic carcinoma. J Urol 1973;110:561–3.

76. Braslis KG, Davi RC, Nelson E, Civantos F, Soloway MS. Squamous cell carcinoma of the prostate: a transformation from adenocarcinoma after the use of a luteinizing hormone-releasing hormone antagonist and flutamide. Urology 1995;45:329–31.

77. Corder MP, Cicmil GA. Effective treatment of metastatic squamous cell carcinoma of the prostate with adriamycin. J Urol 1976;115:222.

78. Devaney DM, Dorman A, Leader M. Adenosquamous carcinoma of the prostate: a case report. Hum Pathol 1991;22:1046–50.

79. Gattuso P, Carson HJ, Candel A, Castelli MJ. Adenosquamous carcinoma of the prostate. Hum Pathol 1995;26:123–6.

80. Gray GF Jr, Marshall VF. Squamous carcinoma of the prostate. J Urol 1975;113:736–8.

81. Kahler JE. Carcinoma of the prostate gland: a pathologic study. J Urol 1939;41:557–74.

82. Konety BR, Lavelle JP, O'Donnell WF, Becich MJ, Bastacky S. Metastatic adenosquamous carcinoma of the prostate. J Urol Pathol 1997;7:33–8.

83. Lager DJ, Goeken JA, Kemp JD, Robinson RA. Squamous metaplasia of the prostate: an immunohistochemical study. Am J Clin Pathol 1988;90:597–601.

84. Little NA, Wiener JS, Walther PJ, Paulson DF, Anderson E. Squamous cell carcinoma of the prostate: 2 cases of a rare malignancy and review of the literature. J Urol 1993;149:137–9.

85. Ma TK, Srigley JR. Adenocarcinoma of prostate and schistosomiasis: a rare association. Histopathology 1995;27:187–9.

86. Mai KT, Leahy CF. Squamous cell carcinoma occurring as a circumscribed nodule in the transition zone of the prostate. J Urol Pathol 1996;5:85–92.

87. Moskovitz B, Munichor M, Bolkier M, Livne PM. Squamous cell carcinoma of the prostate. Urol Int 1993;51:181–3.

88. Mott LJ. Squamous cell carcinoma of the prostate: report of 2 cases and review of the literature. J Urol 1979;121:833–5.

89. Moyana TN. Adenosquamous carcinoma of the prostate. Am J Surg Pathol 1987;11:403–7.

90. Saito R, Davis BK, Ollapally EP. Adenosquamous carcinoma of the prostate. Hum Pathol 1984;15:87–9.

91. Sarma DP, Weilbaecher TG, Moon TD. Squamous cell carcinoma of prostate. Urology 1991;37:260–2.

92. Sieracki JC. Epidermoid carcinoma of the human prostate: report of three cases. Lab Invest 1955;4:232–40.

93. Thompson GJ, Albers DD, Broders AC. Unusual carcinomas involving the prostate gland. J Urol 1953;69:416–25.

94. Wernert N, Goebbels R, Bonkhoff H, Dhom G. Squamous cell carcinoma of the prostate. Histopathology 1990;17:339–44.

Basaloid and Adenoid Cystic Carcinomas

95. Ahn SK, Kim K, Choi IJ, Lee JM. Adenoid cystic carcinoma of the prostate gland—pathological review with a case report. Yonsei Med J 1991;32:74–8.

96. Carpenter AA, Bernardo JR Jr. Adenoid cystic carcinoma of Cowper's gland: case report. J Urol 1971;106:701–3.

97. Cohen RJ, Goldberg RD, Verhaart MJ, Cohen M. Adenoid cyst-like carcinoma of the prostate gland. Arch Pathol Lab Med 1993;117:799–801.

98. Denholm SW, Webb JN, Howard GC, Chisholm GD. Basaloid carcinoma of the prostate gland: histogenesis and review of the literature. Histopathology 1992;20:151–5.

99. Devaraj LJ, Bostwick DG. Atypical basal cell hyperplasia of the prostate. Immunophenotypic profile and proposed classification of basal cell proliferation. Am J Surg Pathol 1993;17:645–59.

100. Epstein JI, Armas OA. Atypical basal cell hyperplasia of the prostate. Am J Surg Pathol 1992;16:1205–14.

101. Frankel K, Craig JR. Adenoid cystic carcinoma of the prostate. Report of a case. Am J Clin Path 1974;62:639–45.

102. Gilmour M, Bell TJ. Adenoid cystic carcinoma of the prostate. Br J Urol 1986;58:105–6.

103. Grignon DJ, Ro JY, Ordoñez NG, Ayala AG, Cleary KR. Basal cell hyperplasia, adenoid basal cell tumor, and adenoid cystic carcinoma of the prostate gland: an immunohistochemical study. Hum Pathol 1988;19:1425–33.

104. Kramer SA, Braedael JJ, Krueger RP. Adenoid cystic carcinoma of the prostate: report of a case. J Urol 1978;120:383–4.

105. Kuhajda FP, Mann RB. Adenoid cystic carcinoma of the prostate. A case report with immunoperoxidase staining for prostate-specific acid phosphatase and prostate-specific antigen. Am J Clin Path 1984;81:257–60.

106. Manrique JJ, Albores-Saavedra J, Orantes A, Brandt H. Malignant mixed tumor of the salivary-gland type primary in the prostate. Am J Clin Path 1978;70:932–7.

107. Reed RJ. Consultation case: prostate (prostatectomy)—adenoid basel-cell tumor—basel-cell hyperplasia. Am J Surg Pathol 1984;18:699–704.

108. Shong-San C, Walters NI. Adenoid cystic carcinoma of the prostate. Report of a case. Pathology 1984;16:337–8.

109. Tannenbaum M. Adenoid cystic or salivary gland carcinomas of the prostate. Urology 1975;6:238–9.

110. van Renterghem K, Mattelaer J, Billiet I. Adenoid cystic carcinoma of the prostate. Acta Urol Belgica 1994;62:69–70.

111. Young RH, Frierson HF, Mills SE, Kaiser JS, Talbot WH, Bhan AK. Adenoid cystic-like tumor of the prostate gland: a report of two cases and review of the literature on adenoid cystic carcinoma of the prostate. Am J Clin Pathol 1988;89:49–56.

Transitional Cell Carcinoma

112. Amin MB, Murphy WM, Reuter VE, et al. Controversies in the pathology of transitional cell carcinoma of the urinary bladder, part II. In: Fechner FE, Rosen PP, eds. ASCP reviews in pathology, Vol. 1. Chicago: ASCP Press, 1997:1–38.

113. Bodner DR, Cohen JK, Resnick MI. Primary transitional cell carcinoma of the prostate. J Urol 1986;92:121–2.

113a. Cheville JC. Urothelial carcinoma of the prostate. An immunohistochemical comparison with high-grade prostatic adenocarcinoma and review of the literature. J Urol Pathol 1998;9:141–54.

114. Cheville JC, Dundore PA, Bostwick DG, et al. Transitional cell carcinoma of the prostate. Clinicopathologic study of 50 cases. Cancer 1998;82:703–7.

115. Ende N, Woods LP, Shelley HS. Carcinoma originating in ducts surrounding the prostatic urethra. Am J Clin Path 1963;40:183–9.

116. Greene LF, Mulcahy JJ, Warren MM, Dockerty MB. Primary transitional cell carcinoma of the prostate. J Urol 1973;110:235–7.

117. Greene LF, O'Dea MJ, Dockerty MB. Primary transitional cell carcinoma of the prostate. J Urol 1976;116:761–3.

118. Johnson DE, Hogan JM, Ayala AG. Transitional cell carcinoma of the prostate. Cancer 1972;29:287–93.

119. Kablain JN, McNeal JE, Price HM, Freiha FS, Stamey TA. Unsuspected adenocarcinoma of prostate in patients undergoing cystoprostatectomy for other causes: incidence, histology and morphometric observations. J Urol 1989;141:1091–4.

120. Karpas CM, Moumgis B. Primary transitional cell carcinoma of prostate gland: possible pathogenesis and relationship to reserve cell hyperplasia of prostatic periurethral ducts. J Urol 1969;101:201–5.

121. Laplante M, Brice M. The upper limits of hopeful application of radical cystectomy for vesical carcinoma: does nodal metastasis always indicate incurability? J Urol 1973;109:261–4.

122. Mahadevia PS, Koss LG, Tar IJ. Prostatic involvement in bladder cancer. Prostate mapping in 20 cystoprostatectomy specimens. Cancer 1986;58:2095–102.

123. Matzkin H, Soloway MS, Hardeman S. Transitional cell carcinoma of the prostate. J Urol 1991;146:1207–12.

124. Montie JE, Wood DP Jr, Pontes JE, Boyett JM, Levin HS. Adenocarcinoma of prostate in cystoprostatectomy specimens removed for bladder cancer. Cancer 1989;63:381–5.

125. Nicolaisen GS, Williams RD. Primary transitional cell carcinoma of prostate. Urology 1984;24:544–9.

126. Razvi M, Fifer R, Berkson B. Occult transitional cell carcinoma of the prostate presenting as skin metastasis. J Urol 1975;113:734–5.

127. Savera AT, Amin MB, Ro JY, Linden MD, Ayala AG. Differential diagnosis of malignant neoplasms in the prostate with large ductal pattern: utility of an immunohistochemical panel [Abstract]. Mod Pathol 1997;10:89A.

128. Sawczuk I, Tannenbaum M, Olsson CA, deVere White R. Primary transitional cell carcinoma of prostatic periurethral ducts. Urology 1985;25:339–43.

129. Schujman E, Mukamel E, Slutzker D, Mor C, Servadio C. Prostatic transitional cell carcinoma: concept of its pathogenesis and classification. Israel J Med Sciences 1983;19:794–800.

130. Smith BD, Flegel G. Primary transitional cell carcinoma of the prostate: report of two cases. J Am Osteopath 1982;82:547–8.

131. Takashi MS, Sakata T, Nagai T, et al. Primary transitional cell carcinoma of prostate: case with lymph node metastasis eradicated by neoadjuvant methotrexate, vinblastine, doxorubicin, and cisplatin (M-vac) therapy. Urology 1990;36:96–8.

132. Tannenbaum M. Transitional cell carcinoma of the prostate. Urology 1975;5:674–8.

133. Ullmann AS, Ross OA. Hyperplasia, atypism and carcinoma in situ in prostatic periurethral glands. J Urol 1967;47:497–504.

Small Cell Carcinoma

134. Abrahamsson PA, Wadstrom LB, Alumets J, Falkmer S, Grimelius L. Peptide-hormone- and serotonin-immunoreactive tumour cells in carcinoma of the prostate. Pathol Res Pract 1987;182:298–307.

135. Amato RJ, Logothetis CJ, Hallinan R, Ro JY, Sella A, Dexeus FA. Chemotherapy for small cell carcinoma of prostatic origin. J Urol 1992;147:935–7.

136. Amin MB, Ro JY, Ayala AG. Clinical relevance of histologic variants of prostate cancer. Cancer Bull 1993;45:403–10.

137. Barkin J, Crassweller PO, Roncari DA, Onrot J. Hypercalcemia associated with cancer of prostate without bony metastases. Urology 1984;24:368–71.

138. Bologna M, Festuccia C, Muzi P, Biordi L, Ciomei M. Bombesin stimulates growth of human prostatic cancer cells in vitro. Cancer 1989;63:1714–20.

139. Bolton DM, Chiu ST, Clarke S, Angus D. Primary small cell carcinoma of the prostate: unusual modes of presentation. Aust N Z Surg 1994;64:91–4.

140. Christopher ME, Seftel AD, Sorenson K, Resnick MI. Small cell carcinoma of the genitourinary tract: an immunohistochemical, electron microscopic and clinicopathological study. J Urol 1991;145:382–8.

141. Ghali VS, Garcia RL. Prostatic adenocarcinoma with carcinoidal features producing adrenocorticotropic syndrome: immunohistochemical study and review of the literature. Cancer 1984;40:773–8.

142. Hindson DA, Knight LL, Ocker JM. Small-cell carcinoma of prostate. Transient complete remission with chemotherapy. Urology 1985;26:182–4.

143. Mnaymneh-Ghandur L, Satterfield S, Block NL. Small cell carcinoma of the prostate gland with inappropriate antidiuretic hormone secretion: morphological, immunohistochemical and clinical expressions. J Urol 1986;135:1263–6.

144. Oesterling JE, Hauzeur CG, Farrow GM. Small cell anaplastic carcinoma of the prostate: a clinical, pathological and immunohistological study of 27 patients. J Urol 1992;147:804–7.

145. Ro JY, Tetu B, Ayala AG, Ordóñez NG. Small cell carcinoma of the prostate, part II: immunohistochemical and electron microscopic study of 18 cases. Cancer 1987;59:977–82.

146. Sarma DP, Weilbaecher TG. Small-cell carcinoma of prostate. Urology 1989;33:332–5.

147. Schron DS, Gipson T, Mendelsohn G. The histogenesis of small cell carcinoma of the prostate: an immunohistochemical study. Cancer 1984;53:2478–80.

148. Smith DC, Tucker JA, Trump DL. Hypercalcemia and neuroendocrine carcinoma of the prostate: a report of three cases and a review of the literature. J Clin Oncol 1992;10:499–505.

149. Tetu B, Ro JY, Ayala AG, Johnson DE, Logothetis CJ, Ordóñez NG. Small cell carcinoma of the prostate, part I. A clinicopathologic study of 20 cases. Cancer 1987;59:1803–9.

150. Tetu B, Ro JY, Ayala AG, Ordóñez NG, Logothetis CJ, von Eschenbach AC. Small cell carcinoma of prostate

151. Wenk RE, Bhagavan BS, Levy R, Miller D, Weisburger W. Ectopic ACTH, prostatic oat cell carcinoma and marked hypernatremia. Cancer 1977;40:733–78.

associated with myasthenic (Eaton-Lambert) syndrome. Urology 1989;33:148–52.

Sarcomatoid Carcinoma and Carcinosarcoma

152. Amin MB, Ro JY, Ayala AG. Clinical relevance of histologic variants of prostate cancer. Cancer Bull 1993;45:403–10.

153. Ashburn LL. New bone formation in a primary carcinoma of the prostate gland. Arch Pathol 1939;28:145–50.

154. Bedrosian SA, Goldman RL, Sung MA. Heterotopic cartilage in prostate. Urology 1983;21:536–7.

155. Coats EC, Lisa JR. Osteogenesis occurring in carcinoma of the prostate. J Urol 1949;62:58–60.

156. Dundore PA, Chevill JC, Nascimento AG, Farrow GM, Bostwick DG. Carcinosarcoma of prostate. Report of 21 cases. Cancer 1995;76:1035–42.

157. Jones EC, Young RH. Non-neoplastic and neoplastic spindle cell proliferation and mixed tumors of the urinary bladder. J Urol Pathol 1994;2:105–34.

158. Kaneko Y, Yoshiki T, Fukumoto M, Oishi K, Yoshida O. Carcinosarcoma of the prostate. Urologia Internationalis 1992;48:105–7.

159. Lauwers GY, Schevchuk M, Armenakas N, Reuter VE. Carcinosarcoma of the prostate. Am J Surg Pathol 1993;17:342–9.

160. Lindboe CF, Jones J. Carcinosarcoma of prostate. Immunohistochemical and ultrastructural observations. Urology 1992;40:376–80.

161. Locke JR, Soloway MS, Evans J, Murphy WM. Osteogenic differentiation associated with x-ray therapy for adenocarcinoma of the prostate gland. Am J Clin Pathol 1986;85:375–8.

161a. Ma TK, Chapman WB, McLean M, Srigley JR. Prostatic carcinosarcoma consisting of the unusual combination of ductal adenocarcinoma with osteogenic sarcoma. J Urol Pathol 1998;8:111–9.

162. Ohtsuki Y, Ro JY, Ordonez NG, Kee KH, Richmond C, Ayala AG. Sarcomatoid carcinoma of the prostate with rhabdomyosarcomatous differentiation. J Urol Pathol 1996;5:157–63.

163. Ordonez NG, Ayala A, von Eschenbach AC, Mackay B, Hanssen G. Immunoperoxidase localization of prostatic acid phosphatase in prostatic carcinoma with sarcomatoid changes. Urology 1982;19:210–4.

164. Shannon RI, Ro JY, Grignon DJ, et al. Sarcomatoid carcinoma of the prostate. A clinicopathologic study of 12 patients. Cancer 1992;69:2676–82.

165. Tannenbaum M. Carcinoma with sarcomatoid changes or carcinosarcoma of prostate. Urology 1975;6:91–3.

166. Wick MR, Young RH, Malvesta R, Beebe DS, Hansen JJ, Dehner LP. Prostatic carcinosarcomas. Clinical, histologic and immunohistochemical data on two cases, with a review of the literature. Am J Clin Pathol 1989;92:131–9.

167. Zenklusen HR, Weymuth G, Rist M, Mihatsch MJ. Carcinosarcoma of the prostate in combination with adenocarcinoma of the seminal vesicles. A case report with immunocytochemical analysis and review of the literature. Cancer 1990;66:998–1001.

Lymphoepithelioma–like Carcinoma

168. Amin MB, Ro JY, Lee KM, et al. Lymphoepithelioma-like carcinoma of the urinary bladder. Am J Surg Pathol 1994;18:466–73.

169. Bostwick DG, Adalkha K. Lymphoepithelioma-like carcinoma of the prostate. J Urol Pathol 1994;2:319–25.

Undifferentiated Carcinoma

170. Mai KT, Burns BF, Morash C. Giant-cell carcinoma of the prostate. J Urol Pathol 1996;5:167–74.

Secondary Carcinoma

171. Amin MB, Murphy WM, Reuter VE, et al. Controversies in the pathology of transitional cell carcinoma of the urinary bladder, part II. In: Fechner FE, Rosen PP, eds. ASCP reviews in pathology, Vol. 1. Chicago: ASCP Press 1997:1–38.

172. Amin MB, Ro JY, Ayala AG. Prostatic intraepithelial neoplasia. Relationship to adenocarcinoma of prostate. Pathol Ann 1994;29 (pt 2):1–30.

173. Arnheim FK. Carcinoma of the prostate. A study of postmortem findings in 176 cases. J Urol 1948;60:599–603.

174. Bretton PR, Herr HW, Whitmore WF, et al. Intravesical bacillus Calmette-Guerin therapy for in-situ transitional cell carcinoma involving the prostatic urethra. J Urol 1989;141:853–6.

174a. Cheville JC. Urothelial carcinoma of the prostate. An immunohistochemical comparison with high-grade prostatic adenocarcinoma and review of the literature. J Urol Pathol 1998;9:141–54.

175. Cheville JC, Dundore PA, Bostwick DG, et al. Transitional cell carcinoma of the prostate: clinicopathologic study of 50 cases. Cancer 1998;82:703–7.

176. Coutts AG, Grigor KM, Fowler JW. Urethral dysplasia and bladder cancer in cystectomy specimens. Br J Urol 1985;57:535–41.

177. Droller MJ, Walsh PC. Intensive intravesical chemotherapy in the treatment of flat carcinoma in situ: is it safe? J Urol 1985;134:1115–7.

178. Esrig D, Freeman JA, Elmajian DA, et al. Transitional cell carcinoma involving the prostate with a proposed staging classification for stromal invasion. J Urol 1996;156:1071–6.

179. Frazier IIA, Robertson JE, Dodge RK, Paulson DF. The value of pathologic factors in predicting cancer–specific survival among patients treated with radical cystectomy for transitional cell carcinoma of the bladder and prostate. Cancer 1993;71:3993–4001.

180. Greene LF, Mulcahy JJ, Warren MM, Dockerty MB. Primary transitional cell carcinoma of the prostate. J Urol 1973;110:235–7.

181. Hardeman SW, Soloway MS: Transitional cell carcinoma of the prostate: diagnosis, staging and management. World J Urol 1988;6:170.

182. Hillyard RW Jr, Ladaga L, Schellhammer PF. Superficial transitional cell carcinoma of the bladder associated with mucosal involvement of the prostatic urethra: results of treatment with intravesicle bacillus Calmette-Guerin. J Urol 1988;139:290–3.

183. Johnson DE, Chalbaud R, Ayala AG. Secondary tumors of the prostate. J Urol 1974;112:507–8.

184. Kabalin JN, McNeal JE, Price HM, Freiha FS, Stamey TA. Unsuspected adenocarcinoma of prostate in patients undergoing cystoprostatectomy for other causes: incidence, histology and morphometric observations. J Urol 1989;141:1091–4.

185. Kahler JE. Carcinoma of the prostate gland: a pathologic study. J Urol 1939;41:557–74.

186. Kirk D, Hinton CE, Shaldon C. Transitional cell carcinoma of the prostate. Br J Urol 1979;51:575–8.

187. Leung CS, Srigley JR, Robertson AR. Metastatic renal cell carcinoma presenting as solitary bleeding prostatic metastasis. J Urol Pathol 1997;7:1–6.

188. Lockhart JL, Chaikin L, Bondhus MJ, Politano VA. Prostatic recurrence in the management of superficial bladder tumors. J Urol 1983;130:256–7.

189. Mahadevia PS, Koss LG, Tar IJ. Prostatic involvement in bladder cancer. Prostate mapping in 20 cystoprostatectomy specimens. Cancer 1986;58:2095–102.

190. Matzkin H, Soloway MS, Hardeman S. Transitional cell carcinoma of the prostate. J Urol 1991;146:1207–12.

191. Montie JE, Wood DP Jr, Mendendorp SV, Levin HS, Pontes JE. The significance and management of transitional cell carcinoma of the prostate. Semin Urol 1990;8:262–8.

192. Pagano F, Bassi P, Ferrante-Drago GL, et al. Is stage pT4a (D1) reliable in assessing transitional cell carcinoma involvement of the prostate in patients with concurrent bladder cancer? A necessary distinction for contiguous or noncontiguous involvement. J Urol 1996;155:244–7.

193. Parr NJ, Grigor KM, Ritchie AW. Metastatic carcinoid tumour involving the prostate. Br J Urol 1992;70:103–4.

194. Prout GR Jr, Griffin PP, Daly JJ, Heney NM. Carcinoma in situ of the urinary bladder with and without associated vesicle neoplasms. Cancer 1983;52:524–32.

195. Rubenstein AB, Rubnitz ME. Transitional cell carcinoma of the prostate. Cancer 1969;24:543–6.

196. Savera AT, Amin MB, Linden MD, Ro JY, Ayala A. Differential diagnosis of malignant neoplasms in the prostate with large ductal pattern: utility of an immunohistochemical panel [Abstract]. Mod Path 1997;10:89A.

197. Schellhammer PF, Bean MA, Whitmore WF Jr. Prostatic involvement by transitional cell carcinoma: pathogenesis, patterns and prognosis. J Urol 1977;118:399–403.

198. Seemayer TA, Knaack J, Thelmo WL, Wang NS, Ahmed MN. Further observations of carcinoma in situ of the urinary bladder: silent but extensive intraprostatic involvement. Cancer 1975;36:514–20.

199. Stein BS, Kendall AR. Malignant melanoma of the genitourinary tract. J Urol 1984;132:859–68.

200. Thompson GJ, Albers DD, Broders AC. Unusual carcinomas involving the prostate gland. J Urol 1953;69:416–25.

201. Wendelken JR, Schellhammer PF, Ladaga LE, El-Mahdi AM. Transitional cell carcinoma: cause of refractory cancer of prostate. Urology 1979;13:557–60.

202. Wishnow KI, Ro JY. Importance of early treatment of transitional cell carcinoma of prostatic ducts. Urology 1988;32:11–2.

203. Wood DP, Montie JE, Pontes JR, Mendendorp SV, Levin HS. Transitional cell carcinoma of the prostate in cystoprostatectomy specimens removed for bladder cancer. J Urol 1989;141:346–9.

204. Zein TA, Huben R, Lane W, Pontes JE, Englander LS. Secondary tumors of the prostate. J Urol 1985;133:615–6.

✧✧✧

6
MISCELLANEOUS TUMORS OF THE PROSTATE

Despite the prevalence of prostatic carcinoma, benign epithelial tumors of the prostate are exceedingly rare, as are mesenchymal proliferations if stromal nodules within the spectrum of benign prostatic hyperplasia are excluded (see chapter 2). The remaining mesenchymal lesions encompass a heterogenous group ranging from the relatively recently described exuberant but benign spindle cell lesions (see chapter 7) to high-grade sarcomas. Mixed epithelial-stromal tumors also occur, and their features have been somewhat clarified by several recent, important studies. In this chapter, benign epithelial, mesenchymal, mixed, hematolymphoid, and miscellaneous other rare primary tumors of the prostate gland are discussed (Table 6-1).

BENIGN EPITHELIAL TUMORS

Cystadenoma (Giant Multilocular Cystadenoma)

General and Clinical Features. This is the only bona fide, benign epithelial neoplasm of the prostate; less than 20 cases have been reported (1–12). Cystadenoma may occur within the gland and extensively replace it (intraprostatic) (1,3,5,10), be attached to it by a pedicle (suprapubic or retrovesical) (4,6–8,12), or be retroperitoneal without a demonstrable attachment to the prostate (parasitic) (2,4a,9,11). The patients are usually elderly, with a mean age of 64.5 years; retroperitoneal cases occur in younger men (mean age, 47 years) (9). The symptoms depend on tumor location: patients with prostatic and retrovesical lesions present with difficulty in voiding, hesitancy, frequency, or obstruction, with or without hematuria (1,3–8,10,12); those with retroperitoneal and suprapubic lesions present with a mass and increasing abdominal girth, with or without micturitional problems (9).

Gross Findings. The specimens are typically large, bosselated, multiloculated cystic masses (fig. 6-1) that have measured up to 45 cm and weighed up to 6500 g (9). The cysts range from a few millimeters to about 4 cm and contain yellowish brown or gray, semi-solid to inspissated

material (6,8,9). Necrosis and hemorrhage are uncommon.

Microscopic Findings. The histology is essentially similar regardless of the location. Glands and cysts are lined by flattened to cuboidal epithelium, with pale cytoplasm and basally located, innocuous nuclei lacking prominent nucleoli (figs. 6-2, 6-3). The lining may occasionally be multilayered with small papillary projections, very rarely forming cribriform structures

Table 6-1

MESENCHYMAL, HEMATOLYMPHOID, AND MISCELLANEOUS TUMORS AND TUMOR-LIKE LESIONS OF THE PROSTATE GLAND

1. Variants of prostatic hyperplasia
   a. Stromal hyperplasia with bizarre nuclei (see chapter 7)
   b. Phyllodes-like hyperplasia (see chapter 2)
   c. Fibroadenoma-like foci in benign hyperplasia (see chapter 2)

2. Other tumor-like lesions
   a. Postoperative spindle cell nodule (see chapter 7)
   b. Inflammatory pseudotumor/pseudosarcomatous fibromyxoid tumor (see chapter 7)

3. Cystadenoma

4. Mixed epithelial-stromal tumor (phyllodes tumor)

5. Stromal tumors
   a. Benign
      1) Leiomyoma
      2) Others
   b. Malignant
      1) Rhabdomyosarcoma
      2) Leiomyosarcoma
      3) Stromal sarcoma
      4) Others

6. Hematolymphoid neoplasms
   a. Malignant lymphoma
   b. Leukemia including granulocytic sarcoma
   c. Plasmacytoma

7. Miscellaneous tumors
   a. Germ cell tumors
   b. Pheochromocytoma (paraganglioma)

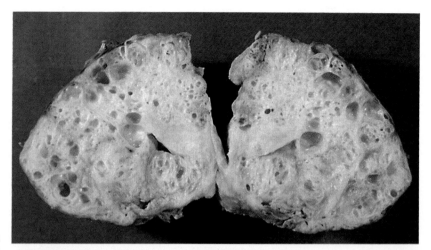

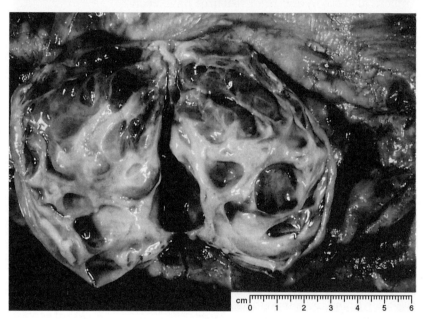

Figure 6-1
CYSTADENOMA

Top: A bivalved specimen shows a large, multiloculated cystic mass with a focally prominent fibrous stroma.

Bottom: Another example. (Fig. 5B from Lim DJ, Hayden RT, Murad T, Nemceck AA, Dalton DP. Multilocular prostatic cystadenoma presenting as a large complex pelvic cystic mass. J Urol 1993;149:856–9.)

(6,8,9). Metaplastic squamous and transitional epithelium may also be seen. The hypocellular stroma may be focally hyalinized and often contains scattered chronic inflammatory cells. Rupture of cysts may result in hemorrhage within the cyst and into the adjacent stroma, with an accompanying granulation tissue reaction. Stromal fibroblasts may demonstrate focal reactive atypia, with vesicular nuclei and prominent nucleoli. Immunohistochemical stains show reactivity for prostate-specific antigen (PSA) and prostatic acid phosphatase (PAP) in the epithelial lining. The stromal cells are negative for desmin and S-100 protein.

Differential Diagnosis. For lesions within the prostatic parenchyma, benign cysts (congenital or acquired) of the prostate (see chapter 7) and mixed epithelial-stromal tumors (phyllodes tumors) enter into the differential diagnosis. The latter has a more cellular, atypical stroma, and often has prominent intraluminal papillary to polypoid structures, features that are absent in cystadenomas. Other entities in the differential for retroperitoneal and retrovesical lesions include multilocular peritoneal cyst, lymphangioma, mullerian duct cyst, and seminal vesicle cyst (see chapter 8) (9). The nature of the cyst lining in all these entities, however, is different from the

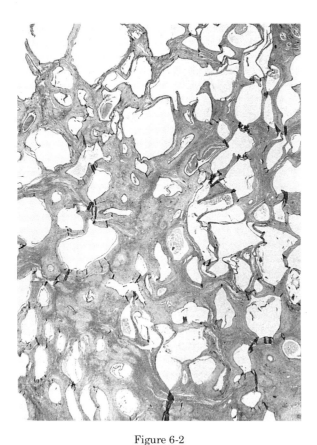

Figure 6-2
CYSTADENOMA
A low-power view shows numerous cystically dilated glands.

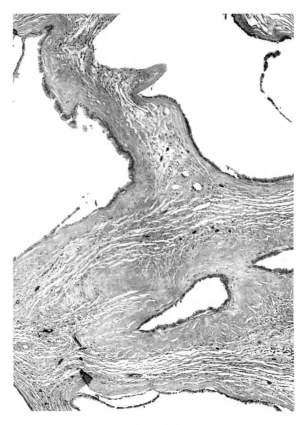

Figure 6-3
CYSTADENOMA
A higher power view shows a single layer of flattened to cuboidal epithelium with features of prostatic secretory epithelium.

prostatic type epithelium of prostatic cystadenoma, and this can be confirmed by negative immunostaining for PSA and PAP in the former in contrast to the positive staining in cystadenoma.

Treatment and Prognosis. All prostatic cystadenomas reported to date have had an uneventful follow-up. Complete primary surgical removal by conservative enucleation of the mass constitutes adequate treatment, but some patients required radical surgery, including anterior pelvic exenteration, because of the large size of the tumor (4,6,7).

BENIGN MESENCHYMAL TUMORS

Leiomyoma

In order to distinguish nodular smooth muscle proliferations of a hyperplastic nature from leiomyoma of the prostate, the latter is arbitrarily defined as a well-circumscribed proliferation of smooth muscle greater than 1 cm in diameter (30). Lesions fitting this definition are rare, and less than 70 cases have been described (13,17,18, 20,21,23,25–27,30). Most occur in men in the sixth and seventh decades (range, 41 to 80 years) who present with prostatism, urinary tract infection, or acute urinary retention. The lesions may be enucleated due to their sharp circumscription, and in prostatectomy specimens their circumscribed nature can be appreciated. The outcome is favorable although recurrence has been reported.

Pathologic Findings. The tumors have measured up to 12 cm (fig. 6-4) and have a firm, whorled, gray-white cut surface (13,23,26). Microscopically, fascicles of smooth muscle cells may be separated by hyalinized connective tissue. The nuclei are blunt-ended and usually lack pleomorphism, with only rare mitoses. Variants similar to uterine tumors include cellular leiomyoma

259

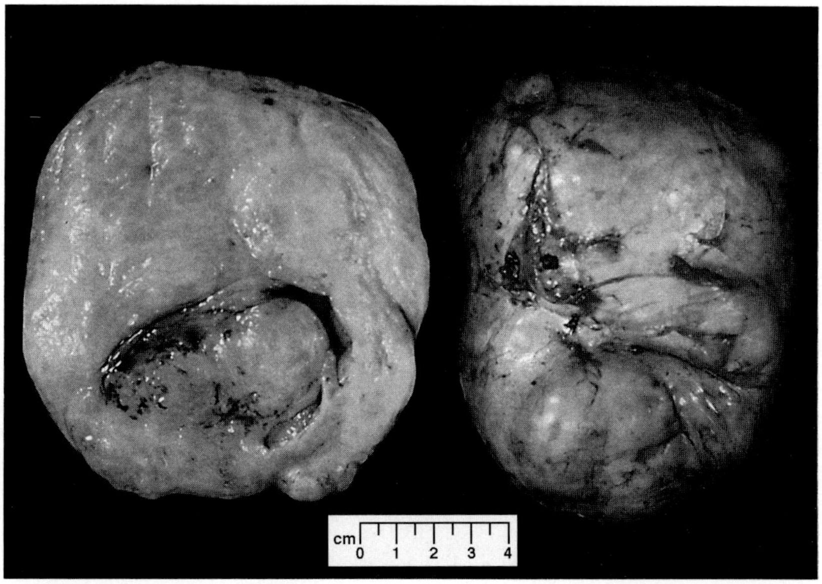

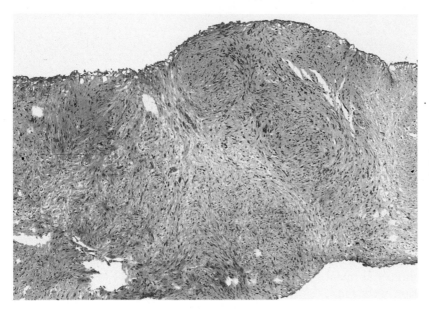

Figure 6-4
LEIOMYOMA
A large well-circumscribed mass has a whorled appearance. (Fig. 2 from Regan JB, Barrett DM, Wold LE. Giant leiomyoma of the prostate. Arch Pathol Lab Med 1987;111:381–3.)

Figure 6-5
LEIOMYOMA IN A TRANSURETHRAL RESECTION SPECIMEN
Numerous prostatic chips showed a similar histology, with fascicles of bland spindle cells with occasional areas of degenerate-type nuclear atypia.

and leiomyoma with bizarre nuclei (symplastic leiomyoma) (figs. 6-5, 6-6) (20,25,27). The atypia of the latter is degenerate in appearance with multinucleation, vacuolated nuclei, and smudged nuclear chromatin, and there is typically no increased mitotic activity. The tumors are immunoreactive for desmin and actin (31).

Differential Diagnosis. Distinction from a large fibromuscular nodule of hyperplasia is aided by the additional fibroblastic component of the latter, which is also sometimes associated with more prominent blood vessels than the usual leiomyoma. The important differential diagnosis is with leiomyosarcoma. Due to the few cases described, it is difficult to give firm criteria to separate benign from malignant smooth muscle lesions of the prostate (30). Most leiomyosarcomas have overt features indicative of malignancy. As in uterine tumors, several features should be sought including hypercellularity, nuclear pleomorphism, significant mitotic activity, necrosis, and infiltrative growth; in general, two or

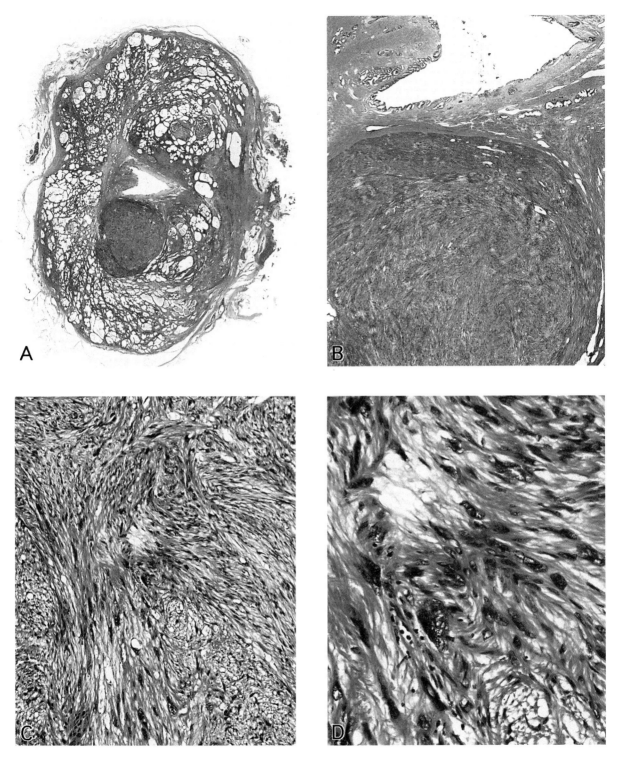

Figure 6-6
LEIOMYOMA

A: A cross section of a whole mount of the prostate shows a distinct, well-circumscribed nodule in the transition zone.

B: This view shows the relationship to the verumontanum (top).

C,D: High-power views show fascicles of spindle cells lacking mitotic activity. The nuclear atypia is degenerate in appearance with occasional multinucleation and smudged nuclear chromatin.

more are necessary to designate a prostatic smooth muscle tumor as leiomyosarcoma. Another problematic differential diagnosis, particularly in limited samples such as from needle biopsies, is the distinction of leiomyoma with bizarre nuclei from prostatic sarcomas and related proliferative lesions of the specialized prostatic stroma (Table 6-2)(15). It is prudent to refrain from making an unequivocally benign diagnosis with only a needle biopsy, even if there is a paucity of mitoses in the presence of degenerate type atypia, because such areas may be focally present in otherwise typical sarcomas (15). For needle biopsies, therefore, terminology such as stromal or smooth muscle lesion of uncertain malignant potential should be used when this circumstance is encountered (15).

Other Benign Stromal Tumors

Rarely, other benign stromal tumors occur in the prostate including fibroma, solitary fibrous tumor (22,29), chondroma, osteochondroma (16), hemangioma (19,28), lymphangioma, ganglioneuroma (24), granular cell tumor (14), neurofibroma (fig. 6-7), and schwannoma. Their pathologic features are similar to those seen in the soft tissues and bone. The ganglioneuroma occurred in a patient with the classic form of neurofibromatosis 1 (24).

MALIGNANT MESENCHYMAL TUMORS

Less than 1 percent of malignant tumors of the prostate are of mesenchymal derivation, and the more common examples involve diametrically opposite age groups. Rhabdomyosarcoma, the most frequent sarcoma, accounts for more than 75 percent of the cases, and it is typically seen in infants, children, and young adults. Leiomyosarcoma, the second most common, characteristically involves adults in the fifth to eighth decades. Stromal sarcomas have generally been the subject of case reports but authors of a recent series of cases that studied hormone receptor positivity, proposed that these tumors arise from the hormonally responsive mesenchymal cells of the prostatic stroma (15). A wide range of other adult soft tissue sarcomas also rarely arise within the prostate, but none has features unique to this site.

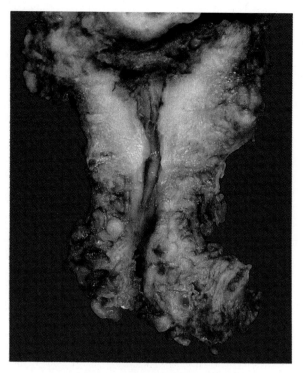

Figure 6-7
NEUROFIBROMATOSIS INVOLVING
PROSTATE AND SOFT TISSUE
SURROUNDING THE PENILE URETHRA
The lesional tissue within the prostatic parenchyma and the periurethral soft tissue has a grayish white nodular appearance. (Courtesy of Dr. J.C. Manivel, Minneapolis, MN.)

Rhabdomyosarcoma

After head and neck rhabdomyosarcomas, genitourinary rhabdomyosarcomas are the most common, with a predilection for the prostate, bladder, and paratesticular region. The overwhelming majority of prostate examples occur in children in the first decade (32–38,40–42,45, 48,49,51), but at least 12 have been described in adults (range, 18 to 80 years; mean, 42.3 years) (33,34,37,43,47,50).

The tumors usually diffusely and extensively involve the prostate and frequently invade into the periprostatic soft tissue, bladder wall, and perirectal and periurethral tissues (37,42,45,47, 49). Large tumors extensively involve this region and it may be difficult to ascertain the precise anatomic origin. Magnetic resonance imaging (MRI) may help determine the dominant site of involvement and the extent of tumor (47).

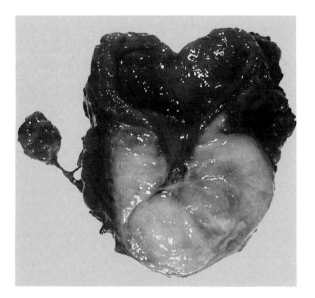

Figure 6-8
EMBRYONAL RHABDOMYOSARCOMA
The prostate gland is replaced by a bulging, fleshy, gray-white mass which had a soft consistency. (Fig. 5-14 from Ro JY, Grignon DJ, Amin MB, Ayala AG. Atlas of surgical pathology of the male reproductive tract. Philadelphia: W.B. Saunders, 1997:88).

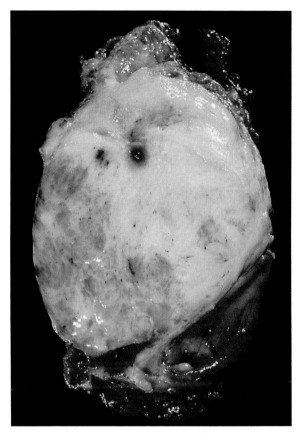

Figure 6-9
EMBRYONAL RHABDOMYOSARCOMA
The cut surface is myxoid.

Gross Findings. The tumors are frequently myxoid, glistening, and soft (figs. 6-8–6-10). They are usually large and extensively involve, sometimes effacing, the prostate. Botryoid examples usually perforate the prostatic urethra and may extend superiorly into the trigone of the urinary bladder, presenting with the typical, multilobulated, grape-like appearance (40).

Microscopic Findings. Most tumors are embryonal, including examples of the botryoid and spindle cell subtypes; rarely, the alveolar variant occurs (33a,43a,45b,47,48a,50). Embryonal rhabdomyosarcoma is composed of sheets of immature, round to oval cells with scant cytoplasm, but rare cells containing abundant eosinophilic cytoplasm are usually detected after careful search (figs. 6-11–6-16). The cellularity varies from dense to hypocellular; tumor cells are separated by a myxoid to edematous stroma. More differentiated tumors show greater numbers of spindle-shaped, tadpole-shaped, or strap cells with abundant, deeply eosinophilic cytoplasm (figs. 6-15, 6-16). Cross striations are more readily appreciable in these differentiated cells. The cells in botryoid tumors often condense to form a densely cellular subepithelial zone (cambium layer).

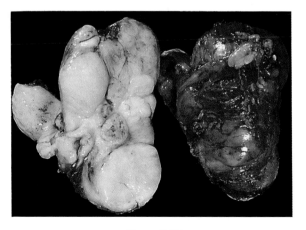

Figure 6-10
EMBRYONAL RHABDOMYOSARCOMA
The tumor is lobulated.

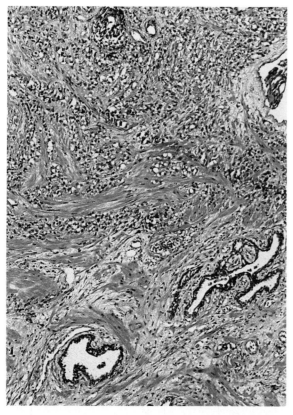

Figure 6-11
EMBRYONAL RHABDOMYOSARCOMA
A small cell neoplasm infiltrates between benign prostatic glands.

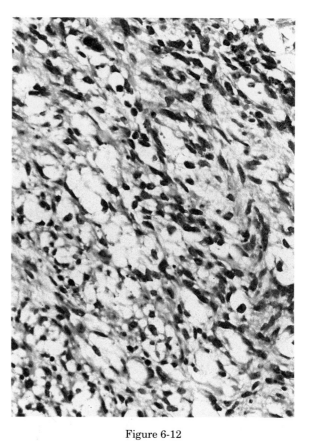

Figure 6-12
EMBRYONAL RHABDOMYOSARCOMA
There are small, round, oval and spindle-shaped cells with scant cytoplasm in a myxoid stroma.

Figure 6-13
EMBRYONAL
RHABDOMYOSARCOMA
Some cells have eosinophilic cytoplasm suggesting rhabdomyoblastic differentiation.

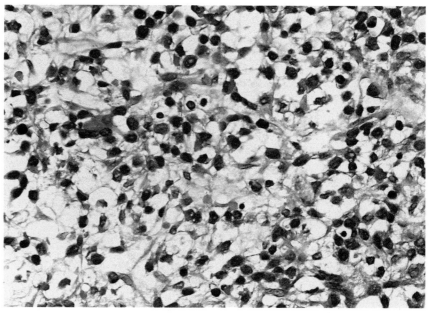

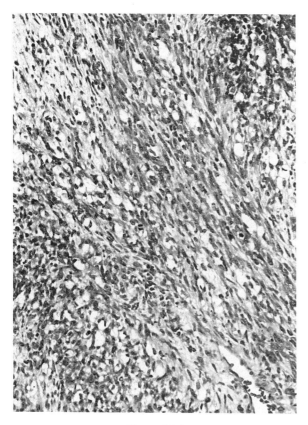

Figure 6-14
EMBRYONAL RHABDOMYOSARCOMA
Primitive round cells and more differentiated spindle cells are present.

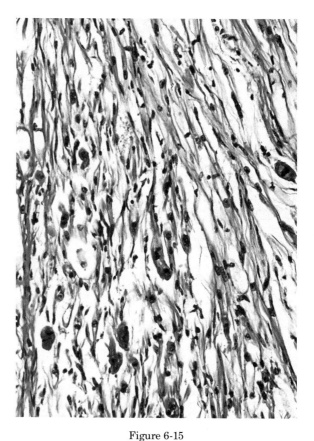

Figure 6-15
EMBRYONAL RHABDOMYOSARCOMA
Many of the cells are spindled with abundant, intensely eosinophilic cytoplasm (strap cells).

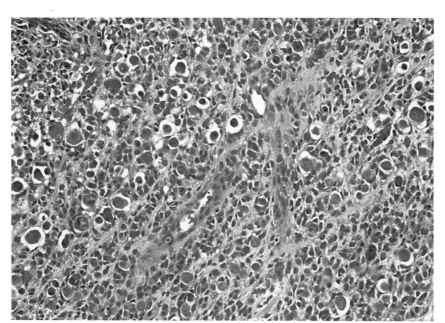

Figure 6-16
EMBRYONAL
RHABDOMYOSARCOMA
The tumor is composed of small, round blue cells interspersed with numerous rhabdomyoblasts. (Fig. 5-16 from Ro JY, Grignon DJ, Amin MB, Ayala AG. Atlas of surgical pathology of the male reproductive tract. Philadelphia: W.B. Saunders, 1997:89.)

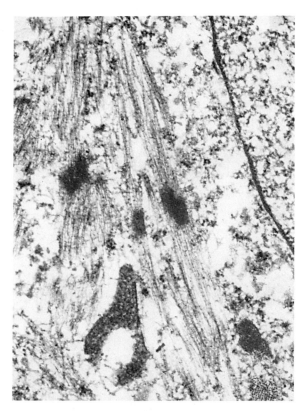

Figure 6-17
EMBRYONAL RHABDOMYOSARCOMA
The cytoplasm shows the characteristic rhabdomyoblastic differentiation with parallel bundles of thick myosin filaments, attached ribosomes, and band-like densities resembling Z bands (X20,000).

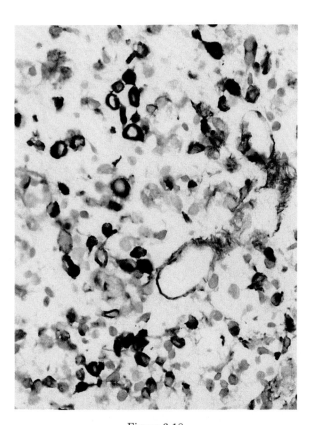

Figure 6-18
EMBRYONAL RHABDOMYOSARCOMA
A desmin stain shows intense cytoplasmic positivity.

Spindle cell rhabdomyosarcoma (leiomyomatous rhabdomyosarcoma) is considered a subtype of embryonal rhabdomyosarcoma. It shows a striking degree of elongated spindle cells with a fascicular arrangement and abundant, fibrillar, eosinophilic cytoplasm. Areas of more conventional embryonal rhabdomyosarcoma are almost invariably present but may be encountered only after thorough sampling.

The *alveolar variant* has the typical morphology of the well-known soft tissue tumor, with tumor cells that are more undifferentiated than in the other variants and whose striated muscle nature may not be apparent by light microscopy. Ultrastructural (fig. 6-17) or immunohistochemical (fig. 6-18) studies may help confirm the diagnosis and, in some cases, are crucial in establishing it; myoglobin, desmin, muscle-specific actin, myogenin, myoD1, and vimentin are positive (33,39,50,51).

Differential Diagnosis. The differential diagnosis in children may include malignant lymphoma or acute leukemia involving the prostate and metastatic neuroblastoma. Clinical information and an appropriate immunohistochemical panel are helpful in arriving at the correct diagnosis, although most cases are straightforward by routine light microscopy. In adults, a diagnosis of rhabdomyosarcoma should be made with extreme caution and only after ruling out other "small cell" malignant tumors such as malignant lymphoma and small cell carcinoma that may simulate it in biopsy specimens with suboptimal cell preservation. Carcinosarcoma, which may show heterologous rhabdomyosarcomatous differentiation and have scant epithelial elements, and inflammatory pseudotumor (see chapter 7) (34a,46) may be considerations. Cytologic characteristics are paramount in distinguishing the latter and the lack of epithelial elements the former.

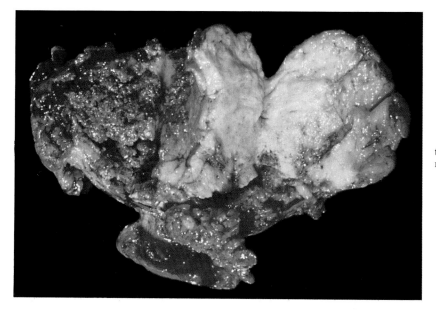

Figure 6-19
LEIOMYOSARCOMA
A fleshy tan-white neoplasm extensively replaces the prostatic parenchyma.

Prognosis. The prognosis of embryonal rhabdomyosarcoma in children has improved greatly with the advent of multimodal therapy (surgery, chemotherapy, radiation). The 3-year survival rate is in the range of 70 to 75 percent (33a). The prognosis remains poor for adults (45a). The reasons for the poor response to therapy in adults are unclear.

Leiomyosarcoma

Leiomyosarcoma accounts for approximately 25 percent of all sarcomas involving the prostate (63). Early series that reported cases in children (54,55,62) were not immunohistochemically proven and likely represent rhabdomyosarcoma; more recent papers document cases only in adults (54,55,60). The reported ages of patients with apparently valid cases range from 23 to 81 years, with a mean of 61 years (54,55,63). Most patients present with symptoms of urinary obstruction or prostatism, but about one quarter present with perineal pain. Other symptoms include hematuria, weight loss, burning on ejaculation, and constipation (54,55).

Gross Findings. The tumors range up to 21 cm (mean, 9 cm), appear fleshy (fig. 6-19) or firm, and may show hemorrhage, necrosis, cystic degeneration (fig. 6-20), and extraprostatic extension (54).

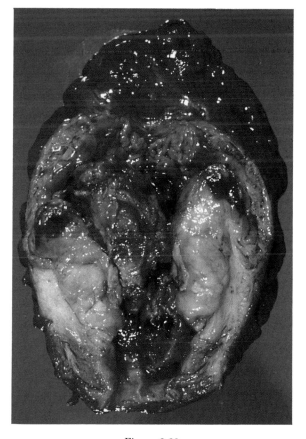

Figure 6-20
LEIOMYOSARCOMA
This neoplasm has a variegated appearance, with grayish white areas which were firm and areas of hemorrhage and necrosis.

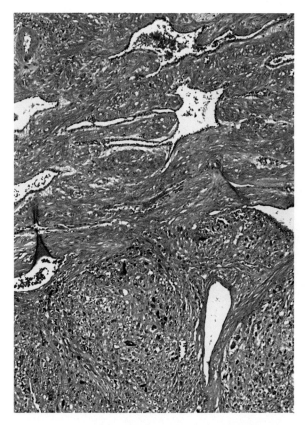

Figure 6-21
LEIOMYOSARCOMA

A low-power view shows the demarcation between the tumor (bottom) and the adjacent prostatic parenchyma.

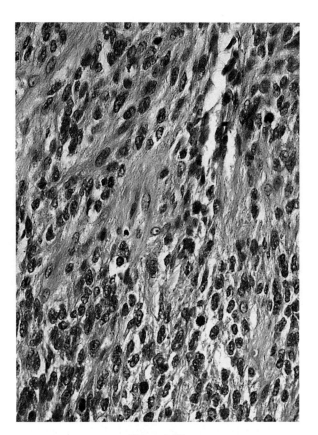

Figure 6-22
LEIOMYOSARCOMA

A high-power view shows oval to spindle-shaped cells with abundant, fibrillar, eosinophilic cytoplasm. Brisk mitotic activity is apparent.

Microscopic Findings. The histologic features are identical to those of their soft tissue and uterine counterparts, with fascicles of interlacing spindle cells with blunt-ended nuclei. Variations in histology include epithelioid cells with abundant clear or eosinophilic cytoplasm, giant cells, and nuclear palisading of the type seen in nerve sheath tumors. Most tumors are intermediate to high grade (figs. 6-21–6-23) (53–62,64). In a series of 23 cases, mitotic figures were identified in all tumors and ranged from 2 to 24 (mean, 8.4) per 10 high-power fields; necrosis was seen in 11 tumors (54). Although the smooth muscle nature of the tumor is usually appreciable by light microscopy, immunohistochemical studies (desmin, smooth muscle actin) (fig. 6-24) and ultrastructural analysis (fig. 6-25) may help confirm the diagnosis (54). Cytokeratin reactivity has been reported in occasional cases, with and without an epithelioid histology (54). Cytogenet-

ics in a single case revealed arrangements involving chromosome numbers 2, 3, 9, 11, and 19. The specificity or significance of these cytogenetic alterations is unclear, since this is the only tumor analyzed (57).

Differential Diagnosis. The differential diagnosis includes benign lesions such as stromal hyperplasia and leiomyoma with bizarre nuclei (see pages 323 and 260, respectively) and other malignant tumors including stromal sarcoma (see below), the spindle cell variant of rhabdomyosarcoma, sarcomatoid carcinoma, and carcinosarcoma. The identification, or history, of adenocarcinoma in cases of sarcomatoid carcinoma and the biphasic heterogenous appearance of carcinosarcoma make distinction generally straightforward. Immunostaining or ultrastructural evaluation may help demonstrate the smooth muscle nature of the neoplastic cells in leiomyosarcomas.

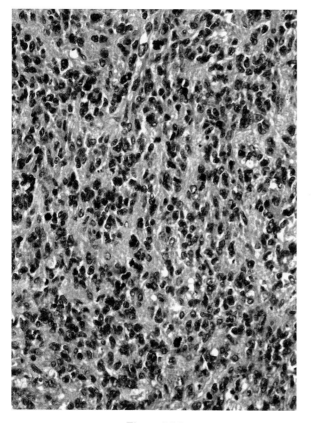

Figure 6-23
LEIOMYOSARCOMA
A high-grade tumor with marked cellularity, pleomorphism, and frequent mitoses.

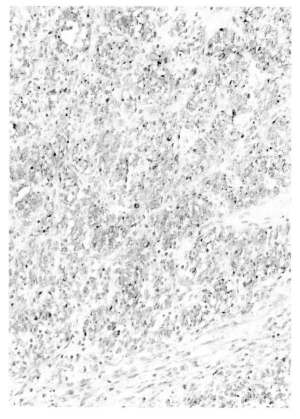

Figure 6-24
LEIOMYOSARCOMA
Diffuse desmin immunoreactivity.

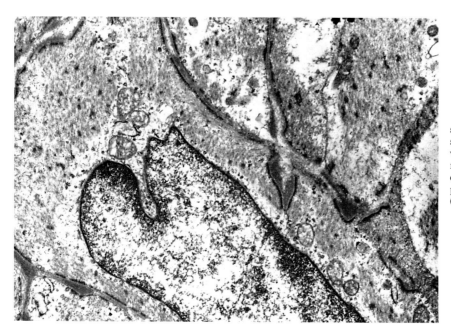

Figure 6-25
LEIOMYOSARCOMA

Ultrastructural features of smooth muscle differentiation are seen, including a basal lamina investing the cell membrane, numerous thin myofilaments with dense bodies, subplasmalemmal plaques, and pinocytotic vesicles (X7000).

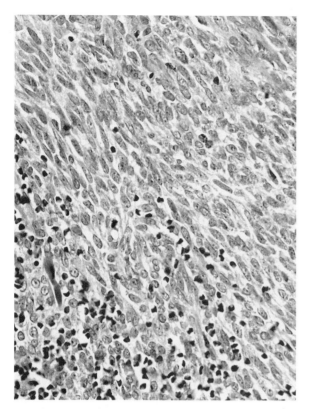

Figure 6-26
STROMAL SARCOMA
The neoplastic cells are fusiform and monotonous.

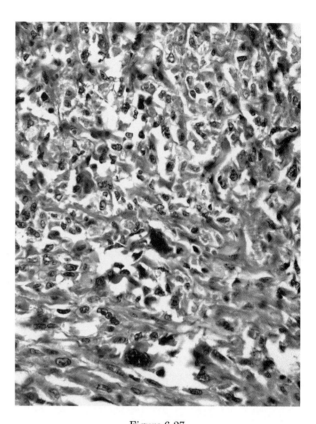

Figure 6-27
STROMAL SARCOMA
There is nuclear pleomorphism. (Courtesy of Dr. A. Ayala, Houston, TX.)

Prognosis. The prognosis of patients with leiomyosarcoma of the prostate is poor, although preliminary recent results with multimodal therapy have been encouraging in a limited number of patients (52,54). Local recurrence and visceral metastases, most commonly to the lungs, typify the aggressive behavior seen in about half the cases (54,55,58).

Stromal Sarcoma

Within the relatively rare category of adult soft tissue sarcomas that occur in the prostate gland, there is a distinct but not yet fully characterized group of spindle cell sarcomas exclusive of the more common leiomyosarcoma. Probable examples of these stromal sarcomas have been reported under other designations, and conversely, cases reported as stromal sarcoma have included examples of sarcomas of other types (70,71,74,75,79,80). These tumors usually occur in middle-aged to older patients.

In a recent series (69), 4 cases of stromal sarcomas and 18 cases of prostatic stromal proliferations of unknown malignant potential were reported. Three of the 4 sarcomas in this series would be classified as high-grade mixed epithelial-stromal tumor (phyllodes tumor) by our criteria (see page 275), and 4 of the stromal tumors of unknown malignant potential would be classified as low-grade mixed epithelial-stromal tumor (phyllodes tumor). Most of the remaining "tumors of unknown malignant potential" in that study would be classified as low-grade stromal sarcoma by us.

Gross Findings. The tumors may be solid and cystic, tan, yellow, pink, or white and are not known to have distinctive gross features (69).

Microscopic Findings. The neoplasm may demonstrate one of several growth patterns: diffuse sheets of primitive, round to oval to spindle cells (figs. 6-26, 6-27) or short fascicles of spindle cells, occasionally with a herringbone pattern. The nuclei are small and round to oval, or elongated and

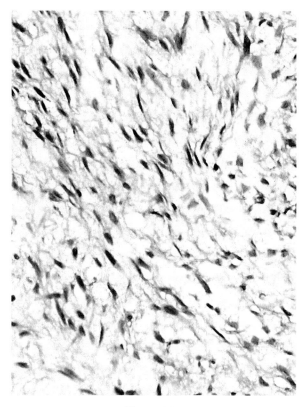

Figure 6-28
STROMAL SARCOMA
The neoplastic cells are spindled, often with a wavy appearance, and the stroma is myxoid.

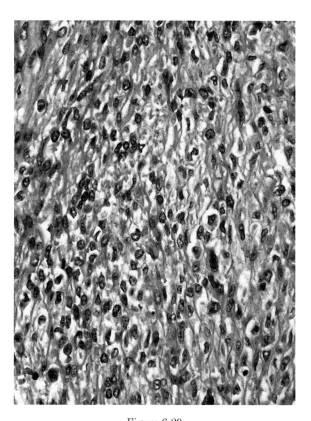

Figure 6-29
STROMAL SARCOMA
The cells are small and separated by delicate collagen.

wavy (fig. 6-28). The cytoplasm may be scant, resulting in an almost small cell appearance (fig. 6-29), but it is occasionally more appreciable and weakly eosinophilic and fibrillar (fig. 6-30). The stroma is variable, sometimes being absent (fig. 6-26), hyalinized (fig. 6-31), or having a pattern identical to sclerosing epithelioid fibrosarcoma (fig. 6-32). The neoplastic cells may obliterate the underlying parenchyma or may percolate between preexisting ducts and acini (figs. 6-33, 6-34), yielding a pattern similar to phyllodes tumor if the glandular structures are dilated or distorted by the stromal proliferation. Rarely, the interglandular infiltrative pattern is exclusive, and this appearance corresponds to patterns 1, 2, and 3 of prostatic stromal tumors of unknown malignant potential reported by Gaudin et al. (69).

Ultrastructural studies show features of a relatively undifferentiated mesenchymal cell with sparse cytoplasmic organelles. From a differential diagnostic point of view, there is no evidence of smooth or striated muscle differentiation (fig. 6-35).

Immunostaining may show some expression of desmin or smooth muscle actin in low-grade tumors, but these markers are usually negative in high-grade tumors. CD34, a progenitor cell marker identified in a subset of mesenchymal tumors, is positive in the majority of cases, indicating that these tumors are immunohistochemically similar to gastric stromal sarcomas (82a). In the study of Gaudin et al. (69), the tumors expressed progesterone receptors and uncommonly expressed estrogen receptors. The authors suggested that stromal tumors, therefore, arise from the hormonally responsive prostatic mesenchymal (stromal) cells.

Stromal sarcomas exhibit a spectrum of anaplasia, and the diagnosis of malignancy is not difficult in high-grade lesions. There is markedly increased cellularity, frequent mitoses, cytologic atypia, necrosis, and stromal overgrowth (absence of glandular elements in a low-power field). For less atypical

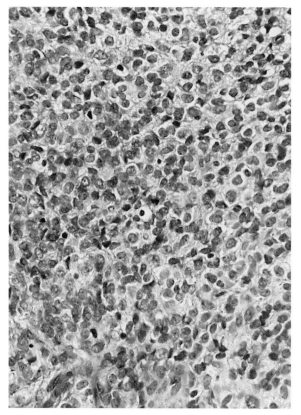

Figure 6-30
STROMAL SARCOMA
Small, round to oval cells with appreciable cytoplasm are seen.

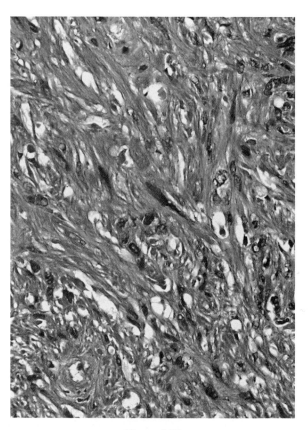

Figure 6-31
STROMAL SARCOMA
There is stromal hyalinization and nuclear atypia.

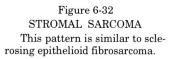
Figure 6-32
STROMAL SARCOMA
This pattern is similar to sclerosing epithelioid fibrosarcoma.

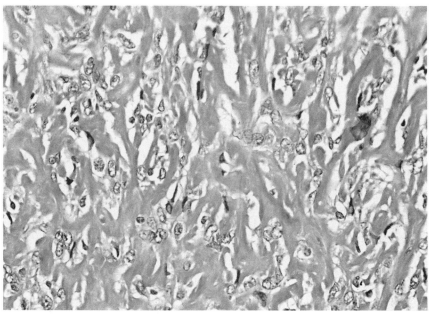

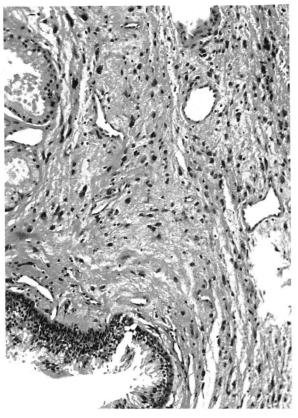

Figure 6-33
STROMAL SARCOMA
The neoplastic cells percolate between ducts and acini.

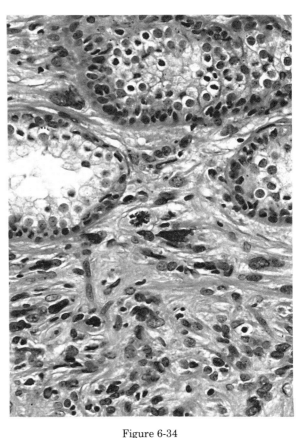

Figure 6-34
STROMAL SARCOMA
Pleomorphism and mitotic activity are evident. (Courtesy of Dr. J.Y. Ro, Houston, TX.)

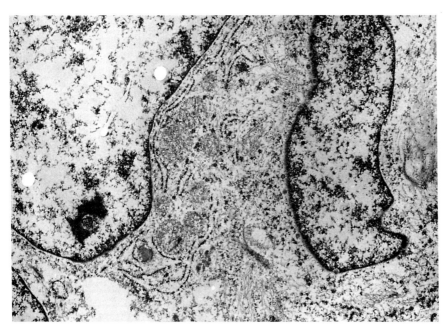

Figure 6-35
STROMAL SARCOMA
This electron micrograph shows an immature multinucleated cell with sparse cytoplasmic organelles, including rough endoplasmic reticulum, mitochondria, and intermediate filaments. No specific ultrastructural features of smooth or striated muscle are seen (X7000).

cases (low-grade tumors) we use traditional criteria such as prominent cellularity, appreciable mitotic activity, nuclear atypia, necrosis, and extraprostatic spread to indicate a malignant nature. Cases not reaching our threshold for outright malignancy are designated "uncertain malignant potential," as recommended by Gaudin et al. (69).

Differential Diagnosis. This includes benign lesions such as stromal hyperplasia with bizarre nuclei, leiomyoma with bizarre nuclei, and malignant tumors (leiomyosarcoma, sarcomatoid carcinoma, and mixed epithelial-stromal [phyllodes] tumor). Thorough sampling is critical, and the above differential diagnoses may be difficult or impossible to resolve in needle biopsy specimens.

When sufficient tissue is available for examination, stromal hyperplasia with bizarre nuclei shows a circumscribed, nodular proliferation with central vascularity; mixed epithelial-stromal tumor is biphasic in its appearance due to intermingled benign glands which may branch and be dilated or narrow, with an architecture resembling a phyllodes tumor of the breast; and sarcomatoid carcinoma may show transition from conventional adenocarcinoma or occur in patients with a history of prostatic carcinoma.

Perhaps the most difficult differential diagnosis is with leiomyosarcoma, but the latter tends to show a fascicular arrangement of tumor cells which have abundant fibrillar cytoplasm and nuclei with blunt ends. Immunoreactivity for CD34 and estrogen and progesterone receptors favors stromal sarcoma over leiomyosarcoma (69). Conversely, strong desmin immunoreactivity favors leiomyosarcoma.

Prognosis. Clinical follow-up is often limited in the reported cases, making it difficult to identify significant pathologic prognostic parameters. Local recurrence is not uncommon and may lead to death in some patients (69).

Other Sarcomas

Many other sarcomas of the prostate such as osteosarcoma, chondrosarcoma, angiosarcoma, malignant fibrous histiocytoma, liposarcoma, and neurogenic sarcoma have rarely been described (65–67,76,78). Thorough sampling of the tumor to rule out a carcinomatous component, a negative past history of prostate cancer, and absence of another primary site are prerequi-

sites before a tumor is considered a primary sarcoma of the prostate of any of these types (72). Rare cases of hemangiopericytoma occurring in the prostate have also been described (73,81). The tumors are large and may invade pelvic structures. They are histologically similar to their soft tissue counterpart; recurrences and metastases have been noted, but are not readily predicted by histology. One case of radiation-induced sarcoma of the prostate has been reported. The patient was treated for prostate cancer with radioactive iodine implants and developed a spindle cell sarcoma after 8 years (77). A case of malignant rhabdoid tumor of the prostate was reported in a 14-year-old boy (68). Negative immunoreactivity for muscle stains and positivity for cytokeratin, as well as ultrastructural studies ruled out rhabdomyosarcoma. At autopsy the patient had widespread metastases.

EPITHELIAL-STROMAL TUMOR (PHYLLODES TUMOR)

General and Clinical Features. Prostatic lesions that resemble the well-known phyllodes tumor of the breast span a wide spectrum, from those seen in the background of typical benign prostatic hyperplasia, in which the pattern is focal, to those that form a clinically significant mass possessing varying degrees of stromal hypercellularity and nuclear atypia. The former have been described as phyllodes type hyperplasia (see chapter 2). The term mixed epithelial-stromal tumor or phyllodes tumor (the first term is preferable, as a phyllodes architecture, although typical, is not invariable) is appropriate for lesions forming a mass.

Patients present with symptoms of urinary obstruction (often with acute retention), hematuria, or dysuria. The age range is 22 to 78 years (mean, 52 years); 40 percent occur in men under 50 years of age (85,86,88–99).

Gross Findings. The tumors range from 4 to 58 cm in size and may occur centrally in the region of the verumontanum (82,92) or in the peripheral zone (91,95,97). They are solid and cystic or multicystic (fig. 6-36), with a sponge-like consistency. If necrotic areas or regions with more solid growth are evident (fig. 6-37), they should arouse suspicion for a higher grade component, and such areas should be sampled liberally.

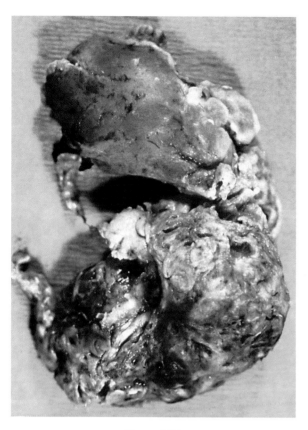

Figure 6-36
EPITHELIAL-STROMAL TUMOR
The tumor is solid and cystic, with focal hemorrhage. (Courtesy of Dr. J.C. Manivel, Minneapolis, MN.)

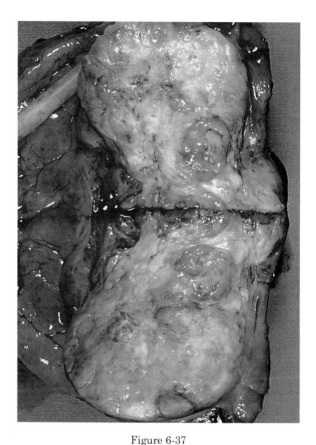

Figure 6-37
EPITHELIAL-STROMAL TUMOR
The mass is grayish white to brown. The stroma showed marked overgrowth which is reflected by the predominantly solid appearance of the neoplasm. (Courtesy of Dr. E.C. Jones, Vancouver, BC, Canada.)

Microscopic Findings. The low-power appearance is characteristically biphasic, with cysts and glands that are often elongated, compressed, and cleft-like amidst and invaginated by an unusually cellular stroma that frequently forms papillary to polypoid projections (figs. 6-38–6-41). The epithelial cells are columnar to low cuboidal and rest on a distinct layer of basal cells (figs. 6-39–6-41). The stromal cells are spindle shaped, often condense around the glands, and occasionally lie in a myxoid matrix (figs. 6-39–6-41) (83,95,97, 99). Heterologous differentiation, such as rhabdomyoblastic, has been noted (98). Like their mammary counterpart, there is a range of cellularity, nuclear atypicality, and mitotic activity in the stromal component. Parallels also exist with the well-known uterine tumors in the mullerian adenofibroma-adenosarcoma spectrum.

It has been suggested that the prostatic tumors be graded as low (fig. 6-42) or high grade (fig. 6-43) based on the stromal-epithelial ratio, stromal cellularity, cytologic atypia, necrosis, and mitotic activity, but their rarity has precluded emergence of definitive criteria for grading these tumors to date. Gaudin et al. (85), using such criteria, have classified lesions with a phyllodes pattern and tumors we recognize as stromal sarcoma (see page 270) as either prostatic stromal proliferations of uncertain malignant potential or prostatic stromal sarcomas. Even in high-grade tumors there is usually an orderly arrangement of glands and stroma, but occasionally there is stromal overgrowth (analogous to some mullerian adenosarcomas of the uterus) which on gross examination may form a distinct nodule, contrasting with the usually regular solid and cystic or multicystic appearance of most cases (95). Microscopically, a designation of

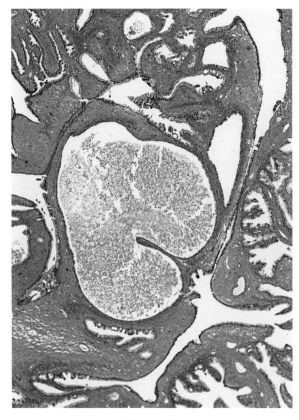

Figure 6-38
EPITHELIAL-STROMAL TUMOR
A low-power view shows the characteristic biphasic appearance with numerous cleft-like glandular spaces.

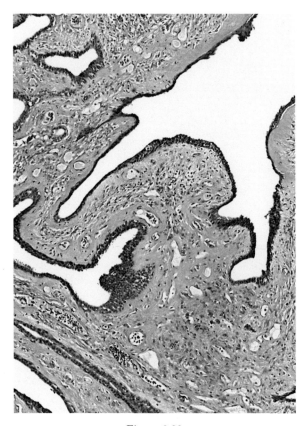

Figure 6-39
EPITHELIAL-STROMAL TUMOR
The stromal component is cellular with nuclear atypia. (Courtesy of Dr. E.C. Jones, Vancouver, BC, Canada.)

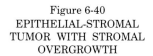

Figure 6-40
EPITHELIAL-STROMAL
TUMOR WITH STROMAL
OVERGROWTH

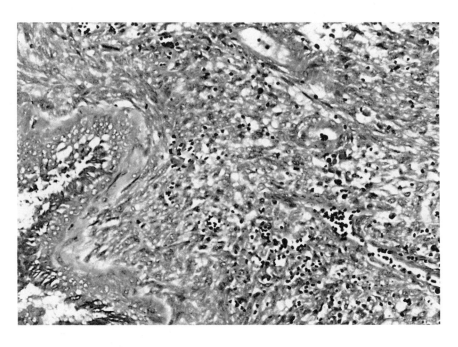

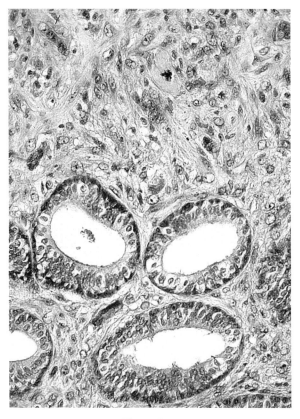

Figure 6-41
EPITHELIAL-STROMAL TUMOR
The epithelial component shows distinct two-cell layers with a conspicuous basal cell layer. The stromal component is cellular with atypical mitotic activity. (Courtesy of Dr. J.F. Young, San Diego, CA.)

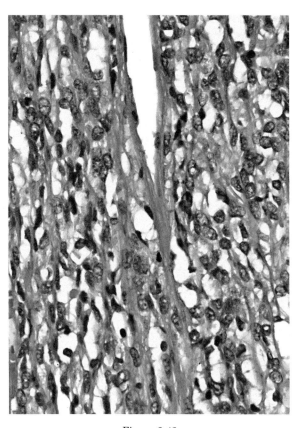

Figure 6-42
EPITHELIAL-STROMAL TUMOR
The stromal component is cytologically low grade.

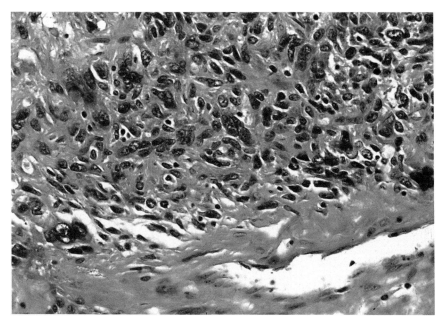

Figure 6-43
EPITHELIAL-STROMAL
TUMOR
There is marked nuclear atypia in the stromal component.

Table 6-2

CLASSIFICATION OF PROSTATIC TUMORS AND TUMOR-LIKE LESIONS WITH CYTOLOGIC ATYPIA OF MESENCHYMAL CELLS

Tumors

A. Leiomyoma with bizarre nuclei*

B. Epithelial-stromal tumors
   1. low grade
   2. high grade

C. Stromal sarcomas
   1. low grade
   2. high grade

D. Other sarcomas

Tumor-Like Lesions

Benign prostatic hyperplasia with bizarre nuclei in stromal cells

---

*Sometimes referred to as symplastic leiomyoma. In biopsy or curettage material it may not be possible to determine if a lesion is a neoplasm or not because of sampling issues. The term "prostatic stromal proliferation of uncertain malignant potential" is recommended in this circumstance.

stromal overgrowth is justified if there is a spindle cell proliferation not associated with glandular elements that exceeds at least one low-power field (85). Sarcomatous "dedifferentiation" may occur in low-grade tumors over time, usually after multiple recurrences (87,99,100).

Immunohistochemical studies have shown PSA and PAP positivity in the epithelial cells. The stromal component is positive for muscle-specific actin and desmin, correlating with the ultrastructural smooth muscle differentiation; the stroma may also be weakly positive for cytokeratin (90). The stromal component also has features consistent with derivation from the specialized prostatic stroma, including immunoreactivity for CD34 and progesterone and estrogen receptors (85).

Differential Diagnosis. The differential diagnosis is with other prostatic lesions with atypical mesenchymal cells (Table 6-2) or biphasic histology and includes hyperplasia with bizarre nuclei (see page 323) and stromal sarcomas (see page 270), as well as phyllodes-type hyperplasia (see page 44), cystadenoma (see page 257), and adenofibroma of the ejaculatory duct (94). Leiomyosarcoma or other sarcomas, sarcomatoid car-

cinoma, and carcinosarcoma may also be considered for high-grade lesions, but the sarcomas are monophasic, while sarcomatoid carcinoma and carcinosarcoma lack the phyllodes type architectural features. Also, the epithelial component in carcinosarcoma has malignant features. Distinction may be particularly difficult in limited material that contains only the stromal component of a mixed epithelial-stromal tumor, and awareness of the gross characteristics may be important in suggesting a mixed epithelial-stromal tumor. Finally, a similar tumor may arise in the seminal vesicle (see chapter 8) (84). Distinction from these is based on knowledge of the exact tumor location and, especially, immunohistochemical studies for PSA and PAP.

Prognosis. Mixed epithelial-stromal tumors must be considered potentially malignant, although complete excision may result in an uneventful follow-up (87,91,92,99,100). Low-grade tumors are prone to recur locally, but distant spread has not been reported. High-grade tumors may metastasize, with the lung being the most frequent site of distant metastasis (86,87,93).

HEMATOLYMPHOID MALIGNANCIES

The prostate gland may be primarily or secondarily involved by the entire spectrum of hematolymphoid malignancies including non-Hodgkin's and Hodgkin's lymphomas, leukemias (acute and chronic, myeloid, and lymphoid), and plasmacytoma.

Leukemic Involvement

Approximately 10 to 20 percent of leukemias involve the prostate gland (103,109,120,128,131). Extensive leukemic involvement of the prostatic parenchyma may cause acute urinary retention (109), or the leukemia may be serendipitously detected in needle biopsies or transurethral resection specimens obtained for the clinical consideration of hyperplasia or carcinoma. Leukemic infiltrates may be incidentally noted in radical prostatectomies performed for cancer in patients with a history of leukemia; rarely, this may be the first sign of a hematolymphoid abnormality which leads to subsequent detection of leukemia (129).

Potentially, a green color could be appreciable on gross examination in cases of myeloid leukemia. Histologically, the prostatic stroma is usually

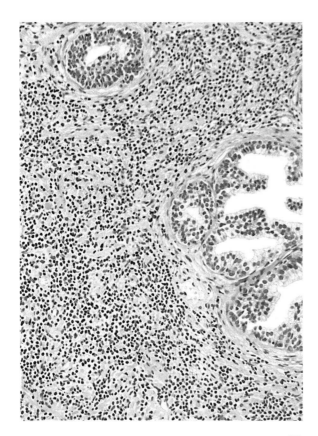 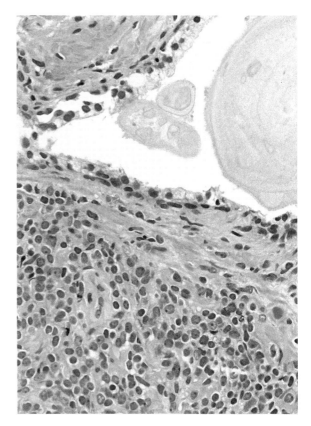

Figure 6-44
LEUKEMIC INVOLVEMENT OF THE PROSTATE
Left: There is extensive infiltration by the small, well-differentiated lymphocytes of chronic lymphocytic leukemia.
Right: Lymphoblastic lymphoma/leukemia involves the prostate.

extensively and diffusely infiltrated by neoplastic cells that typically spare the acini and ducts (fig. 6-44), although there may be focal epithelial involvement (109,120,131). Chronic lymphocytic leukemia is the most common form to secondarily involve the prostate and is characterized by a dense, monomorphic infiltrate of mature-appearing, round lymphocytes (fig. 6-44, left) (109,129). Involvement by acute lymphoid leukemia (precursor T- and B-cell types) and granulocytic sarcoma has been reported (114). The low-power pattern of diffuse infiltration is essentially similar to that of chronic lymphocytic lymphoma; further characterization depends on the cytologic features. Identification of eosinophilic metamyelocytes and myelocytes is helpful in establishing the diagnosis of granulocytic sarcoma and avoiding the misdiagnosis of malignant lymphoma (114, 130). The diagnosis may be confirmed by the naphthol AS-D chloroacetate esterase (Leder's

stain) histochemical reaction and appropriate immunohistochemical staining including lysozyme and myeloperoxidase (113). The cells of acute lymphoid leukemia are monotonous, of small to intermediate size, and contain a round or irregular nucleus with fine chromatin and generally inconspicuous nucleoli. The mitotic rate is usually high (fig. 6-44, right). The tumor cells are positive for terminal deoxynucleotidyl transferase (TdT); most are of T-cell lineage.

Malignant Lymphoma Involving the Prostate

Malignant lymphoma involving the prostate gland is rarer than leukemic involvement (101,102, 108,110,119,122-124,126,127,132). Although the legitimacy of primary lymphoma of the prostate was initially challenged because of the relative scarcity of lymphoid tissue in the gland, subsequent reports of unequivocal solitary involvement of the

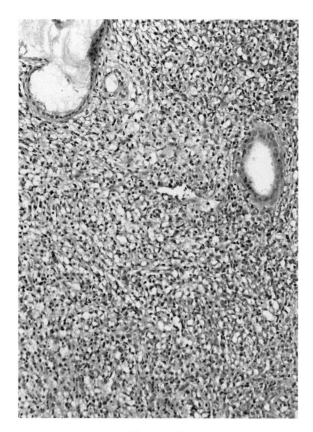

Figure 6-45
DIFFUSE LARGE CELL LYMPHOMA OF PROSTATE
Sheets of atypical cells infiltrate between benign prostatic acini.

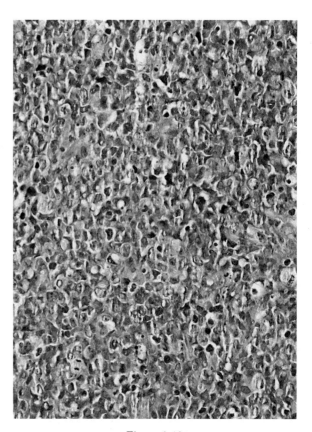

Figure 6-46
DIFFUSE LARGE CELL LYMPHOMA OF PROSTATE
Note the typical cytologic features. (Figures 6-46 and 6-47 are from the same patient.)

gland have established its existence (102,105, 108,112,116). To be designated as a primary lymphoma of the prostate the following criteria should be fulfilled: 1) the lymphoma involves prostatic tissue with absence or minimal involvement of periprostatic tissue; 2) the symptoms of the disease are attributable to enlargement of the prostate; and 3) there is a lack of involvement of the hematopoietic system (peripheral blood, lymph nodes, liver, and spleen) within 1 month of the diagnosis (107,108,120).

About 160 cases of primary and secondary lymphomas involving the prostate have been reported (107). Patients with primary lymphoma of the prostate are somewhat younger (mean, 52 years) than those with secondary involvement (mean, 63 years) (108). Lymphomas have, however, been described in males in the first two decades, with an age range of 5 to 86 years (107). The patients present with urinary obstruction, including

acute retention, or other symptoms of prostatism. When tested, the serum PSA and PAP have been within normal limits (113).

Pathologic Findings. The prostate gland is usually diffusely enlarged, and transurethral resectate specimens may appear yellowish white and firm or rubbery. The entire range of nodal malignant lymphomas occurs in the prostate, although most are diffuse (figs. 6-45–6-47); there are few examples of follicular lymphomas (figs. 6-48–6-50) (107). In the largest series (107) 22 of 62 cases (35 percent) were primary; histologic subtypes included small lymphocytic (4 cases), diffuse small cleaved cell (2 cases), follicular small cell (1 case) (figs. 6-49, 6-50), follicular mixed small and large cell (1 case), diffuse mixed small and large cell (2 cases), diffuse large noncleaved cell (6 cases) (fig. 6-46), diffuse small noncleaved cell (2 cases), and diffuse large cell immunoblastic (4 cases). The histologic types of

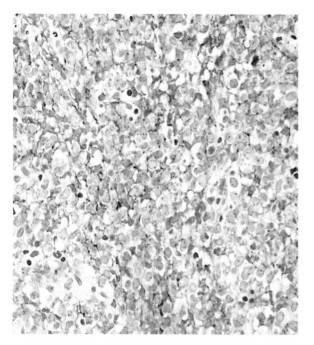

Figure 6-47
DIFFUSE LARGE CELL LYMPHOMA OF PROSTATE
There is immunostaining for leukocyte common antigen.

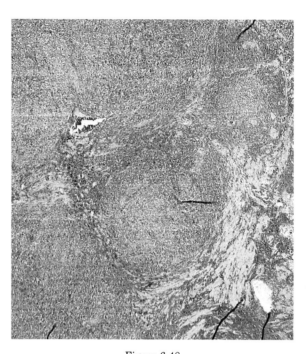

Figure 6-48
FOLLICULAR LYMPHOMA OF PROSTATE
Low-power view of follicular lymphoma. (Courtesy of Dr. B. Osborne, New York, NY.)

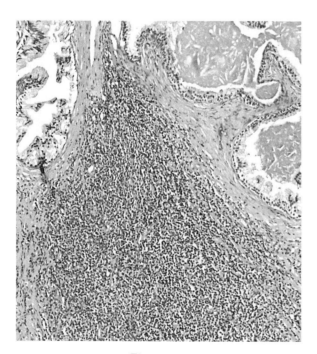

Figure 6-49
FOLLICULAR LYMPHOMA OF PROSTATE
An intermediate-power view of the example depicted in figure 6-48 shows neoplastic cells infiltrating between the duct-acinar framework of the prostate.

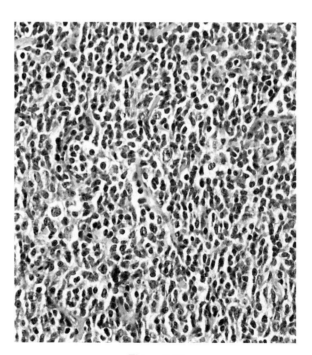

Figure 6-50
FOLLICULAR LYMPHOMA OF PROSTATE
A high-power view of the neoplasm depicted in figure 6-48 shows the features of a small cleaved cell lymphoma.

tumors in 34 patients (55 percent) with previously documented lymphoma at other sites (secondary lymphoma) were small cell lymphocytic (9 cases), diffuse small cleaved cell (2 cases), follicular small cleaved cell (1 case), diffuse mixed small and large cell (2 cases), diffuse large noncleaved cell (8 cases), high-grade diffuse small noncleaved cell, non-Burkitt's (2 cases), large cell immunoblastic (6 cases), Hodgkin's disease (2 cases: nodular sclerosing [1 case] and mixed cellularity [1 case]), and one unknown histologic type. In 6 patients the lymphoma could not be classified as either primary or secondary, and in 8 cases there were foci of conventional adenocarcinoma. Most of the other reports in the literature are case reports and include examples of the above types as well as cases of angiotropic large cell lymphoma, mucosa-associated lymphoid tissue (MALT) lymphoma, monocytoid B-cell lymphoma, Burkitt's lymphoma, and peripheral T-cell lymphoma (102,105,106,115,118,121).

Differential Diagnosis. The differential diagnosis in children includes embryonal rhabdomyosarcoma and, in adults, small cell carcinoma. A clinical history of leukemia or lymphoma and an appropriate panel of immunohistochemical stains, including desmin, cytokeratin, chromogranin, synaptophysin, and PSA, are useful if artifact or small size of the sample makes distinction difficult on routine evaluation. A case of pseudolymphoma, characterized by prominent lymphoid follicular hyperplasia, occurred in a 68-year-old patient who did not have a history of leukemia or lymphoma (125). The presence of mature germinal centers with numerous mitoses helped distinguish this lesion from the rare follicular lymphoma involving the prostate.

Prognosis. The prognosis of malignant lymphoma involving the prostate is generally poor regardless of the type of involvement (primary or secondary: 9.8 months versus 12.7 months, respectively), stage, or histologic classification (107, 108). Prostatic lymphomas affecting young males tend to pursue a more aggressive course (107,108). Almost all cases of primary lymphoma result in extraprostatic disease, most often in pelvic or abdominal lymph nodes. Greater than 60 percent of patients die of disease, although those treated in recent years with combination therapy have survived longer on average (107,108).

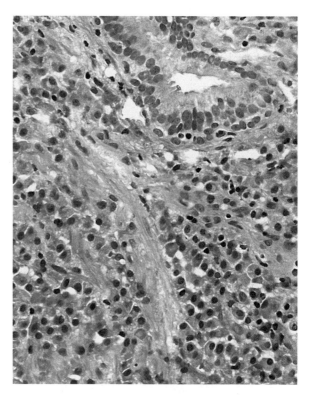

Figure 6-51
PLASMACYTOMA OF THE PROSTATE GLAND

Multiple Myeloma and Plasmacytoma Involving the Prostate

Plasmacytoma of the prostate is very rare; involvement of the prostate is usually recognized after the diagnosis of systemic disease or is made at autopsy (104,111,117,133). Clinically, however, the patients may present with symptoms of prostatism, often attributed to benign prostatic hyperplasia, or with acute urinary retention. There is typically a moderately enlarged, nontender, irregular gland mimicking a primary neoplasm. Production of IgA and IgD M components has been reported. On microscopic examination, sheets of plasma cells diffusely infiltrate the prostatic stroma (fig. 6-51) (117,133).

MISCELLANEOUS TUMORS

Germ Cell Tumors

A few germ cell tumors involving the prostate gland have been reported (135,137,140–143, 145,147,148), some possibly primary, but others with an epicenter in the retroperitoneum or retrovesical space secondarily involving the prostate (138). The tumors predominantly occur in young to middle-aged men. Sequestration of germ cells during migration along the midline, neoplastic transformation of an uncommitted stem cell into germ cells, and metastasis from an occult testicular primary are the proposed explanations for these cases. Two germ cell tumors of the prostate (one primary and one that extended from the retroperitoneum) occurred in patients with Klinefelter's syndrome (140,148).

Pure seminoma, yolk-sac tumor, choriocarcinoma, and mixed germ cell tumors have been documented (134,135,137,138,140–143,145,147,148). Mixed germ cell tumor components have included the first three tumor types, as well as embryonal carcinoma and teratoma components. Involvement of the prostate gland is invariably widespread with frequent extension into the periprostatic space or the urinary bladder.

The exceptional diagnosis of a primary prostatic germ cell tumor should be made only after a testicular primary is excluded. The histologic features are so typical that in most instances the diagnosis is straightforward despite the unusual location. The age of the patient, normal serum PSA levels, absence of coexisting acinar carcinoma, and immunohistochemical staining for PSA, PAP, placental alkaline phosphatase, and alpha-fetoprotein help in difficult cases.

The prognosis is favorable in patients with pure classic seminoma, with remission following therapy (141,142). Patients with mixed germ cell tumors and pure yolk sac tumors have had a less predictable outcome (135,137).

Pheochromocytoma (Paraganglioma)

Paraganglia of the periprostatic soft tissue and prostatic capsule are normal histoanatomic components of the autonomic nervous system (see chapter 7). Neoplasms of paraganglionic tissue in this region are distinctly rare, with only four cases reported in the prostate; the mean patient age was 27 years (range, 8 to 37 years) (139,144,146,149). The presenting signs and symptoms may be due to excretion of norepinephrine and related products (hypertension, headache, blurred vision) or location of the tumor (prostatic mass on digital rectal examination, postmicturition or postdefecation headaches, burning on urination). All cases were locally excised and the tumors have been relatively circumscribed and tan-brown (139,144,146,149). The histologic features are identical to those seen elsewhere, with the characteristic nests ("zellballen") separated by fibrovascular septa. The neoplastic cells may occasionally be arranged in cords and trabeculae, infiltrate the adjacent prostatic stroma, and show scattered cytologic atypia of degenerative type.

In most cases the typical clinical history as well as the supportive laboratory data and imaging studies help achieve the diagnosis preoperatively or at least raise a high index of suspicion for it. In a needle biopsy or transurethral resection specimen of a case lacking a suggestive history, the differential diagnosis with prostatic carcinoma may be difficult, particularly given the rarity of prostatic paraganglioma (figs. 6-52–6-54). Two of the four reported cases were multifocal (144, 149); one extensively involved the prostate and retroperitoneum, and another was limited to the prostate. Only one case, which also involved the retroperitoneum, was malignant, with metastases to pelvic lymph nodes (144). As with paragangliomas at other sites, it is difficult to predict the biologic potential of a tumor on the basis of its histology.

Wilms' Tumor

One case of prostatic Wilms' tumor has been reported (136). It occurred in a 32-year-old who presented with hemospermia. Histologically, the tumor had a typical appearance. The tumor recurred locally and subsequently metastasized to the lungs (136).

Figure 6-52
PROSTATIC
PARAGANGLIOMA
Low-power view of a needle bi-
opsy shows focal cellular areas.

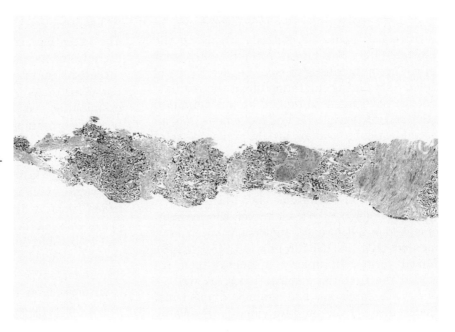

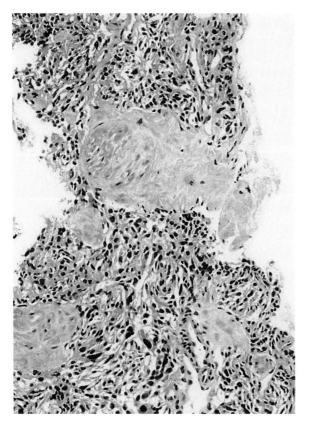

Figure 6-53
PROSTATIC PARAGANGLIOMA

A high-power view of the neoplasm in figure 6-52 shows a
sinusoidal architecture and focal pleomorphism. The PSA
immunostain performed in this case was negative.

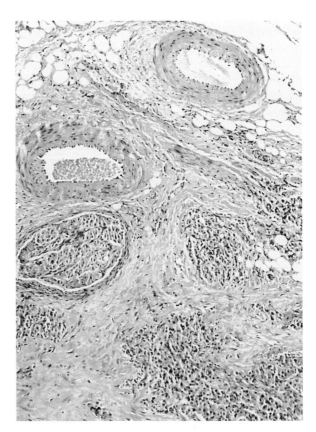

Figure 6-54
PROSTATIC PARAGANGLIOMA

The tumor diffusely infiltrates prostatic parenchyma with
extraprostatic extension and venous invasion. (Courtesy of Dr.
D.J. Grignon, Detroit, MI.)

REFERENCES

Cystadenoma

1. Blum E, Batzenschlager A, Le Gal Y. Adenome prostatique cystico-papillaire a evolution polykystique. J d'Urol 1960;66:411–4.
2. Cummine HG, Johnson AS. Report of a case of retrovesical polycystic tumor of probable prostatic origin. Aust N Z J Surg 1950;19:91–2.
3. Douille MC, Couderc P, Coste M. Cystadenome papillaire de la prostate. J d'Urol Nephrol 1963;69:339–43.
4. Goodale RH. Cystadenoma of the bladder from aberrant prostatic gland. Arch Pathol 1928;6:210–4.
4a. Kanomata N, Eble JN, Ohbayashi C, Yasui N, Tanaka H, Matsumoto O. Ectopic prostate in the retrovesical space. J Urol Pathol 1997;7:121–6.
5. Kirkland KL, Bale PM. A cystic adenoma of the prostate. J Urol 1967;97:324–7.
6. Kirsch AJ, Newhouse J, Hibshoosh H, O'Toole K, Ritter J, Benson MC. Giant multilocular cystadenoma of the prostate. Urology 1996;48:303–5.

7. Levy DA, Gogate PA, Hampel N. Giant multilocular prostatic cystadenoma: a rare clinical entity and review of the literature. J Urol 1993;150:1920–2.
8. Lim DJ, Hayden RT, Murad T, Nemceck AA, Dalton DP. Multilocular prostatic cystadenoma presenting as a large complex pelvic cystic mass. J Urol 1993;149:856–9.
9. Maluf HM, King ME, DeLuca FR, Navarro J, Talerman A, Young RH. Giant multilocular prostatic cystadenoma: a distinctive lesion of the retroperitoneum in men. Am J Surg Pathol 1991;15:131–5.
10. Melen DR. Multilocular cyst of the prostate. J Urol 1932;27:343–9.
11. Pyrah LN. Retrovesical tumours. A report of three cases. Br J Urol 1954;26:75–83.
12. Watanabe J, Konishi T, Takeuchi H, Tomoyoshi T. A case of giant prostatic cystadenoma. Acta Urol Jap 1990;36:1077–9.

Benign Mesenchymal Tumors

13. Cohen MS, McDonald DF, Smith JH. Solitary leiomyoma of the prostate presenting as an encrusted intravesical mass. J Urol 1978;120:641–2.
14. Furihata M, Sonobe H, Iwata J, et al. Granular cell tumor expressing myogenic markers in the prostate. Pathol Int 1996;46:298–300.
15. Gaudin PB, Rosai J, Epstein JI. Sarcomas and related proliferative lesions of specialized prostatic stroma: a clinicopathologic study of 22 cases. Am J Surg Pathol 1998;22:148–62.
16. Goldfarb M, Bertcher RW. Primary osteochondrosarcoma of the prostate gland: a case report. J Urol 1960;84:402–5.
17. Gray C, Thompson GJ. Leiomyoma of the prostate: report of a case. J Urol 1950;64:511–3.
18. Hinman F, Sullivan JJ. Two cases of leiomyoma of the prostate. J Urol 1931;26:475–83.
19. Holtl W, Hruby W, Redtenbacher M. Cavernous hemangioma originating from prostatic plexus. Urology 1982;20:184–5.
20. Károlyi P, Endes P, Krasznai G, Tönkol I. Bizarre leiomyoma of the prostate. Virchows Arch [A] 1988;412:383–6.
21. Leonard A, Baert L, Van Praet F, Van de Voort W, Van Poppel H, Lauweryns J. Solitary leiomyoma of the prostate. Br J Urol 1988;60:184–5.
22. Mentzel T, Bainbridge TC, Katenkamp D. Solitary fibrous tumour: clinicopathological, immunohistochemi-

cal, and ultrastructural analysis of 12 cases arising in soft tissues, nasal cavity and nasopharynx, urinary bladder and prostate. Virchows Arch 1997;430:445–53.
23. Muzafer MH. Large leiomyoma of prostate. Br J Urol 1987;59:192–3.
24. Nassiri M, Ghazi C, Stivers JR, Nadji M. Ganglioneuroma of the prostate. A novel finding in neurofibromatosis. Arch Pathol Lab Med 1994;118:938–9.
25. Persaud V, Douglas LL. Bizarre (atypical) leiomyoma of the prostate gland. West Indian Med J 1982;31:217–20.
26. Regan JB, Barrett DM, Wold LE. Giant leiomyoma of the prostate. Arch Pathol Lab Med 1987;111:381–3.
27. Rosen Y, Ambiavagar PC, Vuletin JC, Macchia RJ. Atypical leiomyoma of the prostate. Urology 1980;15:183–5.
28. Sundarasivarao S, Banerjea S, Nageswararao A, Rao NV. Hemangioma of the prostate: a case report. J Urol 1973;110:708–9.
29. Takeshima Y, Yoneda K, Sanda N, Inai K. Solitary fibrous tumor of the prostate. Pathol Int 1997;47:713–7.
30. Tetu B, Ro JY, Ayala AG, Srigley JR, Begin LR, Bostwick DG. Atypical spindle cell lesions of the prostate. Sem Diagn Pathol 1988;5:284–93.
31. Wang X, Bostwick DG. Prostatic stromal hyperplasia with atypia. A study of 11 cases. J Urol Pathol 1997;6:15–25.

Rhabdomyosarcoma

32. Asmar L, Gehan EA, Newton WA, et al. Agreement among and within groups of pathologists in the classification of rhabdomyosarcoma and related childhood sarcomas. Report of an international study of four pathology classifications. Cancer 1994;74:2579–88.
33. Bos SD, Slaa ET. An adult man with a rhabdomyosarcoma of the prostate. A case report. Scand J Urol Nephrol 1991;25:329–30.

33a. Chin W, Fay R, Ortega P. Malignant fibrous histiocytoma of prostate. Urology 1986;27:363–5.
34. Dupree WB, Fisher C. Rhabdomyosarcoma of prostate in adult. Long-term survival and problem of histologic diagnosis. Urology 1982;19:80–2.
34a. Ekfors TO, Aho HJ, Kekomaki M. Malignant rhabdoid tumor of the prostatic region. Immunohistological and ultrastructural evidence for epithelial origin. Virchows Arch 1985;406:381–8.

35. Fleischmann J, Perinetti EP, Catalona WJ. Embryonal rhabdomyosarcoma of the genitourinary organs. J Urol 1981;126:389–92.

36. Ghavimi R, Herr H, Jereb B, Exelby PR. Treatment of genitourinary rhabdomyosarcoma in children. J Urol 1984;132:313–9.

37. Keenan DJ, Graham WH. Embryonal rhabdomyosarcoma of the prostatic-urethral region in an adult. Br J Urol 1985;57:241.

38. King DG, Finney RP. Embryonal rhabdomyosarcoma of the prostate. J Urol 1977;117:88–90.

39. Kodet R, Kasthuri N, Marsden HB, Coad NA, Raafat F. Gangliorhabdomyosarcoma: a histopathological and immunohistochemical study of three cases. Histopathology 1986;10:181–93.

40. Lemmon WT Jr, Holland JM, Ketcham AS. Rhabdomyosarcoma of the prostate. Surgery 1966;59:736–40.

41. Loughlin KR, Retik AB, Weinstein HJ, et al. Genitourinary rhabdomyosarcoma in children. Cancer 1989;63:1600–6.

42. Loughlin KR, Retik AB, Weinstin HJ, et al. Treatment of genitourinary rhabdomyosarcoma in children. Cancer 1989;63:1600–6.

43. Miettinen M. Rhabdomyosarcoma in patients older than 40 years of age. Cancer 1988;62:2060–5.

43a. Ohtsuki Y, Ro JY, Ordonez NG, Kee KH, et al. Sarcomatoid carcinoma of the prostate with rhabdomyosarcomatous differentiation. J Urol Pathol 1996;5:157–63.

44. Raney RB Jr, Gehan EA, Hays DM, et al. Primary chemotherapy with or without radiation therapy and/or surgery for children with localized sarcoma of the bladder, prostate, vagina, uterus, and cervix. A comparison of the results in Intergroup Rhabdomyosarcoma Studies I and II. Cancer 1990;66:2072–81.

45. Ray EH. Sarcoma of the prostate in infants. Case report and brief review of the literature. J Urol 1935;34:686–91.

45a. Reyes JW, Shinozuka H, Garry P, Putong PB. A light and electron microscopic study of a hemangiopericytoma of the prostate with local extension. Cancer 1977;40:1122–7.

45b. Riba LW, Wheelock MC. Leiomyosarcoma of prostate. J Urol 1950;63:162–4.

46. Ro JY, El-Naggar A, Amin MB, Sahin AA, Ordonez NG. Pseudosarcomatous fibromyxoid tumor of bladder and prostate: an immunohistochemical analysis of 9 cases. Hum Pathol 1993;24:1203–10.

47. Russo P, Demas B, Reuter V. Adult prostatic sarcoma. Abdom Imag 1993;18:399–401.

48. Sarkar K, Tolnai G, McKay DE. Embryonal rhabdomyosarcoma of the prostate. An ultrastructural study. Cancer 1973;31:442–8.

48a. Shehata WM, Kerr AA, Boss HH, Panke TW, Meyer RL. Leiomyosarcoma of the prostate apparently cured by surgery and radical irradiation: report of a case [Letter]. Rad Oncol 1982;8:1814–5.

49. Verga G, Parigi GB. Conservative surgery of bladder-prostate rhabdomyosarcomas in children: results after longterm follow-up. J Ped Surg 1993;28:1016–8.

50. Waring PM, Newland RC. Prostatic embryonal rhabdomyosarcoma in adults. A clinicopathologic review. Cancer 1992;69:755–62.

51. Wijnaendts LC, van der Linden JC, van Unnik AJ, Delemarre JF, Voute PA, Meijer CJ. Histopathological classification of childhood rhabdomyosarcomas: relationship with clinical parameters and prognosis. Hum Pathol 1994;25:900–7.

Leiomyosarcoma

52. Ahlering TE, Weintraub P, Skinner DG. Management of adult sarcomas of the bladder and prostate. Urology 1988;140:1397–9.

53. Aragona F, Serretta V, Marconi A, Spinelli C, Arganini M, Fiorentini L. Leiomyosarcoma of the prostate in adults. Ann Chir Gynaecol 1985;74:191–4.

54. Cheville JC, Dundore PA, Nascimento AG, et al. Leiomyosarcoma of the prostate. Report of 23 cases. Cancer 1995;76:1422–7.

55. Christoffersen J. Leiomyosarcoma of the prostate. Acta Chir Scan 1973;433:75–84.

56. Germiyanoglu C, Özkardes H, Kurt Ü, Öztokatli A, Erol D. Leiomyosarcoma of the prostate. A case report. Intl Urol Nephrol 1994;26:189–91.

57. Limon J, Cin Dal P, Sandberg AA. Cytogenetic findings in a primary leiomyosarcoma of the prostate. Cancer Genet Cytogenet 1986;22:159–67.

58. Mottola A, Selli C, Carini M, Natali A, Gambacorta G. Leiomyosarcoma of the prostate. Eur Urol 1985;11:131–3.

59. Ohmori T, Arita N, Tabei R. Prostatic leiomyosarcoma revealing cytoplasmic virus-like particles and intranuclear paracrystalline structures. Acta Pathol Jpn 1984;34:631–8.

60. Prince CL, Vest SA. Leiomyosarcoma of the prostate. J Urol 1941;46:1129–43.

61. Riba LW, Wheelock MC. Leiomyosarcoma of prostate. J Urol 1950;63:162–4.

62. Shehata WM, Kerr AA, Boss HH, Panke TW, Meyer RL. Leiomyosarcoma of the prostate apparently cured by surgery and radical irradiation: report of a case [Letter]. Rad Oncol 1982;8:1814–5.

63. Smith BH, Dehner LP. Sarcoma of the prostate gland. Am J Clin Pathol 1972;58:43–50.

64. Witherow R, Molland E, Oliver T, Hind C. Leiomyosarcoma of prostate and superficial soft tissue. Urology 1980;15:513–5.

Stromal Sarcoma

65. Bain GO, Danyluk JM, Shnitka TK, Jewell LD, Manickavel V. Malignant fibrous histiocytoma of prostate gland. Urology 1985;26:89–91.

66. Chan KW. Angiosarcoma of the prostate. An immunohistochemical study of a case. Pathology 1990;22:108–10.

67. Chin W, Fay R, Ortega P. Malignant fibrous histiocytoma of prostate. Urology 1986;27:363–5.

68. Ekfors TO, Aho HJ, Kekomaki M. Malignant rhabdoid tumor of the prostatic region. Immunohistological and ultrastructural evidence for epithelial origin. Virchows Arch 1985;406:381–8.

69. Gaudin PB, Rosai J, Epstein JJ. Sarcomas and related proliferative lesions of specialized prostatic stroma: a clinicopathologic study of 22 cases. Am J Surg Pathol 1998;22:148–62.

70. Longley J. Sarcoma of prostate and bladder. J Urol 1955;73:417.

71. Melicow MM, Pelton TH, Fish GW. Sarcoma of the prostate gland: review of literature; table of classification; report of four cases. J Urol 1943;49:675–707.

72. Ohtsuki Y, Ro JY, Ordonez NG, Kee KH, et al. Sarcomatoid carcinoma of the prostate with rhabdomyosarcomatous differentiation. J Urol Pathol 1996;5:157–63.

73. Reyes JW, Shinozuka H, Garry P, Putong PB. A light and electron microscopic study of a hemangiopericytoma of the prostate with local extension. Cancer 1977;40:1122–7.

74. Russo P, Demas B, Reuter V. Adult prostatic sarcoma. Abdom Imaging 1993;18:399–401.

75. Scardino PL, Prince CL. Prostatic sarcoma: survival following radical perineal prostatectomy. Urology 1954;72:729–30.

76. Schuppler J. Malignant neurilemmoma of prostate gland. J Urol 1971;106:903–5.

77. Scully JM, Uno JM, McIntyre M, Mosely S. Radiation-induced prostatic sarcoma: a case report. J Urol 1990;144:746–8.

78. Smith DM, Manivel C, Kapps D, Uecker J. Angiosarcoma of the prostate: report of 2 cases and review of the literature. J Urol 1986;135:382–4.

79. Stevens AR, Barringer BS. Sarcoma of the prostate. J Urol 1940;44:83–108.

80. Stirling WC, Ash JE. Sarcoma of the prostate. J Urol 1939;41:515–40.

81. Wünsch PH, Müller HA. Hemangiopericytoma of the prostate. A light microscopic study of an unusual tumor. Pathol Res Pract 1982;172:334–6.

Mixed Epithelial–Stromal Tumor (Phyllodes Tumor) of the Prostate

82. Attah E, Nkposong E. Phyllodes type of atypical prostatic hyperplasia. J Urol 1976;115:762–4.

83. Cox R, Dawson IM. A curious prostatic tumor: probably true mixed tumor. Br J Urol 1960;32:306–11.

84. Fain JS, Cosnow I, King BF, Zincke H, Bostwick DG. Cystosarcoma phyllodes of the seminal vesicle. Cancer 1993;71:2055–61.

85. Gaudin PB, Rosai J, Epstein JI. Sarcomas and related proliferative lesions of specialized prostatic stroma: a clinicopathologic study of 22 cases. Am J Surg Pathol 1998;22:148–62.

86. Gueft B, Walsh MA. Malignant prostatic cystosarcoma phyllodes. NY State J Med 1975;75:2226–8.

87. Halling AC, Farrow GM, Bostwick DG. Prostatic phyllodes tumor. A report of 6 cases. Am J Clin Pathol 1993;100:320.

88. Ito H, Ito M, Mitsuhata N, Tahara E. Phyllodes tumor of the prostate: a case report. Jpn J Clin Oncol 1989;19:299–304.

89. Kendall AR, Stein BS, Shea FJ, Petersen RO, Senay B. Cystic pelvic mass. J Urol 1986;135:550–3.

90. Kerley SW, Pierce P, Thomas J. Giant cystosarcoma phyllodes of the prostate associated with adenocarcinoma. Arch Pathol Lab Med 1992;116:195–7.

91. Kevwitch MK, Walloch JL, Waters WB, Flanigan RC. Prostatic cystic epithelial-stromal tumors: a report of 2 new cases. J Urol 1993;149:860–4.

92. Lopez-Beltran A, Gaeta J, Huben R, Croghan GA. Malignant phyllodes tumor of prostate. Urology 1990;35:164–7.

93. Lukl P, Baron JA, Gherardi G, Krikorian J. Cystosarcoma phyllodes of the prostate with widespread hematogenous metastases. Pathol Res Pract 1987;182:520.

94. Mai KT, Walley VM. Adenofibroma of the ejaculatory duct. J Urol Pathol 1994;2:301–5.

95. Manivel JC, Shenoy BV, Wick MR, Dehner LP. Cystosarcoma phyllodes of the prostate. A pathologic and immunohistochemical study. Arch Pathol Lab Med 1986;110:534–8.

96. Olson EM, Trambert MA, Mattrey RF. Cystosarcoma phyllodes of the prostate: MRI findings. Abdom Imag 1994;19:180–1.

97. Reese JH, Lombard CM, Krone K, Stamey TA. Phyllodes type of atypical prostatic hyperplasia: a report of 3 new cases. J Urol 1987;138:623–6.

98. Yokota T, Yamashita Y, Okuzono Y, et al. Malignant cystosarcoma phyllodes of prostate. Acta Pathol Jpn 1984;34:663–8.

99. Young JF, Jensen PE, Wiley CA. Malignant phyllodes tumor of the prostate. A case report with immunohistochemical and ultrastructural studies. Arch Pathol Lab Med 1992;116:296–9.

100. Yum M, Miller JC, Agrawal BL. Leiomyosarcoma arising in atypical fibromuscular hyperplasia (phyllodes tumor) of the prostate with distant metastasis. Cancer 1991;68:910–5.

Hematolymphoid Malignancies

101. Banavali SD, Mohandas KM, Iyer R, et al. Non-Hodgkin's lymphoma of prostate: a rare site of primary extranodal presentation (a report of two cases). Indian J Cancer 1991;28:70–4.

102. Banerjee SS, Harris M. Angiotropic lymphoma presenting in the prostate. Histopathology 1988;12:667–83.

103. Barcos M, Lane W, Gomez GA, et al. An autopsy study of 1206 acute and chronic leukemias (1958 to 1982). Cancer 1987;60:827–37.

104. Batts M Jr. Multiple myelomas: review of 40 cases. Arch Surg 1939;39:307.

105. Ben-Ezra J, Sheibani K, Kendrick FE, Winberg CD, Rappaport H. Angiotropic large cell lymphoma of the prostate gland: an immunohistochemical study. Hum Pathol 1986;17:964–6.

106. Boe S, Nielsen H, Ryttov N. Burkitt's lymphoma mimicking prostatitis. J Urol 1981;125:891–2.

107. Bostwick DG, Iczkowski KA, Amin MB, Discigil G, Osborne B. Malignant lymphoma involving the prostate: report of 62 cases. Cancer 1998;83:732–8.

108. Bostwick DG, Mann RB. Malignant lymphomas involving the prostate. A study of 13 cases. Cancer 1985;56:2932–8.

109. Cachia PG, McIntyre MA, Dewar AE, Stockdill G. Prostatic infiltration in chronic lymphatic leukaemia. J Clin Pathol 1987;40:342–5.

110. Cos LR, Rashid HA. Primary non-Hodgkin lymphoma of the prostate presenting as benign prostate hyperplasia. Urology 1984;23:176–9.

111. Estrada PC, Scardino PL. Myeloma of the prostate: a case report. J Urol 1971;106:586–7.

112. Fell P, O'Connor M, Smith JM. Primary lymphoma of prostate presenting as bladder outflow obstruction. Urology 1987;29:555–9.

113. Ferry JA, Young RH. Malignant lymphoma of the genitourinary tract. Curr Diagn Pathol 1997;4:145–69.

114. Frame R, Head D, Lee R, Craven C, Ward JH. Granulocytic sarcoma of the prostate. Two cases causing urinary obstruction. Cancer 1987;59:142–6.

115. Franco V, Florena AM, Quintini G, Ingargiola GB. Monocytoid B-cell lymphoma of the prostate. Pathologica 1992;84:411–7.

116. Fukase N. Hyperplasia of the rudimentary lymph nodes of the prostate. Surg Gynecol Obstet 1922;35:131–6.

117. Hollenberg GM. Extraosseous multiple myeloma simulating primary prostatic neoplasm. J Urol 1978;119:292–4.

118. Isaacson PG, Norton AJ. Extranodal lymphomas. New York: Churchill Livingstone, 1994:280–1.

119. Kerbl K, Pauer W. Primary non-Hodgkin lymphoma of prostate. Urology 1988;32:347–9.

120. King LS, Cox TR. Lymphosarcoma of the prostate. Am J Pathol 1951;27:801–23.

121. Klotz LH, Herr HW. Hodgkin's disease of the prostate: a detailed case report. J Urol 1996;135:1261–2.

122. Masih K, Bhalla S. Primary non-Hodgkin's lymphoma of the prostate gland—a case report. Ind J Pathol Microbiol 1994;37(Suppl):S56–7.

123. Parks RW, Henry PG, Abram WP, Best BG. Primary non-Hodgkin's lymphoma of the prostate mimicking acute prostatitis. Br J Urol 1995;76:409.

124. Patel DR, Gomez GA, Henderson ES, Gamarra M. Primary prostatic involvement in non-Hodgkin lymphoma. Urology 1988;32:96–8.

125. Peison B, Benisch B, Nicora B, Lind E. Acute urinary obstruction secondary to pseudolymphoma of prostate. Urology 1977;10:478–9.

126. Rainwater LM, Barrett DM. Primary lymphoma of prostate: transrectal ultrasonic appearance. Urology 1990;36:522–5.

127. Sarris A, Dimopoulos M, Pugh W, Cabanillas F. Primary lymphoma of the prostate: good outcome with Doxorubicin-based combination chemotherapy. J Urol 1995;153:1852–4.

128. Sridjar KN, Woodhouse CR. Prostatic infiltration in leukaemia and lymphoma. Eur Urol 1983;9:153–6.

129. Terris MK, Hausdorff J, Freiha FS. Hematolymphoid malignancies diagnosed at the time of radical prostatectomy. J Urol 1997;150:1457–9.

130. Thalhammer F, Gisslinger H, Chott A, et al. Granulocytic sarcoma of the prostate as the first manifestation of a late relapse of acute myelogenous leukemia. Ann Hematol 1994;68:97–9.

131. Viadana E, Bross ID, Pickren JW. An autopsy study of the metastatic patterns of human leukemias. Oncology 1978;35:87–96.

132. Williams E, Hanchard B, Brooks SE, Douglas LL. Immunohistochemistry of lymphocyte B-cell lymphoma of the prostate gland. West Indian Med J 1992;41:126–9.

133. Yasuda N, Ohmori SI, Usui T. IgD myelomas involving the prostate. Am J Hematol 1994;47:65–6.

Miscellaneous Tumors

134. Arai Y, Watanabe J, Kounami T, Tomoyoshi T. Retroperitoneal seminoma with simultaneous occurrence in the prostate. J Urol 1988;139:382–5.

135. Benson RC Jr, Segura JW, Carney JA. Primary yolk-sac (endodermal sinus) tumor of the prostate. Cancer 1978;41:1395–8.

136. Casiraghi O, Martinez-Madrigal F, Mostofi FK, Micheau C, Caillou B, Tursz T. Primary prostatic Wilm's tumor. Am J Surg Pathol 1991;15:885–90.

137. Dalla Palma P, Dante S, Guazzieri S, Sperandio P. Primary endodermal sinus tumor of the prostate: report of a case. Prostate 1988;12:255–61.

138. de la Rosette JJ, Debruyne FM. Extragonadal germ cell tumor invading the prostate. Eur Urol 1990;18:77–9.

139. Dennis PJ, Lewandowski AE, Rohner TJ Jr, Weidner WA, Mamourian AC, Stern DR. Pheochromocytoma of the prostate: an unusual location. J Urol 1989;141:130–2.

140. Gohji K, Goto A, Takenaka A, et al. Extragonadal germ cell tumor in the retrovesical region associated with Klinefelter's syndrome: a case report and review of the literature. J Urol 1989;141:133–9.

141. Hayman R, Patel A, Fisher C, Hendry WF. Primary seminoma of the prostate. Br J Urol 1995;76:273–4.

142. Khandekar JD, Holland JM, Rochester D, Christ ML. Extragonadal seminoma involving urinary bladder and arising in the prostate. Cancer 1993;71:3972–4.

143. Marsden HB, Birch JM, Swindell R. Germ cell tumours of childhood: a review of 137 cases. J Clin Pathol 1981;34:879–83.

144. Mehta M, Nadel NS, Lonni Y, Ali I. Malignant paraganglioma of the prostate and retroperitoneum. J Urol 1979;121:376–8.

145. Michel F, Gattegno B, Roland J, Coloby P, Colbert N, Thibault P. Primary nonseminomatous germ cell tumor of the prostate. J Urol 1986;135:597–9.

146. Nielsen VM, Skovgaard O, Kvist N. Phaeochromocytoma of the prostate. Br J Urol 1983;59:478–9.

147. Schriber J, Flax S, Trueau M, et al. Primary yolk sac (endodermal sinus) tumor of the prostate: case report and review of the literature. Prostate 1990;17:137–43.

148. Tay HP, Bidair M, Shabaik A, Gilbaugh JH III, Schmidt JD. Primary yolk sac tumor of the prostate in a patient with Klinefelter's syndrome. J Urol 1995;153:1066–9.

149. Voges GE, Wippermann F, Duber C, Hohenfellner R. Pheochromocytoma in the pediatric age group: the prostate—an unusual location. J Urol 1990;144:1219–21.

7
TUMOR-LIKE LESIONS OF THE PROSTATE

INTRODUCTION

This chapter reviews the diverse mimics of prostatic carcinoma that may be encountered in specimens derived, or thought to be derived, from the prostate gland (1–11). Most of the lesions can lead to a misdiagnosis on microscopic examination and, therefore, may result in inappropriate treatment. Others can cause some confusion with cancer clinically and are also, accordingly, briefly reviewed. Some of these lesions have already been mentioned in the differential diagnosis with other processes, but, excluding atypical adenomatous hyperplasia-adenosis (covered in chapters 3 and 4) and normal prostatic central zone glands (discussed in chapters 1 and 3), they are covered here again to highlight this important category of tumor-like lesions. A classifica-

tion of tumor-like lesions of the prostate and periprostatic tissues is presented in Table 7-1. Ectopic prostatic tissue is also considered here.

ATROPHY

Although the pitfalls associated with it have been recognized for many years, atrophy (figs. 7-1, 7-2), in our experience and that in the literature (17,22,25), is still the benign prostatic lesion most often mistaken for adenocarcinoma in needle biopsy specimens, particularly if atypical adenomatous hyperplasia is excluded. In a review of 535 consecutive needle biopsies of prostate, 7 (1.3 percent) were classified as false positives (16); 5 were atypical adenomatous hyperplasia, and 2 atrophy. In contrast, in transurethral resection specimens other processes such as basal

Table 7-1

TUMOR-LIKE LESIONS OF THE PROSTATE (OTHER THAN NODULAR HYPERPLASIA)

Atypical adenomatous hyperplasia-adenosis (see chapter 3)

Atrophy

Postatrophic hyperplasia, partial atrophy

Sclerosing adenosis

Cribriform hyperplasia

Complex architecture of normal central zone epithelium (see chapter 3)

Mesonephric remnant hyperplasia

Nephrogenic adenoma of prostatic urethra

Squamous metaplasia

Transitional cell metaplasia/hyperplasia

Basal cell hyperplasia

Prostatitis
    Typical
    Nonspecific granulomatous
    Granulomatous, infectious
    Granulomatous, therapy related
    Xanthogranulomatous-xanthoma
    Other forms

Malakoplakia

Inflammatory and miscellaneous other reactive atypias

Radiation atypia

Postoperative spindle cell nodule and post-needle biopsy changes

Inflammatory pseudotumor (pseudosarcomatous fibromyxoid tumor)

Atypical stromal cells

Lipofuscin and melanin pigment in the prostate, including blue nevus

Endometriosis

Normal "nonprostatic" tissue in prostate specimens
    Seminal vesicle/ejaculatory duct
    Cowper's glands
    Verumontanum, including verumontanum mucosal gland hyperplasia
    Paraganglia

Mucinous metaplasia

Benign glands adjacent to nerves and in skeletal muscle

Cysts

Amyloidosis

Collagenous spherulosis

Calculi/calcification/cartilage

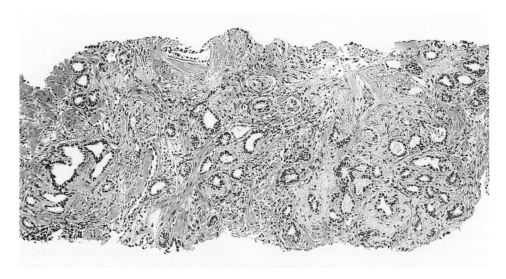

Figure 7-1
LOBULAR ATROPHY
This low-power view of a needle biopsy specimen shows a lobular arrangement of acini, a few of which are slightly dilated.

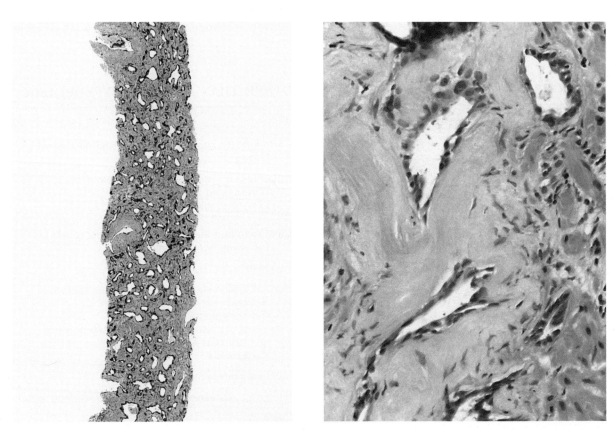

Figure 7-2
SCLEROTIC ATROPHY
Left: A low-power view of a needle biopsy specimen shows haphazardly arranged small acini in a fibrotic stroma. Lobulation is not as conspicuous as in figure 7-1, and the size and spacing of many acini are similar to those of a Gleason grade 3 adenocarcinoma.
Right: This example shows more pronounced stromal sclerosis.

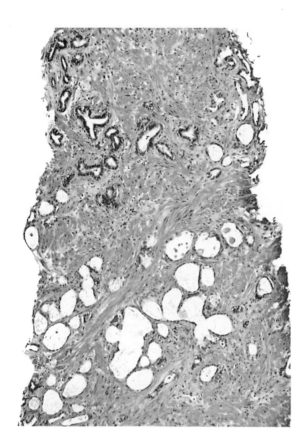 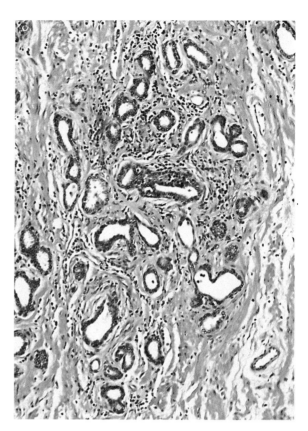

Figure 7-3
LOBULAR ATROPHY
Left: The acini vary from tiny with narrow lumens to those that are cystically dilated.
Right: A lobule from another case shows the typical size and caliber of most atrophic acini and chronic inflammation in the stroma.

cell hyperplasia and cribriform hyperplasia account for the majority of tumor-like lesions, in our experience and that of others (19). Atrophy is most common in "routine" specimens, but has also been described as a frequent finding in men who have received radiation (see page 319) or neoadjuvant hormonal therapy for prostatic carcinoma (15) (see page 186). Atrophy is typically seen in older patients (21), but has been seen in young males (18). Although the focus in this chapter is atrophy mimicking cancer, it is equally important to note that the opposite problem, mistaking small acini of cancer for atrophy, also occurs as pointed out in the older literature (20,24) and reemphasized in recent papers (see page 172).

There are three subtypes of atrophy: lobular (simple), sclerotic, and cystic, but their distinction has no clinical significance. Additionally, there is overlap between the various subtypes (figs. 7-1–7-4), and they are typically combined,

at least if the entire prostate is examined (13). The lobular arrangement seen in the first subtype is a helpful clue to its diagnosis (figs. 7-1, 7-3). Sclerotic atrophy is more problematic because a disorderly arrangement of the glands can simulate infiltrating carcinoma, particularly if the glands are distorted. In cystic atrophy varying degrees of acinar dilatation are seen (fig. 7-4). Regardless of the subtype, the cells lining the atrophic glands lack the cytologic features of malignancy (fig. 7-5).

As with other non-neoplastic acini in the prostate, nucleoli may be visible in the nuclei of the cells lining some atrophic acini (23a). It is therefore important when using nucleolar characteristics as a criterion for diagnosing carcinoma, to require distinctly prominent nucleoli, preferably in many nuclei. Atrophic cells usually have scant cytoplasm, resulting in an increased nuclear to cytoplasmic ratio and apparent hyperchromasia

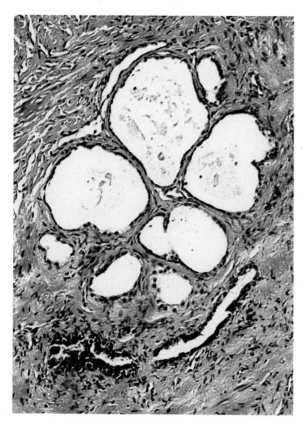

Figure 7-4
CYSTIC ATROPHY

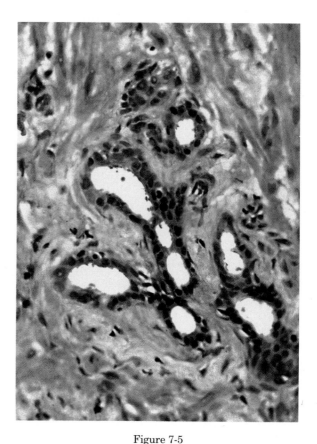

Figure 7-5
PROSTATIC ATROPHY
The characteristic cuboidal cells with scant cytoplasm lining acini are evident.

on low-power examination that causes concern for carcinoma in many cases. In contrast, there is often an appreciable amount of pale or amphophilic cytoplasm in prostatic adenocarcinomas, although this is often focal in cases of so-called atrophic adenocarcinoma. Although atrophic benign acini are usually small and round, they may have irregular contours. In the differential diagnosis with adenocarcinoma, the frequent lobulation and cytologic differences noted above usually facilitate the diagnosis with relative ease. It is also helpful that atrophic acini do not infiltrate between benign glands as is often seen with carcinoma, although when only a few acini are present this feature may not be appreciable. Importantly, in contrast to small neoplastic acini, atrophic benign acini retain a basal cell layer, although it is often difficult to recognize the normal two-cell layer because of the secretory cell atrophy. In a problematic small acinar lesion immunohistochemical stains for high molecular

weight cytokeratin (clone 34βE12) may be indicated to demonstrate the basal cells (fig. 7-6).

Cases from patients treated with radiation or hormonal therapy for carcinoma may be particularly challenging and, indeed, the same specimen may show both atrophic benign acini and neoplastic acini (15). Similar criteria to those used in evaluating specimens from patients without a history of therapy apply. In some such cases the neoplastic acini themselves may appear atrophic, and invasive patterns are paramount in distinguishing them from non-neoplastic atrophic acini.

POSTATROPHIC HYPERPLASIA

The process termed postatrophic hyperplasia (12,14,17), partial atrophy (23), or hyperplastic atrophy (13) (see page 60) is considered again here with regard to the problems it may cause by suggesting the diagnosis of cancer in needle biopsy

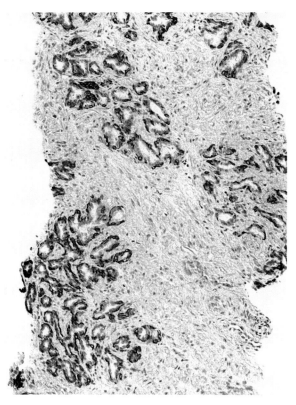

Figure 7-6
LOBULAR ATROPHY
An immunohistochemical stain for high molecular weight cytokeratin (clone 34βE12) shows intense positivity.

material (fig. 7-7). This process is seen in approximately 2 to 3 percent of biopsies (12). Since postatrophic hyperplasia reflects a combination of both atrophic and hyperplastic processes, the glands may be small and closely packed as with conventional atrophy, or may show a neoacinar pattern in which cells with appreciable clear cytoplasm are evident (fig. 7-7). In some instances acini may contain cells with minimal to absent cytoplasm (atrophic) admixed with cells with more abundant cytoplasm (hyperplastic). A clue to the diagnosis on low-power microscopy is the admixture of glands exhibiting variation in size, shape, and cytoplasmic features (fig. 7-7A) (12,14,23). Some glands may be elongated (fig. 7-7B) and cytoplasmic apical blebs may be seen (fig. 7-7C). Features that help distinguish this process from adenocarcinoma are the absence of overt infiltration or gland fusion, bland cytology without (in most cases [23a]) prominent nucleoli, and the

presence, even focally, of a recognizable basal cell layer. In problematic cases, high molecular weight cytokeratin (clone 34βE12) immunostains may demonstrate basal cells in most glands, confirming the benign nature of this proliferation (fig. 7-7D).

SCLEROSING ADENOSIS

In 1983, Chen and Schiff (26) reported a prostatic lesion that was most noteworthy, in their opinion, because of its resemblance to an adenomatoid tumor. We have also noted a resemblance to adenomatoid tumor in some cases (fig. 7-8). Subsequently, Clement (31) noted a resemblance to sclerosing adenosis of the breast and suggested "sclerosing adenosis" an appropriate name for this distinctive prostatic lesion. The first case under this now generally accepted designation was reported in 1987 (31).

The lesion is always an incidental finding, usually in a transurethral resection specimen but occasionally in a needle biopsy (26–31). An initially alarming microscopic appearance caused by cords, clusters, and single cells in a proliferating stroma may suggest carcinoma (fig. 7-9). In some cases the stroma is edematous or myxoid (fig. 7-9, right). These lesions are well circumscribed for the most part (fig. 7-10) but may appear to be focally infiltrative at their periphery. The acini rarely contain mucin or crystalloids, and the nuclei may focally demonstrate prominent nucleoli, compounding the problems in distinction from carcinoma. The presence in some of the cases of a thickened basement membrane-like material enveloping occasional glands (fig. 7-10, right) may suggest this particular non-neoplastic lesion, although the generally circumscribed low-power appearance (fig. 7-10, left), and characteristic features of the stroma are usually diagnostic. Basal cells, which are also diagnostically helpful, are usually discernible on routine light microscopy, but when they are difficult to identify their presence can be confirmed by immunoperoxidase stains for high molecular weight cytokeratin (clone 34βE12). Basal cell hyperplasia may coexist with sclerosing adenosis (29), and the basal cells in sclerosing adenosis are also positive for S-100 protein (fig. 7-11) and actin; ultrastructural studies have confirmed the immunohistochemical features indicative of myoepithelial differentiation. The follow-up in all series has been uneventful.

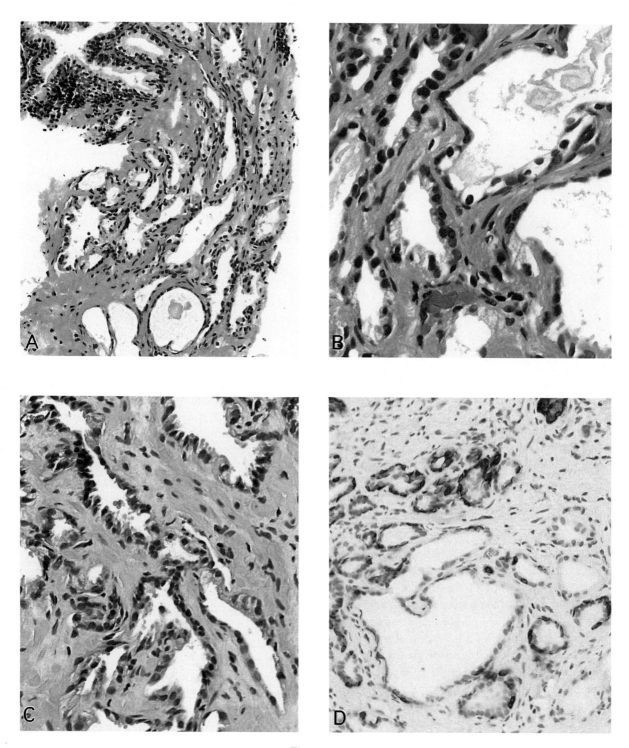

Figure 7-7
POSTATROPHIC HYPERPLASIA

A: A somewhat irregular proliferation of acini, many of which are lined by cells with appreciable cytoplasm, may suggest the diagnosis of adenocarcinoma. Note the cystic glands at the bottom lined predominantly by atrophic epithelium.

B: A higher power view shows some cells lining acini have appreciable clear cytoplasm whereas others are atrophic with scant cytoplasm.

C: A view of another case shows elongated acini and some apical cytoplasmic blebs.

D: An immunostain for cytokeratin (clone 34βE12) shows basal cells investing the acini in most, but not all, regions.

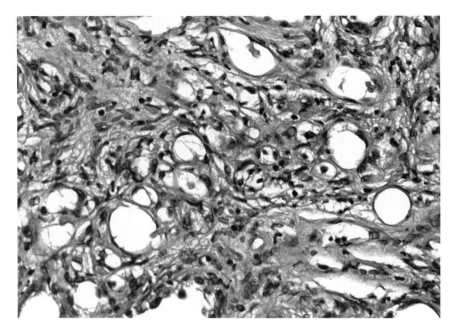

Figure 7-8
SCLEROSING ADENOSIS
The appearance in this area superficially resembles an adenomatoid tumor.

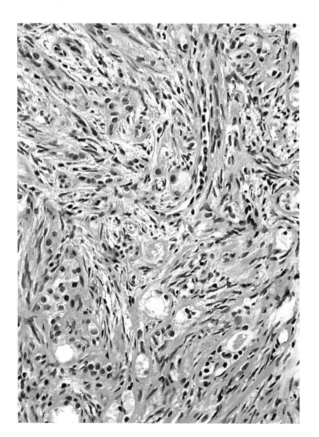
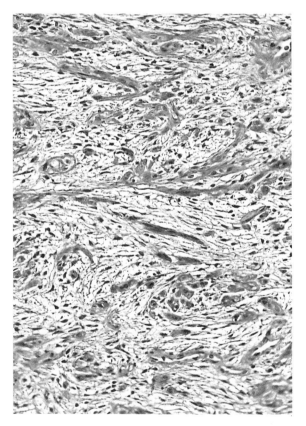

Figure 7-9
SCLEROSING ADENOSIS
Left: The cellular proliferating stroma has extensively obliterated the small acini.
Right: The stroma is conspicuously myxoid.

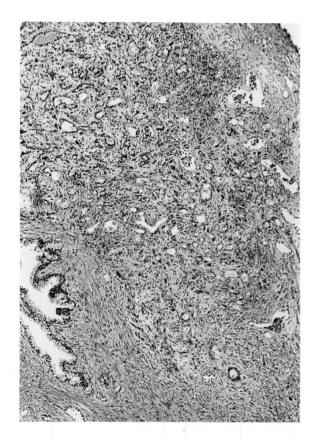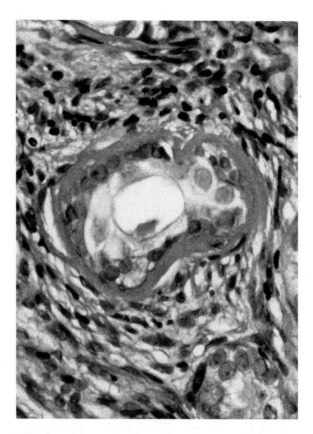

Figure 7-10
SCLEROSING ADENOSIS

Left: The well-circumscribed lesion demonstrates the biphasic nature of this process, characterized by a stromal and glandular proliferation in which the former element compresses the latter in areas.

Right: A high-power view of another case shows dense basement membrane-like material surrounding a tubule.

Figure 7-11
SCLEROSING ADENOSIS

An immunohistochemical stain for S-100 protein highlights basal cells within the lesion, and suggests myoepithelial differentiation.

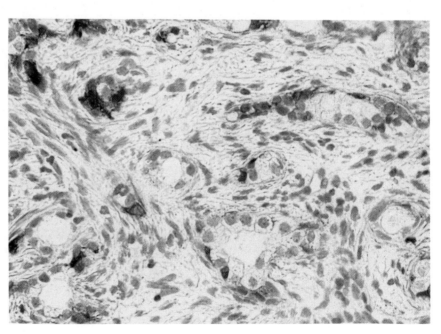

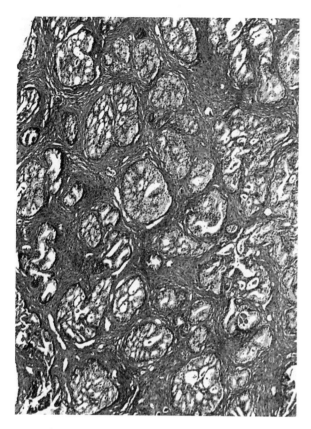 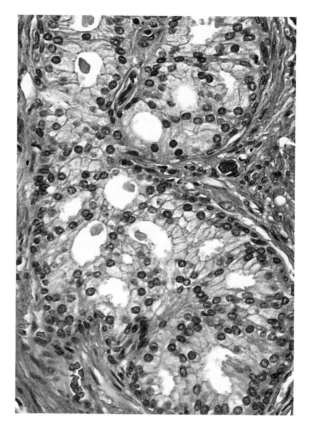

Figure 7-12
CRIBRIFORM HYPERPLASIA

Left: Individual units with a cribriform pattern are separated from one another by unremarkable stroma. There is a lack of confluence of the cribriform foci.

Right: A high-power view shows an absence of malignant cytologic features. Note the easily recognizable basal cells.

CRIBRIFORM HYPERPLASIA

This process falls within the spectrum of benign nodular hyperplasia (see chapter 2), but occasionally the architectural complexity of some cases, with a "back-to-back" proliferation of cribriform glands without accompanying cytologic atypia, warrants a specific diagnosis. This lesion was included as a variant of hyperplasia and illustrated by Dhom in 1979 (33) and in the 1980 World Health Organization classification of tumors and tumor-like lesions of the prostate (37). A series of cases was reported subsequently under the designation "clear cell cribriform hyperplasia" (32). The cells do not always have striking clear cytoplasm, however, and as it is the cribriform pattern that primarily causes concern we do not recommend the prefix "clear cell."

When one group reviewed prostatic cases they had previously termed "suspicious" prior to the description of the lesion, cribriform hyperplasia accounted for 16 percent of the cases (35). Despite the prominent and superficially alarming cribriform pattern in these cases (fig. 7-12), the cribriform units do not exhibit the same degree of confluence seen in most cribriform carcinomas (36), and often the nodularity of conventional nodular hyperplasia can be appreciated. Although usually round to oval, occasional cribriform aggregates are elongated (fig. 7-13). A circumferential basal layer is evident in most cases and is often prominent (fig. 7-13). In some cases this results in an appearance that is a composite of cribriform hyperplasia and basal cell hyperplasia (fig. 7-13, right).

The distinction of cribriform hyperplasia from cribriform prostatic intraepithelial neoplasia and cribriform carcinoma is aided by cytologic differences: the bland cytologic features of cribriform

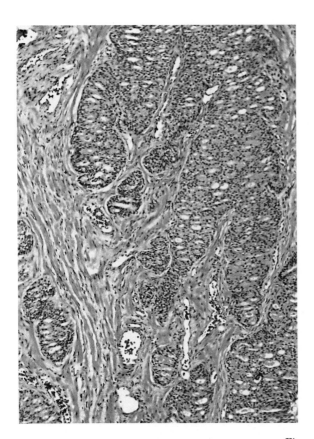 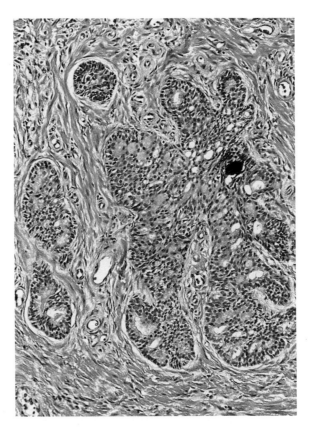

Figure 7-13
CRIBRIFORM HYPERPLASIA WITH BASAL CELL HYPERPLASIA
Left: Elongated formations fuse with each other raising concern for cribriform carcinoma. High-power evaluation is crucial in such cases. Note the prominent basal cells even at this low magnification.
Right: The prominence of basal cells justifies an additional diagnosis of basal cell hyperplasia.

hyperplasia (fig. 7-12, right) contrasts with the at least moderate cytologic atypia and prominent nucleoli in the other two cribriform lesions. A flow cytometric and immunohistochemical study of this lesion showing a diploid DNA content supports its benign nature (34). In contrast, three of four cribriform carcinomas studied were aneuploid. A basal cell layer was confirmed in 15 cribriform hyperplasias using a high molecular weight cytokeratin antibody (clone 34βE12), whereas it was absent in the carcinomas.

MESONEPHRIC REMNANTS AND MESONEPHRIC REMNANT HYPERPLASIA

Mesonephric remnants were found in 0.6 percent of almost 700 transurethral resection specimens reviewed retrospectively (40). It is probable that when few, mesonephric tubules in

prostate specimens go unrecognized unless intraluminal eosinophilic material is conspicuous and suggests their nature. This has no consequence. As in the cervix, cases in which mesonephric tubules are numerous in the prostate warrant the designation "mesonephric hyperplasia" and may cause concern for carcinoma (38).

Gikas and associates (39) described two cases of mesonephric hyperplasia in the prostate and periprostatic tissue in transurethral resection specimens that led, in one case, to an unnecessary radical prostatectomy because of the misdiagnosis of carcinoma. The typically small acini of this process are usually similar in size and shape to those of prostatic carcinoma and are lined by a single layer of epithelium (fig. 7-14). The tubules may be dilated in some areas. Features that may compound the potential diagnostic difficulty include the florid small acinar architecture

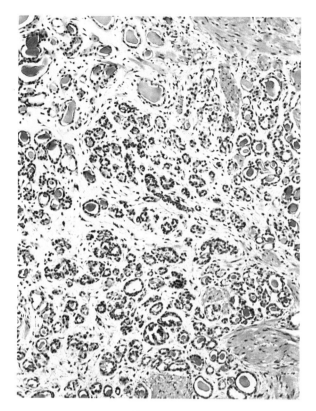

Figure 7-14
MESONEPHRIC HYPERPLASIA
The tubules are small and regular, and many contain dense, uniform, eosinophilic luminal material. A rare tubule has micropapillae.

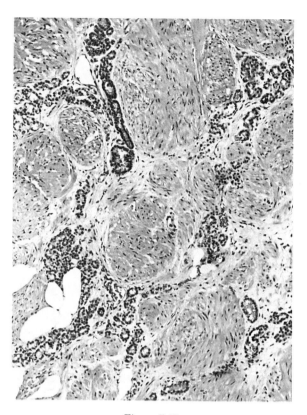

Figure 7-15
MESONEPHRIC HYPERPLASIA
Note the lobular arrangement of the acini.

(fig. 7-15), the occasional presence of prominent nucleoli, intraluminal eosinophilic material (fig. 7-14), and even "perineural invasion" and extraprostatic extension (39a). The occasional epithelial tufting or micropapillary formations (fig. 7-16) are helpful diagnostic features of mesonephric hyperplasia. Also, the intraluminal material in mesonephric hyperplasia typically has a dense, hyaline appearance, contrasting with the more flocculent nature of the intraluminal eosinophilic material in cases of prostatic cancer. The cells lining the mesonephric tubules fail to stain immunohistochemically for prostate-specific antigen (PSA) and prostatic acid phosphatase (PAP), proving the nonprostatic lineage of the lesion and ruling out neoplastic prostatic acini. The high molecular weight cytokeratin (clone 34βE12) stain is positive in the single layer of lesional cells of mesonephric hyperplasia (39), in contrast to carcinoma where staining is lacking due to an absence of basal cells.

NEPHROGENIC ADENOMA OF URETHRA INVOLVING PROSTATE

Nephrogenic adenoma of the urethra is typically either exophytic or, if flat, confined to a narrow zone immediately beneath the urethral epithelium. Rarely, however, it extends to involve the subjacent prostate gland and is identified in a prostatic transurethral resection or biopsy specimen (fig. 7-17) (41-44). In such cases the tubules of the nephrogenic adenoma may be mistaken for the acini of a prostatic adenocarcinoma. The usual initial clue to the diagnosis is an appreciation that the "acini" are not characteristic of prostatic adenocarcinoma. In general, they are even smaller (fig. 7-18) than those of small acinar prostatic adenocarcinoma and have cells with scantier cytoplasm. However, there are exceptions to the latter, as one case of nephrogenic adenoma involving the prostate did have cells with conspicuous clear cytoplasm (44). Paramount in this differential diagnosis is an appreciation of the typical histopathology

299

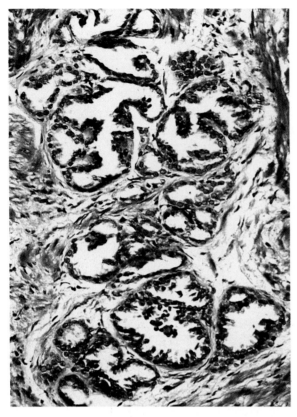

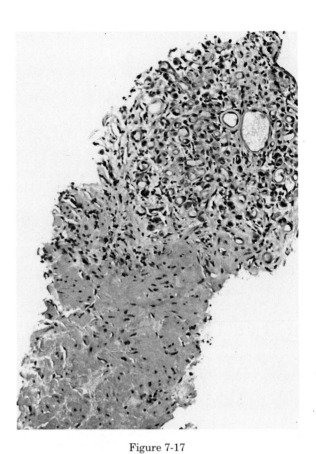

Figure 7-16
MESONEPHRIC HYPERPLASIA
Small micropapillae protrude into the lumens, a feature that may be diagnostically helpful. (Courtesy of Dr. J.I. Epstein, Baltimore, MD.)

Figure 7-17
NEPHROGENIC ADENOMA IN
NEEDLE BIOPSY OF PROSTATE
The closely packed small tubules raise a suspicion of prostatic adenocarcinoma. (Courtesy of Dr. G.G. Bassil, Passaic, NJ.)

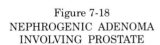

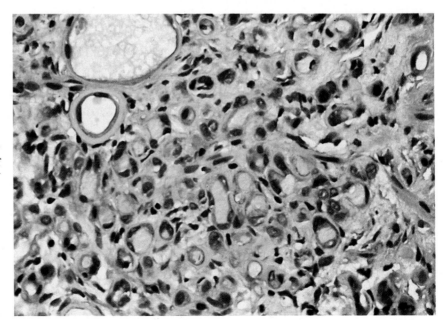

Figure 7-18
NEPHROGENIC ADENOMA
INVOLVING PROSTATE
High-power view of figure 7-17 shows the typical tiny tubules of nephrogenic adenoma. (Courtesy of Dr. G.G. Bassil, Passaic, NJ.)

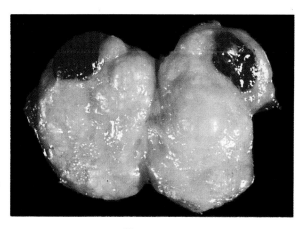

Figure 7-19
PROSTATIC INFARCT
A hemorrhagic nodule is present.

of nephrogenic adenoma (43): the distinctive appearance of at least some of the small tubules which often undergo focal cystic change, the occasional presence of hobnail cells (unlike prostatic adenocarcinoma acini), and the frequently edematous or inflamed stroma. Negative immunohistochemical staining of the lesional cells for PSA and PAP is also important, but use of these stains depends on suspecting nephrogenic adenoma on the basis of examination of routine slides.

SQUAMOUS METAPLASIA

Squamous metaplasia is a common finding in cases of prostatic infarct (fig. 7-19), and is usually most striking at the periphery (fig. 7-20). In the past this has led to an erroneous diagnosis of squamous cell carcinoma of the prostate (46,48, 51). Squamous metaplasia is also found with increased frequency in patients who have undergone a recent transurethral resection and is commonly found in the benign areas of the glands of patients who received hormonal therapy for prostatic carcinoma (fig. 7-21) (45,47,49,50). Minor foci in which the cells appear squamoid sometimes accompany chronic prostatitis, but overt squamous metaplasia in this setting is rare. Squamous metaplasia is rarely found without any predisposing factors.

Squamous cell carcinoma of the prostate is so rare (see chapter 5) that such a diagnosis should only be made after metaplasia has been excluded. Although associated inflammation and

some stromal alterations due to the accompanying infarct may result in regenerative epithelial atypia (fig. 7-20C), the lack of severe cytologic atypia, the absence of an infiltrative pattern, and the associated findings, either pathologic or clinical, are important clues to a benign process.

Adenosquamous carcinoma most commonly occurs in patients with a history of prostatic carcinoma treated by hormonal or radiation therapy. The obvious invasive architecture and the accompanying cytologic atypia make separation of adenosquamous carcinoma from squamous metaplasia straightforward.

TRANSITIONAL CELL METAPLASIA AND HYPERPLASIA

Although transitional epithelium normally lines the prostatic urethra and extends for a variable distance into the underlying prostatic ducts, it is generally accepted that transitional cells are not seen more peripherally, unless there is "transitional cell metaplasia" (fig. 7-22). When the transitional cells form stratified layers and involve several acini the designation "transitional cell hyperplasia" is appropriate (fig. 7-23), although the distinction between metaplasia and hyperplasia is arbitrary. The transitional cells are distinguished from basal cells by their more appreciable cytoplasm, which is usually eosinophilic, or rarely clear, and elongated fusiform nuclei, many of which have longitudinal grooves (figs. 7-22, right, 7-23, right). The metaplastic nature of this process is substantiated by the frequent presence of normal prostatic secretory cells overlying the transitional cells.

A review of 103 consecutive biopsies showed a 34 percent frequency of transitional cell metaplasia that was nearly equally associated with benign and malignant processes (52). Although the precise histogenesis appears unclear, in that study one third of the cases were associated with inflammation, suggesting that at least some examples may be secondary to that process. The cells of infarction-associated metaplasia may have transitional features, but squamous features invariably dominate.

Occasionally, transitional cell hyperplasia may be so exuberant as to suggest transitional cell carcinoma involving the prostate, but there is a marked contrast between the cytologic features of

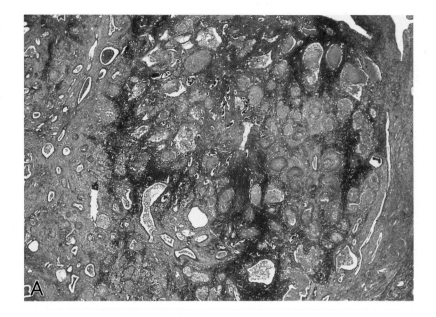

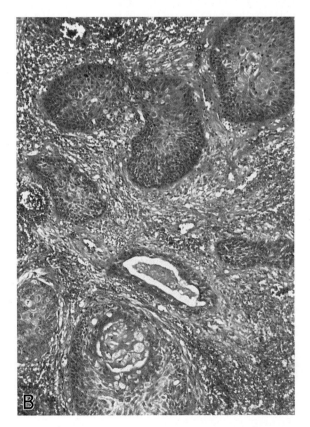

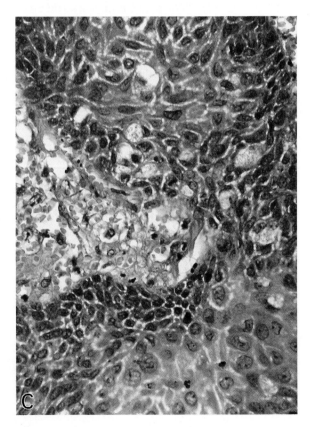

Figure 7-20
PROSTATIC INFARCT

A: A low-power view shows hemorrhage and foci of squamous metaplasia.

B: The squamous metaplasia is more apparent at higher magnification.

C: Reactive atypia of the squamous epithelium is seen, with a mitotic figure just above the center.

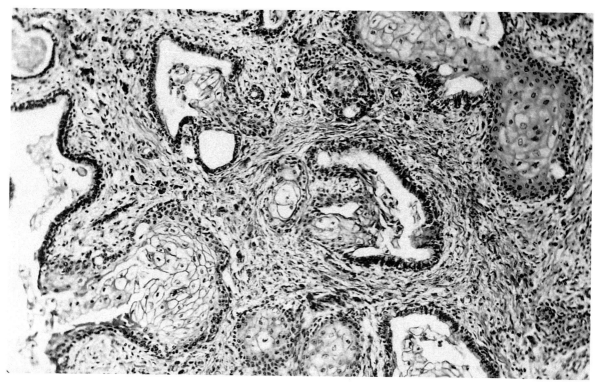

Figure 7-21
SQUAMOUS METAPLASIA OF THE PROSTATE IN A PATIENT RECEIVING ESTROGEN
(Fig. 17 from Fascicles 31b and 32, 1st Series.)

the cells of hyperplasia and those of carcinoma (see chapter 5). In one case the misinterpretation of florid transitional cell hyperplasia of both the periurethral glands and prostatic ducts resulted in a misdiagnosis of transitional cell carcinoma and subsequent radical prostatectomy (52). In less pronounced cases, where the designation of transitional cell metaplasia is more appropriate, confusion with prostatic intraepithelial neoplasia may occur (fig. 7-22, left). In contrast to the latter, which frequently shows complex architectural patterns including micropapillae and epithelial tufting, transitional cell metaplasia, although multilayered, usually lacks similar degrees of architectural complexity, but there is architectural overlap (fig. 7-22, left). The cells of metaplasia, although they may appear hyperchromatic, are noticeably oriented perpendicular to and streaming toward the glandular lumens. High-grade prostatic intraepithelial neoplasia is characterized by prominent nucleoli, a feature not encountered in the usual case

of transitional cell metaplasia. Cases of transitional cell metaplasia may potentially show superimposed dysplastic changes, however.

BASAL CELL HYPERPLASIA

Like cribriform hyperplasia, basal cell hyperplasia falls within the spectrum of benign nodular hyperplasia. It is only since 1983 (54) that attention in the English language literature has been focused on the extent to which a striking proliferation of prostatic basal cells may be confused with carcinoma (figs. 7-24–7-26). However, the cells usually appear cytologically bland (fig. 7-24, right) (although there are exceptions as discussed below), and the patterns differ significantly from those of typical prostatic adenocarcinoma, enabling one to avoid a misinterpretation. Cases reported as embryonal hyperplasia of the prostate (53) appear similar to basal cell hyperplasia except for the presence of a loose, myxoid stroma (fig. 7-25C). Basal cell hyperplasia has recently

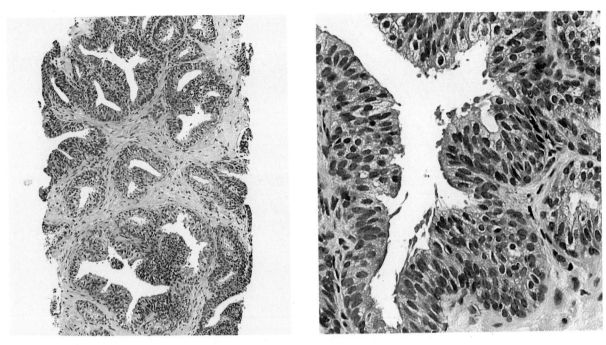

Figure 7-22
TRANSITIONAL CELL METAPLASIA

Left: A low-power view shows cellular stratification imparting a picture that suggests the possibility of prostatic intraepithelial neoplasia.

Right: High-power examination shows pale nuclei, several with visible nuclear grooves, surrounded by pale cytoplasm with perinuclear clearing. There is a lack of the cytologic atypia required to make a diagnosis of prostatic intraepithelial neoplasia.

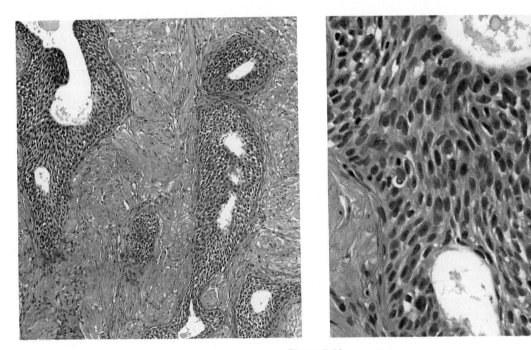

Figure 7-23
TRANSITIONAL CELL HYPERPLASIA
A number of the fusiform nuclei have longitudinal nuclear grooves (right).

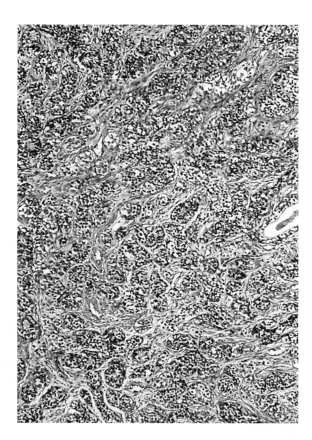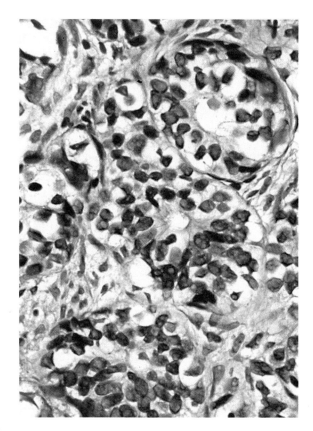

Figure 7-24
BASAL CELL HYPERPLASIA
In this florid example, an orderly arrangement of the epithelial units is still apparent. Note the bland cytologic features (right).

been described as a frequent finding in patients treated for prostate cancer by luteinizing hormone–releasing hormone agonists and flutamide (59). Basal cell hyperplasia usually arises in the central region of the gland and, as a result, is typically encountered in simple prostatectomy or transurethral resection specimens (fig. 7-26A,B) rather than needle biopsy specimens, although it is occasionally seen in the latter (fig. 7-26C).

Basal cell hyperplasia may be incomplete or complete. In its complete form, there is a lack of secretory (luminal) differentiation and the presence of solid nests of basaloid cells (fig. 7-25B). In the more common, incomplete form, there are typically small lumina occasionally lined by secretory cells that are underlain by proliferating basal cells (figs. 7-24, left, 7-25A). Each of these two patterns, the complete and incomplete, contrasts markedly with the appearance of most carcinomas. In most cases of basal cell hyperpla-

sia the cells have scant cytoplasm, another contrast with most prostate carcinomas, but occasionally there is abundant pale cytoplasm (fig. 7-26D). Although normal basal cells may have discernible nucleoli, it is our experience that in typical basal cell hyperplasia nucleolar prominence is rare; however, it may be seen in "atypical" examples of this process (see below). Some cases of basal cell hyperplasia may be associated with calcification (fig. 7-25A). Distinction between basal cell hyperplasia and transitional cell metaplasia/hyperplasia is not always easy, and the two processes may merge with each other, and also with squamous metaplasia; occasional cases have features of each of these processes together (fig. 7-25D).

Incomplete basal cell hyperplasia may result in a confusing, cribriform pattern of pseudocysts that resembles adenoid cystic carcinoma (fig. 7-27)(57,58,60). The cribriform spaces surround

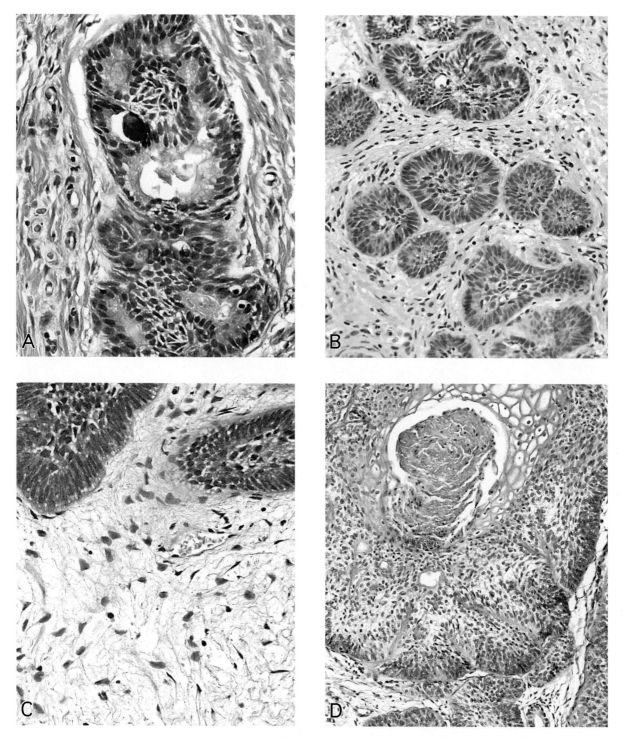

Figure 7-25
BASAL CELL HYPERPLASIA

A: When luminal differentiation is seen, it has been referred to as incomplete basal cell hyperplasia. Some nuclei are fusiform suggesting a transitional nature, but nuclear grooves are inconspicuous. A small focus of calcification is seen.

B: There is minimal luminal differentiation (complete basal cell hyperplasia).

C: There is a myxoid stroma.

D: The cells at the base appear basaloid but merge imperceptibly with cells that appear more transitional, which in turn become squamous with keratin production (top).

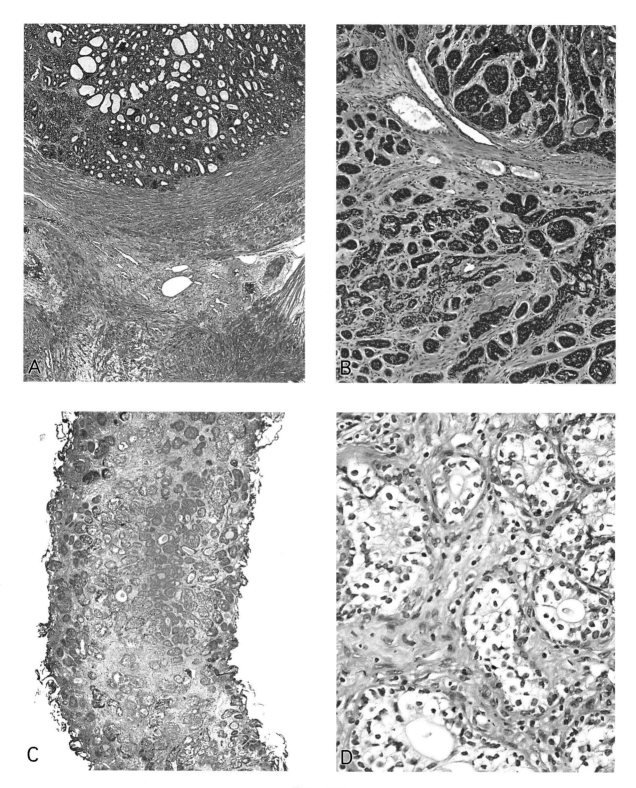

Figure 7-26
BASAL CELL HYPERPLASIA

A,B: The picture is reminiscent of a basal cell adenoma because of the background adenomatous nodule.

C: A needle biopsy specimen is massively involved by basal cell hyperplasia.

D: The cells have abundant pale cytoplasm, an occasional feature of this lesion.

Table 7-2

**COMPARISON OF ADENOID CYSTIC CHANGE IN
BASAL CELL HYPERPLASIA AND ADENOID CYSTIC CARCINOMA**

	Adenoid Cystic-Like Basal Cell Hyperplasia	Adenoid Cystic Carcinoma
Areas of conventional basal cell hyperplasia	complete and incomplete	no
Growth	usually lobular	diffuse infiltrative
Cribriform architecture	focal	prominent
Necrosis	–	+/–
Perineural invasion	–	+/–
Extraprostatic extension	–	+/–
Mitoses	absent	occasional
Apoptosis	absent	common
Sebaceous differentiation	absent	may be seen
Immunophenotype	high molecular weight cytokeratin +	high molecular weight cytokeratin +

basophilic secretion or hyalinized, eosinophilic material. Squamous metaplasia may occur in some cases. Adenoid cystic carcinoma of the prostate is exceedingly rare (see chapter 5) and several of the previously reported cases (slides from some of which one of us has reviewed [60]), appear to represent basal cell hyperplasia with an adenoid cystic-like change. Crucial to the differential diagnosis with carcinoma in these cases are foci of typical basal cell hyperplasia without prominent atypia or mitotic activity, and the absence of infiltrative growth, necrosis, or extraprostatic extension. The features of these processes are contrasted in Table 7-2.

Some cases of basal cell hyperplasia may show atypical cytologic features (fig. 7-28), such as nucleomegaly, prominent nucleoli (fig. 7-29), and mitotic activity, which cause concern but do not justify a diagnosis of either prostatic intraepithelial neoplasia or carcinoma (55,56). In one series, nucleolar prominence was present in 11 of 12 cases; 2 cases exhibited hyperchromatism and nuclear pleomorphism, and 6 had rare mitotic figures (56). In atypical basal cell hyperplasia a normal architecture is still retained, whereas architectural abnormalities indicative of stromal invasion are necessary to establish a diagnosis of basal cell carcinoma. Although some authors include a category of basal cell adenoma

(55) or adenoid basal tumor (57) in their classification of basaloid lesions of the prostate, we favor the interpretation of these cases as basal cell hyperplasia extensively involving adenomatous nodules (fig. 7-26A,B).

In one report on atypical basal cell hyperplasia there was a frequent association with inflammation, and the authors proposed that the atypia was reactive (55). However, in another major series inflammation was not prominent (56). Hence, the precise nature of the cytologic atypia in these cases is uncertain, but, from the practical viewpoint, there is no current evidence to suggest that this lesion is premalignant.

PROSTATITIS

"Typical" Prostatitis

Occasionally, needle biopsies from a case of "typical" prostatitis (63,66,68,70) are difficult to distinguish from carcinoma when the specimen exhibits "squeeze" artifact (fig. 7-30, left). However, appreciation of the inflammatory nature of at least a few well-preserved cells usually helps distinguish the two. Rarely, immunohistochemical stains may be indicated to show that the cells in question are not prostatic epithelial cells. In some cases lymphoid aggregates with germinal

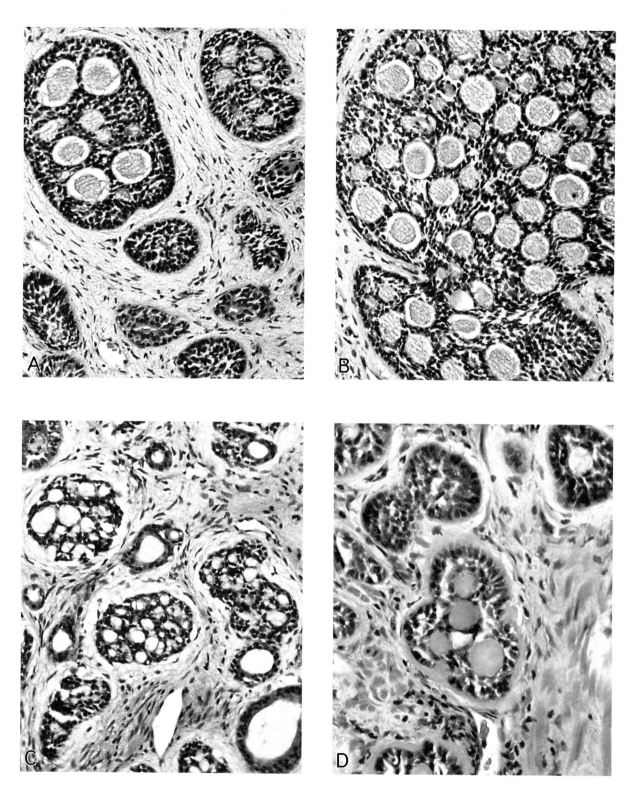

Figure 7-27
BASAL CELL HYPERPLASIA WITH ADENOID CYSTIC-LIKE PATTERN
Low-power view (A) shows many solid foci of conventional basal cell hyperplasia and nests with a punched out cribriform pattern (B). Two other cases show the variable material that may be seen in the spaces: wispy basophilic material (C) and dense, eosinophilic, hyaline-like material (D).

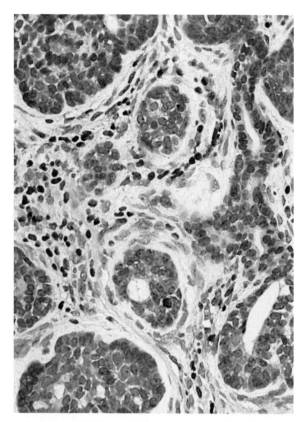

Figure 7-28
ATYPICAL BASAL CELL HYPERPLASIA
There is cytologic atypia and an occasional mitotic figure.

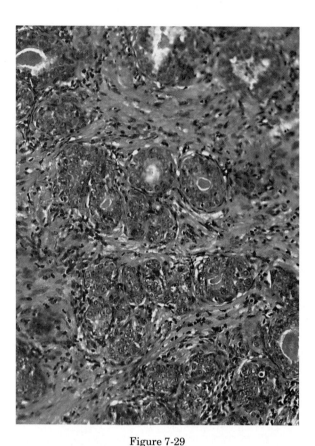

Figure 7-29
ATYPICAL BASAL CELL HYPERPLASIA
Many of the nuclei of the proliferating basal cells have prominent nucleoli.

centers are conspicuous (fig. 7-30, right) and should be distinguished from the rare follicular lymphoma involving the prostate using conventional criteria. Chronic prostatitis may be associated with inflammatory atypia that can potentially be misinterpreted as neoplastic atypia (see page 317). Degenerative changes within lymphocytes and stromal cells that cause them to resemble signet ring cells have been described in prostate specimens (61,76). In one needle biopsy series of 47 cases, such cells were rare in 11 cases and more prominent in 3 cases (76). Immunohistochemical stains confirm the nonepithelial nature of these cells, and help exclude carcinoma in problematic cases.

Nonspecific Granulomatous Prostatitis

The most common form of prostatitis that is clinically suspicious for carcinoma is nonspecific granulomatous prostatitis, a subtype that ac-

counts for approximately 3 percent of cases of prostatitis (67,72–74,75,79–81). In one series, nonspecific granulomatous prostatitis caused clinical suspicion of cancer in 55 percent of the cases (73).

On gross inspection, firm, yellow nodules and cystically dilated ducts containing inspissated material may be visible. The characteristic microscopic appearance is that of a mixed inflammatory cell infiltrate containing histiocytes, neutrophils, eosinophils, lymphocytes, plasma cells, and giant cells (fig. 7-31). The "granulomatous" nature of the infiltrate is not always pronounced; discrete tuberculoid granulomas are exceptional. Multinucleate giant cells are absent or rare in approximately two thirds of cases (74). The inflammatory cells often surround dilated ducts which typically have an eroded lining and contain inspissated secretion with neutrophils, eosinophils, and desquamated epithelial cells. In older lesions the ducts are often obliterated by the

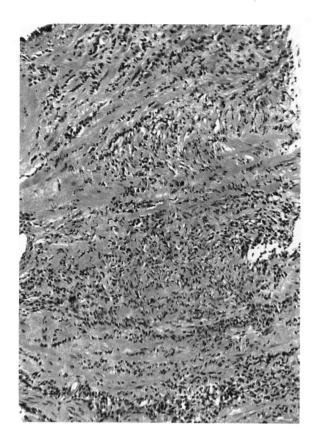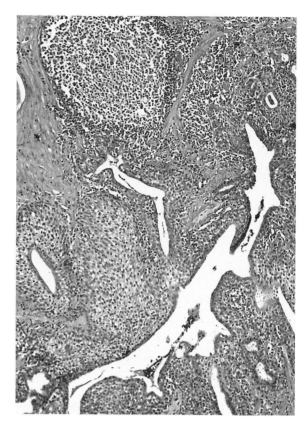

Figure 7-30
CHRONIC PROSTATITIS
Left: This biopsy specimen exhibits considerable squeeze artifact, and at this magnification the possibility of carcinoma is raised.
Right: A lymphoid follicle with a germinal center is conspicuous (follicular prostatitis).

inflammatory process, and there may be extensive fibrosis. This condition is thought to result from duct obstruction with stasis, leading to rupture and a granulomatous inflammatory reaction to the extruded material. Unless the picture approaches that of an infectious granulomatous process to at least some degree, special stains are not indicated.

In needle biopsies, nonspecific granulomatous prostatitis is more difficult to differentiate from carcinoma than in prostatectomy or transurethral resection specimens where the diagnostically helpful architecture is more easily appreciated. In needle core material the association with ducts is rarely obvious and, because of a frequently diffuse pattern, the suspicion of high-grade cancer may result, a problem that occurred in 4 percent of the cases in one series (74). Although high-grade carcinomas usually have cytologic features that indicate a neoplastic nature, some lack conspic-

uous atypia. Appreciation of the inflammatory nature of the cells, the presence of giant cells, and a fibrotic appearance are all helpful. Negative immunostains for prostatic and other epithelial markers may help resolve the occasional problematic case (75).

Granulomatous Prostatitis, Infectious

Tuberculosis and a variety of other infections may cause abnormalities within the prostate gland that are suspicious for carcinoma on clinical examination (62,69,71,78). Tuberculosis is usually encountered in patients with established disease in other areas of the genitourinary system (71), and there is also often lung disease, although rarely the prostatic involvement is apparently isolated.

In his classic account of tuberculosis of the prostate, Moore (71) described the gross characteristics as "grayish yellow or yellow and rubbery or

311

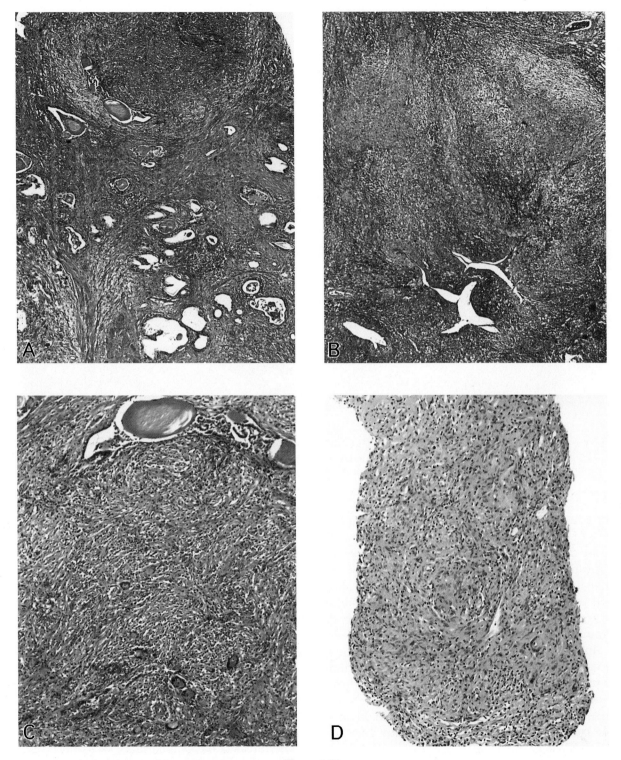

Figure 7-31
NONSPECIFIC GRANULOMATOUS PROSTATITIS
A: The process is focal within a transurethral resection specimen.
B: Several residual ducts are seen at the bottom, but at the top the ducts are effaced by the inflammatory infiltrate.
C: A high-power view of A shows sheets of histiocytes with admixed lymphocytes, giant cells, and fibroblasts.
D: A needle biopsy shows replacement of normal parenchyma by the granulomatous infiltrate.

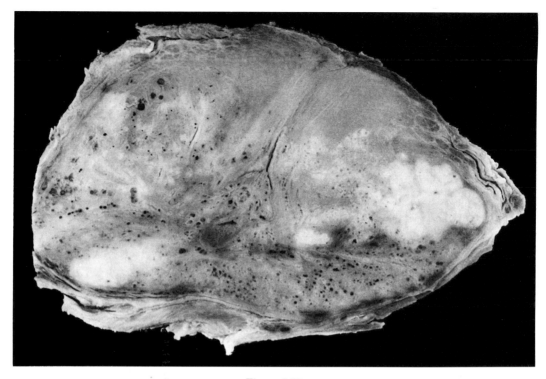

Figure 7-32
TUBERCULOUS PROSTATITIS
The tuberculous lesion involves primarily the peripheral zone of the right side. Note the tumor-like appearance. (Fig. 2 from Moore RA. Tuberculosis of the prostate gland. J Urol 1937;37:372–84.)

crumbly in consistency" (fig. 7-32). He also commented on the scalloped border of the tuberculous lesion which he contrasted with that of carcinoma, which is also typically firmer in consistency. On microscopic examination the distinction is straightforward, and the infectious nature of the granulomas can often be suspected (fig. 7-33). In these cases special stains are indicated, in contrast to nonspecific granulomatous prostatitis.

Granulomatous Prostatitis, Therapy Related

A form of granulomatous prostatitis that is increasing in frequency results from the use of bacillus Calmette-Guérin (BCG) as therapy for transitional cell carcinoma of the bladder. In one series, these cases caused clinical suspicion of carcinoma more frequently (almost 75 percent) than cases of nonspecific granulomatous prostatitis (74). Correlation with the clinical history is helpful, and the microscopic identification of granulomas is diagnostic. An eosinophilic infiltrate is less common in the BCG-associated pro-

cess than with nonspecific granulomatous prostatitis, whereas multinucleate giant cells are more frequent (74).

Xanthogranulomatous Prostatitis (Xanthoma)

Localized collections of lipid-laden histiocytes in the prostate may cause diagnostic difficulty (64,72,77), although the presence of other admixed inflammatory cells usually facilitates the diagnosis. The xanthomatous histiocytes have small, uniform nuclei and inconspicuous nucleoli (fig. 7-34). These bland cytologic features, the foamy nature of the cytoplasm, and the associated inflammatory cells of other types are clues to the diagnosis, but the first two features, in particular, are seen in some cancers of the "foamy gland" group (see page 148); furthermore, some cases of xanthogranulomatous prostatitis are almost purely composed of xanthoma cells ("prostatic xanthoma"[77]), and the lack of other associated inflammatory cells may be diagnostically confusing. However, the cancers

313

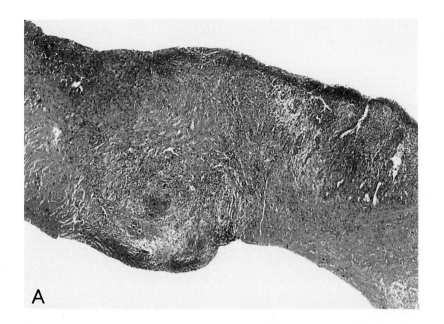

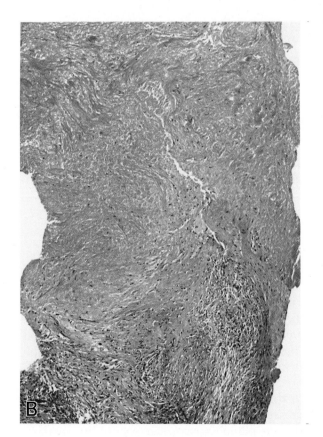

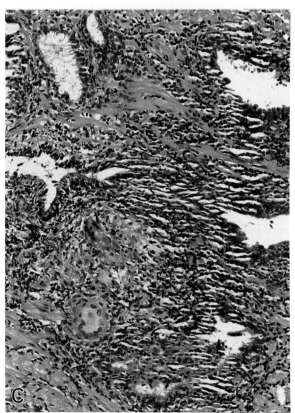

Figure 7-33
TUBERCULOUS PROSTATITIS

A: A needle biopsy shows replacement of normal parenchyma by the infectious process.

B: There is focal extensive caseous necrosis.

C: In other areas residual prostatic glands and stroma are seen with granulomas in the stroma. (Case 43 from Case Records of the Massachusetts General Hospital. N Engl J Med 1972;287:872–8.)

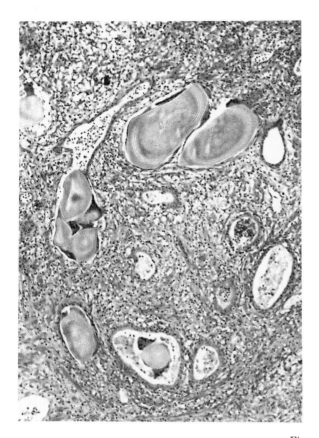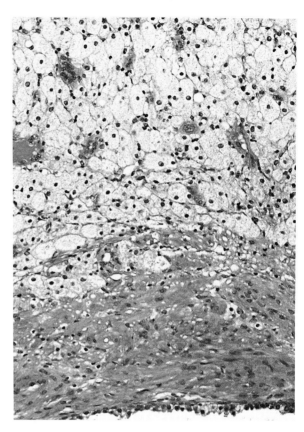

Figure 7-34
XANTHOGRANULOMATOUS PROSTATITIS (XANTHOMA)
Left: The mixed inflammatory infiltrate is helpful for diagnosis.
Right: Histiocytes with abundant foamy cytoplasm and small shrunken nuclei predominate. (Courtesy of Dr. D.J. Grignon, Detroit, MI.)

may show either acinar differentiation or invasive architectural features that are diagnostic. Immunohistochemical stains highlighting the histiocytic nature of the cells are helpful in a particularly difficult case, usually one in which the tissue sample is so small that associated findings to aid in the diagnosis are lacking.

Other Forms of Granulomatous Prostatitis Including Procedure Related

A complete list of the miscellaneous causes of granulomatous prostatitis is presented in Table 7-3 (85a). Many of these are infectious, but some are iatrogenic (82–88) or associated with systemic diseases (85a). Although these may be challenging diagnoses, both clinically and pathologically, and some may mimic a neoplasm on clinical or gross evaluation, their non-neoplastic nature is usually straightforward on microscopic examination.

The granulomas that occur after a recent procedure, usually a transurethral resection but occasionally a biopsy, have a characteristic central region of fibrinoid necrosis surrounded by palisading, epithelioid histiocytes and often a very characteristic, irregular, serpiginous shape (fig. 7-35) (82–88). The latter is helpful in distinguishing them from infectious granulomas, as is the history of a prior procedure. Nonspecific foreign body giant cell granulomas may also be seen in these cases, and, when the procedure is recent, eosinophils may be conspicuous. The latter should not lead to confusion with cases of granulomatous prostatitis that have an allergic basis. In contrast to the latter, the procedure-related granulomas have eosinophils localized around the granuloma rather than diffusely infiltrating the stroma. Nonetheless, clinical correlation may be required in occasional cases with overlapping

315

Table 7-3
CLASSIFICATION OF GRANULOMATOUS PROSTATITIS*

Infectious
  Bacterial
    Tuberculosis
    Brucellosis
    Syphilis
  Fungal
    Coccidioidomycosis
    Cryptococcosis
    Blastomycosis
    Histoplasmosis
    Paracoccidioidomycosis
  Parasitic
    Schistosomiasis
    Echinococcosis
    Enterobiasis
  Viral
    Herpes virus infection

Iatrogenic
  Postsurgical
  Postradiation
  BCG**-induced
  Teflon-associated

Malakoplakia

Systemic granulomatous disease
  Allergic ("eosinophilic")
  Sarcoidosis
  Rheumatoid arthritis
  Autoimmune-vascular
    Wegener's granulomatosis
    Polyarteritis nodosa
    Benign lymphocytic angiitis and granulomatosis
  Churg-Strauss disease

Idiopathic ("nonspecific")
  Typical nonspecific granulomatous prostatitis
  Xanthoma - xanthogranulomatous prostatitis

---

*Modified from Table 2-1 from reference 85a.
**Bacille Calmette-Guérin.

features. Stains for organisms are not indicated in these cases.

Rarely, granulomatous prostatitis is due to foreign material. Teflon was the causative agent in two cases which were clinically suspicious for cancer (86a). Foreign material is recognizable in such cases, and its identification may be aided by viewing with polarized light (fig. 7-36).

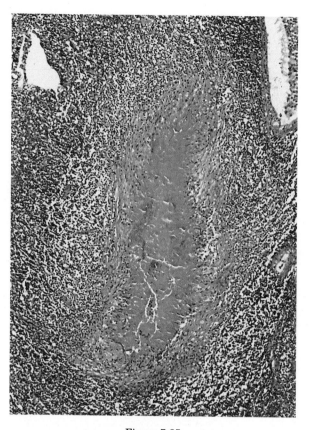

Figure 7-35
NECROTIZING GRANULOMA
POST–TRANSURETHRAL RESECTION
A necrobiotic focus is surrounded by focally palisading epithelioid histiocytes.

MALAKOPLAKIA

Patients with malakoplakia of the prostate gland (89–92) usually have an enlarged gland. As with granulomatous prostatitis, the diffuse arrangement of the cells on microscopic examination may lead to a misdiagnosis of high-grade carcinoma. The level of diagnostic difficulty depends on the phase of the disease. In classic and late stages of the process there is generally no difficulty because in the former there is an admixture of inflammatory cells (lymphocytes, plasma cells, neutrophils, and histiocytes) whereas in the latter the fibrosis imparts a picture dissimilar to that of prostatic carcinoma. However, in the so-called early phase of malakoplakia, where there are numerous histiocytes with eosinophilic cytoplasm (von Hansemann histiocytes; fig. 7-37), the appearance of a carcinoma, particularly of Gleason grade 4, may be simulated. The admixed

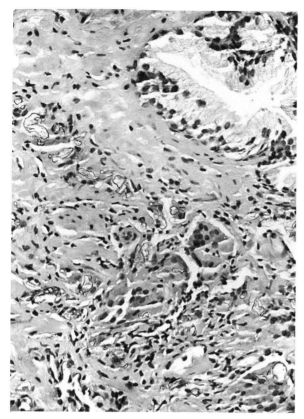

Figure 7-36
TEFLON GRANULOMA
Note the foreign material. (Courtesy Dr. R. Orozco, Oklahoma City, OK.)

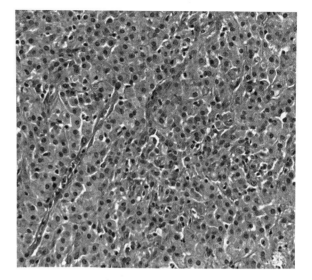

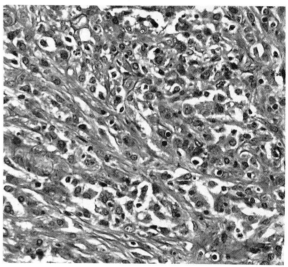

Figure 7-37
MALAKOPLAKIA
Top: There is a sheet-like proliferation of histiocytes with abundant eosinophilic cytoplasm. Michaelis-Gutmann bodies are inconspicuous, potentially resulting in a misdiagnosis of carcinoma.

Bottom: In another case typical targetoid Michaelis-Gutmann bodies are highlighted by a periodic acid-Schiff stain.

inflammatory infiltrate, at least focally, lack of small acinar differentiation, and identification of the typical Michaelis-Gutmann bodies (fig. 7-37, bottom) are all helpful. The immunohistochemical demonstration of histiocytic markers (CD68) and absence of cytokeratins in malakoplakia may resolve this differential diagnosis but are rarely required.

INFLAMMATORY AND MISCELLANEOUS OTHER REACTIVE ATYPIAS

Reactive epithelial atypia in association with acute or chronic prostatitis may be seen but is not, in general, as frequent an interpretative problem in prostatic specimens as it is with specimens from other sites, such as the uterine cervix. Nonetheless, both architectural and cytologic abnormalities are encountered (93,95) which, if the association with inflammation or ischemia is not appreciated, may lead to misinterpretation as carcinoma (fig. 7-38) or the rendering of a nondefinitive opinion. In one series of cases interpreted as "atypical but not diagnostic of cancer" associated inflammation was present in 8 of 200 cases (94). From the architectural viewpoint the prostatic acini may appear atrophic and, in some cases, may be packed together, having a pseudocribriform

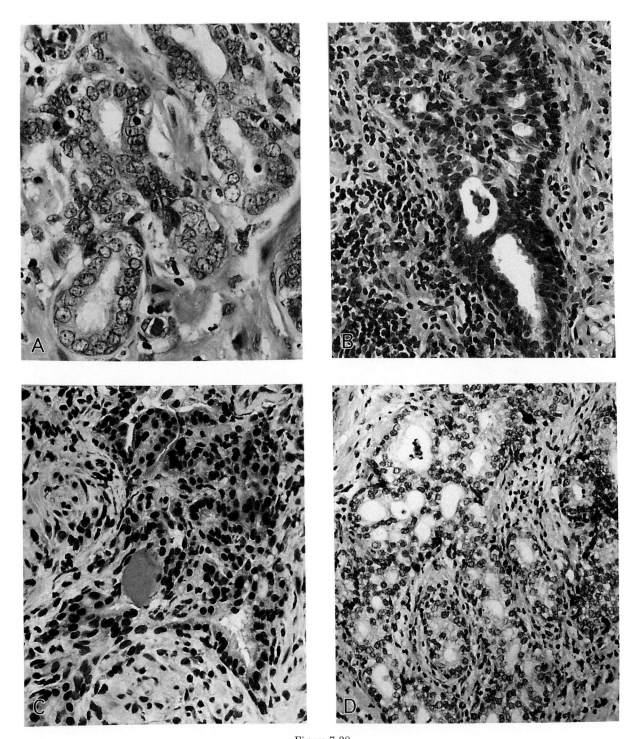

Figure 7-38
INFLAMMATORY ATYPIA IN PROSTATE

A: The closely packed small acini, which show some reactive atypia, may suggest adenocarcinoma. Although nucleoli are easily visible, they are not prominent.

B: There is a component of basal cell-transitional cell hyperplasia. Note the numerous inflammatory cells within the stroma.

C: There is distortion of the architecture which may be confusing, but the lack of cytologic features of carcinoma is apparent in the acinar lining cells.

D: There is a prominent "back-to-back" arrangement. (A–D: Figs. 31.1, 31.2, 31.3, and 31.4 from Epstein JI. Differential diagnosis in pathology. Urologic disorders. New York: Igaku-Shoin, 1992:83.)

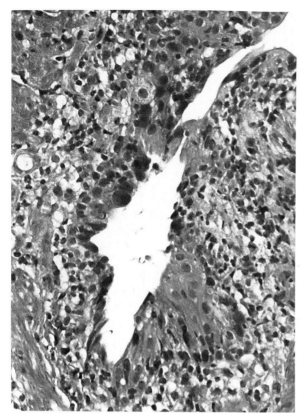

Figure 7-39
INFLAMMATORY ATYPIA IN PROSTATE
The nucleus of one cell is markedly larger than most of the other nuclei. Some of the epithelial cells have an appearance which suggests abortive squamous differentiation. Note the mantle of inflammatory cells around the duct.

appearance (95). From the cytologic viewpoint there may be mild to moderate nuclear enlargement (fig. 7-39) and some degree of nucleolar prominence, although the latter usually does not reach that typically seen in carcinoma. Some degree of basal cell and transitional cell hyperplasia is a relatively frequent finding in cases of reactive atypia, and in some cases a squamoid appearance is seen (fig. 7-39). The presence of basal cells, failure of the cytologic abnormalities to reach a degree usually seen in carcinoma, and the association with inflammation should help avoid a misdiagnosis. Despite the foregoing comments, carcinoma may, of course, coexist with inflammation, but clear-cut architectural or cytologic features are required for its diagnosis. The possibility that lesser degrees of atypia are attributable to inflammation should be carefully evaluated.

RADIATION EFFECT

This is probably the most common form of "reactive atypia" in the prostate, but has a particular etiology and features meriting separate coverage from those in the prior section. Cytologic atypia of non-neoplastic glands, including enlarged and hyperchromatic nuclei with prominent nucleoli, was present in approximately three quarters of radiated prostates in two studies (96,97). The architectural arrangement of atypical but non-neoplastic glands remains relatively normal, a helpful feature in excluding carcinoma. When other obvious changes of radiation injury are present, the cytologic atypia should be conservatively interpreted. In benign glands cytologic atypia involves both secretory and basal cells, resulting in an atypia that has a more heterogeneous appearance than usual in carcinoma. The "spotty" nature of the atypia, being seen in some acini and not in others, is also often helpful (fig. 7-40). Architecture is usually more reliable than cytology in recognizing residual tumor postradiation. In diagnostically difficult cases a high molecular weight cytokeratin immunostain may be useful as it shows retention of the basal cell layer in benign glands; a concurrent pan cytokeratin stain may help highlight rare infiltrating single neoplastic cells.

Other radiation-induced changes in the prostate include a decrease in the ratio of neoplastic glands to stroma, atrophy, squamous metaplasia and basal cell hyperplasia (that may be atypical), stromal fibrosis with atypical fibroblasts, occasional foreign body giant cells, intimal proliferation of arteries, and foam cells in vessel walls (96,96a,97).

POSTOPERATIVE SPINDLE CELL NODULE AND POST–NEEDLE BIOPSY CHANGES

The designation "postoperative spindle cell nodule" was given in 1984 (101) to a proliferative spindle cell lesion that developed in the lower urinary tract of five men and the lower genital tract of four women. All of the lesions developed within 3 months after a surgical procedure at the same site. Three of the lesions in men were found in transurethral resections of the prostate following a similar procedure.

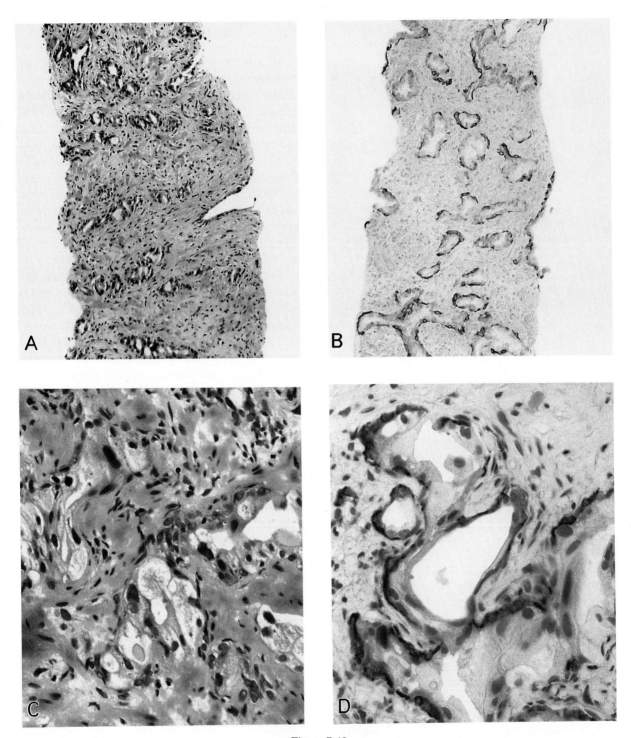

Figure 7-40
RADIATION ATYPIA

A: Low-power examination of a needle biopsy specimen shows shrunken acini with hyperchromatic nuclei that suggest the possibility of adenocarcinoma.

B: High molecular weight cytokeratin (clone 34βE12) shows circumferential staining of basal cells in the acini, supporting a benign diagnosis.

C: The irregular angulated glands, abundant cytoplasm, and nuclear atypia suggest carcinoma.

D: Basal cells are prominently displayed in the same case as C using the high molecular weight cytokeratin immunostain (clone 34βE12).

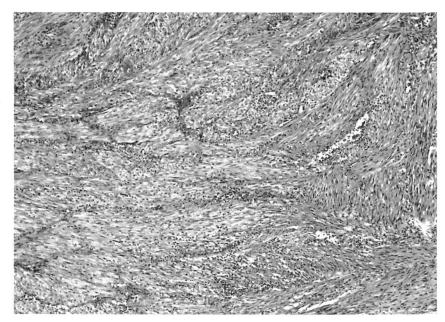

Figure 7-41
POSTOPERATIVE
SPINDLE CELL NODULE
The interlacing fascicles of spindle-shaped cells raise concern for sarcoma, particularly leiomyosarcoma.

Microscopic examination reveals intersecting fascicles of spindle cells (fig. 7-41) which often show striking mitotic activity (up to 25 mitotic figures per 10 high-power fields), resulting in a marked resemblance to a sarcoma. The cells, however, do not exhibit high-grade cytologic atypia (fig. 7-42). Additional microscopic features include prominent blood vessels, which are often small; scattered acute and chronic inflammatory cells; small foci of hemorrhage; mild to moderate edema; and focal myxoid change in the stroma. In some cases the stigmata of a previous procedure may be seen in the form of a granulomatous process with fibrinoid change, and this is a helpful circumstantial finding.

The clinical association with a recent operation is the major initial clue that these lesions represent an exuberant reactive proliferation, an interpretation supported by the benign outcome after conservative management of most of the initially and subsequently reported cases (99–101). In spite of the great number of cases of genitourinary instrumentation, this pathologic complication remains rare but may be diagnostically treacherous.

Although other sarcomas, such as Kaposi's sarcoma, occasionally are suggested, leiomyosarcoma is usually the major consideration in the differential diagnosis. Distinction from a moderate to poorly differentiated leiomyosarcoma is not difficult since the atypia in these

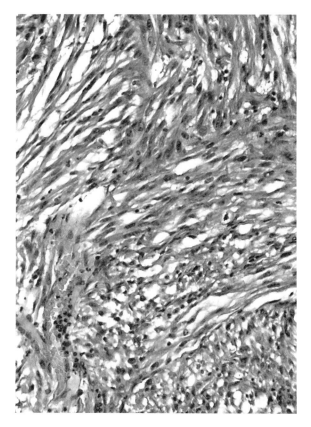

Figure 7-42
POSTOPERATIVE SPINDLE CELL NODULE
High-power evaluation shows prominent nucleoli in occasional cells but a lack of high-grade cytologic atypicality and, in this area, a paucity of mitotic figures, although the latter may be conspicuous in this process.

cases exceeds that seen in a postoperative spindle cell nodule. However, some well-differentiated leiomyosarcomas are not much more atypical than a postoperative spindle cell nodule and may be less mitotically active. Although leiomyosarcomas may be vascular, they lack the often prominent delicate network of small blood vessels that is seen in many postoperative spindle cell nodules. Necrosis, infiltrative growth, and cytologic anaplasia favor the diagnosis of sarcoma. Often the distinction between these two processes is dependent on the clinical history of a recent operative procedure.

Rarely, an exuberant spindle cell proliferation may be seen in the prostate after a recent needle biopsy procedure, but the presence of such change along a recognizable biopsy tract as well as other obvious reactive changes facilitate its diagnosis. A variety of changes were observed in 62 needle tracts encountered in 37 radical prostatectomy specimens (98). The tracts typically consisted of partially collapsed cavities, often filled with red blood cells and rimmed by a mixed acute and chronic inflammatory infiltrate including eosinophils, lymphocytes, and macrophages. Granulation tissue, hemosiderin pigment, and fibrosis were usually restricted to the edge of the cavities. Multinucleated giant cells were seen in 10 percent of the cases.

INFLAMMATORY PSEUDOTUMOR (PSEUDOSARCOMATOUS FIBROMYXOID TUMOR)

This rare lesion of the prostate gland is similar to the more common inflammatory pseudotumor of the urinary bladder. In reports on the prostate, the term "pseudosarcomatous fibromyxoid tumor" has been used, but we prefer the designation "inflammatory pseudotumor" to highlight the resemblance to the urinary bladder lesion and similar lesions at various sites in the body. Only a few prostatic examples have been encountered to date, all in adults (102,103). There may be significant enlargement of the prostate gland, mimicking a neoplasm. On microscopic examination there is a proliferation of spindle cells in a loose, edematous to myxoid stroma that is prominently vascular and typically contains many acute and chronic inflammatory cells (fig. 7-43). In many areas the process has an appearance reminis-

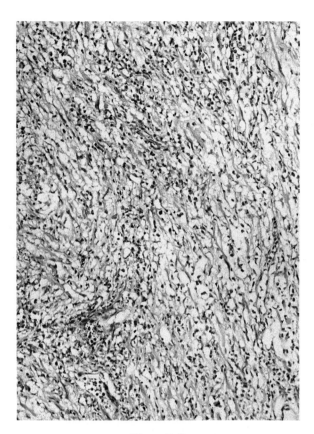

Figure 7-43
INFLAMMATORY PSEUDOTUMOR
(PSEUDOSARCOMATOUS FIBROMYXOID TUMOR)
Note the relatively acellular pale background and many inflammatory cells.

cent of very exuberant granulation tissue. The nuclei of the spindle-shaped cells may be moderately hyperchromatic with a mild degree of pleomorphism, and there is often abundant eosinophilic cytoplasm (fig. 7-44); these features could potentially lead to confusion with rhabdomyoblasts. Mitoses are usually seen, but atypical mitotic figures are not. Immunohistochemical and ultrastructural examination has shown features of myofibroblasts.

Although this process is, in some ways, similar to the postoperative spindle cell nodule, it tends to have a looser, dispersed, less compact arrangement of spindle cells, and the lack of a history of a recent operative procedure is a defining difference between the two entities. The differential diagnosis with sarcoma is aided by the inflammatory, granulation tissue-like background and lack of severe pleomorphism.

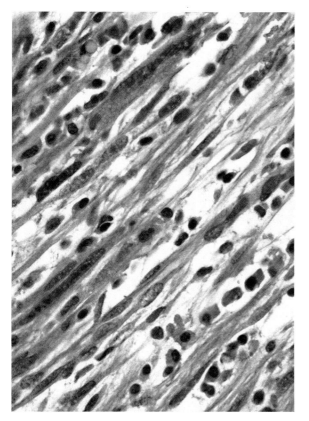

Figure 7-44
INFLAMMATORY PSEUDOTUMOR
(PSEUDOSARCOMATOUS FIBROMYXOID TUMOR)
The spindle cells have features consistent with myofibroblasts and are separated by inflammatory cells.

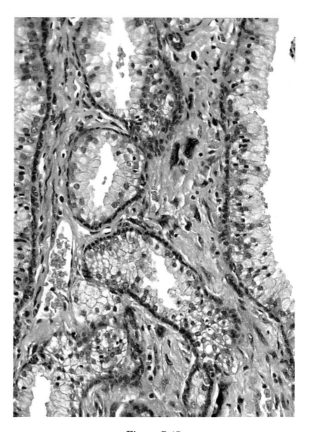

Figure 7-45
BENIGN PROSTATIC HYPERPLASIA
WITH ATYPICAL STROMAL CELLS
Note the bizarre hyperchromatic nuclei with smudged nuclear chromatin and lack of mitotic figures in the atypical cells.

ATYPICAL STROMAL CELLS

Pleomorphic, hyperchromatic nuclei may be seen in the prostatic stromal cells between the epithelial elements in otherwise unremarkable cases of benign prostatic hyperplasia (fig. 7-45) (104,106,109–112), in circumscribed benign fibromuscular nodules in which smooth muscle typically predominates, in leiomyomas, and in frank sarcomas and mixed epithelial-stromal tumors (107) (see page 277). In one study of 11 cases of stromal hyperplasia with atypia, 4 occurred in the first setting, referred to as the "infiltrative pattern," and 7 in the second setting, the "leiomyomal-like pattern" (111). In the latter cases immunoreactivity for desmin was typically intense, confirming the smooth muscle nature of the majority of the cells in the nodules.

It is important to be aware that malignant neoplasms of the prostate (see Table 6-2) may contain atypical cells similar to those that occur either in nodular hyperplasia or fibromuscular nodules. The distinction of the latter two entities from the former, however, depends on the absence of a mass, the lack of stromal hypercellularity or phyllodes-type architecture, the degenerative nuclear appearance with smudged chromatin, and the lack of mitoses. Distinction of degenerative stromal atypia from the atypicality seen within neoplasms may be very difficult in a limited sampling, and, as recommended by Gaudin and colleagues (107), the designation "prostatic stromal proliferation of uncertain malignant potential" is justified in such cases to alert the clinician to this uncertainty.

MISCELLANEOUS OTHER STROMAL ABNORMALITIES

An exceptionally rare consideration in the differential diagnosis of unusual stromal lesions is *extramedullary hematopoiesis* which has been described in the prostate in one case (108). It contained, as characteristic of this disorder, atypical megakaryocytes that could conceivably be mistaken for atypical stromal cells. The association of these cells with immature granulocytes and normoblasts facilitates the correct diagnosis.

In one patient who underwent radical prostatectomy and received collagen injections for subsequent urinary incontinence, the injected material resulted in a mass in the prostatic fossa that was suspicious for recurrent carcinoma on clinical evaluation. Histologic examination showed nodules of dense collagen easily distinguishable from carcinoma (105).

In occasional cases of prostatic hyperplasia the stroma is the predominant or sole hyperplastic component (see chapter 2). Nodules can be seen on gross examination, but the overall background is that of conventional hyperplasia, for the most part. On microscopic examination the bland appearance of the lesional cells, the frequently prominent, delicate vascularity, and the usual presence of multiple nodules of conventional hyperplasia permit distinction from a mesenchymal neoplasm. True leiomyomas of the prostate do occur but are rare in our experience, and it is largely a matter of personal preference whether one considers some dominant leiomyomatous nodules to represent nodular hyperplasia or true leiomyoma. This distinction has no clinical significance.

LIPOFUSCIN AND MELANIN PIGMENT IN THE PROSTATE, INCLUDING BLUE NEVUS

The prostate gland can show two distinct types of pigment: lipofuscin and melanin (113–124). The latter is seen in true melanocytic lesions involving the prostate, blue nevus and malignant melanoma, but the former is more common and seen chiefly in prostatic epithelium.

There is some confusion in the literature regarding the terminology of both types of pigment, as they have been interchangeably described under various terms including melanosis, epithelial melanosis, melanin-like pigment, lipochrome, and lipofuscin. The term melanosis has been used for grossly apparent pigmented lesions (often blue nevi) or for pigment within the epithelium and stroma (most often lipofuscin). Other authors have used the term melanosis for epithelial pigment only. We recommend that the pigment in the prostate be classified according to the type—that is, either melanin or lipofuscin.

Blue nevus of the prostate histologically resembles its cutaneous counterpart in several aspects and is characterized by a spindle cell proliferation, often with long dendritic processes. Grossly, the pigment may impart a striking black discoloration to the prostatic parenchyma (fig. 7-46), potentially leading to the consideration of malignant melanoma. The pigment is usually abundant within the spindle cells, often obscuring them (fig. 7-47), but may also be dispersed extracellularly within and between collagen fibers. The exuberant pigmentation may be imbibed by adjacent epithelial cells. Histologically, the pigment is granular and brown or black, and histochemically it is identical to melanin (Fontana-Masson positive, bleached by permanganate reaction, and negative for Luxol fast blue, oil red O, or Ziehl Neelsen stain). Immunohistochemical studies show S-100 protein positivity (123). Ultrastructural studies have shown melanosomes in different stages of maturation in the lesional cells, and only mature melanosomes in the epithelial cells (123,124). Less than 30 cases have been described.

Lipofuscin pigment (fig. 7-48) has been reported in benign epithelium (up to 100 percent of cases), high-grade prostatic intraepithelial neoplasia (30 to 78 percent), and occasional prostatic adenocarcinomas (13 reported cases) (113, 115,119). The variation in the reported frequency of lipofuscin pigment in various benign, premalignant, and neoplastic lesions of the prostate may be explained by a lack of uniform methods of detection (light microscopy versus histochemical staining) and the samples studied (autopsy material, transurethral resection material, or radical prostatectomy). Lipofuscin pigment differs from melanin pigment in being finely granular and yellow, yellow-brown (fig. 7-48A), or blue (fig. 7-48B); it is seen predominantly in epithelial cells. Sometimes the pigment has a

Table 7-4

**CONTRASTING FEATURES OF PROSTATIC
AND SEMINAL VESICULAR LIPOFUSCIN PIGMENT**

	Pigment in Seminal Vesicle	**Pigment in Prostatic Epithelium**
Frequency	Common, usually prominent (increases with age)	Common, usually inconspicuous and focal
Location	Throughout epithelium	Usually basal, throughout when florid
Granularity	Usually coarse, droplet-like, refractile	Usually finely granular, rarely coarse
Color	Golden yellow to brown	Yellow-brown, yellow, or blue

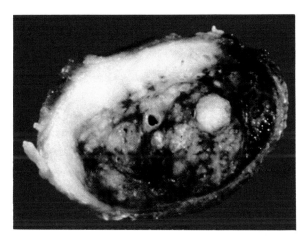

Figure 7-46
BLUE NEVUS OF PROSTATE
A cross section of a prostatectomy specimen shows local-ized, extensive, jet black discoloration of the parenchyma. (Courtesy of Dr. L. Lu, Winnipeg, Canada.)

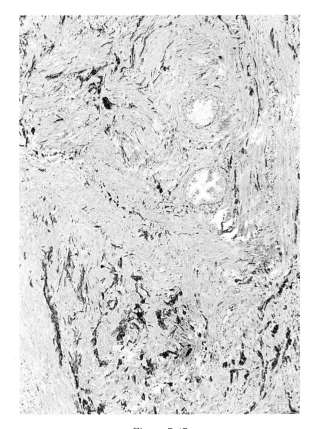

Figure 7-47
BLUE NEVUS OF PROSTATE
A photomicrograph of the specimen in figure 7-46 shows extensive golden brown, granular, melanocytic pigment within elongated cells.

central pallor with an accentuated rim. It can be found in all zones of the prostate (113), although one study has shown predominance in the cen-tral zone (119). Lipofuscin pigment may also be found in oval to spindled cells in the stroma (6 to 78 percent of cases) (fig. 7-48D), but the pigment deposition is typically very focal and by immu-nohistochemistry has been demonstrated to be within macrophages (KP-1 positive). Lipofuscin pigment of the prostate, like that of the seminal vesicle, is positive for Fontana-Masson stain, bleached by the permanganate reaction, and posi-tive for Ziehl Neelsen, Luxol fast blue, and oil red O stains (fig. 7-48C) (115). It is negative immuno-histochemically for S-100 protein (113). It is also ultrastructurally similar to lipofuscin pigment of

the seminal vesicle (115). The pigment is be-lieved to represent an "aging pigment" in which "wear and tear" leads to endogenous lipofuscin-cellular byproducts within the cell. Features of lipofuscin in the prostate and seminal vesicle are contrasted in Table 7-4.

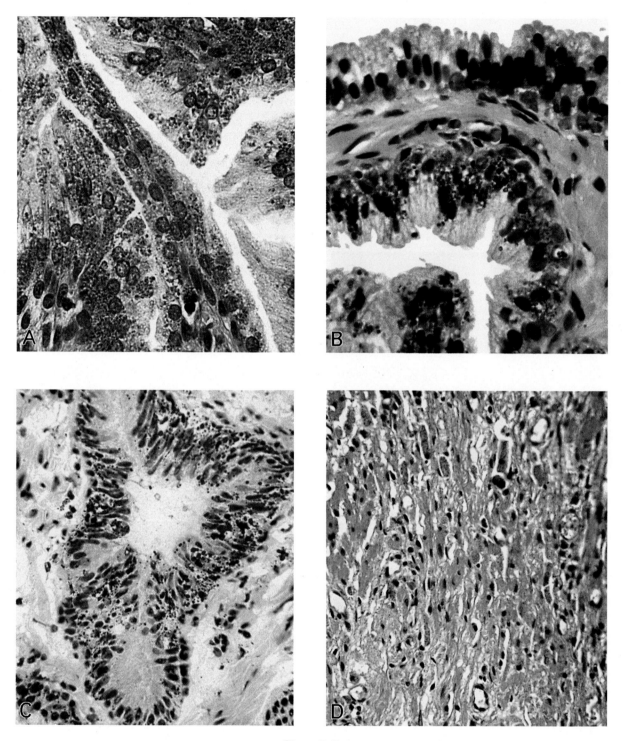

Figure 7-48
LIPOFUSCIN PIGMENT IN PROSTATE

A: Abundant, granular, yellow-brown pigment is present within benign prostatic epithelial cells.

B: Subnuclear, 1 to 3 µm diameter, intraepithelial, grayish blue granules, many with a dark blue rim, are present within benign prostatic epithelial cells.

C: Lipofuscin granules stain with oil red O.

D: Oval to elongated stromal macrophages contain lipofuscin. (Fig. 2E from Brennick JB, O'Connell JX, Dickersin GR, Young RH. Lipofuscin pigmentation (so-called "melanosis") of the prostate. Am J Surg Pathol 1994;18:446–54.)

ENDOMETRIOSIS

Beckman and colleagues (125) described a unique case in which endometriosis involved the prostate of a 78-year-old man who had received estrogen for almost 6 years for treatment of adenocarcinoma of the prostate. The patient developed gross hematuria, and investigation disclosed a small raised area proximal to the internal urethral orifice that was clinically suspicious for a neoplasm. A transurethral resection disclosed involvement of prostatic tissue by endometriosis with the typical glandular and stromal components (fig. 7-49).

NORMAL NONPROSTATIC TISSUE IN PROSTATE SPECIMENS

Seminal Vesicle/Ejaculatory Duct

Seminal vesicle tissue is present in approximately 10 percent of transurethral resection specimens of the prostate and is occasionally seen in needle biopsies (126,132,133,138). The acini of this organ may be closely apposed (see chapter 8), and, as their cells typically exhibit striking nuclear hyperchromasia (fig. 7-50) and pleomorphism, a neoplasm may be simulated. However, although atypical, the nuclei do not show mitotic activity and are paradoxically less uniform and larger than those seen in prostatic carcinoma. Appreciation of these features and the frequent intranuclear inclusions and abundant cytoplasmic golden-brown lipofuscin pigment in the seminal vesical epithelium (fig. 7-50) should help avoid a potentially serious diagnostic error. As noted above, lipofuscin is not rare in prostatic epithelium and its presence should not be considered diagnostic of seminal vesicle, although it is rarely abundant in the prostate. In problematic cases, the absence of PSA and PAP, as well as the presence of basal cells as demonstrated by high molecular weight keratin immunostains, can distinguish seminal vesicle from prostatic carcinoma. This problem is discussed further in chapter 8. Cytologic atypia of the type seen in the seminal vesicle also occurs in the ejaculatory duct. When carcinoma abuts the seminal vesicle or ejaculatory duct the formations of the normal structure may be misconstrued as representing a pattern of the neoplasm (fig. 7-51).

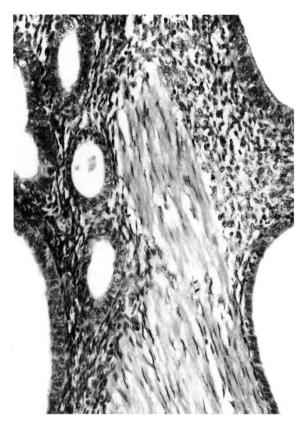

Figure 7-49
ENDOMETRIOSIS OF PROSTATE
Note the endometrioid type glands and stroma. (Courtesy of Dr. E.N. Beckman, New Orleans, LA.)

Cowper's Glands

Cowper's (bulbourethral) glands are rarely seen within a prostatic specimen (127,134,137), and, because of their closely packed acini, can potentially be misinterpreted as prostatic adenocarcinoma. The acini of Cowper's glands resemble minor salivary glands with a lobular arrangement (128) and are associated with excretory ducts and skeletal muscle (fig. 7-52). The cells lining the acini are not atypical, and their small regular nuclei lack prominent nucleoli; the cytoplasm is typically voluminous, frothy, and mucinous. Although well-differentiated prostatic adenocarcinomas typically have glands that are closely packed and may occur in lobular aggregates, their organization is not as strikingly uniform as that exhibited by Cowper's glands, and they have atypical cytologic features. Proving the mucinous nature of the abundant cytoplasm

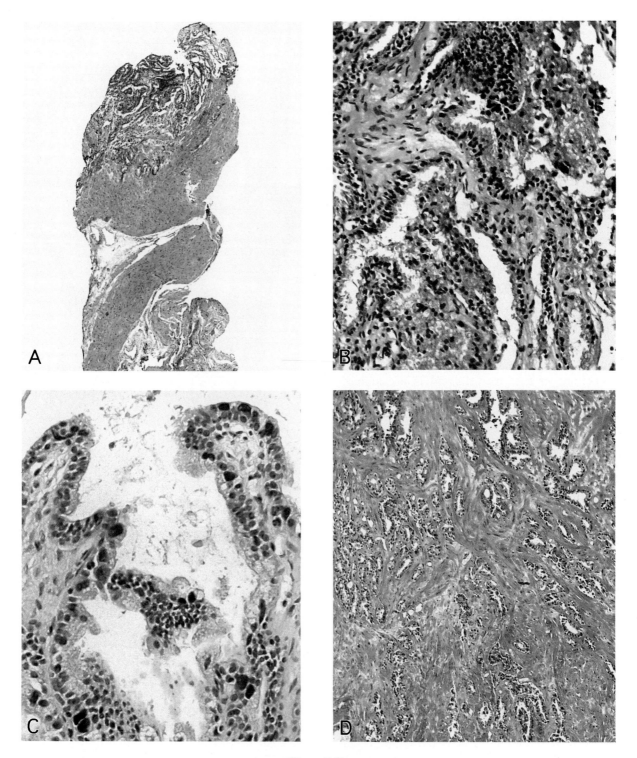

Figure 7-50
POTENTIALLY PROBLEMATIC ASPECTS OF NORMAL SEMINAL VESICLE
OBTAINED WHEN EVALUATING THE PROSTATE GLAND
A: Seminal vesicle tissue in prostatic needle biopsy.
B: Spotty atypical epithelial cells and cytoplasmic pigmentation.
C: High-power photomicrograph shows enlarged hyperchromatic nuclei with degenerative atypia.
D: Adenotic pattern of seminal vesicle simulating small acinar carcinoma.

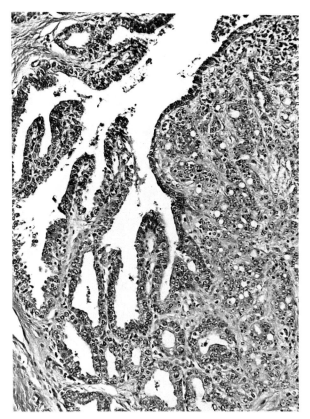

Figure 7-51
EJACULATORY DUCT WITH
ADJACENT PROSTATIC CARCINOMA

There is abundant lipofuscin pigment in the ejaculatory duct epithelium. The association with carcinoma may potentially lead to the normal structure being considered part of the neoplastic proliferation.

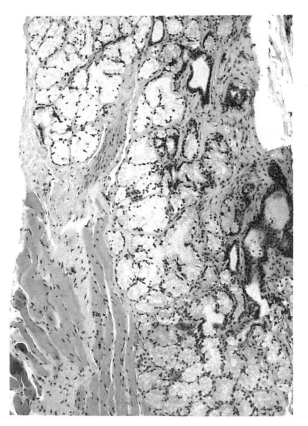

Figure 7-52
COWPER'S GLANDS IN
PROSTATIC NEEDLE BIOPSY SPECIMEN

Note the excretory duct; uniform, voluminous, pale cytoplasm; and nearby skeletal muscle.

by appropriate special stains is also helpful in the differential diagnosis with prostatic adenocarcinoma. Recent studies have provided conflicting results concerning staining of Cowper's glands for high molecular weight cytokeratin (127,137); PSA and PAP are negative.

Verumontanum

Verumontanum mucosal glands are infrequently encountered in prostate needle biopsy specimens (131). In a study of over 30 radical prostatectomy specimens, 14 percent contained one or more foci of hyperplasia of the glands of the verumontanum (130). Because of the closely packed small acini (fig. 7-53A), the process can be confused with prostatic adenocarcinoma on needle biopsy. Findings helpful in indicating the

non-neoplastic nature of this process include awareness of the histologic features of the glands of the verumontanum, including the distinctive orange-brown luminal secretions (fig. 7-53B), the presence of basal cells (fig. 7-53C), the lack of prominent nucleoli, and the frequent lipofuscin pigment. Criteria for the distinction between the appearance of the normal verumontanum mucosal glands and verumontanum mucosal gland "hyperplasia" are arbitrary.

Paraganglia

Paraganglia may be present in prostate specimens and may result in a misdiagnosis of cancer (129,135,136). Paraganglia appear as small clusters or nests of cells with clear to eosinophilic or amphophilic cytoplasm and may display a "zellballen" arrangement (fig. 7-54). They usually occur in the periprostatic soft tissue but may

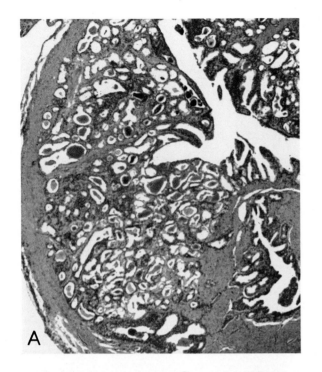

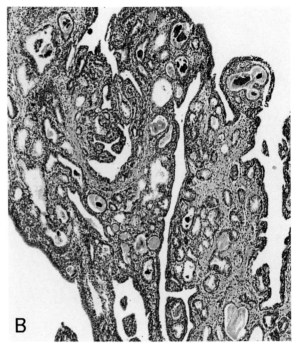

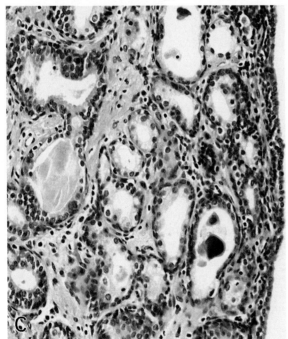

Figure 7-53
VERUMONTANUM MUCOSAL
GLAND HYPERPLASIA

A: Note the closely packed glands and the orange-brown luminal concretions. (Courtesy of Dr. T.M. Wheeler, Houston, TX.)

B: There is a papillary pattern and also abundant, characteristic, orange-brown luminal concretions.

C: Basal cells are evident.

rarely be present in the lateral prostatic stroma. Nuclear atypia may provoke concern for carcinoma, but the atypia has the dense chromatin quality and focality typical of degenerative atypia. Paraganglia should be recognizable on routine stains, but a positive immunoreaction for chromogranin (fig. 7-54C) and negativity for PSA and PAP help in the differential with carcinoma, particularly in needle biopsy specimens. In prostatectomy specimens mistaking paraganglia for carcinoma may result in overstaging an organ-confined cancer as having extraprostatic spread.

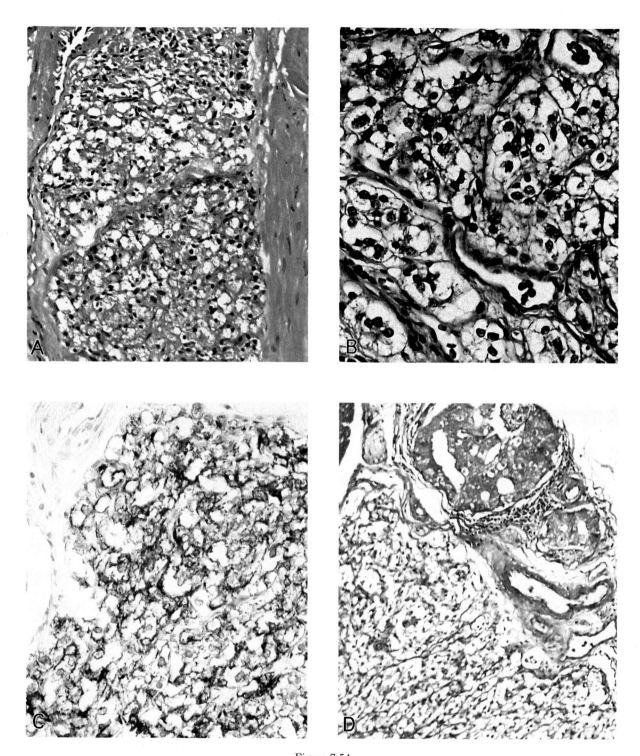

Figure 7-54

PARAGANGLIA IN PROSTATECTOMY SPECIMENS

A: Note the circumscription, bland nuclear features, and abundant dusky cytoplasm.

B: A high-power view shows the characteristic "zellballen" arrangement with sustentacular cells at their periphery. A delicate capillary network is present.

C: A chromogranin immunostain is positive.

D: In another case the juxtaposition of adenocarcinoma (top) with a paraganglion whose cells have striking clear cytoplasm could lead to the latter being considered carcinoma with clear cell features. Note the delicate vascular pattern of the paraganglion.

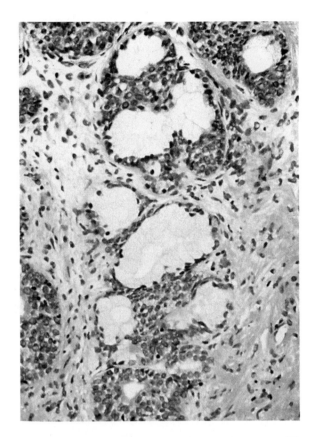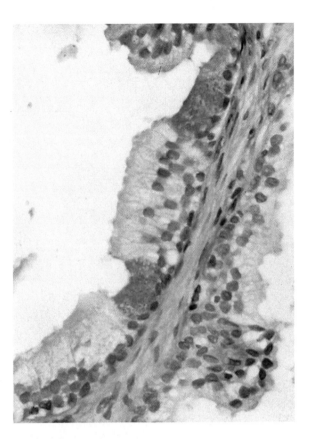

Figure 7-55
MUCINOUS METAPLASIA OF PROSTATE

Left: Prostatic acini showing basal cell hyperplasia also exhibit prominent mucinous metaplasia in the form of tall columnar epithelial cells.

Right: A mucin stain is positive. (Figs. 2-3, 2-4 from Ro JY, Grignon DJ, Amin MB, Ayala A. Atlas of surgical pathology of the male reproductive tract. Philadelphia: WB Saunders, 1997:15.)

MUCINOUS METAPLASIA

Mucinous metaplasia may rarely be seen in the prostate, usually only partially involving acini (fig. 7-55) but infrequently completely replacing the secretory epithelium of a group of acini. This appearance may be mistaken for that of Cowper's glands. It is a finding of no known clinical consequence (139).

BENIGN GLANDS ADJACENT TO NERVES AND IN SKELETAL MUSCLE

Occasionally, benign prostatic glands may be immediately adjacent to nerves (fig. 7-56), without appreciable intervening stroma (140,141,146). The glands rarely completely surround the nerve and are not seen in endothelium-lined spaces. This phenomenon should be distinguished by cyto-

logic criteria from the perineural invasion by malignant glands that occurs with prostatic carcinoma. In our experience, the presence of circumferential perineural invasion is almost invariably diagnostic of adenocarcinoma, and intraneural invasion is diagnostic. The presence of benign glands within the skeletal muscle that occurs normally in the prostate (fig. 7-57), particularly in the region of the apex and anterior fibromuscular stroma, should also not lead to an erroneous diagnosis of malignancy (142–145).

CYSTS

Although never a mimic of a neoplasm on microscopic examination, brief mention of prostatic cysts is appropriate in this chapter since physical examination and imaging studies may be misleading regarding their nature. It has always been

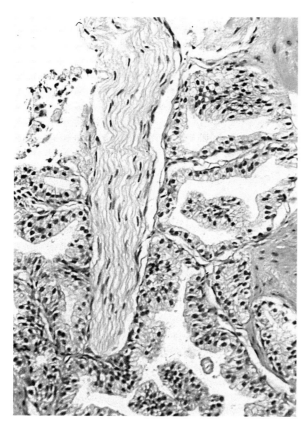

Figure 7-56
BENIGN PROSTATIC GLANDS
PARTIALLY ENVELOPING A NERVE

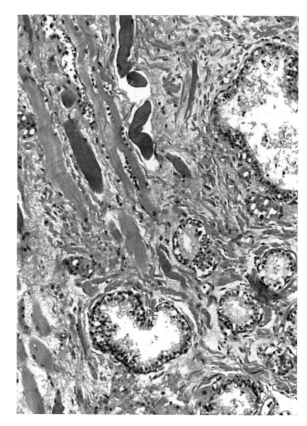

Figure 7-57
BENIGN PROSTATIC GLANDS
ADMIXED WITH SKELETAL MUSCLE

difficult to discriminate between a true cyst and cystic dilations of the prostatic acini which may be seen both as part of a hyperplastic process in the transition zone or an atrophic process in the peripheral zone. Some of the better descriptions are encountered in the older literature, by Wesson in 1924 (153), Magri in 1960 (151), and Emmett and Braasch in 1936 (148). This group, faced with the above problem of distinguishing cysts from cystic dilatations, suggested an arbitrary definition of 0.75 cm, although we feel that realistically a size limit of 3 to 4 cm may be more appropriate.

Wesson (153) classified cysts of the prostate and urethra as congenital cysts, retention cysts, cystic dilation of the utricle (fig. 7-58) and ejaculatory ducts, cysts in connection with cancer, echinococcal cysts (147,150), cysts of Cowper's glands, and Littre gland cysts. A more recent report documents a case of prostatic utricle cyst in a patient with unilateral renal agenesis (149). Dermoid cysts occur rarely in the prostate. One was 10 cm, in

the left lobe, and contained brown paste and hair (152). Most cystic lesions of the prostate occur in the midline and do not contain spermatozoa (a feature of distinction from seminal vesicle cysts; see Table 8-1). They often have a flattened lining, particularly when large (fig. 7-59).

AMYLOIDOSIS

Involvement of the prostate is common in patients with primary amyloidosis, less common but still relatively frequent in patients with secondary amyloidosis, and even sporadically identified in routine specimens from patients without either primary amyloidosis or any chronic illness that would be likely to cause secondary amyloidosis (154–160). There are, however, exceptional cases in which the amyloid deposition in the prostatic stroma has apparently been considered the cause of an abnormality on rectal examination of the prostate, but discerning whether this has been

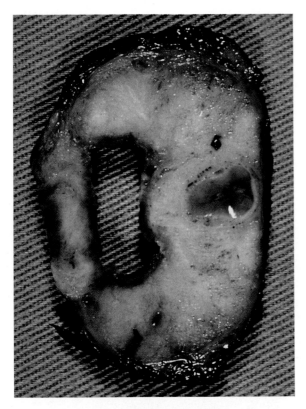

Figure 7-58
CYST OF THE PROSTATIC UTRICLE
The cyst is seen in the posterior midline beneath the verumontanum. Evidence of a prior transurethral resection is seen anteriorly. (Courtesy of Dr. E.C. Jones, Vancouver, BC, Canada.)

due to the amyloidosis or the almost invariable coexisting nodular hyperplasia is difficult if not impossible (159). Microscopic examination shows the typical features (fig. 7-60) and should not be problematic. Corpora amylacea shows a similar staining reaction to that of amyloid (155).

COLLAGENOUS SPHERULOSIS

Very rarely the prostatic ducts contain hyaline spherules with an appearance that has been likened to that of collagenous spherulosis of the breast (fig. 7-61) (161).

CALCULI, CALCIFICATION, CARTILAGINOUS METAPLASIA

Calculi and calcification within the prostate (165,169,172,177) may produce a firm area suspicious for carcinoma clinically (177), but neither poses difficulty in pathologic interpretation. Benign cartilaginous metaplasia of the prostatic stroma has been reported rarely (163).

ECTOPIC PROSTATIC TISSUE

Prostatic tissue itself may form an enigmatic tumor-like lesion when seen beyond the confines of the prostate gland. The most common site for

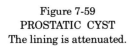

Figure 7-59
PROSTATIC CYST
The lining is attenuated.

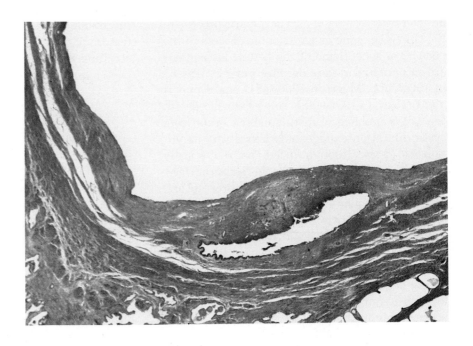

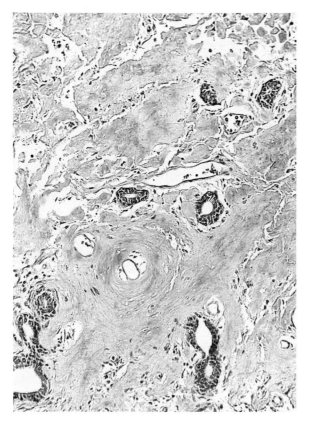

Figure 7-60
AMYLOIDOSIS INVOLVING PROSTATE
The stroma is replaced by homogeneous, eosinophilic, glassy deposits. The prostate gland in this case was clinically suspicious for carcinoma.

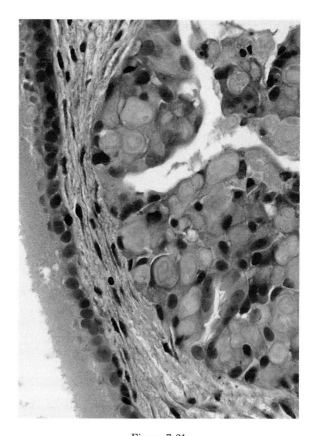

Figure 7-61
COLLAGENOUS SPHERULOSIS OF PROSTATE
Eosinophilic spherical bodies, some with concentric lamellae, are intermixed with epithelial cells in a duct/acinar structure. (Courtesy of Dr. M.R. Melamed, Valhalla, NY.)

such tissue is the urethra, where it often forms a polyp, the so-called prostatic-type polyp (see page 392). These lesions are usually seen in the prostatic urethra but rarely are present in the penile urethra (167). Ectopic prostate may also be found in the wall of the urinary bladder and sometimes in the retrovesicle space, occasionally forming a sizable mass (fig. 7-62) (170). Ectopic prostatic tissue also, rarely, involves the seminal vesicle (176). It should be noted that the seminal vesicle itself may be within the prostate, something that is much more common than prostate within the seminal vesicle. The epididymis (164), testis (174), root of the penis (179), and even pericolic fat (168) have also been documented to harbor prostatic tissue. Surprisingly, although still rare, there are more reported cases of benign prostatic tissue in the uterine cervix (fig. 7-63) than in most genitourinary sites in males. We

know of five cases (166,171,175a), in one of which the process apparently caused a cervical mass.

The most common situation in which benign prostatic tissue is seen beyond the confines of the prostate gland is when it is part of a teratoma; a modest number of examples have been documented in ovarian teratomas (fig. 7-64) (173, 175,178). We have seen one example in a testicular teratoma. The appearance of the prostatic tissue in these cases ranges from relatively normal to having the features of prostatic hyperplasia (fig. 7-62C), and the prostatic nature of the epithelial cells can be confirmed by the appropriate immunohistochemical stains (fig. 7-63C). In one case of a retrovesicle mass of prostatic tissue, foci were considered to represent low-grade prostatic intraepithelial neoplasia (170), and even prostatic adenocarcinoma is documented in ectopic prostate tissue (162).

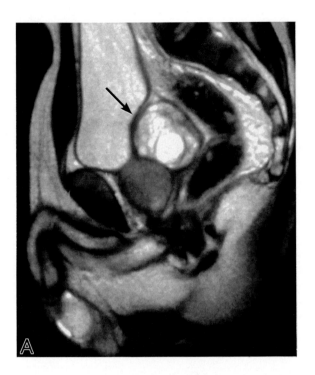

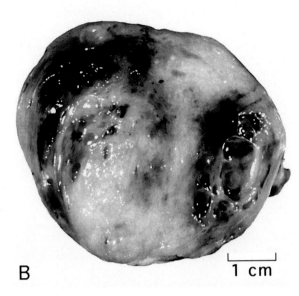

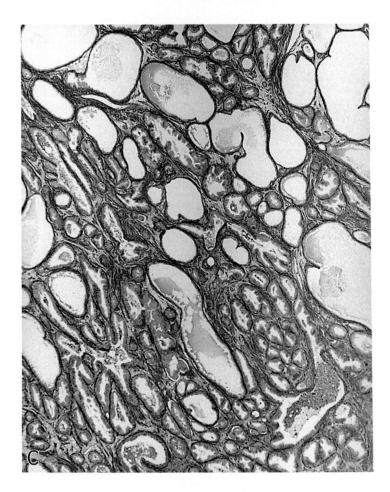

Figure 7-62
ECTOPIC PROSTATIC TISSUE IN RETROVESICLE SPACE

A: A magnetic resonance imaging technique (T2-weighted image) demonstrates the retrovesicle mass (arrow). (Fig. 1 from Kanomata N, Eble JN, Ohbayashi C, Yasui N, Tanaka H, Matsumoto O. Ectopic prostate in the retrovesicle space. J Urol Pathol 1997;7:121–6.)

B: The well-circumscribed, 5 cm mass was yellow-white, with small foci of hemorrhage and contains small cysts. (Fig. 2 from Kanomata N, Eble JN, Ohbayashi C, Yasui N, Tanaka H, Matsumoto O. Ectopic prostate in the retrovesicle space. J Urol Pathol 1997;7:121–6.)

C: Microscopic examination shows hyperplastic dilated glands of prostatic type. (Fig. 3 from Kanomata N, Eble JN, Ohbayashi C, Yasui N, Tanaka H, Matsumoto O. Ectopic prostate in the retrovesicle space. J Urol Pathol 1997;7:121–6.)

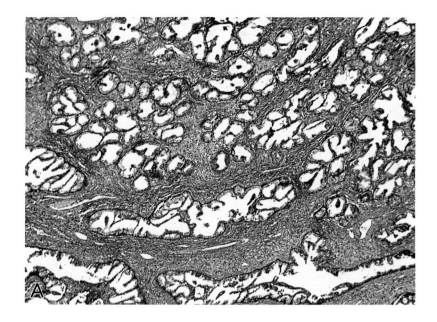

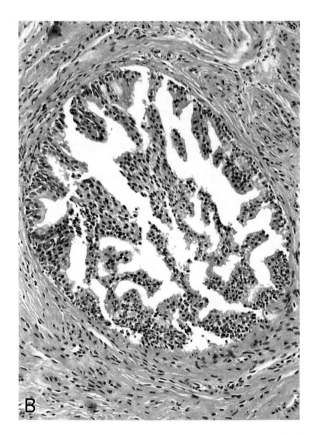

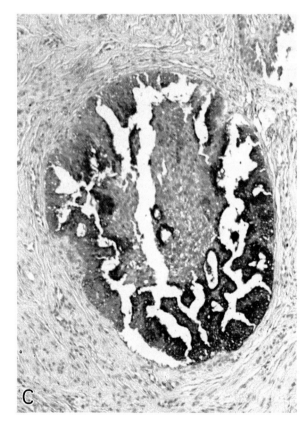

Figure 7-63

ECTOPIC PROSTATIC TISSUE IN UTERINE CERVIX

A: This is a low-power view of a lesion that formed a cervical mass.

B: A high-power view of an incidentally discovered microscopic focus of prostate in another case shows the characteristic features of normal prostate.

C: Immunostaining for the case in B is positive for prostate-specific antigen.

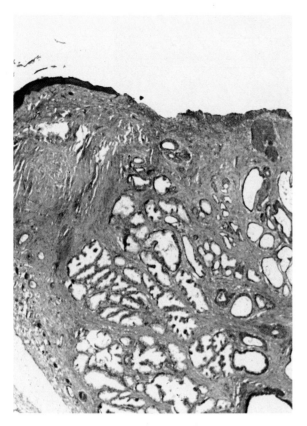
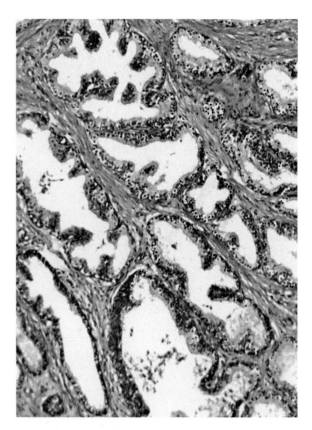

Figure 7-64
PROSTATIC TISSUE IN OVARIAN DERMOID CYST
Left: A squamous epithelial lining is seen at the top.
Right: Higher magnification of the prostatic tissue seen on the left.

REFERENCES

General References

1. Bostwick DG, Dundore PA. Biopsy pathology of the prostate. New York: Chapman and Hall, 1997.
2. Bostwick DG, Iczkowski KA. Minimal criteria for the diagnosis of prostate cancer on needle biopsy. Ann Diagn Pathol 1997;1:104–29.
3. Epstein JI. Diagnostic criteria of limited adenocarcinoma of the prostate on needle biopsy. Hum Pathol 1995;26:223–9.
4. Epstein JI. Differential diagnosis in pathology: urologic disorders. Igaku-Shoin, New York, 1992.
5. Foster CS, Bostwick DG. Pathology of the prostate. In: LiVolsi VA, ed. Major problems in pathology, vol. 34. Philadelphia: WB Saunders, 1998.
6. Jones EC, Young RH. The differential diagnosis of prostatic carcinoma. Its distinction from premalignant and pseudocarcinomatous lesions of the prostate gland. Am J Clin Pathol 1994;101:48–64.
7. Kovi J. Microscopic differential diagnosis of small acinar adenocarcinoma of prostate. Pathol Annu 1985;20(Pt. I):157–96.
8. Mostofi FK, Sesterhenn IA, Davis CJ. Prostatic carcinoma: problems in the interpretation of prostatic biopsies. Hum Pathol 1992;23:223–41.
9. Srigley JR. Small-acinar patterns in the prostate gland with emphasis on atypical adenomatous hyperplasia and small-acinar carcinoma. Semin Diagn Pathol 1988;5:254–72.
10. Totten RS, Heinemann MW, Hudson PB, Sproul EE, Stout AP. Microscopic differential diagnosis of latent carcinoma of prostate. Arch Pathol 1953;55:131–41.
11. Young RH. Pseudoneoplastic lesions of the prostate gland. Pathol Annu 1988;23(Pt. 1):105–28.

Atrophy and Postatrophic Hyperplasia

12. Amin MB, Tamboli P, Varma M, Srigley JR. Post-atrophic hyperplasia of the prostate gland. a detailed analysis of its morphology in needle biopsy specimens. Am J Surg Pathol 1999;8:925–31.
13. Billis A. Prostatic atrophy: an autopsy study of a histologic mimic of adenocarcinoma. Mod Pathol 1998;11:47–54.
14. Cheville JC, Bostwick DG. Post-atrophic hyperplasia of the prostate. A histologic mimic of prostatic adenocarcinoma. Am J Surg Pathol 1995;19:1068–76.
15. Civantos F, Marcial MA, Banks ER, et al. Pathology of androgen deprivation therapy in prostate carcinoma. Cancer 1995;75:1634–41.
16. Epstein JI, Walsh PC, Sanfilippo F. Clinical and cost impact of second-opinion pathology. Review of prostate biopsies prior to radical prostatectomy. Am J Surg Pathol 1996;20:851–7.
17. Franks LM. Atrophy and hyperplasia in the prostate proper. J Path Bact 1954;68:617–21.
18. Gardner WA Jr, Culberson DE. Atrophy and proliferation in the young adult prostate. J Urol 1987;137:53–6.
19. Keane PF, Ilesley IC, O'Donoghue EP, Parkinson MC. Pathological classification and follow-up of prostatic lesions initially diagnosed as "suspicious of malignancy." Br J Urol 1990;66:306–11.
20. Lewis LG. Precancerous lesions of the prostate. Surg Clin N Am 1950;30:1777–82.
21. Liavag I. Atrophy and regeneration in the pathogenesis of prostatic carcinoma. Acta Pathol Microbiol Scand 1968;73:338–50.
22. Moore RE. The evolution and involution of the prostate gland. Am J Pathol 1936;12:599–624.
23. Oppenheimer JR, Wills ML, Epstein JI. Partial atrophy in prostate needle cores: another diagnostic pitfall for the surgical pathologist. Am J Surg Pathol 1998;22:440–5.
23a. Ruska KM, Sauvageot J, Epstein JI. Histology and cellular kinetics of prostatic atrophy. Am J Surg Pathol 1998;22:1073–7.
24. Totten RS, Heinemann MW, Hudson PB, Sproul EE, Stout AP. Microscopic differential diagnosis of latent carcinoma of prostate. Arch Pathol 1953;55:131–41.
25. Young RH. Pseudoneoplastic lesions of the prostate gland. Pathol Annu 1988;23(Pt. 1):105–28.

Sclerosing Adenosis

26. Chen KT, Schiff JJ. Adenomatoid prostatic tumor. Urology 1983;21:88–9.
27. Grignon DJ, Ro JY, Srigley JR, Troncoso P, Raymond AK, Ayala AG. Sclerosing adenosis of the prostate gland. A lesion showing myoepithelial differentiation. Am J Surg Pathol 1992;16:383–91.
28. Jones EC, Clement PB, Young RH. Sclerosing adenosis of the prostate gland. A clinicopathological and immunohistochemical study. Am J Surg Pathol 1991;15:1171–80.
29. Ronnett BM, Epstein JI. A case showing sclerosis adenosis and an unusual form of basal cell hyperplasia of the prostate. Am J Surg Pathol 1989;13:866–72.
30. Sakamoto N, Tsuneyoshi M, Enjoji M. Sclerosis adenosis of the prostate. Histopathologic and immunohistochemical analysis. Am J Surg Pathol 1991;15:660–7.
31. Young RH, Clement PB. Sclerosing adenosis of the prostate. Arch Pathol Lab Med 1987;111:363–6.

Cribriform Hyperplasia

32. Ayala AG, Srigley JR, Ro JY, Abdul-Karim FW, Johnson DE. Clear cell cribriform hyperplasia of prostate. Report of 10 cases. Am J Surg Pathol 1986;10:665–71.
33. Dhom G. Frühe neoplastiche veranderungen der prostata (early neoplastic changes in the prostate) Verh Dtsch Ges Pathol 1979;63:218–31.
34. Frauenhoffer EE, Ro JY, El-Naggar AK, Ordonez NG, Ayala AG. Clear cell cribriform hyperplasia of the prostate. Immunohistochemical and DNA flow cytometric study. Am J Clin Pathol 1991;95:446–53.
35. Keane PF, Ilesley IC, O'Donoghue EP, Parkinson MC. Pathological classification and follow-up of prostatic lesions initially diagnosed as "suspicious of malignancy." Br J Urol 1990;66:306–11.
36. McNeal JE, Reese JH, Redwine EA, Freiha FS, Stamey TA. Cribriform adenocarcinoma of the prostate. Cancer 1986;58:1714–9.
37. Mostofi FK, Sesterhenn I, Sobin LH. Histological typing of prostatic tumors. International Histological Classification of Tumours, No. 22. Geneva: World Health Organization, 1980.

Mesonephric Remnants and Mesonephric Hyperplasia

38. Amin MB. Florid hyperplasia of mesonephric remnants: yet another differential diagnostic consideration under "small acinar proliferations of the prostate." Adv Anat Pathol 1995;2:108–13.
39. Gikas PW, Del Buono EA, Epstein JI. Florid hyperplasia of mesonephric remnants involving prostate and periprostatic tissue. Possible confusion with adenocarcinoma. Am J Surg Pathol 1993;17:454–60.
39a. Jimenez RE, Raval MF, Spanta R, Sakr W, Grignon DJ. Mesonephric remnants hyperplasia. Pitfall in the diagnosis of prostatic adenocarcinoma. J Urol Pathol 1998;9:83–92.
40. Muir TE, Pacelli A, Farrow GM, Bostwick DG. Mesonephric remnants of the prostate: incidence and clinical significance [Abstract]. Mod Pathol 1997;10:83A.

Nephrogenic Adenoma

41. Daroca PJ, Martin AA, Reed RJ, Krenger SS, Hellstrom WJ. Nephrogenic adenoma of the prostatic urethra. A report of these cases including a case with infiltration of the prostatic stroma. J Urol Pathol 1993;1:157–72.
42. Malpica A, Ro JY, Troncoso P, et al. Nephrogenic adenoma of the prostatic urethra involving the prostate gland: a clinicopathologic and immunohistochemical study of eight cases. Hum Pathol 1994;25:390–5.
43. Oliva E, Young RH. Nephrogenic adenoma of the urinary tract: a review of the microscopic appearance of 80 cases with emphasis on unusual features. Mod Pathol 1995;8:722–30.
44. Young RH. Nephrogenic adenomas of the urethra involving the prostate gland: a report of two cases of a lesion that may be confused with prostatic adenocarcinoma. Mod Pathol 1992;5:617–20.

Squamous Metaplasia

45. Bainborough AR. Squamous metaplasia of prostate following estrogen therapy. J Urol 1952;68:329–36.
46. Culp OS. Squamous metaplasia simulating carcinoma associated with prostatic infarction. Bull John Hopkins Hosp 1939;65:239–49.
47. Fergusson JD, Franks LM. The response of prostatic carcinoma to oestrogen treatment. Br J Surg 1953;40:422–8.
48. Mostofi FK, Morse WH. Epithelial metaplasia in "prostatic infarction." Arch Pathol 1951;51:340–5.
49. Nanson EM. Squamous metaplasia of the prostate gland. Br J Urol 1950;22:394–403.
50. Rezek PR, Coplan MM, Woods FM, Melvin PD. Histological studies of carcinoma of the prostate treated by estrogen. J Urol 1951;66:379–92.
51. Sutton EB, McDonald JR. Metaplasia of the prostatic epithelium: a lesion sometimes mistaken for carcinoma. Am J Clin Pathol 1943;13:607–15.

Transitional Cell Metaplasia/Hyperplasia

52. Yantiss RK, Young RH. Transitional cell "metaplasia" in the prostate gland: a survey of its frequency and features based on over 100 consecutive prostatic biopsy specimens. J Urol Pathol 1997;7:71–80.

Basal Cell Hyperplasia

53. Bennett BD, Gardner WA. Embryonal hyperplasia of the prostate. Prostate 1985;7:411–7.
54. Cleary KR, Choi HY, Ayala AG. Basal cell hyperplasia of the prostate. Am J Clin Pathol 1983;80:850–4.
55. Devaraj LT, Bostwick DG. Atypical basal cell hyperplasia of the prostate. Immunophenotypic profile and proposed classification of basal cell proliferations. Am J Surg Pathol 1993;17:645–59.
56. Epstein JI, Armas OA. Atypical basal cell hyperplasia of the prostate. Am J Surg Pathol 1992;16:1205–14.
57. Grignon DJ, Ro JY, Ordonez NG, Ayala AG, Cleary KR. Basal cell hyperplasia, adenoid basal cell tumor, and adenoid cystic carcinoma of the prostate gland: an immunohistochemical study. Hum Pathol 1988;19:1425–33.
58. Reed RJ. Consultation case: prostate (prostatectomy)—adenoid basal-cell tumor—multifocal basal-cell hyperplasia. Am J Surg Pathol 1984;8:699–704.
59. Tetu B, Srigley JR, Boivin JC, et al. Effect of combination endocrine therapy (LHRH agonist and flutamide) on normal prostate and prostatic adenocarcinoma. Am J Surg Pathol 1991;15:111–20.
60. Young RH, Frierson HF, Mills SE, Kaiser JS, Talbot WH, Bhan AK. Adenoid cystic-like tumor of the prostate gland. A report of two cases and review of the literature on "adenoid cystic carcinoma" of the prostate. Am J Clin Pathol 1988;89:49–56.

Prostatitis (Including Xanthoma)

61. Alguacil-Garcia A. Artifactual changes mimicking signet ring cell carcinoma in transurethral prostatectomy specimens. Am J Surg Pathol 1986;10:795–800.
62. Baker WJ, Graf EC. Tuberculosis in the obstructive prostate gland. J Urol 1951;66:254–62.
63. Bennett BD, Richardson PH, Gardner WA. Histopathology and cytology of prostatitis. In: Lepor H, Lawson R, eds. Prostate diseases. Philadelphia: WB Saunders 1993:399–413.
64. Epstein JI, Hutchins GM. Granulomatous prostatitis: distinction among allergic, nonspecific, and post-transurethral resection lesions. Hum Pathol 1984;15:818–25.
65. Fox H. Nodular histiocytic prostatitis. J Urol 1966;96:372–4.
66. Helpap B. Histological and immunohistochemical study of chronic prostatic inflammation with and without benign prostatic hyperplasia. J Urol Pathol 1994;2:49–64.
67. Kelalis PP, Greene LF, Harrison EG. Granulomatous prostatitis. A mimic of carcinoma of the prostate. JAMA 1965;191:287–9.
68. Lopez-Plaza I, Bostwick DG. Prostatitis. In: Bostwick DG, ed. Pathology of prostate. New York: Churchill Livingstone, 1990:15–30.
69. Menville JG, Priestley JT. Tuberculosis of the male genital tract. A pathologic study. J Urol 1938;40:66–73.

70. Moore RA. Inflammation of the prostate gland. J Urol 1937;38:173–82.

71. Moore RA. Tuberculosis of the prostate gland. J Urol 1937;37:372–84.

72. Myhre E. Chronic inflammation of the urinary tract resembling neoplastic growth. Acta Path Microbiol Scand 1963;59:189–94.

73. O'Dea MJ, Hunting DB, Greene LF. Non-specific granulomatous prostatitis. J Urol 1977;118:58–60.

74. Oppenheimer JR, Kahane H, Epstein JI. Granulomatous prostatitis on needle biopsy. Arch Pathol Lab Med 1997;121:724–9.

75. Presti B, Weidner N. Granulomatous prostatitis and poorly differentiated prostate carcinoma. Their distinction with the use of immunohistochemical methods. Am J Clin Pathol 1991;95:330–4.

76. Schned AR. Artifactual signet ring cells. Am J Surg Pathol 1987;11:736–7.

77. Sebo TJ, Bostwick DG, Farrow GM, Eble JN. Prostatic xanthoma: a mimic of prostate adenocarcinoma. Hum Pathol 1994;25:386–9.

78. Sporer A, Oppenheimer G. Tuberculosis of prostate and seminal vesicles. J Urol 1957;78:278–86.

79. Tanner FH, McDonald JR. Granulomatous prostatitis. A histologic study of a group of granulomatous lesions collected from prostate glands. Arch Pathol 1943;36:358–70.

80. Taylor EW, Wheelis RF, Correa RJ, Gibbons RP, Mason JT, Cummings KB. Granulomatous prostatitis: confusion clinically with carcinoma of the prostate. J Urol 1977;117:316–8.

81. Thompson GJ, Albers DD. Granulomatous prostatitis: a condition which clinically may be confused with carcinoma of prostate. J Urol 1953;69:530–8.

Granulomas Subsequent to Procedure

82. Eyre RC, Aaronson AG, Weinstein BJ. Palisading granulomas of the prostate associated with prior prostatic surgery. J Urol 1986;136:121–2.

83. Hedelin H, Johansson S, Nilsson S. Focal prostatic granulomas. A sequel to transurethral resection. Scand J Urol Nephrol 1981;15:193–6.

84. Helpap B, Vogel J. TUR-prostatitis. Histological and immunohistochemical observations on a special type of granulomatous prostatitis. Pathol Res Pract 1986;181:301–7.

85. Lee G, Shepherd N. Necrotizing granulomata in prostatic resection specimens–a sequel to previous operation. J Clin Pathol 1983;36:1067–70.

85a. Lopez-Plaza I, Bostwick DG. Prostatitis. In: Bostwick DG, ed. Pathology of prostate. New York: Churchill Livingstone, 1990:15–30.

86. Mies C, Balogh K, Stadecker M. Palisading prostate granulomas following surgery. Am J Surg Pathol 1984;8:217–21.

86a. Orozco RE, Peters RL. Teflon granulosa of the prostate mimicking adenocarcinoma. Report of two cases. J Urol Pathol 1995;3:365–8.

87. Pieterse AS, Aarons I, Jose JS. Focal prostatic granulomas rheumatoid like—probably iatrogenic in origin. Pathology 1984;16:174–7.

88. Yamada Y. Focal palisading granuloma in the prostate and bladder. A clinicopathologic study of 88 total cystectomy specimens. Acta Pathol Jpn 1986;36:1813–22.

Malakoplakia

89. Damjanov I, Katz SM. Malakoplakia. Pathol Annu 1981;16:103–28.

90. Koga S, Arakaki Y, Matsuoka M, Ohyama C. Malakoplakia of prostate. Urology 1986;27:160–1.

91. McClure J. Malakoplakia of the prostate: a report of two cases and a review of the literature. J Clin Pathol 1979;32:629–32.

92. Nonomura A, Kono N, Takazakura E, Ohta G. Renal and prostatic malakoplakia associated with submassive hepatic necrosis. A case report with immunocytochemical, ultrastructural and x-ray analytical observations. Acta Pathol Jpn 1986;36:1251–62.

Inflammatory and Other Reactive Atypias

93. Bennett BD, Richardson PH, Gardner WA. Histopathology and cytology of prostatitis. In: Lepor H, Lawson R, eds. Prostate diseases. WB Saunders, Philadelphia, 1993:399–413.

94. Chan TY, Epstein JI. Follow up of atypical prostate needle biopsies suspicious for cancer. Urology 1999;53:351–5.

95. Epstein J. Inflammatory atypia vs prostate adenocarcinoma with inflammation. In: Epstein J. Differential diagnosis in pathology, urologic diseases. New York: Igaku-Shoin, 1992:82–3.

Radiation Changes

96. Bostwick DG, Egbert BM, Fajardo LF. Radiation injury of the normal and neoplastic prostate. Am J Surg Pathol 1982;6:541–51.

96a. Cheng L, Cheville JC, Bostwick DG. Diagnosis of prostate cancer in needle biopsies after radiation therapy. Am J Surg Pathol 1999;23:1173–83.

97. Sheaff MT, Baithun SI. Effects of radiation on the normal prostate gland. Histopathology 1997;30:341–8.

Postoperative Spindle Cell Nodule and Post-Needle Biopsy Changes

98. Bostwick DG, Vonk JB, Picado A. Pathologic changes in the prostate following contemporary 18-gauge needle biopsy. J Urol Pathol 1994;2:203–11.

99. Guillou L, Costa J. Pseudosarcomes post-opératoires du tractus génito-urinaire. Un piége diagnostique. Présentation de 4 observations dont 2 avec tude immunohistochimique et revue de la littérature. Ann Pathol 1989;9:340–5.

100. Huang WL, Ro JY, Grignon DJ, Swanson D, Ordonez NG, Ayala AG. Postoperative spindle cell nodule of the prostate and bladder. J Urol 1990;143:824–6.

101. Proppe KH, Scully RE, Rosai J. Postoperative spindle cell nodules of genitourinary tract resembling sarcomas. A report of eight cases. Am J Surg Pathol 1984;8:101–8.

Inflammatory Pseudotumor (Pseudosarcomatous Fibromyxoid Tumor)

102. Hafiz MA, Toker C, Sutula M. An atypical fibromyxoid tumor of the prostate. Cancer 1984;54:2500–4.

103. Ro JY, El-Naggar AK, Amin MB, Sahin AA, Ordonez NG, Ayala AG. Pseudosarcomatous fibromyxoid tumor of the urinary bladder and prostate: immunohistochemical, ultrastructural, and DNA flow cytometric analyses of nine cases. Hum Pathol 1993;24:1203–10.

Atypical Stromal Cells and Miscellaneous Other Stromal Abnormalities

104. Attah EB, Powell ME. Atypical stromal hyperplasia of the prostate. Am J Clin Pathol 1977;67:324–7.

105. Bejarano PA, Nestok B, Bracken RB. Collagen. A new cause for mass in the prostatic fossa after radical prostatectomy. J Urol Pathol 1996;4:99–105.

106. Eble JN, Tejada E. Prostatic stromal hyperplasia with bizarre nuclei. Arch Pathol Lab Med 1991;115:87–9.

107. Gaudin PB, Rosai J, Epstein JI. Sarcomas and related proliferative lesions of specialized prostatic stroma: a clinicopathologic study of 22 cases. Am J Surg Pathol 1998;22:148–62.

108. Humphrey PA, Vollmer RT. Extramedullary hematopoiesis in the prostate. Am J Surg Pathol 1991;15:486–90.

109. Leong SS, Vogt PJ, Yu GS. Atypical stromal smooth muscle hyperplasia of prostate. Urology 1988;31:163–7.

110. Tetu B, Ro JY, Ayala AG, Srigley JR, Begin LR, Bostwick DG. Atypical spindle cell lesions of the prostate. Semin Diagn Pathol 1988;5:284–93.

111. Wang X, Bostwick DG. Prostatic stromal hyperplasia with atypia. A study of 11 cases. J Urol Pathol 1997;6:15–26.

112. Young RH, Scully RE. Pseudosarcomatous lesions of the urinary bladder, prostate gland, and urethra. A report of three cases and review of the literature. Arch Pathol Lab Med 1987;111:354–8.

Melanosis

113. Amin MB, Bostwick DG. Pigment in prostatic epithelium and adenocarcinoma: a potential source of diagnostic confusion with seminal vesicular epithelium. Mod Pathol 1996;9:791–5.

114. Botticelli AR, DiGregorio C, Losi L, Fano RA, Manenti A. Melanosis (pigmented melanocytosis) of the prostate gland. Eur Urol 1989;16:229–32.

115. Brennick JB, O'Connell JX, Dickersin GR, Pilch BZ, Young RH. Lipofuscin pigmentation (so-called "melanosis") of the prostate. Am J Surg Pathol 1994;18:446–54.

116. Gardner WA Jr, Spitz WU. Melanosis of the prostate gland. Am J Clin Pathol 1971;56:762–4.

117. Jao W, Fretzin DF, Christ ML, Prinz LM. Blue nevus of the prostate gland. Arch Pathol 1971;91:187–91.

118. Kovi J, Jackson AG, Jackson MA. Blue nevus of the prostate: ultrastructural study. Urology 1977;9:576–8.

119. Leung CS, Srigley JR. Distribution of lipochrome pigment in the prostate gland: biological and diagnostic implications. Hum Pathol 1995;26:1302–7.

120. Lew S, Richter S, Jelin N, Siegal A. A blue naevus of the prostate: a light microscopic study including an investigation of S-100 protein positive cells in the normal and in the diseased gland. Histopathology 1991;18:443–8.

121. Martinez Martinez CJ, Garcia Gonzalez R, Castaneda Casanova AL. Blue nevus of the prostate: report of two new cases with immunohistochemical and electron-microscopic studies. Eur Urol 1992;22:339–42.

122. Nigogosyan G, De La Pava S, Pickren JW, Woodruff MW. Blue nevus of the prostate gland. Cancer 1963;16:1097–9.

123. Ro JY, Grignon DJ, Ayala AG, Hogan SF, Tetu B, Ordonez NG. Blue nevus and melanosis of the prostate. Electron-microscopic and immunohistochemical studies. Am J Clin Pathol 1988;90:530–5.

124. Ryan J, Crow J. Melanin in the prostate gland. Br J Urol 1988;61:455–6.

Endometriosis

125. Beckman EN, Pintado SO, Leonard GL, Sternberg WH. Endometriosis of the prostate. Am J Surg Pathol 1985;9:374–9.

Seminal Vesicle, Cowper's Gland, and Paraganglia in Prostate Specimens; Verumontanum Mucosal Gland Hyperplasia

126. Arias Stella J, Takano-Moron J. Atypical epithelial changes in the seminal vesicle. Arch Pathol 1958;66:761–6.

127. Cina SJ, Silberman MA, Kahane H, Epstein JI. Diagnosis of Cowper's glands on prostate needle biopsy. Am J Surg Pathol 1997;21:550–5.

128. Dikman SH, Toker C. Seromucinous gland ectopia within the prostatic stroma. J Urol 1973;109:852–4.

129. Freedman SR, Goldman RL. Normal paraganglia in the human prostate. J Urol 1975;113:874–5.

130. Gagucas RJ, Brown RW, Wheeler TM. Verumontanum mucosal gland hyperplasia. Am J Surg Pathol 1995;19:30–6.

131. Gaudin PB, Wheeler TM, Epstein JI. Verumontanum mucosal gland hyperplasia (VMGH) in prostatic needle biopsy specimens: a mimic of low-grade prostatic adenocarcinoma. Am J Clin Pathol 1995;104:620–6.

132. Jensen KM, Sonneland P, Madsen PO. Seminal vesicle tissue in "resectate" of transurethral resection of prostate. Urology 1983;22:20–3.

133. Kuo TT, Gomez LG. Monstrous epithelial cells in human epididymis and seminal vesicles. A pseudomalignant change. Am J Surg Pathol 1981;5:483–90.

134. Melcher MP. Bulbourethral glands of Cowper [Letter]. Arch Pathol Lab Med 1986;110:991.

135. Ostrowski ML, Wheeler TM. Paraganglia of the prostate. Location, frequency, and differentiation from prostatic adenocarcinoma. Am J Surg Pathol 1994;18:412–20.

136. Rode J, Bentley A, Parkinson C. Paraganglial cells of urinary bladder and prostate: potential diagnostic problem. J Clin Pathol 1990;43:13–6.

137. Saboorian MH, Huffman H, Ashfaq R, Ayala AG, Ro JY. Distinguishing Cowper's glands from neoplastic and pseudoneoplastic lesions of prostate. Immunohistochemical and ultrastructural studies. Am J Surg Pathol 1997;21:1069–74.

138. Tsuang MT, Weiss MA, Evans AT. Transurethral resection of the prostate with partial resection of the seminal vesicle. J Urol 1981;126:615–7.

Mucinous Metaplasia

139. Grignon DJ, O'Malley FP. Mucinous metaplasia in the prostate gland. Am J Surg Pathol 1993;17:287–90.

Benign Glands Adjacent to Nerves and in Skeletal Muscle

140. Carstens PH. Perineural glands in normal and hyperplastic prostates. J Urol 1980;123:686–8.

141. Cramer SF. Benign glandular inclusion in prostatic nerve. Am J Clin Pathol 1981;75:854–5.

142. Graversen PH, England DM, Madsen PO, Bruskewitz RC. Significance of striated muscle in curettings of the prostate. J Urol 1988;139:751–3.

143. Hasui Y, Shinkawa T, Osada Y, Sumiyoshi A. Striated muscle in the biopsy specimen of the prostate. Prostate 1989;14:65–9.

144. Kost LV, Evans GW. Occurrence and significance of striated muscle within the prostate. J Urol 1964;92:703–4.

145. Manley CB. The striated muscle of the prostate. J Urol 1966;95:234–40.

146. McIntire TL, Franzini DA. The presence of benign prostatic glands in perineural spaces. J Urol 1986;135:507–9.

Cysts

147. Deklotz RJ. Echinococcal cyst involving the prostate and seminal vesicles: a case report. J Urol 1976;115:116–7.

148. Emmett JN, Braasch WF. Cysts of the prostate gland. J Urol 1936;36:236–49.

149. Holm L, Forsberg L. Computed tomography and ultrasound studies of prostatic utricle cyst associated with unilateral renal agenesis. A case report. Scand J Urol Nephrol 1984;18:87–9.

150. Kimbell NK. Two cases of hydatid disease at the site of the prostate. Br J Urol 1938;10:55–9.

151. Magri J. Cysts of the prostate gland. Br J Urol 1960;32:295–301.

152. Uthmann U, Terhorst B. Dermoid cyst of the prostate with contralateral renal agenesis. Br J Urol 1981;53:479.

153. Wesson MB. Cysts of the prostate and urethra. J Urol 1925;13:605–32.

Amyloidosis

154. Carris CK, McLaughlin AP III, Gittes RF. Amyloidosis of the lower genitourinary tract. J Urol 1976;115:423–6.

155. Cross PA, Bartley CJ, McClure J. Amyloid in prostatic corpora amylacea. J Clin Pathol 1992;45:894–7.

156. Dahlin DC. Secondary amyloidosis. Ann Intern Med 1949; 31:105–19.

157. Lupovitch A. The prostate and amyloidosis. J Urol 1972;108:301–2.

158. McDonald JH, Heckel NJ. Primary amyloidosis of the lower genitourinary tract. J Urol 1956;75:122–32.

159. Tripathi VN, Desautels RE. Primary amyloidosis of the urogenital system: a study of 16 cases and brief review. J Urol 1969;102:96–101.

160. Wilson SK, Buchanan RD, Stone WJ, Rhamy RK. Amyloid deposition in the prostate. J Urol 1973;110:322–3.

Collagenous Spherulosis

161. Melamed MR. Neoplastic lesions [Letter]. Am J Surg Pathol 1998;22:903.

Calculi/Calcification/Cartilaginous Metaplasia/Ectopic Prostatic Tissue

162. Adams JR Jr. Adenocarcinoma in ectopic prostatic tissue. J Urol 1993;150:1253–4.
163. Bedrosian SA, Goldman RL, Sung MA. Heterotopic cartilage in prostate. Urology 1983;21:536–7.
164. Bromberg WD, Kozlowski JM, Oyasu R. Prostate-type gland in the epididymis. J Urol 1991;145:1273–4.
165. Clark JB. Calculus replacement of the prostate. Report of a case. J Urol 1934;32:495–500.
166. Clement PB, Young RH. Tumors and tumor-like lesions of the uterine corpus and cervix. In: Roth LM, ed. Contemporary issues in surgical pathology, 1993:44.
167. Congleton L, Thomason WB, McMullan DT, Worsham GF. Painless hematuria and urethral discharge secondary to ectopic prostate. J Urol 1989;142:1554–5.
168. Gledhill A. Ectopic prostatic tissue. J Urol 1985;133:110–1.
169. Jones WA, Miller EW, Sullivan LD, Chapman WH. Severe prostatic calcification after radiation therapy for cancer. J Urol 1979;121:828–30.
170. Kanomata N, Eble JN, Ohbayashi C, Yasui N, Tanaka H, Matsumoto O. Etopic prostate in the retrovesicle space. J Urol Pathol 1997;7:121–6.
171. Larraza-Hernandez O, Molberg KH, Lindberg G, Albores-Saavedra J. Ectopic prostatic tissue in the uterine cervix. Int J Gynecol Pathol 1997;16:291–3.
172. MacKenzie DW, Seng MI. Calcification of the prostate. J Urol 1924;12:243–9.
173. McLachlin CM, Srigley JR. Prostatic tissue in mature cystic teratomas of the ovary. Am J Surg Pathol 1992;16:780–4.
174. Milburn JM, Bluth EI, Mitchell WT. Ectopic prostate in the testicle: an unusual case of a solid testicular mass on ultrasonography. J Ultrasound Med 1994;13:578–80.
175. Nogales FF, Vergara E, Medina MT. Prostate in ovarian mature cystic teratoma. Histopathology 1995;26:373–5.
175a.Nucci MR, Ferry JA, Young RH. Ectopic prostatic tissue in the uterine cervix: a report of four cases and review of ectopic prostatic tissue. Am J Surg Pathol 2000;24:1224–30.
176. Salem CE, Gibbs PM, Highshaw RA, Reuter VE, Cote RJ. Benign ectopic prostatic tissue involving the seminal vesicle in a patient with prostate cancer: recognition and implication for staging. Urology 1996;48:490–3.
177. Suarez GM, Roberts JA. Ochronosis of prostate presenting as advanced carcinoma. Urology 1983;22:168–71.
178. Vadmal M, Hajdu SI. Prostatic tissue in benign cystic ovarian teratomas. Hum Pathol 1996;27:428–9.
179. Willis RA. Developmentally heterotopic tissues. In: The borderland of embryology and pathology, 2nd ed. London: Butterworths, 1962:339.

❖❖❖

8

THE SEMINAL VESICLE

ANATOMY AND HISTOLOGY

The seminal vesicles, accessory sex glands derived from outpouchings of the lower mesonephric ducts, are highly coiled, paired, tubular structures located along the posterolateral aspect of the external surface of the base of the urinary bladder, superior to the posterior surface of the prostate (figs. 8-1–8-5) (3). Occasionally they are present within or adherent to the posterior prostatic capsule. In adults, they average about 6 cm in length and 2 cm in width (2), and contain 2 to 5 ml of milky fluid which composes the majority of the ejaculatory volume. The excretory duct of the seminal vesicle joins the ampullary portion of the vas deferens to form the ejaculatory duct, which then penetrates the posterior superior aspect of the prostate, in the central zone of the gland, to empty into the prostatic urethra at the verumontanum.

First and second degree ducts branch from the main seminal vesicle duct into the thick coat of smooth muscle that constitutes the wall of the seminal vesicle. This wall has a relatively thin, longitudinal external layer and a thicker, inner circular layer and in areas is very close to the prostatic base (fig. 8-2). With puberty, the ductal structures develop complex mucosal folds, so that a cross section of an adult seminal vesicle shows complex papillary structures (fig. 8-3) and small glands arranged in a somewhat lobular fashion (fig. 8-5) around sizable ducts that typically have an elongated, slit-like appearance (figs. 8-1, 8-2). The elongated papillae have a thin

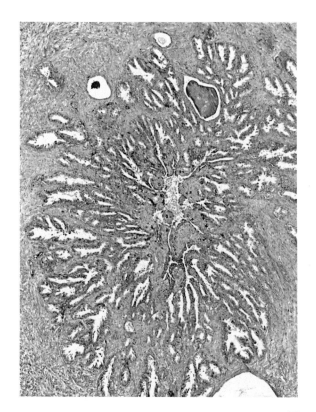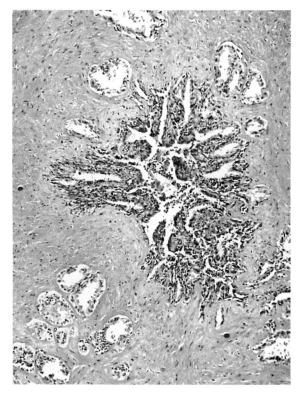

Figure 8-1

NORMAL ADULT SEMINAL VESICLE

These illustrations show the classic central, slit-like glandular pattern with a few papillae. Less distinctive peripheral small acini are seen on the right which also shows two stromal hyaline bodies.

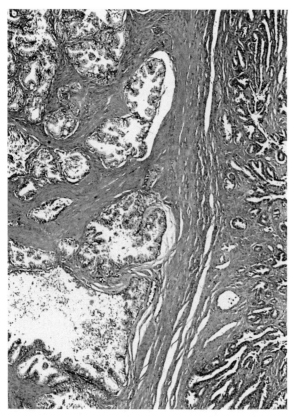

Figure 8-2
NORMAL ADULT SEMINAL VESICLE
The typical elongated, slit-like glandular pattern is seen at the right, separated from the prostate by a relatively narrow zone of fibromuscular tissue.

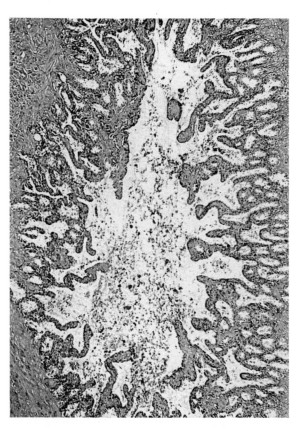

Figure 8-3
NORMAL ADULT SEMINAL VESICLE
There are prominent intraluminal papillae.

Figure 8-4
NORMAL ADULT
SEMINAL VESICLE

Vacuolated, faintly staining, pigmented epithelium lines the papillae and glands. Basal cells are inconspicuous. An eosinophilic hyaline body is present in the smooth muscle stroma at the top left.

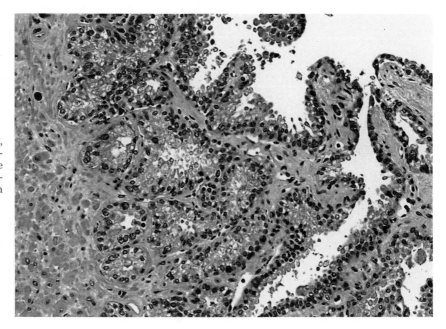

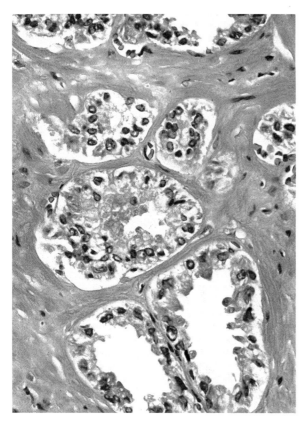

Figure 8-5
NORMAL ADULT SEMINAL VESICLE

A high-power view of the small peripheral acini in figure 8-1, right, shows lipofuscin pigment. Note the bland cytologic features and lack of prominent nucleoli that help distinguish these acini from neoplastic prostatic acini.

Table 8-1

HISTOLOGIC CLASSIFICATION OF TUMORS AND TUMOR-LIKE LESIONS OF THE SEMINAL VESICLE

Primary Tumors
    Carcinoma
        Adenocarcinoma
            Mucinous
            Clear cell
            Not otherwise specified
        Undifferentiated
    Cystadenoma
    Epithelial-Stromal Tumors
        Fibroadenoma
        Adenomyoma
        Not otherwise specified
            Low grade
            High grade
    Benign mesenchymal tumors
    Malignant mesenchymal tumors
    Others

Secondary Tumors

Tumor-like Lesions
    Cysts
        Developmental
        Acquired
    Epithelial atypia
    Amyloid deposits
    Fibromuscular hyperplasia
    Mesonephric hamartoma
    Adenomyomatous nodule
    Megavesicles
    Calcification

core of fibromuscular tissue; the papillae and glands are lined by a layer of columnar to cuboidal secretory cells and basal cells. Lipofuscin granules and small droplets of lipid are often prominent in the cytoplasm of the secretory cells after puberty (fig. 8-5) (1). Nucleomegaly, hyperchromasia, and multinucleation, creating a "pseudomalignant" appearance, are common in the secretory cells, especially in older patients (see page 360).

The basal cells, as in the prostate, stain for high molecular weight cytokeratin (clone 34βE12), whereas the secretory cells are negative. In contrast to the prostate, the secretory cells do not stain for prostate-specific antigen (PSA), prostatic acid phosphatase (PAP), and androgen receptors. Round, eosinophilic and fuchsinophilic hyaline bodies are sometimes seen in the muscular wall of the seminal vesicle; they are thought to be derived from degenerate smooth muscle cells (figs. 8-1, 8-4).

PRIMARY TUMORS

Primary tumors of the seminal vesicle are rare. Their classification and that of other lesions considered here is presented in Table 8-1. Four major categories of primary tumors are included: carcinoma, cystadenoma, combined epithelial and stromal tumors, and miscellaneous, even rarer benign and malignant tumors. Much of the information about these tumors is derived from individual case reports and is limited.

Carcinomas

General and Clinical Features. The seminal vesicle is commonly involved by prostatic carcinoma and less commonly by bladder carcinoma, but primary seminal vesicle carcinoma is one of the rarest primary tumors in the body. Dalgaard and Giersten (6) accepted only cases in which the histologic appearance was that of a papillary or anaplastic carcinoma, mainly localized in the seminal vesicle and with no other known primary tumor. Benson et al. (4) identified 37 acceptable cases in 1984 (updated to 48 cases in 1996 by Ormsby and co-workers [16]) and insisted that prostatic and rectal carcinomas be excluded and that new cases have negative immunoreactivity for PSA and PAP. We agree with these recommendations, having seen more cases thought clinically to be seminal vesicle carcinoma than we have bona fide examples of pathologically verified primary carcinoma.

The mean patient age is 62 years, with a range of 24 to 90 years (4–7,9,11–14,16–19); at least 10 patients were less than 40 years of age (4,5,12). The usual symptoms are those of urinary obstruction (4,19), although hematuria (13,16,17), perineal pain (7), and hemospermia (4,6) may also occur; 30 percent have ureteral obstruction (4,17). A nontender mass superior to, or in continuity with, the prostate is usually apparent on rectal examination. Imaging studies, including ultrasound, computerized tomographic scans, and seminal vesiculography, are helpful in demonstrating that the lesion involves, and is centered in, the seminal vesicle. Most patients have metastatic disease at the time of diagnosis (8), and the prognosis is poor: in 95 percent of cases with follow-up the survival was less than 3 years (16). Only five patients are known to have survived more than 18 months, all of whom were treated either with estrogen therapy, orchiectomy, and/or antiandrogen therapy (4,16).

Gross Findings. The tumor often consists of irregular nodules of firm, gray-white to brown, sometimes gritty tissue (7,8,12,18). Bilateral involvement occurs in 8 percent of cases (16). Most of the reported tumors have been large (12,13), and even less bulky tumors typically measure at least several centimeters (4,18,19). Pale tan, granular material may be present in the tubules of the seminal vesicle, and necrosis may be prominent (7,19).

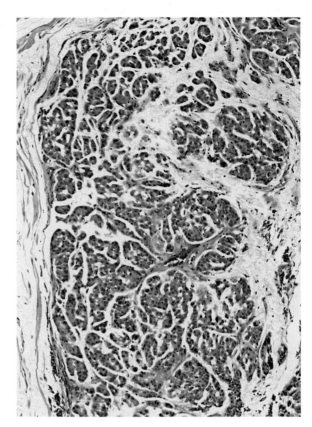

Figure 8-6
PAPILLARY ADENOCARCINOMA

Microscopic Findings. The tumors overall have nonspecific features (10), sometimes being papillary (figs. 8-6, 8-7) (5), and often poorly differentiated, with solid, nested, and cord-like patterns (5,7,12,16,18). Others produce prominent extracellular mucin, similar to colloid carcinoma at other sites (fig. 8-8) (4). One papillary adenocarcinoma occurred in a congenital cyst that was associated with renal agenesis (15). One tumor had a tubulopapillary pattern with clear and hobnail cells (fig. 8-7) (14) resembling a clear cell adenocarcinoma of the female genital tract, and occasional tumors in the older literature had such an appearance to some degree (17). The clear cell carcinoma and another reported papillary carcinoma (16) stained for the tumor-associated antigen, CA125. Mucin and carcinoembryonic antigen (CEA) stains may be positive in seminal vesicle carcinoma, but, by definition, PSA and PAP are negative (4,16,18).

Differential Diagnosis. The main lesions in the differential diagnosis are adenocarcinomas

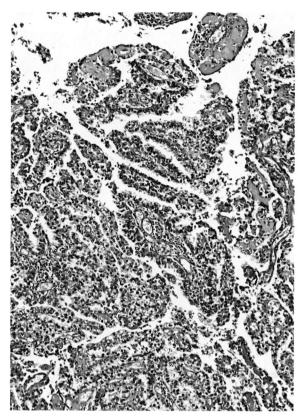

Figure 8-7
ADENOCARCINOMA, CLEAR CELL TYPE
Neoplastic papillae are lined by malignant epithelium with clear cytoplasm. There is focal hyalinization of the papillary cores. (Courtesy of Dr. T. Ohmori, Shigenobu-cho, Japan.)

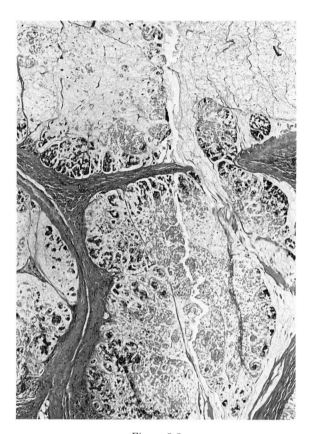

Figure 8-8
MUCINOUS ADENOCARCINOMA, COLLOID TYPE
(Courtesy of Dr. G.M. Farrow, Rochester, MN.)

that spread from adjacent structures, particularly the prostate, bladder, and intestinal tract. General clinical evaluation and knowledge of the distribution of tumor, in addition to the gross and microscopic features, are variably important in establishing the diagnosis of primary seminal vesicle carcinoma which, because of its rarity, is a diagnosis of exclusion. The presence of a current or previous cancer in any of the organs mentioned above should cast suspicion on this diagnosis. Comparison of the morphology of the seminal vesicle neoplasm with that of prior or concurrent tumors of other sites is crucial. On gross inspection the diagnosis of a seminal vesicle primary is supported if the neoplasm has its epicenter in the seminal vesicles, with no or minimal extension into adjacent structures. On microscopic examination, the tumor must have a morphology consistent with that seen with

seminal vesicle carcinoma and should, as noted, stain negatively for prostate immunomarkers; positivity for CEA, CA125, and cytokeratin 7, and negativity for cytokeratin 20, support a seminal vesicle primary (15a). In situ involvement of the seminal vesicle epithelium might be helpful but has rarely been documented, and the features of in situ disease may be mimicked by secondary spread.

The paramount importance of clinical and gross findings in establishing the diagnosis of primary seminal vesicle carcinoma was elegantly demonstrated in a case of an adenocarcinoma arising in a mullerian duct cyst (8), with two normal seminal vesicles on either side of a large intracystic neoplasm (figs. 8-9, 8-10). On microscopic examination, the tumor was a typical tubulocystic clear cell adenocarcinoma of mullerian type (fig. 8-11), a histology that may be seen with primary seminal vesicle carcinoma, as noted above.

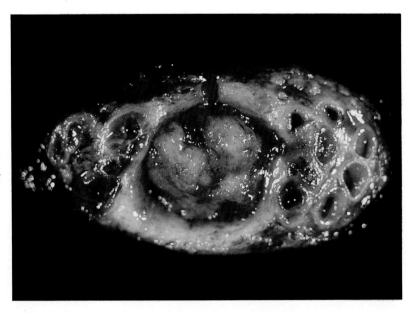

Figure 8-9
CLEAR CELL ADENOCARCINOMA
ARISING WITHIN A
MULLERIAN DUCT CYST
The polypoid intracystic neoplasm
(center) is bounded on either side by un-
involved seminal vesicles. (Courtesy of
Dr. J. Ibarra, Long Beach, CA.)

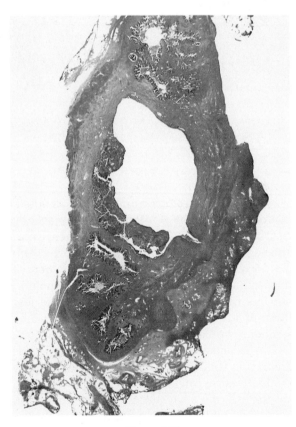

Figure 8-10
CLEAR CELL ADENOCARCINOMA ARISING
WITHIN A MULLERIAN DUCT CYST
Whole mount of the specimen in figure 8-9 shows a
central mullerian duct cyst with focal carcinoma. Note the
lack of involvement of the seminal vesicles. (Courtesy of Dr.
J. Ibarra, Long Beach, CA.)

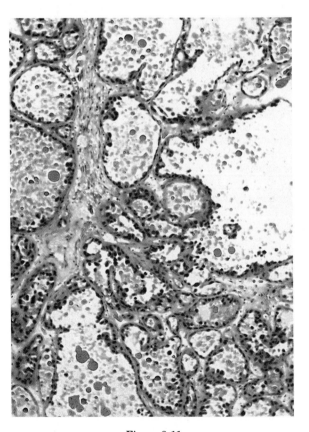

Figure 8-11
CLEAR CELL ADENOCARCINOMA ARISING
WITHIN A MULLERIAN DUCT CYST
The tumor has a tubulocystic pattern with hobnail cells.
(Courtesy of Dr. J. Ibarra, Long Beach, CA.)

Cystadenoma

Clinical Features. These lesions may be incidentally discovered on rectal examination or at autopsy in middle-aged men, or the patients may present with hemospermia or nonspecific suprapubic pain (20-23). Recurrence may follow incomplete excision (20), but the outcome is benign.

Gross Findings. Multilocular, cystic lesions, measuring up to 14 cm in diameter and containing clear to brown-yellow gelatinous fluid, are typical (fig. 8-12) (20,21,23).

Microscopic Findings. The cysts (fig. 8-13, left) are lined by flattened to cuboidal, bland epithelium and contain abundant, eosinophilic, mucoid secretion with an intervening, non-neoplastic, muscular or fibromuscular stroma (fig. 8-13, right). The epithelial cells may contain lipofuscin pigment similar to that of the non-neoplastic seminal vesicle.

Differential Diagnosis. Cystadenoma is primarily distinguished from fibroadenoma, adenomyoma, and other epithelial-stromal tumors by its non-neoplastic, usually relatively scant, nonspecific appearing stroma. Distinction from a multiloculated developmental cyst may not be possible, but the presence of associated urinary tract anomalies points to the latter.

Epithelial-Stromal Tumors

Epithelial-stromal tumors of the seminal vesicle include a spectrum of tumors that grossly and microscopically resemble the similarly named tumor of the prostate (see chapter 6), and fibroadenoma and phyllodes tumor of the breast. They are also similar to the müllerian adenofibroma and adenosarcoma of the uterus. The nomenclature used for these neoplasms has been inconsistent in the literature, most often reflecting, at least recently, their resemblance to phyllodes tumors. However, the typical appearance of that lesion is not always seen, and we recommend the term "epithelial-stromal tumor" which emphasizes the presence of both neoplastic epithelial and stromal elements. These tumors can be further subclassified as listed in Table 8-1.

Some tumors in this category have been reported as "cystadenoma" because of their cystic nature and a hypocellular stroma which was not considered neoplastic (27,29,31). We, and others (25,28), regard some of these "cystadenomas" as low-grade tumors in the epithelial-stromal, not otherwise specified, category. The distinction between cystadenoma and an epithelial-stromal tumor of the seminal vesicle hinges upon whether or not the stroma is neoplastic. For cases in which the stroma is limited in amount and appears to represent the normal or possibly reactive smooth muscle of the seminal vesicle, the term "cystadenoma" is preferred, whereas for cases with a conspicuous, presumably neoplastic stroma, "fibroadenoma" or "adenomyoma" is appropriate (24,30), depending on whether the stroma is clearly benign and fibrous or myomatous; "epithelial-stromal tumor, not otherwise specified" is preferable if the stromal cellularity, atypia, or other features suggest the possibility of recurrence or metastasis.

Fibroadenoma/Adenomyoma. Three fibroadenomas and one adenomyoma have occurred in patients from 39 to 66 years of age who presented with pain, voiding difficulty, or a palpable, asymptomatic mass (27,29–31).

The tumors were solid and cystic, ranging from 3 to 15 cm in greatest dimension, and were centered on the seminal vesicle. In one case, the cysts contained chocolate-brown fluid (30).

Microscopically, glands that may be slit-like or cystically dilated are lined by a layer of flattened to columnar, bland-appearing, sometimes pigmented epithelium and separated by fibrous to muscular stroma (27,29–31). Focal stromal hypercellularity of a mild degree was present in one case (29), and in another there was nodular growth of smooth muscle stroma (adenomyoma) (30).

These tumors are distinguished from cystadenomas by their more conspicuous stromal component and from low-grade epithelial-stromal tumors, not otherwise specified (NOS) by the bland appearance and inconspicuous mitotic activity of the stroma which contrasts with that of epithelial-stromal tumors, NOS. Similar appearing tumors of the prostate are distinguished from those of seminal vesicle origin by location or, if large size prevents accurate determination of the site of origin, by the absence of PSA staining in the latter.

Epithelial-Stromal Tumors, Not Otherwise Specified (Low Grade and High Grade). Three reported epithelial-stromal tumors of the seminal vesicle were malignant or possibly malignant (25,26,28), and we have seen

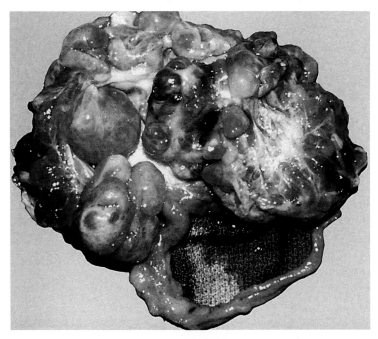

Figure 8-12
CYSTADENOMA
Multiple cysts are evident on the sectioned surface of this tumor that measured 8 cm in maximum dimension. The cysts contained thick mucinous fluid. The vas deferens is seen at the bottom of the illustration. (Fig. 2 from Peker KR, Hellman BH Jr, McCammom KA, Bui TT, Schlossberg SM. Cystadenoma of the seminal vesicle. J Urol Pathol 1997;6:213–21.)

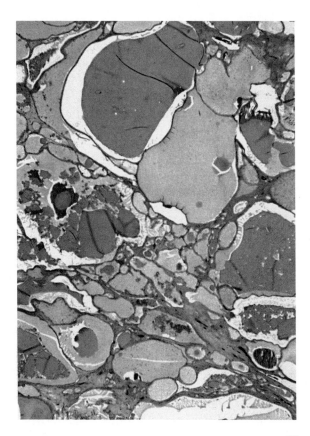

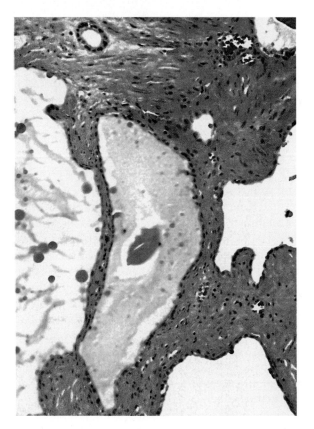

Figure 8-13
CYSTADENOMA
Left: Multiple cysts of varying size are lined by bland, flattened to cuboidal epithelium.
Right: Note the hypocellular fibrous stroma. (Left and right: courtesy of Dr. D.G. Bostwick, Rochester, MN.)

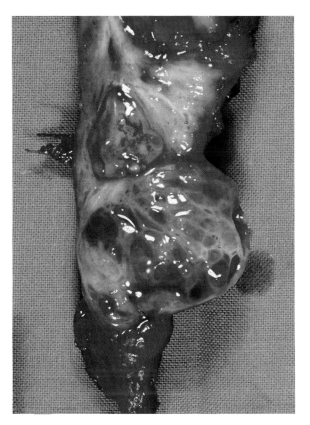

Figure 8-14
EPITHELIAL-STROMAL TUMOR, LOW GRADE
The sectioned surface is multicystic. (Courtesy of Dr. E. C. Jones, Vancouver, BC, Canada.)

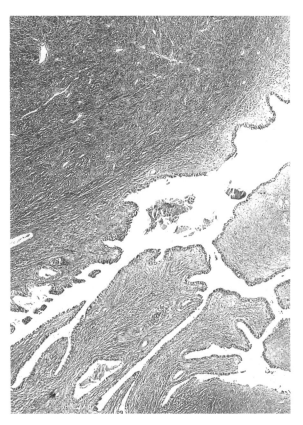

Figure 8-15
EPITHELIAL-STROMAL TUMOR, LOW GRADE
Spaces are lined by bland epithelium and contain phyllodes-like protrusions of a moderately cellular stroma. (Courtesy of Dr. R. Orozco, Oklahoma City, OK.)

several additional unpublished examples (figs. 8-14–8-19). They occurred in middle-aged to elderly men who presented with urinary retention and had a pelvic mass which at operation appeared to arise from a seminal vesicle (25,26,28).

The tumors are grossly either multicystic (fig. 8-14) or solid and cystic, sometimes with intracystic polypoid masses (fig. 8-16). Microscopically, irregular glands that may be cystically dilated are lined by focally stratified, usually nonpigment-containing epithelium surrounded by a variably cellular stroma whose cells may have enlarged, atypical nuclei (figs. 8-17, 8-18) and can exhibit scant or brisk mitotic activity. A phyllodes-type appearance may be seen (fig. 8-15). There may be evidence of smooth muscle differentiation of the stroma, either by ultrastructure or immunohistochemistry (26,28). Immunostains for PAP, PSA, and carcinoembryonic antigen (CEA) are negative (25,26,28).

Although clinicopathologic studies have not yet been conducted to validate their prognostic usefulness, we consider the following features sufficient to place a tumor in the high-grade group: 1) stromal overgrowth and 2) anaplasia with marked cellularity, necrosis, pleomorphism, and frequent mitoses. However, it is probable that, as with the similar tumors of the uterus in the adenofibroma-adenosarcoma category, rare tumors without worrisome features might recur or even metastasize. One low-grade tumor recurred 2 years after initial resection, but the patient was disease free 18 months after a second excision (28). An overtly malignant tumor (fig. 8-19) that grossly invaded the rectal wall metastasized to the lung 4 years after resection (25).

Lack of staining for PAP and PSA may be crucial in distinguishing an epithelial-stromal tumor of the seminal vesicle from one of prostatic origin (which is more common; see chapter 6), if the

Figure 8-16
EPITHELIAL-STROMAL TUMOR,
LOW GRADE
Dark brown hemorrhagic nodules project into the lumen of a multi-loculated, cystic mass. (Courtesy of Dr. M.T. Mazur, Syracuse, NY.)

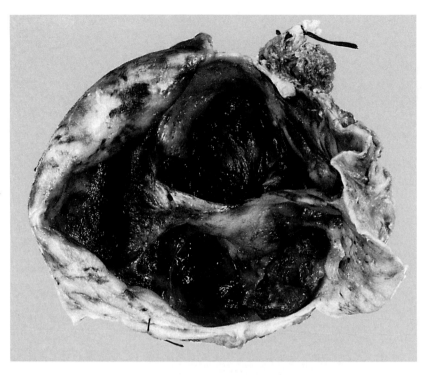

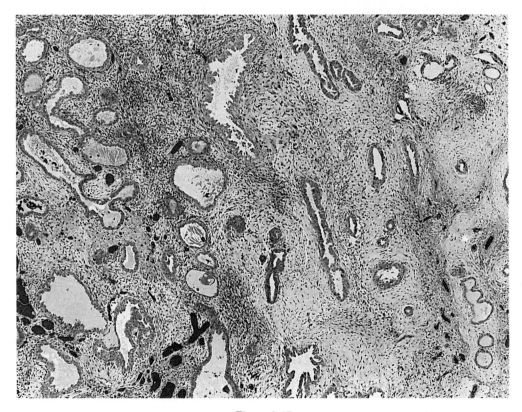

Figure 8-17
EPITHELIAL-STROMAL TUMOR, LOW GRADE
Irregularly shaped glands are separated by stroma that is densely cellular in some areas and shows a tendency to condense around glands. (Courtesy of Dr. M.T. Mazur, Syracuse, NY.)

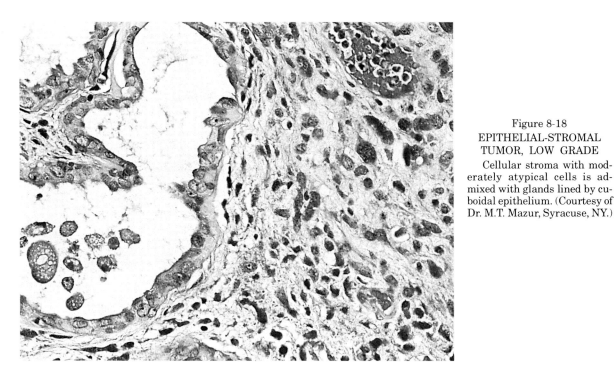

Figure 8-18
EPITHELIAL-STROMAL
TUMOR, LOW GRADE
Cellular stroma with moderately atypical cells is admixed with glands lined by cuboidal epithelium. (Courtesy of Dr. M.T. Mazur, Syracuse, NY.)

Figure 8-19
EPITHELIAL-STROMAL
TUMOR, HIGH GRADE
There is a densely cellular stromal component and "leaf-like" pattern. There were 5 mitotic figures per 10 high-power fields, and pulmonary metastases occurred 4 years after excision. (Courtesy of Dr. D.G. Bostwick, Rochester, MN.)

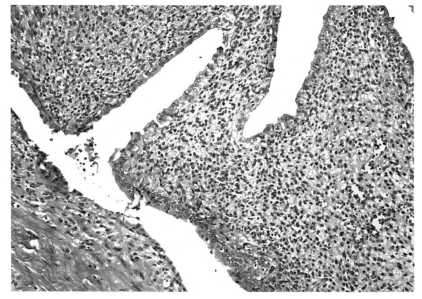

location of the lesion is indefinite in ascribing a primary site (as it may when the tumors are large), as the tumors of the different organs are indistinguishable on routine stains in our admittedly limited experience. The tumors are distinguished from cystadenomas on the basis of their biphasic nature. The phyllodes type nature of the epithelial component in many cases is another distinguishing feature. The differential with fibroadenomas and adenomyomas has been discussed on page 351. Direct extension from a prostatic stromal sarcoma may also be a consideration and distinction depends largely on the clinical and gross findings.

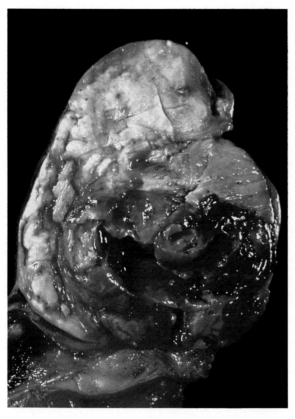

Figure 8-20
LEIOMYOSARCOMA
There is cystic degeneration with prominent necrosis and hemorrhage. (Courtesy of Dr. K.H. Molberg, Dallas, TX.)

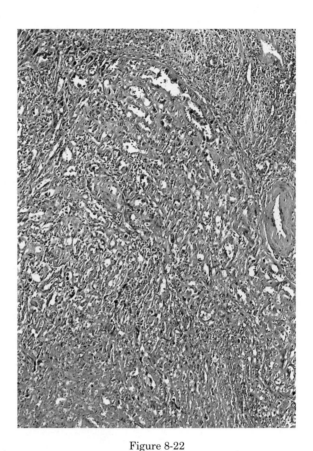

Figure 8-22
EPITHELIOID ANGIOSARCOMA
Malignant epithelioid endothelial cells form nests and vessel-like structures, with focal necrosis. (Courtesy of Dr. A. De las Morenas, Boston, MA.)

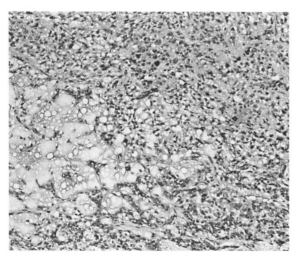

Figure 8-21
LEIOMYOSARCOMA
Highly atypical spindle to polygonal cells have a solid and cord-like arrangement. There is focal myxoid change. (Courtesy of Dr. K.H. Molberg, Dallas, TX.)

Other Benign and Malignant Tumors. There are sporadic reports of leiomyoma (34,35, 38) and miscellaneous other benign mesenchymal tumors (39,41,47). Malignant mesenchymal tumors have also been described but are equally rare. They include: fibrosarcoma (35,48), leiomyosarcoma (figs. 8-20, 8-21) (33,44,46), a pleomorphic sarcoma consistent with malignant fibrous histiocytoma (43), liposarcoma (40), and angiosarcoma (fig. 8-22) (36,42). Sometimes it is difficult to determine if such tumors arose from the seminal vesicle or the adjacent pelvic soft tissues and then grew into the seminal vesicle (43), although occasional cases in which the tumor is small and centered in the seminal vesicle with little involvement of adjacent structures provide good evidence for a seminal vesicle origin (44). Their pathologic features are as observed at other sites.

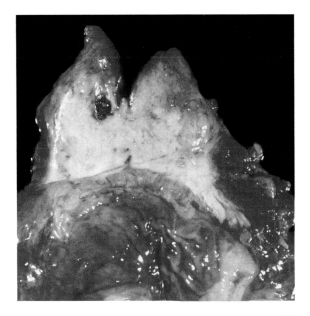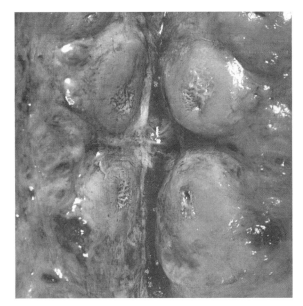

Figure 8-23
PROSTATIC ADENOCARCINOMA INVOLVING THE SEMINAL VESICLE
Left: An autopsy specimen shows massive replacement of both seminal vesicles by contiguous spread from prostatic adenocarcinoma.
Right: Another case shows encasement of the seminal vesicles by tumor with preservation of the central ducts.

One tumor replaced the seminal vesicle of a 29-year-old man and resembled the female adnexal tumor of probable wolffian origin (43a). It recurred twice over a 23-year interval following surgical excision.

A "primary" choriocarcinoma of the seminal vesicle occurred in a 28-year-old man who presented with widespread metastatic choriocarcinoma (37); autopsy failed to show abnormalities in the testis, including the absence of regressive changes such as scars and calcifications. It remains possible, however, that this case represented a metastatic lesion with an undetected, regressed primary choriocarcinoma of the testis. A "seminoma" of the seminal vesicle is questionable because of failure to examine the testes microscopically (32). A "primary" carcinoid tumor of the seminal vesicle is also questionable, given bilateral involvement and extensive peritoneal metastases; metastasis to the seminal vesicles appears more likely (45).

SECONDARY TUMORS

Radical prostatectomy specimens for prostatic carcinoma may show spread to one or both seminal vesicles, defined as at least involvement of the muscularis (figs. 8-23, 8-24) (50,54). This may occur by contiguous spread from the adjacent prostatic parenchyma, by extracapsular spread with involvement of the seminal vesicles from extraprostatic tumor, or as deposits in the seminal vesicle that are not contiguous with prostatic or other extraprostatic tumor and that presumably represent spread by lymphatics or blood vessels (51). The latter form of involvement may be associated with a better prognosis than the other types (51).

Less commonly, carcinoma of the bladder may involve the seminal vesicles (fig. 8-25). Ro et al. (52) reported seminal vesicle involvement by transitional cell carcinoma in 6 of 187 (3.2 percent) cystoprostatectomy specimens obtained from patients with bladder carcinoma. Such involvement may either be in the form of spread along the mucosa or by direct stromal invasion. The latter form of involvement indicates a high-stage bladder carcinoma, but the prognostic significance of mucosal spread is not clear (52).

Rectal adenocarcinoma may spread directly to the seminal vesicles, and we have seen a case of metastatic mucinous adenocarcinoma of the

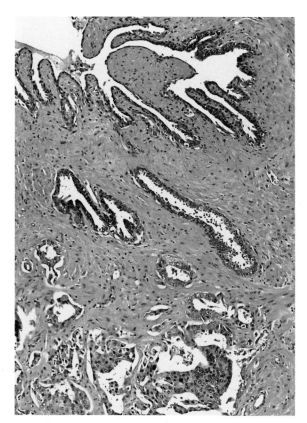

Figure 8-24
PROSTATIC ADENOCARCINOMA
INVOLVING THE SEMINAL VESICLE
Carcinoma (bottom) invades the smooth muscle of the seminal vesicle.

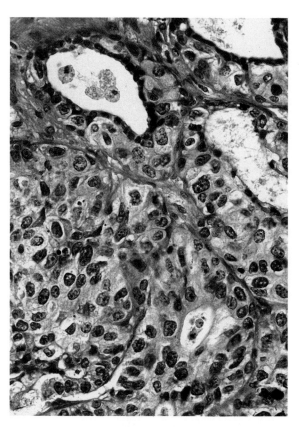

Figure 8-25
TRANSITIONAL CELL CARCINOMA
OF BLADDER WITH SECONDARY
INVOLVEMENT OF SEMINAL VESICLE
The normal seminal vesicle epithelium is focally present (top) and undermined by the carcinoma.

appendix to the seminal vesicle which was initially confused clinically with a primary seminal vesicle carcinoma (figs. 8-26, 8-27). There is a report of seminoma metastasizing to the seminal vesicle (49), and, as noted above, a probable metastatic carcinoid (53). Despite the rarity of this diagnostic problem, most cases of secondary spread are readily distinguished from primary neoplasia, although the clinical history and findings are often key in this regard.

TUMOR-LIKE LESIONS

Cysts

A variety of cysts may be seen in, or adjacent to, the seminal vesicles (Table 8-2), and imaging studies are important in establishing whether the cyst originated from the seminal vesicles or other sites, including vestiges of the mullerian duct.

Developmental Cysts. These usually communicate with the lumen of the seminal vesicle and the vas deferens (67) and are associated with ipsilateral abnormalities of the urinary tract, including renal, ureteral, and hemitrigone agenesis (55–57,59–62,64–66,68). Occasionally a blind-ending ureter enters the cyst (60), and usually the vas deferens can be seen communicating with the cyst (57,64). Such cysts are identified most commonly in young men in the third decade of life who present with perineal pain, painful ejaculation, urinary frequency, or constipation (59,67).

The cysts often measure several centimeters in diameter (55-57,59–62,65), and may be huge (68). They frequently contain amber to dark brown fluid with degenerating spermatozoa, leukocytes, and bacteria (55,57,60–62,65,68). Typically, the cysts are unilocular but may be multilocular; areas of

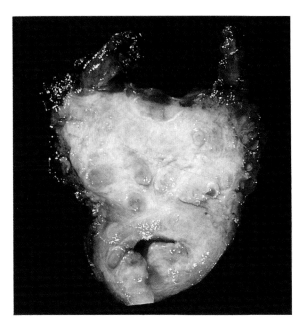

Figure 8-26
MUCINOUS ADENOCARCINOMA OF APPENDIX
INVOLVING THE SEMINAL VESICLE
The residual architecture of the seminal vesicle can be appreciated in the midst of a mucoid mass.

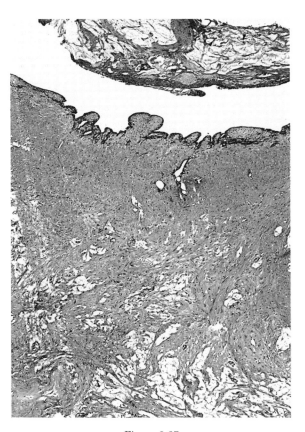

Figure 8-27
MUCINOUS ADENOCARCINOMA OF APPENDIX
INVOLVING THE SEMINAL VESICLE
Pools of extracellular mucin containing malignant glandular epithelium invade the smooth muscle of the seminal vesicle. Tumor is also present in the lumen (top).

red, yellow, and brown mottling are noted on the internal surface (fig. 8-28) (57).

Microscopically, the fibromuscular walls are lined by flattened to cuboidal to columnar epithelium (fig. 8-29) that resembles that of the seminal vesicle (57,59,60,65). Secondary inflammation may occur in some cases (65).

Acquired Cysts. Acquired seminal vesicle cysts generally occur secondary to inflammation and outflow obstruction (63). Patients may present with perineal pain, bloody ejaculate, or irritative urinary symptoms, or the lesions may be incidentally discovered on rectal examination (63). They are usually unilocular, are several centimeters in diameter, have a thick fibrous wall, and generally contain amber to bloody fluid (63). On microscopic examination there is typically a low cuboidal epithelial lining that may be largely denuded, and the lumen may contain leukocytes, sloughed epithelium, and degenerating spermatozoa. Resolution may occur if the obstruction is relieved; one 14-cm cyst involuted after removal of a small stone from the ejaculatory duct (58). Occasional specific infectious cysts are encountered.

Table 8-2

**DIFFERENTIAL DIAGNOSIS
OF SEMINAL VESICLE CYST***

Type of Cyst	Location	Size	Contains Sperm?
Seminal vesicle cyst	Lateral	Large	Yes
Diverticulum of ejaculatory duct of ampulla	Lateral	Variable	Yes
Prostatic cyst	Lateral	Variable	No
Mullerian duct cyst	Midline	Large	No

*Table 8-1 from: Bostwick DG, Eble JN, eds. Urologic surgical pathology. St. Louis: Mosby, 1997:425.

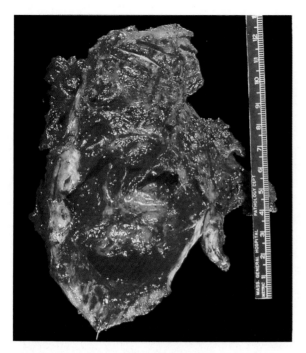

Figure 8-28
SEMINAL VESICLE CYST
The large cyst has a mottled, hemorrhagic lining.

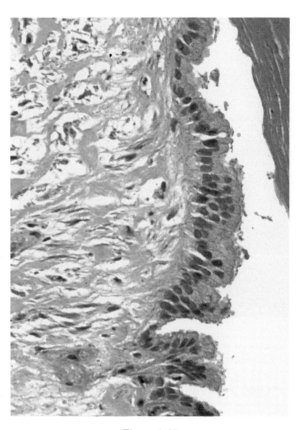

Figure 8-29
SEMINAL VESICLE CYST
The lining epithelium is simple to pseudostratified columnar.

Pseudomalignant Features of Normal Seminal Vesicle

The best known pseudomalignant feature of this organ is the common cytologic atypia of the epithelium, a phenomenon that increases in frequency with age (70,71,73). Arias-Stella and Takano-Moron (70) noted marked cytologic atypia of the seminal vesicle epithelium in 13 percent of men over 45 years of age. Kuo and Gomez (73) noted some degree of atypia in the seminal vesicles of 75 percent of males ranging in age from 3 days to 83 years; the median age of patients having atypia was 63.5 years, whereas the median age of patients lacking atypia was 23.5 years. Scattered cells display nuclear enlargement, hyperchromasia, and prominent nucleoli; intranuclear cytoplasmic inclusions may also be seen (fig. 8-30) (70,73). Mitoses, however, are not identified (72). Cytophotometric analysis of such cases has demonstrated polyploid DNA contents (72), whereas a flow cytometric study of 30 seminal vesicles from older men yielded a 7 percent frequency of aneuploidy, with diploidy in the remaining cases (69). There is no evidence that this atypia is premalignant.

Another feature of the normal histology of the seminal vesicle that may be problematic is the arrangement of regular small acini (fig. 8-5) that are usually peripheral to the more characteristic central, slit-like glands of the organ. These acini typically do not show the degenerative nuclear atypia that is usually recognizable as a characteristic feature of seminal vesicle epithelium. Indeed, procurement of such small acini in occasional needle biopsy specimens probably goes unappreciated as being seminal vesicle epithelium because of the lack of such features, and the small acini are distinguished from neoplastic prostatic acini by the absence of the cytologic features of carcinoma. We have seen radical prostatectomy specimens in which adenocarcinoma involved the seminal vesicles, and distinction of carcinomatous acini from the normal, small acini of the seminal vesicle depended on the cytologic criteria used in needle biopsy material. We have, however, rarely needed to immunostain

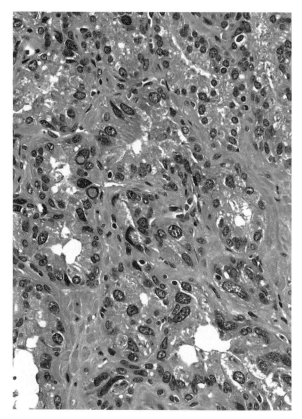

Figure 8-30
ATYPICAL CELLS IN THE SEMINAL VESICLE
The cells have enlarged, hyperchromatic, irregularly shaped nuclei and occasional intranuclear cytoplasmic inclusions. Note the crowded appearance of the glands which may contribute to diagnostic difficulty if seen in a needle biopsy.

for prostate markers to aid in this differential and to establish the benign nature of the problematic glands.

Although the above described variably complex and closely packed glands that represent the normal histology of the seminal vesicle may be problematic, the elongated shape, pigment, and cytologic atypia aid in the recognition of the distinctive, central, slit-like areas. In prostate needle biopsies, these features plus negative staining for PSA and positive staining for basal cells in the less distinctive small acinar foci can help prevent misinterpretation as prostatic adenocarcinoma (71). In one series, 5 percent of prostatic needle biopsy specimens contained fragments of seminal vesicle epithelium (71). The differential diagnosis of adenocarcinoma of the prostate and seminal vesicle tissue is discussed further in chapter

7 which also considers differences in the nature of the lipofuscin pigment in the seminal vesicle and prostate (Table 7-1).

Miscellaneous Tumor-Like Lesions

Several other non-neoplastic conditions may clinically mimic tumor in the seminal vesicle. Amyloid deposits are identified at autopsy in the subepithelial region of the seminal vesicles, as well as within blood vessels, in 4 to 12 percent of males (75,78,81). The frequency increases with age: 32 percent of patients 75 years of age or older have amyloid deposits. They are usually incidental findings (fig. 8-31), but amyloidosis of the seminal vesicles may be associated with hematospermia, raising concern for tumor (81), or mimic spread of prostatic carcinoma on magnetic resonance imaging studies (84). One recent report suggests a higher frequency of amyloid deposits in patients treated with anti-androgen therapy (88). Most cases of seminal vesicle amyloidosis are not associated with systemic amyloidosis, and the protein may be locally derived from the seminal vesicle (84,86). Rarely, amyloid in the seminal vesicle reflects systemic involvement by AA amyloid (75).

A case of fibromuscular hyperplasia causing tumorous enlargement of the wall of the left seminal vesicle presented as perineal pain in a 27-year-old man (79). A case of "mesonephric hamartoma" of the seminal vesicle may represent the same finding, although the pathologic details are scant (80). We have seen occasional, small, adenomyomatous nodules as incidental findings in the wall of the seminal vesicle; these consist of a circumscribed proliferation of bland-appearing smooth muscle cells arranged in short fascicles with occasional intermixed seminal vesicle–type acini (fig. 8-32) (74). It is probable that these represent either small leiomyomas or smooth muscle hyperplasias with entrapped, non-neoplastic acini. Their relationship to clinical leiomyomas and tumors in the epithelial-stromal category is unknown.

Bilateral enlargement of the seminal vesicles with marked cystic dilatation may mimic tumor. Such megavesicles occur for unknown reasons but appear to be associated with diabetes (83).

Calcification in the seminal vesicle is unusual (85). Most cases are described in elderly men and

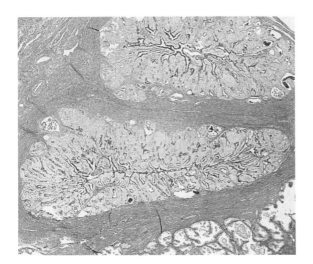
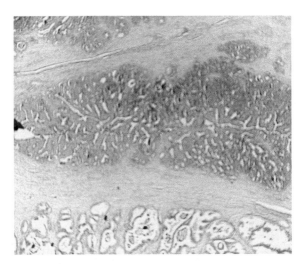

Figure 8-31
AMYLOIDOSIS
A positive Congo red reaction is illustrated on the right.

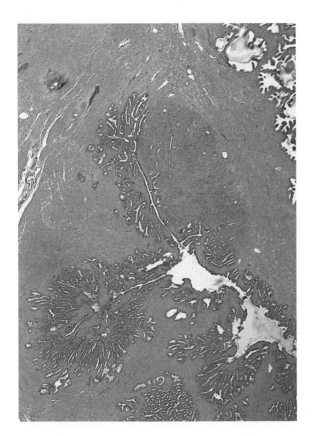
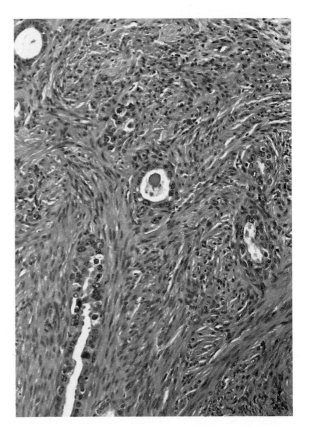

Figure 8-32
ADENOMYOMATOUS NODULE

Left: Note the small, circumscribed, unencapsulated nodule within the wall of the seminal vesicle just above center on the right side of the slit-like lumen.

Right: Entrapped seminal vesicle acini showing prominent cytoplasmic lipofuscin are separated by haphazardly arranged smooth muscle fascicles.

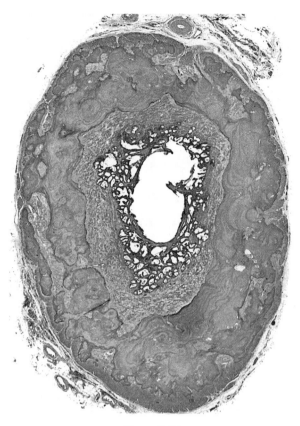

Figure 8-33
CALCIFICATION OF SEMINAL VESICLE
There is concentric calcification of the muscular wall.
(Courtesy of Dr. J.N. Eble, Indianapolis, IN.)

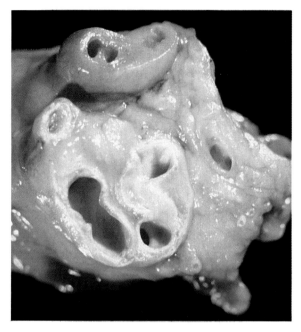

Figure 8-34
CALCIFICATION OF SEMINAL VESICLE

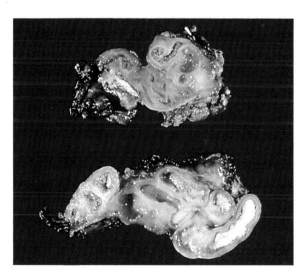

Figure 8-35
CALCIFICATION OF SEMINAL VESICLE
Note the prominent inspissated secretion in seminal vesicles, with thickening of their walls.

occur in the muscularis (figs. 8-33, 8-34) (77), although radiographically demonstrated seminal vesicle calcification is described in young patients with inflammatory disease (tuberculosis) and uremia (82,87). Rarely, inspissation of secretion within the seminal vesicles may be striking, and may be associated with calcification and thickening of the walls (fig. 8-35). Diabetes mellitus may also predispose to seminal vesicle calcification (87), but there is a stronger association of diabetes with calcification of the vas deferens (76,89).

REFERENCES

Anatomy and Histology

1. Herbut PA. Urological pathology, Vol II. Philadelphia: Lea & Febiger, 1952:980–1010.
2. Spring-Mills E. The seminal vesicles. In: Spring-Mills E, Hafez ES, eds. Male accessory sex glands: biology and pathology. Amsterdam: Elsevier/North Holland Biomedical Press, 1980:63–77.
3. Watson EM. The developmental stages of the human seminal vesicles. J Urol 1918;2:129–39.

Carcinoma

4. Benson RC, Jr, Clark WR, Farrow GM. Carcinoma of the seminal vesicle. J Urol 1984;132:483–5.
5. Chinoy RF, Kulkarni JN. Primary papillary adenocarcinoma of the seminal vesicle. Indian J Cancer 1993;30:82–4.
6. Dalgaard JB, Giertsen JC. Primary carcinoma of the seminal vesicle. Acta Pathol Microbiol Scand 1956;39:255–67.
7. Ewell GH. Seminal vesicle carcinoma. J Urol 1963;89:908–12.
8. Gilbert RF, Ibarra J, Tansey LA, Shanberg AM. Adenocarcinoma in a mullerian duct cyst. J Urol 1992;148:1262–4.
9. Hajdu SI, Faruque AA. Adenocarcinoma of the seminal vesicle. J Urol 1968;99:798–801.
10. Herbut PA. Urological pathology, Vol II. Philadelphia: Lea & Febiger, 1952:980–1010.
11. Kawahara M, Matsuhashi M, Tajima M, et al. Primary carcinoma of seminal vesicle. Diagnosis assisted by sonography. Urology 1988;32:269–72.
12. Kindblom LG, Pettersson G. Primary carcinoma of the seminal vesicle. Case report. Acta Pathol Microbiol Scand [A] 1976;84:301–5.
13. Oguchi K, Takeuchi T, Kuriyama M, Tanaka T. Primary carcinoma of the seminal vesicle (cross-imaging diagnosis). Br J Urol 1988;62:383–4.
14. Ohmori T, Okada K, Tabei R, et al. CA 125-producing adenocarcinoma of the seminal vesicle. Pathol Int 1994;44:333–7.
15. Okada Y, Tanaka H, Takeuchi H, Yoshida O. Papillary adenocarcinoma in a seminal vesicle cyst associated with ipsilateral renal agenesis. A case report. J Urol 1992;148:1543–5.
15a. Ormsby AH, Haskell R, Jones D, Goldblum JR. Primary seminal vesicle carcinoma: an immunohistochemical analysis of four cases. Mod Pathol 2000;13:46–51.
16. Ormsby AH, Haskell R, Ruthven SE, Mylne GE. Bilateral primary seminal vesicle carcinoma. Pathology 1996;28:196–200.
17. Smith BA, Webb EA, Price WE. Carcinoma of the seminal vesicle. J Urol 1967;97:743–50.
18. Tanaka T, Takeuchi T, Oguchi K, Niwa K, Mori H. Primary adenocarcinoma of the seminal vesicle. Hum Pathol 1987;18:200–2.
19. Williamson RC. Seminal vesicle tumours. J Roy Soc Med 1978;71:286–8.

Cystadenoma

20. Bullock KN. Cystadenoma of the seminal vesicle. J R Soc Med 1988;81:294–5.
21. Damjanov I, Apic R. Cystadenoma of seminal vesicles. J Urol 1974;111:808–9.
22. Peker KR, Hellman BH Jr, McCammon KA, Bui TT, Schlossberg SM. Cystadenoma of the seminal vesicle: a case report and review of the literature. J Urol Pathol 1997;6:213–21.
23. Soule EH, Dockerty MB. Cystadenoma of the seminal vesicle, a pathologic curiosity: report of a case and review of the literature concerning benign tumors of the seminal vesicle. Proc Staff Meetings Mayo Clinic 1951;26:406–14.

Epithelial–Stromal Tumor

24. Damjanov I, Apic R. Cystadenoma of seminal vesicles. J Urol 1974;111:808–9.
25. Fain JS, Cosnow I, King BF, Zincke H, Bostwick DG. Cystosarcoma phyllodes of the seminal vesicle. Cancer 1993;71:2055–61.
26. Laurila P, Leivo I, Makisalo H, Ruutu M, Miettinen M. Mullerian adenosarcoma-like tumor of the seminal vesicle. Arch Pathol Lab Med 1992;116:1072–6.
27. Lundhus E, Bundgaard N, Sorensen FB. Cystadenoma of the seminal vesicle: a case report. Scand J Urol Nephrol 1984;18:341–2.
28. Mazur MT, Myers JL, Maddox WA. Cystic epithelial-stromal tumor of the seminal vesicle. Am J Surg Pathol 1987;11:210–7.
29. Mazzucchelli L, Studer UE, Zimmermann A. Cystadenoma of the seminal vesicle: case report and literature review. J Urol 1992;147:1621–4.
30. Plaut A, Standard S. Cystomyoma of the seminal vesicle. Ann Surg 1944;119:253–61.
31. Soule EH, Dockerty MB. Cystadenoma of the seminal vesicle, a pathologic curiosity: report of a case and review of the literature concerning benign tumors of the seminal vesicle. Proc Staff Meetings Mayo Clinic 1951;26:406–14.

Other Primary Tumors

32. Adachi Y, Rokujyo M, Kojima H, Nagashima K. Primary seminoma of the seminal vesicle: report of a case. J Urol 1991;146:857–9.

33. Amirkhan RH, Molberg KH, Wiley EL, Nurenberg P, Sagalowsky AI. Primary leiomyosarcoma of the seminal vesicle. Urology 1994;44:132–5.

34. Bahn DK, Brown RK, Shei KY, White DB. Sonographic findings of leiomyoma in the seminal vesicle. J Clin Ultrasound 1990;18:517–9.

35. Buck AC, Shaw RE. Primary tumours of the retro-vesical region with special reference to mesenchymal tumours of the seminal vesicles. Br J Urol 1972;44:47–50.

36. Chiou RK, Limas C, Lange PH. Hemangiosarcoma of the seminal vesicle: case report and literature review. J Urol 1985;134:371–3.

37. Fairey AE, Mead GM, Murphy D, Theaker J. Primary seminal vesicle choriocarcinoma. Br J Urol 1993;71:756–7.

38. Gentile AT, Moseley HS, Quinn SF, Franzini D, Pitre TM. Leiomyoma of the seminal vesicle. J Urol 1994;151:1027–9.

39. Islam M. Benign mesenchymoma of seminal vesicles. Urology 1979;13:203–5.

40. Juhasz J, Kiss P. A hitherto undescribed case of "collision" tumour: liposarcoma of the seminal vesicle and prostatic carcinoma. Int Urol Nephrol 1978;10:185–93.

41. Kan DV. Benign tumors of seminal vesicles. Urologia 1963;28:27.

42. Lamont JS, Hesketh PJ, de las Morenas A, Babayan RK. Primary angiosarcoma of the seminal vesicle. J Urol 1991;146:165–7.

43. Lazarus JA. Primary malignant tumors of the retrovesical region with special reference to malignant tumors of the seminal vesicles; report of a case of retrovesical sarcoma. J Urol 1946;55:190–205.

43a. Middleton LP, Merino MJ, Popok SM, Ordonez NG, Ayala AG, Ro JY. Male adnexal tumour of probable wolffian origin occurring in a seminal vesicle. Histopathology 1998;33:269–74.

44. Schned AR, Ledbetter JS, Selikowitz SM. Primary leiomyosarcoma of the seminal vesicle. Cancer 1986;57:2202–6.

45. Soyer P, Rougier P, Gad M, Roche A. Primary carcinoid tumor of the seminal vesicles: CT and MR findings. J Belge Radiol 1991;74:117–9.

46. Tripathi VN, Dick VS. Primary sarcoma of the urogenital system in adults. J Urol 1969;101:898–904.

47. Weitzer M, Cohen RJ. Benign peripheral nerve sheath tumor of the seminal vesicle. Pathology 1998;30:80.

48. Williamson RC. Seminal vesicle tumours. J Roy Soc Med 1978;71:286–8.

Secondary Tumors

49. Bostwick DG. Seminal vesicle. In: Bostwick DG, Eble JN, eds. Urologic surgical pathology. St. Louis: Mosby, 1997:422–33.

50. Epstein JI, Carmichael M, Walsh PC. Adenocarcinoma of the prostate invading the seminal vesicle: definition and relation of tumor volume, grade and margins of resection to prognosis. J Urol 1993;149:1040–5.

51. Ohori M, Scardino PT, Lapin SL, Seale-Hawkins C, Link J, Wheeler TM. The mechanisms and prognostic significance of seminal vesicle involvement by prostate cancer. Am J Surg Pathol 1993;17:1252–61.

52. Ro JY, Ayala AG, El-Naggar A, Wishnow KI. Seminal vesicle involvement by in-situ and invasive transitional cell carcinoma of the bladder. Am J Surg Pathol 1987;11:951–8.

53. Soyer P, Rougier P, Gad M, Roche A. Primary carcinoid tumor of the seminal vesicles: CT and MR findings. J Belge Radiol 1991;74:117–9.

54. Villers AA, McNeal JE, Redwine EA, Freiha FS, Stamey TA. Pathogenesis and biological significance of seminal vesicle invasion in prostatic adenocarcinoma. J Urol 1990;143:1183–7.

Cysts

55. Beeby DI. Seminal vesicle cyst associated with ipsilateral renal agenesis: case report and review of the literature. J Urol 1974;112:120–2.

56. Carvalho HA, Paiva JL, Santos VH, Andrade M, Galvao-Teles A. Ultrasonic recognition of a cystic seminal vesicle with ipsilateral renal agenesis. J Urol 1986;135:1267–8.

57. Case Records of the Massachusetts General Hospital. Case 21-1980. N Engl J Med 1980;302:1246–51.

58. Conn IG, Peeling WB, Clements R. Complete resolution of a large seminal vesicle cyst—evidence for an obstructive aetiology. Br J Urol 1992;69:636–9.

59. Ejeckam GC, Govatsos S, Lewis AS. Cyst of the seminal vesicle associated with ipsilateral renal agenesis. Urology 1984;24:372–4.

60. Fuselier HA Jr, Peters DH. Cyst of seminal vesicle with ipsilateral renal agenesis and ectopic ureter: case report. J Urol 1976;116:833–5.

61. Hart JB. A case of cyst of the seminal vesicle. J Urol 1966;96:247–9.

62. Heetderks DR Jr, Delambre LC. Cyst of the seminal vesicle. J Urol 1965;93:725–8.

63. Heller E, Whitesel JA. Seminal vesicle cysts. J Urol 1963;90:305–7.

64. Knudsen JB, Brun B, Emus HC. Familial agenesis of urogenital malformations: seminal vesicle cyst and vaginal cyst with bicornuate uterus in sibling. Scand J Urol Nephrol 1979;13:109–12.

65. Linhares Furtado AJ. Three cases of cystic seminal vesicle associated with unilateral renal agenesis. Br J Urol 1973;45:536–40.

66. Okada Y, Tanaka H, Takeuchi H, Yoshida O. Papillary adenocarcinoma in a seminal vesicle cyst associated with ipsilateral renal agenesis: a case report. J Urol 1992;148:1543–5.

67. Reddy YN, Winter CC. Cyst of the seminal vesicle: a case report and review of the literature. J Urol 1972;108:134–5.

68. Roehborn CG, Schneider H-J, Rugendoff W, Hamann W. Embryological and diagnostic aspects of seminal vesicle cysts associated with upper urinary tract malformation. J Urol 1986;135:1029–32.

Pseudomalignant Lesions

69. Arber DA, Speights VO. Aneuploidy in benign seminal vesicle epithelium: an example of the paradox of ploidy studies. Mod Pathol 1991;4:687–9.

70. Arias-Stella J, Takano-Moron J. Atypical epithelial changes in the seminal vesicle. Arch Pathol 1958;66:761–6.

71. Coyne JD, Kealy WF, Annis P. Seminal vesicle epithelium in prostatic needle biopsy specimens. J Clin Pathol 1987;40:932.

72. Karolyi P, Szentirmay Z, Krasznai G. Cytophotometric investigations on atypical epithelial cells of the human seminal vesicle. Int Urol Nephrol 1989;21:399–402.

73. Kuo T, Gomez LG. Monstrous epithelial cells in human epididymis and seminal vesicles. A pseudomalignant change. Am J Surg Pathol 1981;5:483–90.

Miscellaneous Lesions

74. Bostwick DG, Dundore PA. Biopsy pathology of the prostate. London: Chapman & Hall, 1997.

75. Coyne JD, Kealy WF. Seminal vesicle amyloidosis: morphological, histochemical and immunohistochemical observations. Histopathology 1993;22:173–6.

76. Culver GJ, Tannenhaus J. Calcification of the vas deferens in diabetes. JAMA 1960;173:645–51.

77. George S. Calcification of the vas deferens and the seminal vesicles. JAMA 1906;47:103–5.

78. Goldman H. Amyloidosis of seminal vesicles and vas deferens. Arch Pathol 1963;75:94–8.

79. Hatcher PA, Tucker JA, Carson CC. Fibromuscular hyperplasia of the seminal vesicle. J Urol 1989;141:957–8.

80. Kinas H, Kuhn MJ. Mesonephric hamartoma of the seminal vesicle: a rare cause of a retrovesical mass. N Y State J Med 1987;87:48–9.

81. Krane RJ, Klugo RC, Olsson CA. Seminal vesicle amyloidosis. Urology 1973;2:70–2.

82. Kretschmer HL. Calcification of the seminal vesicles. J Urol 1922;7:67–71.

83. Pryor JP, Hendry WF. Ejaculatory duct obstruction in subfertile males: analysis of 87 patients. Fertil Steril 1991;56:725–30.

84. Ramchandani P, Schnall MD, LiVolsi VA, Tomaszewski JE, Pollack HM. Senile amyloidosis of the seminal vesicles mimicking metastatic spread of prostatic carcinoma on MR images. Am J Radiol 1993;161:99–100.

85. Schned AR, Cozzolino DJ. Idiopathic dense calcification of the seminal vesicles. J Urol 1997;157:2263.

86. Seidman JD, Shmookler BM, Connolly B, Lack EE. Localized amyloidosis of seminal vesicles: report of three cases in surgically obtained material. Mod Pathol 1989;2:671–5.

87. Silber SJ, McDonald FD. Calcification of the seminal vesicles and vas deferens in a uremic patient. J Urol 1971;105:542–4.

88. Unger PD, Wang Q, Gordon RE, Stock R, Stone N. Localized amyloidosis of the seminal vesicle: possible association with hormonally treated prostatic adenocarcinoma. Arch Pathol Lab Med 1997;121:1265–8.

89. Wilson JL, Marks JH. Calcification of the vas deferens: its relation to diabetes mellitus and arteriosclerosis. N Engl J Med 1951;245:321–5.

9
THE MALE URETHRA

ANATOMY AND HISTOLOGY

The male urethra consists of prostatic and membranous segments (the proximal [posterior] urethra), and bulbous and penile (pendulous) segments (the distal [anterior] urethra) (fig. 9-1) (1-4). The bulbous and membranous portions are often considered together as the "bulbo-membranous" urethra because, from the practical viewpoint, tumors of these regions have similar clinical features. The approximately 3 to 4 cm prostatic urethra originates at the bladder neck from the internal urethral orifice. It consists of proximal and distal portions divided by the verumontanum (colliculus seminalis) (fig. 9-2) (6), a longitudinal ridge on the dorsal aspect of the prostatic urethra. The prostatic urethra merges with the membranous urethra at the urogenital diaphragm. The prostatic utricle, an epithelium-lined sac that represents a mullerian vestige, and the distal portions of the ejaculatory ducts that lie lateral to the utricle, open into the prostatic urethra through the verumontanum on the posterior wall (5). Microscopically, the verumontanum is

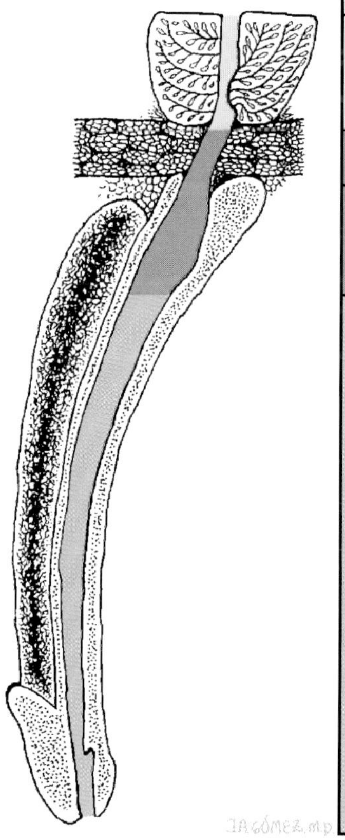

REGION	HISTOLOGY	CARCINOMA
Prostatic	Transitional	Prostatic (7%) Transitional 86% Squamous 14%
Membranous Bulbous	Stratified / Pseudostratified Columnar	Bulbomembranous (59%) Squamous 82% Transitional 8% Adenocarcinoma 8% Undifferentiated 2%
Penile	Non-Keratinizing Squamous	Penile (34%) Squamous 90% Transitional 10%

Figure 9-1
NORMAL MALE URETHRA
Line drawing illustrating the anatomy and histology of the male urethra and showing the relative frequencies of various histologic subtypes of carcinoma at different sites. (Modified from fig. 12.1 from Srigley JR, Hartwick RW. Surgical pathology of the male urethra and seminal vesicles. In: Bostwick DG, ed. Contemporary issues in surgical pathology, vol. 15. Pathology of the prostate. New York: Churchill Livingstone, 1990.)

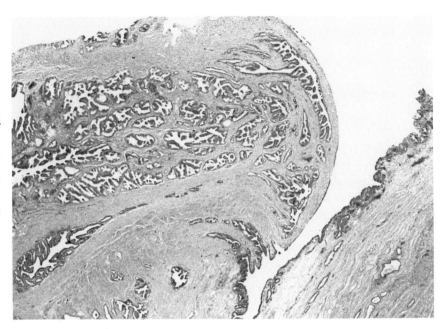

Figure 9-2
NORMAL VERUMONTANUM
This low-power view shows the eminence on the dorsal aspect of the prostatic urethra that represents the verumontanum. In this photomicrograph only a few verumontanum mucosal glands are seen at the top. The complex glandular pattern is composed of periurethral glands and ducts, and prostatic acini.

normally composed of rather closely apposed small glands which often contain eosinophilic to brown concretions. Periurethral prostatic glands consisting of short ducts and acini are present along the proximal segment of the prostatic urethra. These structures are normally variably enveloped by transitional cells (see page 394).

The membranous urethra, usually 2 to 2.5 cm long, is the shortest segment. It traverses the urogenital diaphragm, is surrounded by muscle fibers, and extends to the posterior margin of the penile bulb. Cowper's (bulbourethral) glands are paired tubuloalveolar glands that lie in the skeletal muscle of the urogenital diaphragm. Their secretory ducts enter the posterior aspect of the bulbous urethra. The acini of Cowper's glands are composed of cuboidal to columnar cells with dark basal nuclei and abundant mucinous cytoplasm. The 3- to 4-cm long bulbous urethra, which is of larger caliber than the prostatic and membranous urethra segments, begins immediately distal to the urogenital diaphragm at the root of the penis.

The penile urethra extends from the distal aspect of the bulbous urethra to the fossa navicularis where it merges with the external urethral meatus. The penile urethra lies in the corpus spongiosum, below the paired corpora cavernosa; Buck's fascia surrounds the three cylinders of erectile tissue (see figs. 10-7, 10-8).

The penile urethra measures approximately 15 cm in length (2) and opens externally at the tip of the glans penis as the urethral meatus. The mucosa has numerous recesses, called the lacunae of Morgagni (fig. 9-3), which extend deeper into the mucin secreting glands of Littré (figs. 9-3, 9-4) that are present in the lateral walls of the penile and bulbous urethra.

The lamina propria of the urethra is composed of loose fibroconnective tissue containing numerous elastic bundles and scattered smooth muscle that is mainly oriented longitudinally. Circular bundles are also present in the outer layers. Striated muscle from the urogenital diaphragm envelops the membranous urethra. The lymphatics of the prostatic and bulbomembranous urethra drain to the obturator and external iliac nodes, and those of the penile urethra drain to the superficial inguinal nodes.

The proximal prostatic urethra is lined predominantly by transitional epithelium (fig. 9-4) in which superficial (umbrella) cells can be identified. This epithelium merges imperceptibly with pseudostratified or stratified columnar epithelium lining the distal prostatic, bulbomembranous, and most of the penile urethra. Interspersed mucinous cells may be seen in this region (fig. 9-4). The distal penile urethra, including the fossa navicularis, is lined by ciliated stratified columnar epithelium or stratified, nonkeratinizing,

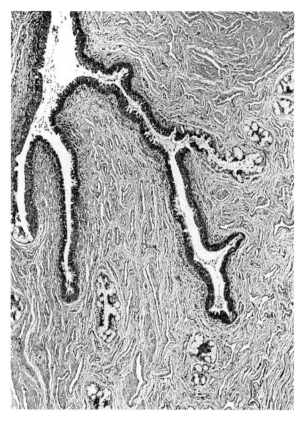

Figure 9-3
NORMAL URETHRA
A section taken from mid-penile urethra shows the recesses known as the lacunae of Morgagni. In close proximity are several clusters of glands of Littré.

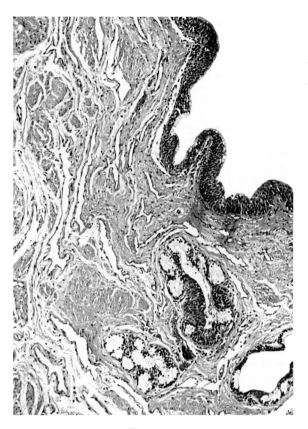

Figure 9-4
NORMAL URETHRA
A section of the proximal penile urethra shows the transitional lining and the glands of Littré composed mainly of mucinous cells but with scattered foci of transitional epithelium. Note the rare mucinous cells within the mucosa.

squamous epithelium (fig. 9-5), that is continuous with the mucosa of the external meatus. Patchy foci of squamous epithelium may also be seen more proximally, and there may be focal mucous cells within the perimeatal squamous epithelium of the glans.

MALIGNANT TUMORS

Carcinomas

General and Clinical Features. Urethral carcinoma accounts for most urethral malignant tumors and has traditionally been considered unique among genitourinary neoplasms by being less common in men than women (7–48). Analysis of the overall literature, including many relatively large series, has shown a three to four times greater frequency in women; however, a large study from the Surveillance Epidemiology

and End Results (SEER) program had a male predominance (31). The reason for this discrepancy is unclear. The tumors usually occur in patients in the sixth and seventh decades with a median age of about 58 years (26), although there are occasional cases documented in patients in the second and third decades (33).

Urethral stricture was present in approximately one third of the patients in one review of cases reported prior to 1967, and a history of venereal disease was also common (37 percent of the cases) (26). Symptoms are often related to urinary tract obstruction, particularly with tumors of the posterior urethra, and there may be a purulent urethral discharge, hematuria, or both. If the tumor is in the anterior urethra, the patient may palpate a mass. Difficulty in urination is also quite common as is pain during erection

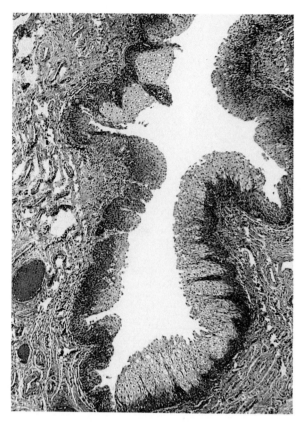

Figure 9-5
NORMAL URETHRA
A section of the penile urethra shows a lining of non-keratinizing glycogenated squamous epithelium.

Table 9-1

ANATOMIC CLASSIFICATION OF PRIMARY EPITHELIAL TUMORS OF MALE URETHRA

1. Tumors of penile urethra
2. Tumors of bulbomembranous urethra
3. Tumors of prostatic urethra
4. Tumors of "paraurethral tissue" presenting as a urethral mass
   a. Littré's glands
   b. Cowper's glands

(15). Physical examination may disclose a palpable mass, evidence of a periurethral or perineal abscess, often combined with sinus tracts and multiple fistulae, or an enlarged prostate. A combination of urinary tract obstruction and an enlarged prostate often leads to a clinical diagnosis of prostatic hyperplasia. Rare tumors are associated with paraneoplastic hypercalcemia (20,40), and a few patients have had pseudohyperparathyroidism (13). One case of squamous cell carcinoma of the distal urethra arose in a patient with congenital hypospadias (16).

In a comprehensive review of 232 cases, the tumors were considered primary in the bulbomembranous urethra (the most common site of urethral stricture) in 133 patients, in the penile urethra in 83, and in the prostatic urethra in 16 (Table 9-1) (26). Other "urethral" carcinomas actually arise in paraurethral tissues, and some have questioned the validity of considering

these, particularly those of Cowper's gland origin, "urethral"; in our opinion they are appropriately grouped with urethral tumors.

Squamous cell carcinomas account for approximately 75 percent of male urethral carcinomas (Table 9-2) (26). The remainder are transitional cell carcinomas, adenocarcinomas, adenosquamous carcinomas, and occasional undifferentiated or other carcinomas. Transitional cell carcinomas are twice as common as adenocarcinomas in males. Transitional cell tumors predominate in the prostatic urethra and only occasionally occur in the distal urethra, including the fossa navicularis (7). Many tumors of the prostatic urethra arise in patients with a history of transitional cell carcinoma of the urinary bladder. Approximately 10 percent of patients with bladder cancer subsequently develop a tumor of similar cell type in the prostatic urethra (45). Dysplasia, in situ carcinoma, or rarely, invasive carcinoma of the prostatic urethra may be found synchronously with a bladder tumor (14); pagetoid spread to the urethra from a bladder tumor may also occur. In situ transitional cell carcinoma of the urethra is much more often encountered in a patient with a prior or concomitant carcinoma of the bladder than as a de novo phenomenon. The latter obviously occurs, but biopsies are rarely performed early enough to detect only in situ changes. In situ changes, and occasionally, papillary or frankly invasive transitional cell carcinomas, are sometimes discovered during evaluation of a transurethral resection specimen performed for prostatic disease, and the overlying prostatic urethral epithelium in such specimens, when present, should be carefully evaluated (12). Most

Table 9-2

HISTOLOGIC CLASSIFICATION OF MALIGNANT TUMORS OF MALE URETHRA

Primary Tumors
Carcinomas
    Squamous cell carcinoma
    Transitional cell carcinoma
    Adenocarcinoma
        Colloid (mucinous) carcinoma
        Signet ring cell carcinoma
        Clear cell carcinoma
        Adenocarcinoma, not otherwise specified
    Adenoid cystic carcinoma
    Adenosquamous carcinoma
    Undifferentiated carcinoma
Malignant melanoma
Malignant lymphoma/plasmacytoma
Sarcomas
    Leiomyosarcoma
    Rhabdomyosarcoma
    Malignant fibrous histiocytoma
    Others
Carcinosarcoma
Miscellaneous
    Yolk sac tumor
    Carcinoid tumor
    Salivary gland type tumors
    Others
Secondary Tumors

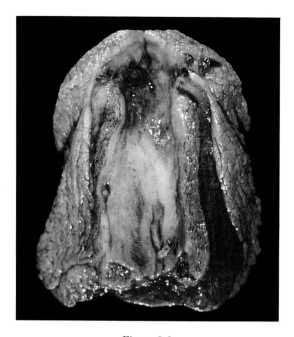

Figure 9-6
SQUAMOUS CELL CARCINOMA, DISTAL URETHRA
The neoplastic area is represented by irregular, erythematous mucosa just proximal to the meatus.

of the adenocarcinomas occur in the bulbomembranous urethra.

The spectrum of cell types of urethral carcinoma is understandable since the epithelium of the prostatic urethra is transitional, that of the membranous and penile (cavernous) portions is pseudostratified or stratified columnar, and that of the fossa navicularis is squamous; additionally, patches of squamous epithelium may be found anywhere throughout the penile urethra. The higher frequency of squamous tumors is probably due to their origin from squamous epithelium that has occurred on a metaplastic basis at sites where the native epithelium is not squamous. This is consistent with the frequent background of chronic irritation that is known to predispose to squamous metaplasia throughout the urinary tract.

At endoscopy there may be a roughened or reddened mucosa, an exophytic cauliflower-like or papillary tumor, or ulceration. In some cases the findings are relatively unimpressive. By the time the patient presents, tumors of the anterior urethra are often a few centimeters in diameter and may have invaded the corpus cavernosum; those of the posterior urethra may invade into or even beyond the prostate or the base of the bladder. Periurethral or perineal abscesses with sinus tracts, fistulae, or both are usually associated with tumors of the membranous urethra. Patients who delay seeking medical attention may have extensive local spread of the tumor.

Gross Findings. The variations in gross morphology seen by the pathologist in resected specimens parallel those seen at endoscopy. The appearance varies from lesions which may be subtle to massive destructive tumors with extensive spread into adjacent tissues (figs. 9-6–9-12). There are variations in appearance according to the different cell types. Squamous lesions may be pearly white, transitional cell lesions papillary, and adenocarcinomas mucoid, but many have nondistinctive features. Carcinomas of Cowper's gland characteristically present as ulcerated perineal lesions (fig. 9-13).

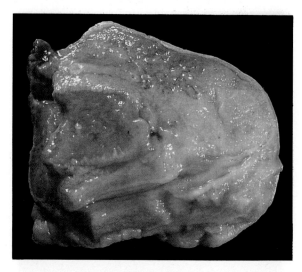

Figure 9-7
SQUAMOUS CELL CARCINOMA, DISTAL URETHRA

The normal urethral mucosa merges with yellow-white granular neoplastic tissue which diffusely infiltrates the adjacent glans.

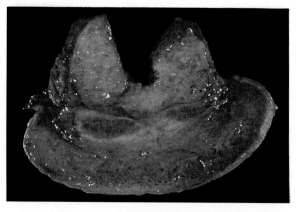

Figure 9-9
SQUAMOUS CELL CARCINOMA, DISTAL URETHRA

A cross section of the tumor in figure 9-8 shows effacement of the corpus spongiosum but sparing of the corpora cavernosa.

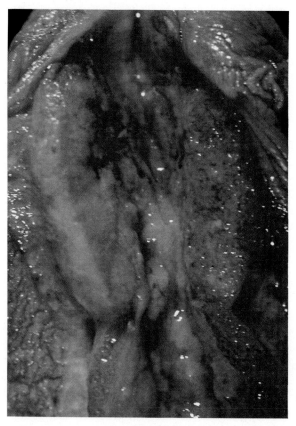

Figure 9-8
SQUAMOUS CELL CARCINOMA, DISTAL URETHRA

This tumor formed an annular constricting mass. The mucosa has a cobblestone appearance.

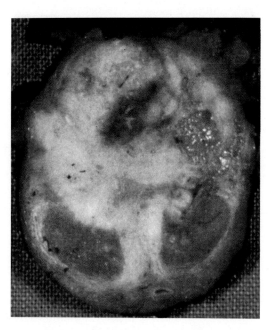

Figure 9-10
SQUAMOUS CELL CARCINOMA,
BULBOMEMBRANOUS URETHRA

A large destructive mass has spread to involve a portion of each corpus cavernosum. (Courtesy of Dr. E.C. Jones, Vancouver, B.C., Canada.)

Microscopic Findings. The microscopic features and spectrum of differentiation of squamous cell carcinomas (figs. 9-14–9-16) are as seen elsewhere. Most are well or moderately differentiated. Rarely, a squamous cell carcinoma has a "pseudosarcomatous" component as seen more commonly in carcinomas of the head and neck, or

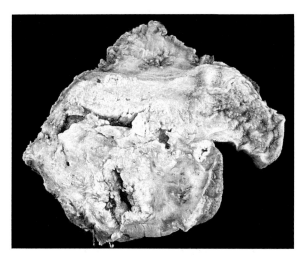

Figure 9-11
SQUAMOUS CELL CARCINOMA
OF PENILE URETHRA

There is massive local spread with destruction of the scrotal contents and extension to scrotal skin. Note the pearly white appearance of the neoplasm and the prominent cyst formation. (Courtesy of Dr. F. Algaba, Barcelona, Spain.)

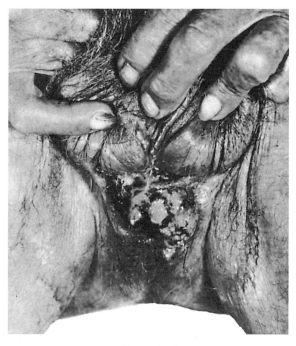

Figure 9-13
COWPER'S GLAND CARCINOMA

Carcinoma of Cowper's gland extensively ulcerates the perineal skin. (Fig. 112 from Fascicles 31B and 32, 1st Series.)

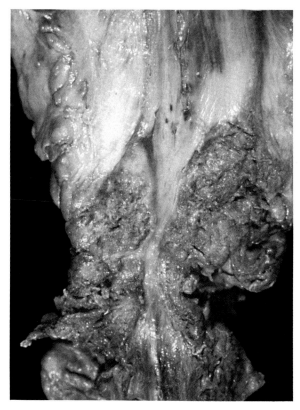

Figure 9-12
TRANSITIONAL CELL CARCINOMA OF URETHRA

The mass has a granular surface. (Courtesy of Dr. C.D. M. Fletcher, Boston, MA.)

basaloid features leading to occasional usage of the term "cloacogenic carcinoma" (17), a term we do not recommend. One squamous cell carcinoma we saw had large areas with features of a so-called lymphoepithelioma-like carcinoma.

The microscopic spectrum exhibited by transitional cell tumors (fig. 9-17) parallels that seen in the urinary bladder, and, as in the bladder, there may be adjacent transitional cell carcinoma in situ (fig. 9-17D). Some transitional cell tumors exhibit squamous or glandular differentiation, or both. Papillomavirus type 6 has been identified in a few low-grade transitional cell carcinomas and in one squamous cell carcinoma (21,35).

The adenocarcinomas may be deeply infiltrative or exophytic papillary lesions that are noninvasive (8). They frequently have a nonspecific microscopic appearance but may resemble colonic adenocarcinoma of typical (41), colloid (fig. 9-18) (8,30,46), or signet ring cell types (37), either partially or predominantly, and may have a villoglandular papillary pattern (29,48). Some tumors have a surface component that resembles a villous adenoma (11a,46). However, interpretation

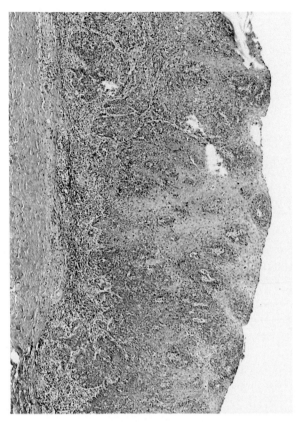

Figure 9-14
SQUAMOUS CELL CARCINOMA, PENILE URETHRA
This tumor is only superficially invasive.

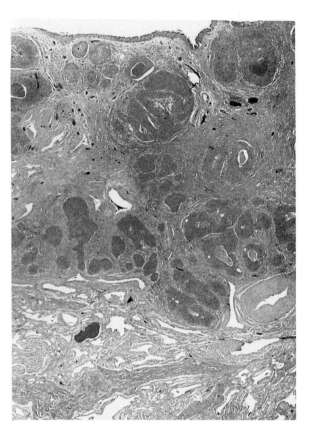

Figure 9-15
SQUAMOUS CELL CARCINOMA,
PENILE URETHRA
This tumor has spread to involve the corpus spongiosum.

Figure 9-16
SQUAMOUS CELL CARCINOMA
OF URETHRA, GRADE 2/3
Note the in situ carcinoma of the overlying epithelium which merges with the invasive tumor at the right. Note also the focal acantholysis, which should not be misinterpreted as representing glandular differentiation.

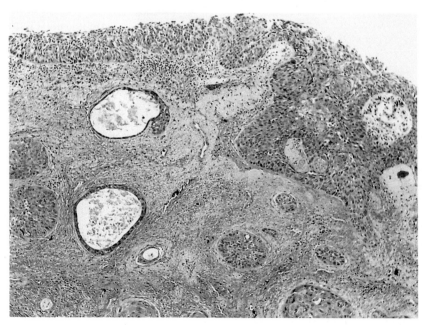

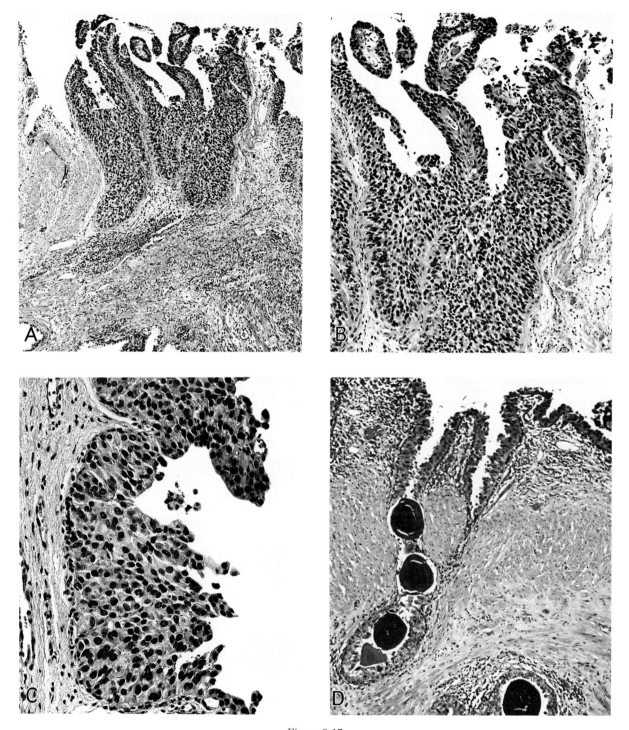

Figure 9-17
TRANSITIONAL CELL CARCINOMA OF PROSTATIC URETHRA

A: Typical low-power view of noninvasive papillary transitional cell carcinoma.

B: Higher power view of tumor in A showing the smooth contour of the base of the tumor.

C: Noninvasive transitional cell carcinoma. At the top and bottom there are foci of stromal hypervascularity with early papilla formation.

D: Nonpapillary transitional cell carcinoma. Carcinoma in situ is seen at the top. There is involvement of periurethral glands by the malignant cells. The smooth contour of those foci indicates a lack of stromal invasion, analogous to the picture that may be seen in the bladder when in situ carcinoma cells involve von Brunn's nests.

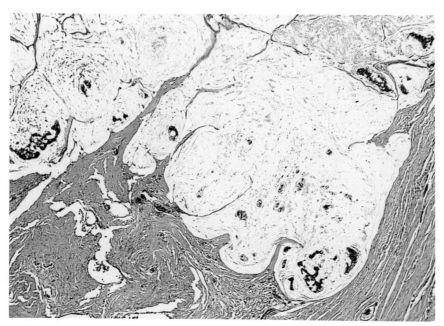

Figure 9-18
COLLOID
ADENOCARCINOMA
OF URETHRA
(Courtesy of Dr. M.L. Silverman,
Burlington, MA.)

of a surface component as villous adenoma should be carefully restricted to tumors with a very regular villous architecture and cytologic atypia that falls short of that of adenocarcinoma. In tumors with a surface component of papillary adenocarcinoma potentially confusable with villous adenoma the surface component is more irregular and has greater cytologic atypia than in the latter. Adenocarcinomas may be associated with adjacent urethritis glandularis (37,46) which may show premalignant changes (8) and is a plausible origin for the tumor in such cases; in other cases adenocarcinoma is presumed to arise from the periurethral glands of Littré (39) or from the scattered mucinous cells that may be present in the urethral epithelium. The exceptionally rare malignant tumors of Cowper's gland are usually pure adenocarcinomas (fig. 9-19A), but two adenoid cystic carcinoma have been reported (fig. 9-19B,C) (11,43).

Occasional adenosquamous carcinomas occur (25,40) and have features similar to those seen elsewhere (fig. 9-20). In some cases the glandular and squamous components are relatively discrete (fig. 9-21), whereas in others there is a more intimate admixture of the two components. Some of these tumors, like occasional squamous or transitional cell carcinomas, may have a conspicuous component of spindled epithelial cells, "sarcomatoid carcinoma" (fig. 9-20). Ad-

enosquamous carcinoma should be distinguished from the more common transitional cell carcinoma with gland differentiation in which transitional cells are seen surrounding the glandular cells in at least some areas. We have seen one urethral tumor that had the features of a low-grade mucoepidermoid carcinoma.

Only three clear cell adenocarcinomas have been reported in the urethra of males (fig. 9-22) (10,24,36); this subtype is much more common in females. One tumor was thought to have possibly arisen from a nephrogenic adenoma (24); another was considered of probable periurethral gland origin (10).

One small cell carcinoma of neuroendocrine type has been described, having the typical cell type and dense core granules on ultrastructural examination (47).

Differential Diagnosis. The distinction of primary carcinoma from secondary spread to the urethra is often difficult or impossible on histologic grounds alone, but the clinical findings and distribution of disease generally aid in these cases. Definite mucosal involvement of the urethral neoplasm on gross and microscopic examination, with apparent "in situ" changes, suggests a primary neoplasm, but secondary tumors may produce a picture that simulates that of primary neoplasia (see page 387). Distinction from secondary involvement by a ductal carcinoma of the

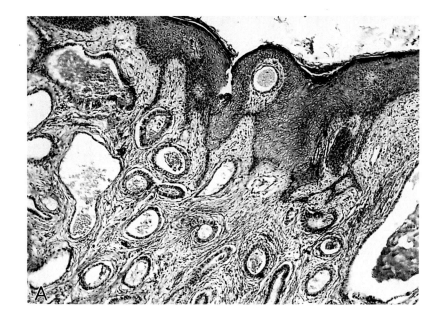

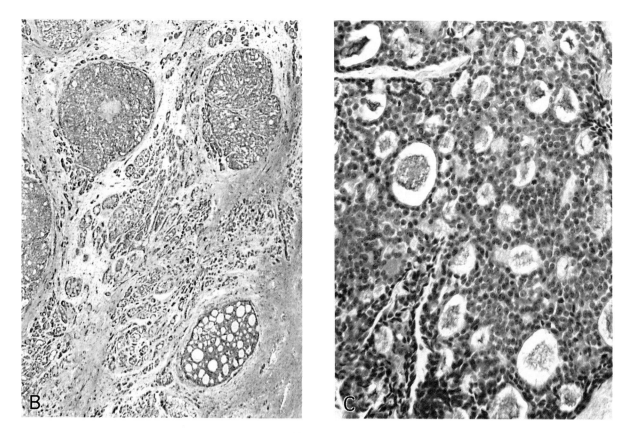

Figure 9-19
CARCINOMAS OF COWPER'S GLAND

A: Adenocarcinoma. Acini of varying sizes are lined by atypical cells which contain intraluminal mucin. (Fig. 113 from Fascicles 31B and 32, 1st Series.)

B,C: Adenoid cystic carcinoma. Note the infiltrative growth in B and the typical punched-out spaces with basophilic luminal material in C. (Courtesy of Dr. D. Gnepp, Providence, RI.) (Case illustrated is that reported in reference 11.)

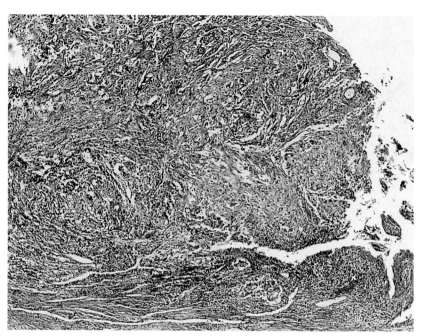

Figure 9-20
ADENOSQUAMOUS
CARCINOMA
This tumor forms a striking poly-
poid intraluminal mass. Note a com-
ponent of spindled epithelial cells.

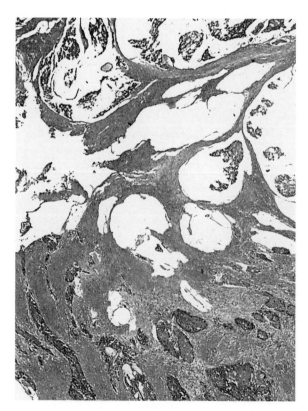

Figure 9-21
ADENOSQUAMOUS CARCINOMA,
BULBOMEMBRANOUS URETHRA
Both colloid adenocarcinoma (top) and conventional
squamous cell carcinoma (bottom) are present. (Courtesy of
Dr. E.C. Jones, Vancouver, BC, Canada.)

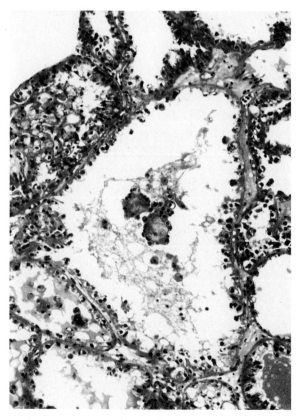

Figure 9-22
CLEAR CELL ADENOCARCINOMA OF URETHRA
Note the characteristic tubulocystic pattern with hobnail
cells. (Courtesy of the late Dr. J. Eggleston, Baltimore, MD.)

prostate may be particularly difficult, and stains for prostate-specific antigen and prostatic acid phosphatase are often indicated to investigate this possibility.

The differential diagnosis of urethral carcinoma with entities other than secondary carcinoma is limited; most of the squamous, transitional, and glandular neoplasms are readily recognized as such and are clearly neoplastic based on a combination of architecture and cytology. Within the adenocarcinomas the greatest difficulty occurs with the clear cell variant, although these tumors are extremely rare in the male urethra. Some clear cell carcinomas may be focally innocuous appearing, making distinction from nephrogenic adenoma difficult in a limited biopsy specimen. When there is clinical evidence of a mass it is strong evidence that the lesion is carcinoma. The most crucial cytologic difference between nephrogenic adenoma and clear cell carcinoma is the paucity of mitotic figures in the former and their relative frequency in the latter (36). Finally, some transitional cell carcinomas have cells with clear cytoplasm (27) which should not lead to their misdiagnosis as clear cell carcinoma in the absence of the typical patterns and other cell types of the latter neoplasm. There is one documented case of transitional cell carcinoma of the urethra initially misdiagnosed as clear cell carcinoma (27) because of clarity of the cytoplasm, admittedly in a female, but this problem could be encountered in a male. The differential diagnosis of adenocarcinoma and villous adenoma has already been considered (see page 376) and is further aided in many cases by identifying definite invasion in the carcinomas.

Behavior. Extensive local invasion is the rule with urethral carcinomas that are not eradicated at an early stage. Invasion of the prostate and base of the bladder occurs with tumors of the prostatic urethra, which may also extend along the mucosa to involve the trigone. Invasion of lymphatics and regional lymph nodes is also frequent. Tumors of the anterior urethra usually spread to inguinal and external iliac lymph nodes, and tumors of the posterior urethra tend to metastasize to the deeper internal iliac and hypogastric nodes, but there are many exceptions. Despite early invasion of the corpus cavernosum, distant bloodborne metastases are rare with either anterior or posterior tumors.

Table 9-3

STAGING OF MALE URETHRAL CANCER*

Stage 0	In situ (limited to mucosa)
Stage A	Submucosal (not beyond submucosa)
Stage B	Into but not beyond the corpus spongiosum or prostate
Stage C	Direct extension into tissue beyond the corpus spongiosum (corpora cavernosum, muscle, fat, fascia, skin, direct skeletal involvement) or beyond the prostatic capsule
Stage D	Metastasis 1) Inguinal lymph nodes 2) Pelvic lymph nodes below the bifurcation of the aorta 3) Lymph nodes above the bifurcation of the aorta 4) Distant

*Modified from reference 28.

Distant visceral metastases, seen in just 29 of 232 patients (13 percent) in a pre-1970 literature review (26), usually occur only in patients who have survived for appreciable periods of time.

The stage is an important prognostic factor for tumors of any site, and the major current staging systems are presented in Tables 9-3 and 9-4. The prognosis for patients with tumors of the anterior urethra is much better than for those with tumors of the posterior urethra. This difference is due to the earlier presentation of anterior tumors and their greater amenability to surgical cure by penile amputation. While local recurrence after excision is not uncommon for tumors of the anterior urethra, it is almost the rule for posterior tumors. Death often results from complications of local disease rather than from metastases. Radical surgical procedures necessary to remove posterior tumors and resultant complications, including morbidity due to urinary tract obstruction and infection with subsequent debilitation, all contribute to the poor outcome.

Malignant Melanoma

General and Clinical Features. Although rare, malignant melanoma accounts for the single greatest number of malignant urethral tumors other than carcinoma (4 percent) (49–55). When only genitourinary tract sites are considered, the

379

Table 9-4

TNM STAGING SYSTEM OF THE AMERICAN JOINT COMMITTEE ON CANCER FOR MALE AND FEMALE URETHRAL CANCER*

Stage	TX	Primary tumor cannot be assessed
	T0	No evidence of primary tumor
	Ta	Noninvasive papillary, polypoid, or verrucous carcinoma
	Tis	Carcinoma in situ
	T1	Tumor invades subepithelial connective tissue
	T2	Tumor invades any of the following: corpus spongiosum, prostate, periurethral muscle
	T3	Tumor invades any of the following: corpus cavernosum, beyond prostatic capsule, anterior vagina, bladder neck
	T4	Tumor invades other adjacent organs
	NX	Regional lymph nodes cannot be assessed
	N0	No regional lymph node metastasis
	N1	Metastasis in a single lymph node, 2 cm or less in greatest dimension
	N2	Metastasis in a single node more than 2 cm in greatest dimension, or in multiple nodes
	MX	Distant metastasis cannot be assessed
	M0	No distant metastasis
	M1	Distant metastasis

*Data from AJCC Cancer Staging Manual, 5th ed. Philadelphia: Lippincott Raven, 1997:248.

urethra is a relatively frequent primary site for melanoma. It is, however, less common than penile melanoma (50) and less common in the male urethra than in the female urethra. Of the approximately 160 cases of primary urethral melanoma in the world literature, 37 percent have been in males.

The tumors almost always occur in patients over 50 years of age, with an average age at diagnosis of 61 years; no cases have been reported in patients in the first three decades. They are exceptionally rare in black men. The presenting symptoms are similar to those of other urethral cancers, except for occasional patients who have melanuria. The majority of the cases have involved the fossa navicularis (55 percent), but the prostatic urethra (15 percent), pendulous urethra (15 percent), bulbous urethra (10 percent), and meatus (5 percent) may also be primary sites. The prognosis is very poor, but occasional patients, usually those with tumors invasive to less than 2 mm, have survived 5 or more years (51a).

Gross Findings. Like melanomas elsewhere, the lesion is frequently noteworthy grossly because of its black color, but amelanotic tumors are not rare. The tumors usually are polypoid masses but occasionally are papules or macules. They may be multifocal (fig. 9-23).

Microscopic Findings and Differential Diagnosis. The tumors often resemble their counterparts in the skin (figs. 9-24, 9-25) but, in our experience, are sometimes not readily classifiable into the well-known cutaneous subtypes. The melanin content is variable, and its absence may make the diagnosis difficult. A prominent spindle cell component may also cause problems. Rare cases have had a prominent papillary pattern and mimicked a papillary transitional cell carcinoma (51a,52a). In one series of three urethral melanomas, one was initially misdiagnosed as a sarcoma and another as a transitional cell carcinoma (51).

Pagetoid spread of primary carcinomas of the urethra and paraurethral glands, and pagetoid spread to the urethra from the bladder, may simulate a malignant melanoma. Mucin stains should aid in the case of adenocarcinomas, and immunohistochemical stains, particularly HMB-45, may also be indicated to assist in this differential diagnosis. For cases with a papillary pattern cytoplasmic melanin pigment may be an important clue and appropriate immunostains (cytokeratin, S-100 protein, HMB-45) can resolve the differential with papillary transitional cell carcinoma if the possibility of melanoma is considered (52a). Immunostains also aid in the differential diagnosis

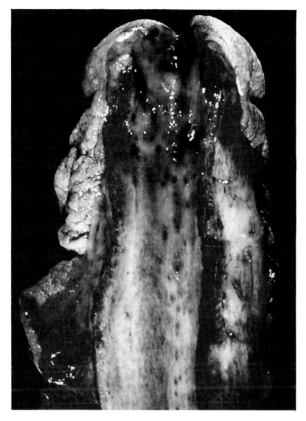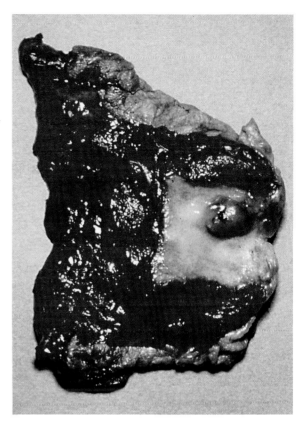

Figure 9-23
MALIGNANT MELANOMA OF URETHRA
Left: The distal urethra shows a variably pigmented lesion with irregular edges. Figure 2 from Oliva E, Quinn TR, Amin MB, et al. Primary malignant melanoma of the urethra: a clinicopathological analysis of 15 cases. Am J Surg Pathol 2000;24:785–96.
Right: In another case the lesion is polypoid. (Courtesy of Dr. J.C. Manivel, Minneapolis, MN.)

between overtly invasive melanoma and a poorly differentiated carcinoma or sarcoma. Before the diagnosis of a primary malignant melanoma is rendered, the possibility of spread to the urethra should be excluded by obtaining a detailed clinical history and suggesting clinical evaluation for an overlooked primary tumor elsewhere.

Other Malignant Primary Tumors

Malignant urethral tumors of other types are rare and include occasional sarcomas (56). A rhabdomyosarcoma of the posterior urethra has been described in a 10-year-old boy (57). We have seen a case of primary malignant fibrous histiocytoma at the meatus (fig. 9-26). One carcinosarcoma of the penile urethra has been reported (67).

Non-Hodgkin's lymphoma has occasionally been reported to present with manifestations in the male urethra (58,60,61,63), and we have seen an unpublished example in a 30-year-old man that was a diffuse large cell lymphoma of B-cell lineage (fig. 9-27). One T-cell lymphoma was the initial manifestation in a patient with acquired immunodeficiency syndrome (AIDS) (59). Plasmacytomas have also rarely presented in the urethra (62,66).

Single cases of yolk sac tumor (64) and carcinoid tumor (65), both apparently primary in the male urethra, have been reported. We have seen an additional unpublished example of a primary yolk sac tumor in the prostatic urethra of a 20-month-old boy (fig. 9-28). The lesion could not be surgically excised and the patient received both chemotherapy and radiation therapy but died with extensive local recurrence and pulmonary metastases within a few months (Professor H. B. Marsden, personal communication). We have also seen a primary tumor, apparently

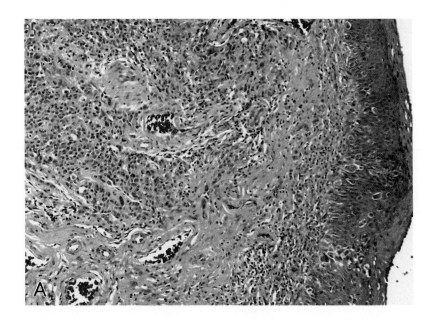

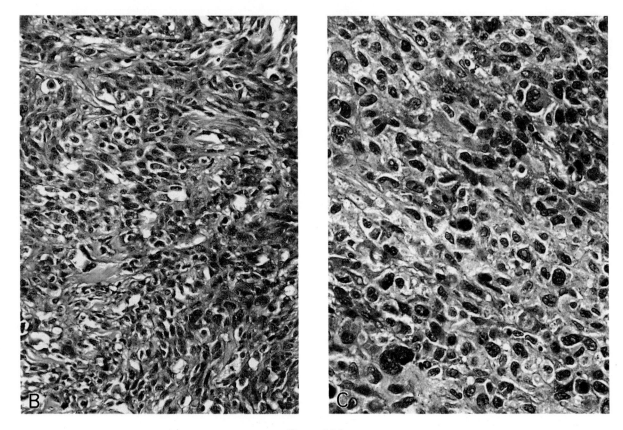

Figure 9-24
MALIGNANT MELANOMA OF URETHRA
A: An invasive component is associated with an intraepithelial component (right). Pigment is not apparent.
B: This tumor has epithelioid and spindled areas.
C: The same case as in B shows focal pigmentation.

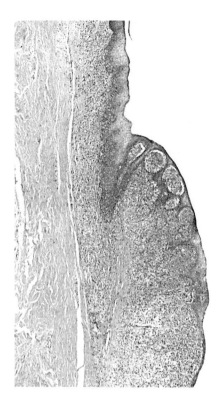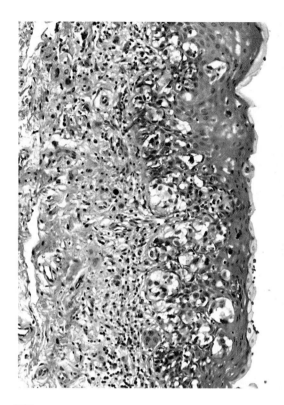

Figure 9-25
MALIGNANT MELANOMA OF URETHRA
Left: There are radial and vertical growth phases.
Right: An intraepithelial component with pagetoid spread is apparent.

derived from Cowper's glands, which resembled a low-grade malignant mixed tumor of salivary gland type (fig. 9-29). If the urethra is involved by a huge tumor, estimation of the primary site may be difficult or impossible.

Secondary Tumors

The possibility of a secondary neoplasm of the urethra is an important consideration, particularly with posterior tumors. As mentioned earlier, transitional cell carcinomas of the prostatic urethra frequently occur in patients with a history of transitional cell carcinoma of the bladder (69,70, 73,80). Many probably represent independent neoplasms, reflecting the propensity of the urothelium to undergo multifocal neoplasia; accordingly, they are not conventionally considered secondary neoplasms. In occasional cases transitional cell carcinoma of the bladder involves the urethra in a pagetoid fashion, sometimes involving the periurethral glands, or extending to the meatus

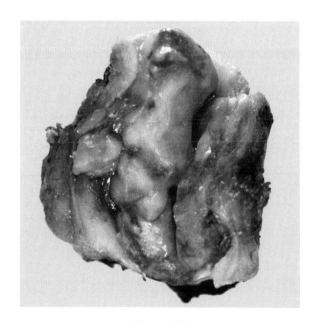

Figure 9-26
MALIGNANT FIBROUS HISTIOCYTOMA
A large mass envelops and protrudes into the urethra.
(Courtesy of Dr. A. Levine, Royal Oak, MI.)

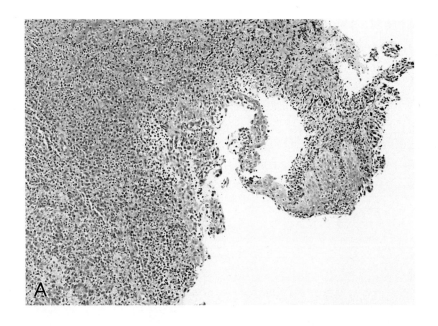

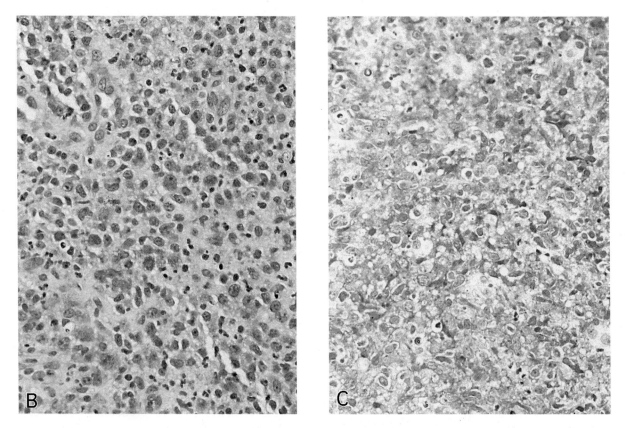

Figure 9-27
MALIGNANT LYMPHOMA OF URETHRA

This mass involved the urethra of a 30-year-old man and accounted for the clinical presentation. The tumor was of B-cell type. The urethral epithelium is seen at the right in A, the neoplastic lymphoid cells with prominent nucleoli in B, and positive immunoreactivity for leukocyte common antigen in C.

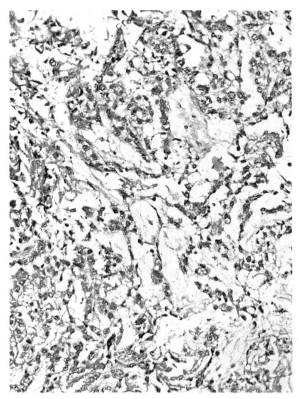

Figure 9-28
YOLK SAC TUMOR OF PROSTATIC URETHRA
There is a characteristic reticular pattern in this case from a 20-month-old boy. (Courtesy of Professor H. B. Marsden, Manchester, UK.)

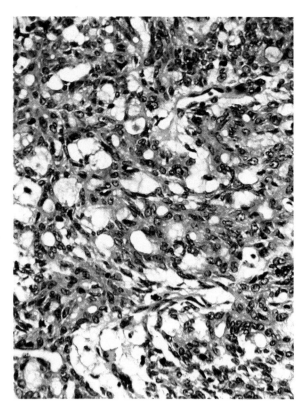

Figure 9-29
MALIGNANT MIXED TUMOR OF SALIVARY GLAND TYPE OF PROBABLE COWPER'S GLAND ORIGIN
This cellular tumor shows myoepithelial differentiation (spindled and epithelioid cells) as well as epithelial differentiation in the form of small tubules, some containing mucinous material.

(68,74–79). Any malignant tumor of the bladder may involve the urethra by direct extension, and occasionally striking cases of urethral recurrence of bladder tumors of various types are seen (figs. 9-30, 9-31) (82,83). Rarely, tumors of the upper urinary system, including Wilms' tumor, involve the urethra (71a,81).

Prostatic adenocarcinoma is an important category of true secondary neoplasia of the prostatic urethra (fig. 9-32); it accounted for one third of proximal urethral tumors in one large series (72). Prostatic adenocarcinoma of ductal type is particularly prone to present as an intraurethral mass (fig. 9-33), and it is important to consider it in the differential of a urethral adenocarcinoma because of its clinical implications (fig. 9-34). Immunohistochemical stains for PSA and PAP usually assist in the diagnosis of a prostatic neoplasm. Less often, the conventional small acinar adenocarcinoma presents as an intraurethral mass and may be confused with a prostatic-type polyp (see page 392) when there is a relatively orderly growth of small glands without high-grade atypia. Careful evaluation, however, shows the cytologic features of prostatic adenocarcinoma and the expected absence of basal cells. The penile urethra is less often involved by prostatic carcinoma and in such cases it has been suggested that implantation after a prior catheterization or transurethral resection may explain this phenomenon (76,77).

Spread from more distant sites may also be problematic; in particular, colorectal adenocarcinoma may resemble occasional primary urethral adenocarcinomas by light microscopy, histochemistry, and immunohistochemistry (71). The clinical history and overall clinical evaluation are important in such cases.

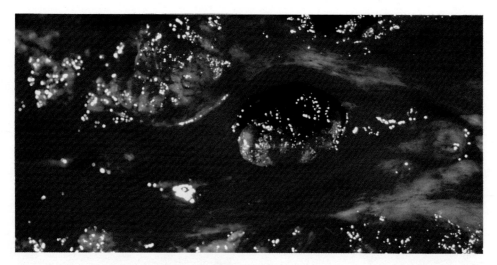

Figure 9-30
SECONDARY INVOLVEMENT OF URETHRA BY TRANSITIONAL CELL CARCINOMA OF URINARY BLADDER
There is a discrete polypoid intraluminal mass. Less obvious foci of tumor are seen in the urethral wall.

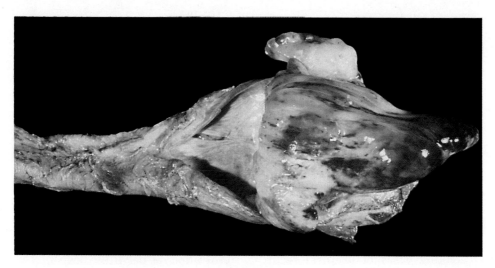

Figure 9-31
SECONDARY INVOLVEMENT OF URETHRA BY CARCINOSARCOMA OF BLADDER
A large polypoid mass projects from the urethral mucosa.

BENIGN TUMORS

Transitional Cell Papillomas

Both typical (fig. 9-35) and inverted (fig. 9-36) types of transitional cell papilloma occur in the urethra (Table 9-5) and account for a subset of urethral "polyps" (88). We restrict the diagnosis of typical papilloma to rare lesions that meet the criteria of Eble and Young (84) and distinguish them from grade 1 papillary transitional cell carcinoma by their lesser degree of hyperplasia and absence of dysplasia. Only 3.5 percent of inverted papillomas occur in the urethra, almost always in the prostatic segment (86,87), although rare cases are also described in the penile and bulbomembranous urethra (85). The description of both typical and inverted papillomas of the urethra in the literature is limited, but there is no evidence from these reports or our own experience that they differ grossly or microscopically from those in the urinary bladder. It should be noted that, as in the bladder, some urethral papillomas are of mixed

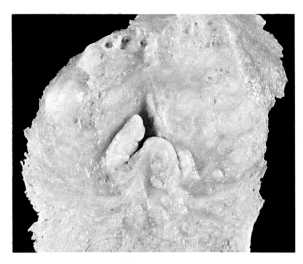

Figure 9-32
SECONDARY INVOLVEMENT OF URETHRA
BY PROSTATIC ADENOCARCINOMA

A polypoid white focus of tumor projects into the urethral lumen in the region of the verumontanum. (Courtesy of Dr. J.N. Eble, Indianapolis, IN.)

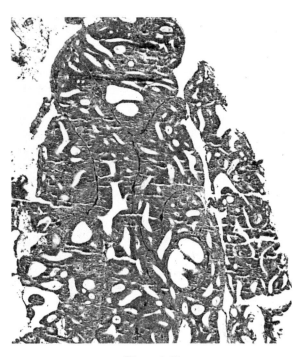

Figure 9-33
SECONDARY INVOLVEMENT OF URETHRA
BY PROSTATIC DUCTAL ADENOCARCINOMA

A polypoid focus of tumor forms an intraluminal mass.

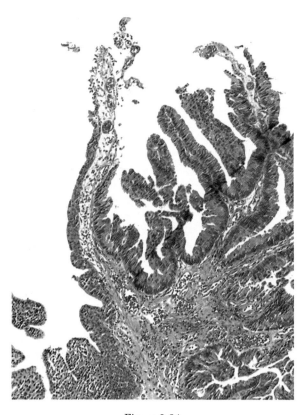

Figure 9-34
SECONDARY INVOLVEMENT OF URETHRA
BY PROSTATIC DUCT ADENOCARCINOMA

The mucosal involvement simulates a primary urethral adenocarcinoma.

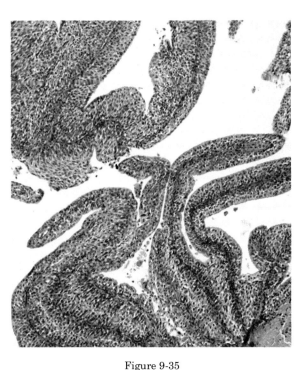

Figure 9-35
TRANSITIONAL CELL PAPILLOMA, TYPICAL TYPE

Tall finger-like papillae lined by hyperplastic transitional cells project from the urethral mucosa.

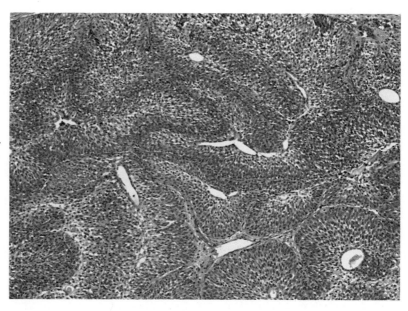

Figure 9-36
TRANSITIONAL CELL
PAPILLOMA, INVERTED TYPE
There is a compact arrangement of trabeculae of transitional cells focally punctuated by glandular spaces.

Table 9-5

HISTOLOGIC CLASSIFICATION OF BENIGN TUMORS AND TUMOR-LIKE LESIONS OF THE MALE URETHRA

Benign Tumors

Typical papilloma
Inverted papilloma
Villous adenoma
Hemangioma
Leiomyoma
Others

Tumor-Like Lesions

Von Brunn's nests, urethritis glandularis, urethritis cystica
Polypoid-papillary urethritis
Nonspecific chronic urethritis
Nephrogenic adenoma
Fibroepithelial polyp
Prostatic-type polyp
Condyloma acuminatum
Squamous papilloma
Transitional cell hyperplasia
Malakoplakia
Amyloidosis
Radiation change
Verumontanum gland hypertrophy
Cowper's gland hyperplasia
Others, including infectious diseases

type, having an exophytic (typical) component and an endophytic (inverted) component.

Villous Adenoma

A single example of this lesion occurring in pure form has been reported in detail in the male urethra (89), and another example is mentioned in an older paper on glandular metaplasia in the urinary tract (90). The case described in detail occurred in a 70-year-old and involved the prostatic urethra. Follow-up at 1 year was uneventful. The lesion appeared similar to the typical colonic lesion. Because of the rarity of urethral villous adenoma and because some urethral adenocarcinomas are predominantly papillary (see page 376) and may be only focally invasive, the diagnosis of villous adenoma should be made cautiously and only after the lesion has been entirely resected and examined, with particular attention to the base. Some adenocarcinomas have been interpreted as arising from a villous adenoma (89a,91).

Benign Mesenchymal Tumors

Benign mesenchymal tumors, such as leiomyomas and hemangiomas (92–95), occur rarely in the male urethra, the former being much more common in women. Their pathologic features, and those of other benign mesenchymal tumors, do not differ from those seen elsewhere.

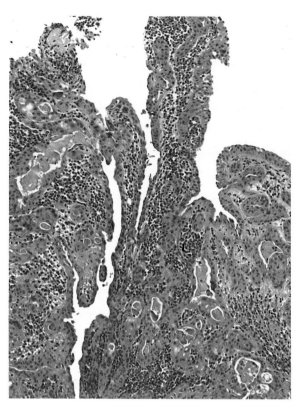

Figure 9-37
PAPILLARY URETHRITIS
Papillae project from a prominently inflamed urethra.

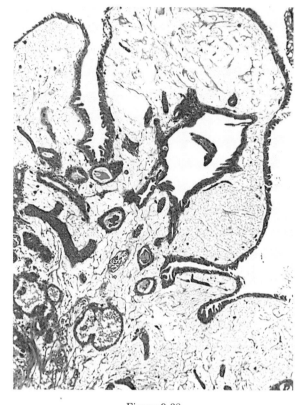

Figure 9-38
POLYPOID URETHRITIS
Edematous polyps project into the urethral lumen.

TUMOR-LIKE LESIONS

Von Brunn's Nests, Urethritis Glandularis, and Urethritis Cystica

These well-known, common proliferations of bladder urothelium may also be seen in the prostatic urethra. In a study of the proximal prostatic urethra, either von Brunn's nests or urethritis glandularis were found in 72 percent of the specimens (96). In a series of patients with schistosomiasis, "urethritis cystica" (a term apparently used for the triad of von Brunn's nests, urethritis glandularis, and urethritis cystica), was found in 80 percent of the cases (102). The features of these lesions are similar to those seen in the bladder, and they are usually not a source of diagnostic difficulty. Intestinal metaplasia is rarely seen in urethritis glandularis and may also be seen in the mucosa lining the urethra (97). There may be associated dysplasia (97) and even adenocarcinoma (99).

Polypoid-Papillary Urethritis and Nonspecific Chronic Urethritis

Papillary (fig. 9-37) or more commonly polypoid (fig. 9-38) inflammatory lesions may occur in any portion of the male urethra (98,100). These lesions typically have a prominently vascular stroma with varying degrees of inflammation and edema (granulation tissue-like) (98). The covering epithelium may be hyperplastic or attenuated and is usually transitional but may exhibit squamous or, rarely, mucinous metaplasia. The stroma in cases of polypoid-papillary urethritis is typically more abundant, vascular, and inflamed than that of either a transitional cell papilloma or carcinoma, and the epithelium of the latter two lesions shows more uniform hyperplasia than seen in papillary-polypoid urethritis.

The proximal urethral mucosa and the underlying periurethral glands and ducts may, in the setting of prominent chronic inflammation, exhibit hyperplastic and metaplastic changes

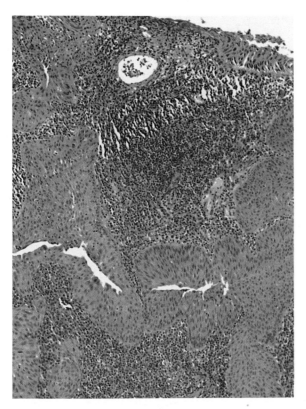

Figure 9-39
CHRONIC URETHRITIS
There is prominent hyperplasia of periurethral gland epithelium and associated marked chronic inflammation producing a superficially worrisome picture.

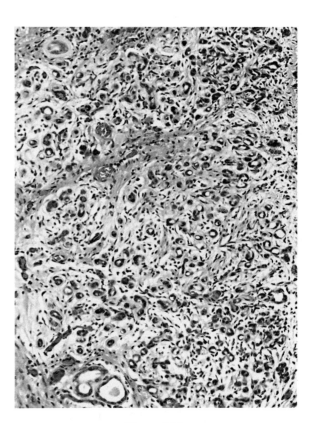

Figure 9-40
NEPHROGENIC ADENOMA OF URETHRA
Note the characteristic tiny tubules.

(fig. 9-39) with reactive atypia that produce a striking picture and raise concern for carcinoma. The usual retention of an orderly architecture, lack of high-grade cytologic atypia, and associated inflammation should enable distinction of particularly florid examples from carcinoma, but the interpretation can be difficult.

The urethritis that occurs in patients with Reiter's syndrome is usually obviously of inflammatory type, although gray-white elevated lesions that may be grossly confused with a neoplasm are rarely encountered (101). The non-neoplastic nature of the lesion is readily apparent on microscopic examination.

Nephrogenic Adenoma

Approximately 10 percent of nephrogenic adenomas occur in the urethra. In men, nephrogenic adenoma involves either the bulbous or, more often, the prostatic urethra (103,104,106–

108). There is usually a history of transurethral resection consistent with the known association of nephrogenic adenoma with trauma. The lesions may be exophytic or flat and on microscopic examination exhibit the spectrum of tubular (figs. 9-40, 9-41), cystic (fig. 9-42), and papillary to polypoid patterns (fig. 9-43) seen in the examples encountered more commonly in the bladder. The lesion is usually confined to the mucosa or a relatively narrow zone immediately beneath it, but occasionally the tubules may extend downward for some distance and rarely involve the prostate (104,106,108) (see chapter 7). One case was interpreted as nephrogenic adenoma of the male urethra associated with clear cell adenocarcinoma (105).

Fibroepithelial Polyps

Urethral fibroepithelial polyps are less common than ureteral examples. Most have been reported in males younger than 10 years, but a

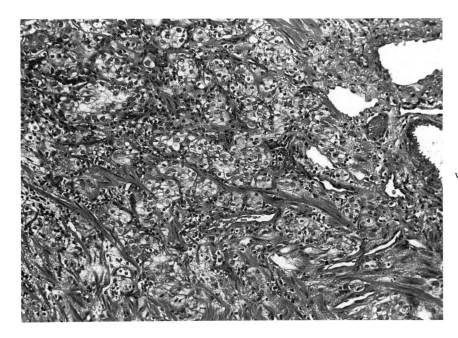

Figure 9-41
NEPHROGENIC ADENOMA
OF URETHRA
Small solid tubules are some-
what irregularly distributed.

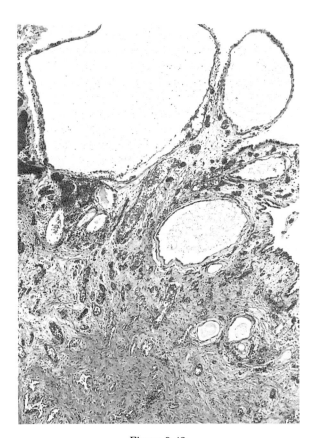

Figure 9-42
NEPHROGENIC ADENOMA OF URETHRA
There is a typical cystic pattern.

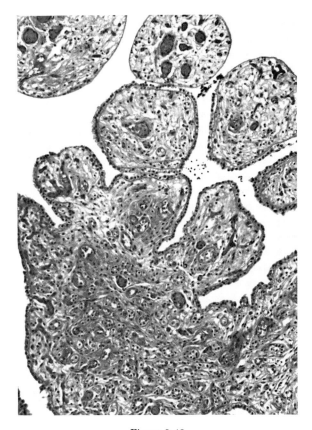

Figure 9-43
NEPHROGENIC ADENOMA OF URETHRA
A characteristic polypoid pattern is present.

Table 9-6

DIFFERENTIAL DIAGNOSIS OF POLYPOID URETHRAL LESIONS IN MALES*

Type	Usual Age Range (yrs)	Usual Location	Proposed Pathogenesis
Fibroepithelial polyp	<10	P**	Developmental (? postinflammatory)
Polypoid urethritis	Wide range	P	Inflammatory
Nephrogenic adenoma	Wide range	P	Metaplastic
Condyloma acuminatum	20–40	D	Virus-associated
Prostatic-type polyp	20–40	P	Developmental ectopia
Squamous papilloma	20–40	D	Neoplastic
Transitional cell papilloma	>40	P	Neoplastic
Papillary carcinoma	>40	P,D	Neoplastic
Prostatic carcinoma	>60	P	Neoplastic

*Modified from Table 12-1 from Srigley JR, Hartwick RW. Surgical pathology of the male urethra and seminal vesicles. In: (Bostwick DG, ed. Pathology of the prostate. Vol. 15. Contemporary issues in surgical pathology. New York: Churchill Livingstone, 1990:213.)
**P = proximal urethra; D = distal urethra.

few have arisen in adults (111). A series of 17 cases occurring in the posterior urethra close to the verumontanum has been reported in children from 4 months to 12 years of age (110); they have also been reported in the anterior urethra (111). The childhood polyps range from 4 to 27 mm (110). In children these lesions may reflect a developmental anomaly whereas in adults they are probably the result of longstanding polypoid urethritis. One polyp that may have been of fibroepithelial type had prominent vascularity of granulation tissue type and was likened to a pyogenic granuloma (109). Conventional fibroepithelial polyps are covered by transitional epithelium that may be ulcerated or show squamous metaplasia. Sometimes, ulcerated polyps show marked reactive epithelial atypia which can result in atypical cells being shed in the urine and lead to a false positive cytology. The stroma is composed of loose connective tissue.

Prostatic-Type Polyp

This is an important benign papillary lesion of the prostatic urethra (Table 9-6) (112–122) containing prostatic type epithelium. Most are found in young men who characteristically present with hematuria or hematospermia, but they may be seen in older patients. They were especially common around the verumontanum in one large series (117). They are generally 1 cm or less in size and appear as sessile, papillary lesions. Microscopic examination shows delicate papillae or occasionally thicker polypoid fronds covered by cuboidal to columnar cells, similar to those lining prostatic acini (fig. 9-44), with underlying basal cells. Verumontanum mucosal glands may also be present. Prostatic-type glands are present in the stroma. A component of transitional epithelium may also be present, particularly on the surface (114). The prostatic nature of the epithelium can be confirmed by immunohistochemical staining for PSA and PAP.

Because they are often found in young men, the differential diagnosis with polypoid protrusion of prostatic adenocarcinoma into the urethra rarely arises, but in older patients it may, and the clinical presentation may be similar (119). Thus, the diagnosis of a prostatic-type polyp in an elderly male should be made only after carcinoma has been ruled out by careful microscopic evaluation. The prostatic-type polyp must also be differentiated from papillary adenocarcinoma of the prostatic urethra and metastatic adenocarcinomas from other sites, but this is rarely difficult because of the bland cytologic features of the former.

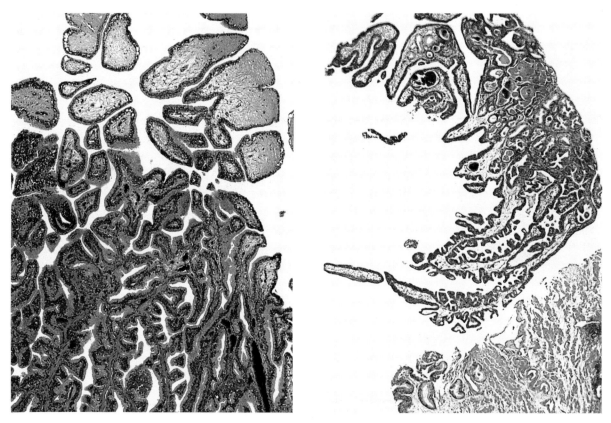

Figure 9-44
URETHRAL POLYPS
Left: Prostatic-type polyp of urethra. Polypoid structures are present superficially, with prostatic type glands beneath them.
Right: Prostatic-type polyp of verumontanum. An exophytic lesion contains verumontanum glands, many of which contain concretions (upper left). Prostatic type epithelium is seen towards the bottom.

Condyloma Acuminatum and Squamous Papilloma

Condylomata acuminata involve the urethra in 5 to 25 percent of cases in which there is involvement of the male genital system, usually in patients from 15 to 40 years of age (123–137). The symptoms are those of a urethral mass: frequency, hematuria, urethral bleeding or discharge, and difficulty voiding. Typically only the distal urethra is involved (129a) since the majority of lesions are just inside the urethral meatus (fig. 9-45) (124), but occasionally there is extension to the proximal urethra, and rarely the bladder and ureter are involved (123). In one study of 27 cases, 13 were located just inside the meatus, 8 from 2 to 2.9 cm from the meatus, 3 from 3 to 3.9 cm from the meatus, and 3 involved the entire urethra (135). No lesions involved the prostatic and membranous urethra alone. There are often multiple lesions (126), and in some cases they are numerous (130). Grossly (fig. 9-45) and microscopically (fig. 9-46) these lesions are similar to those of the genital mucosa. Like the genital lesions, human papilloma virus (HPV) has been detected in up to 96 percent of male urethral condyloma acuminata, using in situ hybridization with biotinylated HPV DNA probes on formalin-fixed, paraffin-embedded tissues; both HPV 6/11 and 16/18 DNA have been detected (131). In another study using polymerase chain reaction evaluation of urine specimens the most common subtypes of HPV were 6 and 11 (133). As elsewhere, an occasional case is associated with carcinoma, which may have arisen from the condyloma (137). At least one case reported in the older literature as a "condyloma"

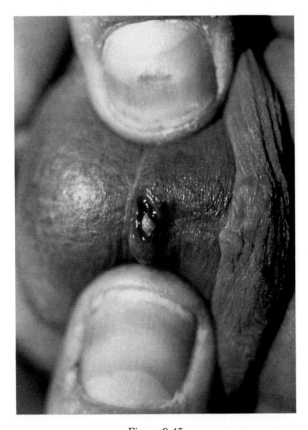

Figure 9-45
CONDYLOMA ACUMINATUM OF URETHRA

The urethral meatus has been everted to disclose a small white papillary lesion. (Fig. 18.19 from Weiss MA, Mills SE. Atlas of genitourinary tract disorders. Philadelphia: JB Lippincott, 1988:18.11.)

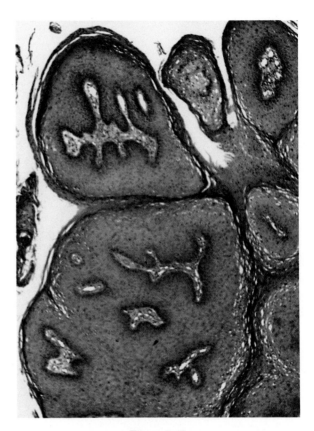

Figure 9-46
CONDYLOMA ACUMINATUM

Note the typical low-power histologic appearance. (Courtesy of Dr. A. Huvos, New York, NY.)

with extensive local spread represented a warty (condylomatous) carcinoma (134).

In the region of the meatus one may see squamoproliferative lesions with an inflammatory stromal component that have some of the clinical, gross (fig. 9-47), and microscopic characteristics of the urethral caruncle of females, although the general convention in the literature has been not to designate these lesions as "caruncles." There is a spectrum from lesions resembling squamous papillomas, with absent to marked inflammation (fig. 9-48), to inflammatory polyps. Huvos and Gradstald (132) described 18 examples in this general category (including a few condylomas) which were usually solitary polypoid lesions of the distal penile urethra and periurethral area (fig. 9-47). The clinical findings were the usual ones associated with a urethral abnormality, and on microscopic examination there was

usually a papillary proliferation of squamous epithelium with hyperkeratosis and a variably prominent inflammatory stromal component (fig. 9-48).

Transitional Cell Hyperplasia of Periurethral Glands

Transitional cells of the periurethral glands are often prominent and the point at which they become "hyperplastic" is unclear. In a series of autopsies of young men, "conspicuous hyperplasia" was found in almost 20 percent (138). This process is sometimes so striking (fig. 9-49) that a misdiagnosis of transitional cell carcinoma is possible, particularly if associated with a similar change in the underlying prostatic ducts (139). However, the transitional cells in this benign phenomenon lack cytologic atypia.

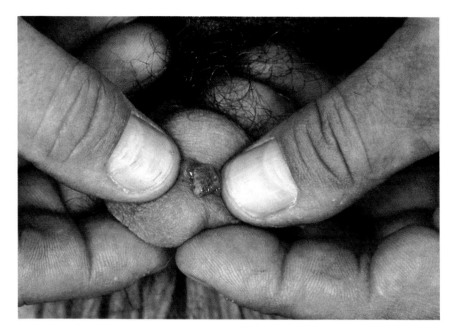

Figure 9-47
SQUAMOUS PAPILLOMA
OF URETHRAL MEATUS
The polypoid lesion is some-
what reminiscent of the well-known
caruncle of females. (Courtesy of Dr.
A. Huvos, New York, NY.)

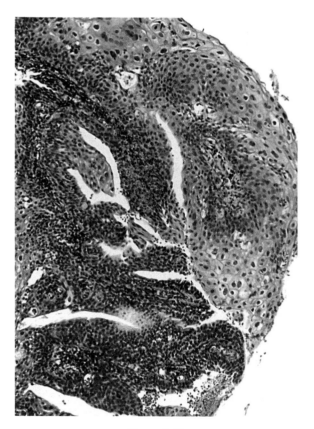

Figure 9-48
SQUAMOUS PAPILLOMA OF URETHRAL MEATUS
WITH PROMINENT STROMAL INFLAMMATION
(Courtesy of Dr. A. Huvos, New York, NY.)

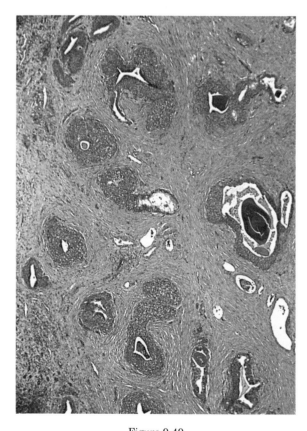

Figure 9-49
TRANSITIONAL CELL HYPERPLASIA
OF PERIURETHRAL GLANDS
On high-power examination there was no cytologic atypicality.

395

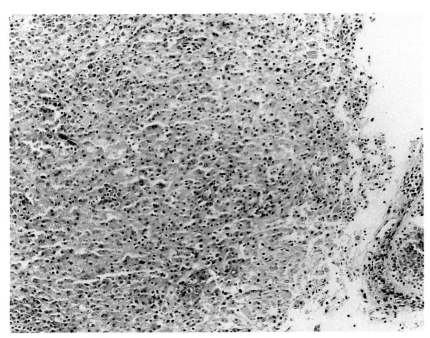

Figure 9-50
MALAKOPLAKIA OF URETHRA
There is a diffuse proliferation of histiocytes with abundant cytoplasm that was eosinophilic, and scattered chronic inflammatory cells. Michaelis-Gutmann bodies are visible in the cytoplasm of a number of cells on close scrutiny. Note fragments of detached urethral epithelium on the right.

Malakoplakia

The male urethra is a very infrequent site of involvement by malakoplakia, particularly when compared to other sites in the urogenital system, with less than 30 examples described (140). In one case from a 64-year-old man, a firm mass extended 5 cm distally from the prostatic urethra and clinically was thought to represent carcinoma (141). Microscopic examination showed the characteristic von Hansemann histiocytes of malakoplakia with the pathognomonic Michaelis-Gutmann bodies. Similar features were present in one unpublished example of malakoplakia of the male urethra we have seen (fig. 9-50).

Amyloidosis

Almost 30 examples of primary localized amyloidosis of the urethra have been reported in males 21 to 82 years of age, most of whom were over 40 years (142–150). In many of the cases the urethral involvement simulated carcinoma clinically, and it was only pathologic examination that clarified the diagnosis by showing the characteristic features of amyloidosis. Involvement of the penile urethra has been most common, but the bulbous and prostatic segments have also been involved (149). On gross examination, ill-defined ulceration and plaque-like or nodular lesions may be present. The process is usually amenable to conservative surgical therapy, but in one patient amyloidosis behaved like a locally invasive tumor and required extensive urethral reconstruction (142).

Radiation Change

As elsewhere in the body, radiation therapy may cause architectural distortion, metaplasia, cytologic atypia, and stromal changes producing a picture that may be confusing (fig. 9-51), particularly if the history is unavailable.

Verumontanum Gland Hypertrophy

Hypertrophy of the verumontanum was the subject of some interest in the older literature but has received little attention recently. It should be noted that this term is used for gross enlargement of the verumontanum and is distinct from the mucosal gland hyperplasia that has been recently emphasized as a rare cause of problems in the differential diagnosis of prostate carcinoma (see chapter 7). As summarized by Herbut (151), hypertrophy of the verumontanum is characterized by enlargement that usually does not exceed 2 cm in diameter and may appear as a regular elevation into the urethra or a

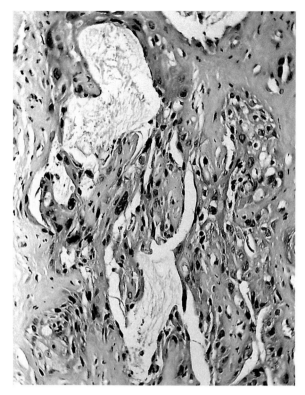

Figure 9-51
RADIATION CHANGE INVOLVING URETHRA
Periurethral glands are distorted and show squamous metaplasia with cytologic atypicality. There is marked hyaline fibrosis of the intervening stroma.

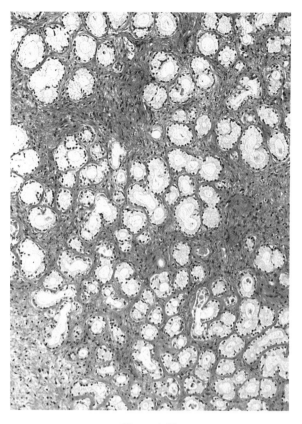

Figure 9-52
LOBULAR HYPERPLASIA OF COWPER'S GLAND
The benign-appearing acini are closely packed and arranged in lobules separated by bland fibrous stroma.

more pedunculated lesion. There is typically a smooth surface, and on microscopic examination one sees the normal complex histology of the verumontanum. Clinically, this lesion may result in symptoms similar to those associated with an enlarged "median lobe" of the prostate.

Cowper's Gland Hyperplasia

We have observed an apparently unique case that we have designated lobular hyperplasia of Cowper's gland. It presented as an approximately 6 cm perineal mass in the Cowper's gland region of a 46-year-old man (fig. 9-52). On microscopic

examination the typical mucinous acini and ducts of Cowper's gland were greatly expanded but maintained a normal lobular architecture.

Infectious Disease Mimicking Neoplasia

As at other locations in the body, and particularly in some geographic regions, infectious diseases may produce a mass suspicious for a neoplasm. Clinical evaluation by an experienced observer is often definitive, however, and light microscopy with appropriate special studies resolves the differential in clinically ambiguous cases.

REFERENCES

Anatomy and Histology

1. Bloom A, Fawcett DW. A textbook of histology, 10th ed. Philadelphia: WB Saunders, 1975:799–804.
2. Herbut P. The urethra. In: Urological pathology, vol I, Philadelphia: Lea and Febiger, 1952:20–6.
3. Johnson FP. The later development of the urethra in the male. J Urol 1920;4:447–501.
4. McCallum RW. The adult male urethra: normal anatomy, pathology and method of urethrography. Radiol Clin North Am 1979;17:227–44.

5. McCarthy JF, Ritter JS, Klemperer P. Anatomical and histological study of the verumontanum with especial reference to the ejaculatory ducts. J Urol 1927;17:1–16.
6. Rytina AG. The verumontanum, with special reference to the sinus pocularis: its anatomy, histology, and physiology. J Urol 1917;1:231–43.

Carcinoma of Male Urethra

7. Bans LL, Eble JN, Lingeman JE, Maynard BR. Transitional cell carcinoma of the fossa navicularis of the male urethra. J Urol 1983;129:1055–6.
8. Bostwick DG, Lo R, Stamey TA. Papillary adenocarcinoma of the male urethra. Case report and review of the literature. Cancer 1984;54:2556–63.
9. Bryan RL, Newman J, Suarez, W, Kadow C, O'Brien JM. The significance of prostatic urothelial dysplasia. Histopathology 1983;22:501–3.
10. Cantrell BB, Leifer G, DeKlerk DP, Eggleston JC. Papillary adenocarcinoma of the prostatic urethra with clear-cell appearance. Cancer 1981;48:2661–7.
11. Carpenter AA, Bernardo JR Jr. Adenoid cystic carcinoma of Cowper's gland: case report. J Urol 1971;106:701–3.
11a. Cheng L, Montironi R, Bostwick DG. Villous adenoma of the urinary tract: a report of 23 cases, including 8 with coexistent adenocarcinoma. Am J Surg Pathol 1999;23:764–71.
12. Cohen RJ, Nixon JM, Robinson E, Edgar SG, Allison L, McRae CU. Transitional cell carcinoma diagnosed at transurethral prostatectomy in patients with prostatic adenocarcinoma. J Urol Pathol 1996;5:29–37.
13. Colapinto V, Evans DH. Primary carcinoma of the male urethra developing after urethroplasty for stricture. J Urol 1977;118:581–4.
14. Coutts AG, Grigor KM, Fowler JW. Urethral dysplasia and bladder cancer in cystectomy specimens. Br J Urol 1985;57:535–41.
15. Dean AL. Carcinoma of the male and female urethra: pathology and diagnosis. J Urol 1956;75:505–3.
16. Dodd M, Lawson P, Hayman J. Squamous cell carcinoma of the distal urethra in a patient with congenital hypospadias. Pathology 1996;28:96–7.
17. Diaz-Cano SJ, Rios JJ, Rivera-Hueto F, Galera-Davidson H. Mixed cloacogenic carcinoma of male urethra. Histopathology 1992;20:82–4.
18. Dinney CP, Johnson DE, Swanson DA, Babaian RJ, von Eschenbach AC. Therapy and prognosis for male anterior urethral carcinoma: an update. Urology 1994;43:506–14.
19. Gowing NF. Urethral carcinoma associated with cancer of the bladder. Br J Urol 1960;32:428–38.
20. Grabstald H. Tumors of the urethra in men and women. Cancer 1973;32:1236–55.
21. Grussendorf-Conen EI, Deutz FJ, De Villiers EM. Detection of human papilloma virus-6 in primary carcinoma of the urethra in men. Cancer 1987;60:1832–5.

22. Guinn GA, Ayala AG. Male urethral cancer: report of 15 cases including a primary melanoma. J Urol 1970;103:176–9.
23. Hopkins SC, Nag SK, Soloway MS. Primary carcinoma of male urethra. Urology 1984;23:128–33.
24. Ingram EA, Depauw P. Adenocarcinoma of the male urethra with associated nephrogenic metaplasia. Case report and review of the literature. Cancer 1985;55:160–4.
25. Kageyama S, Ueda T, Kushima R, Sakamoto T. Primary adenosquamous carcinoma of the male distal urethra: magnetic resonance imaging using a circular surface coil. J Urol 1997;158:1913–4.
26. Kaplan GW, Bulkley GJ, Grayhack JT. Carcinoma of the male urethra. J Urol 1967;98:365–71.
27. Kotliar SN, Wood CG, Schaeffer AJ, Oyasu R. Transitional cell carcinoma exhibiting clear cell features. A differential diagnosis for clear cell adenocarcinoma of the urinary tract. Arch Pathol Lab Med 1995;119:79–81.
28. Levine RL. Urethral cancer. Cancer 1980;45:1965–72.
29. Lieber MM, Malek RS, Farrow GM, McMutry J. Villous adenocarcinoma of the male urethra. J Urol 1983;130:1191–3.
30. Loo KT, Chan JK. Colloid adenocarcinoma of the urethra associated with mucosal in situ carcinoma. Arch Pathol Lab Med 1992;116:976–7.
31. Lynch CF, Cohen MB. Urinary system. Cancer 1995;75:316–29.
32. Mandler JI, Pool TL. Primary carcinoma of the male urethra. J Urol 1966;96:67–72.
33. McCrea LE, Furlong JH. Primary carcinoma of the male urethra. Urol Survey 1951;1:1–30.
34. Melicow MM, Roberts MM. Pathology and natural history of urethral tumors in males. Review of 142 cases. Urology 1978;11:83–9.
35. Mevorach RA, Cos LR, Di Sant'Agnese PA, Stoler M. Human papillomavirus type 6 in Grade 1 transitional cell carcinoma of the urethra. J Urol 1990;143:126–8.
36. Oliva E, Young RH. Clear cell adenocarcinoma of the urethra: a clinicopathologic analysis of 19 cases. Mod Pathol 1996;9:513–20.
37. Posso MA, Berg GA, Murphy AI, Totten RS. Mucinous adenocarcinoma of the urethra: report of a case associated with urethritis glandularis. J Urol 1961;85:944–8.

38. Ray B, Canto AR, Whitmore WF Jr. Experience with primary carcinoma of the male urethra. J Urol 1977;117:591–4.

39. Sacks SA, Waisman J, Appelbaum HB, Lake P, Goodwin WE. Urethral adenocarcinoma (possibly originating in the glands of Littre). J Urol 1975;113:50–5.

40. Saito R. An adenosquamous carcinoma of the male urethra with hypercalcemia. Hum Pathol 1981;12:383–5.

41. Scott EV, Barelare B. Adenocarcinoma of the male urethra. J Urol 1952;68:311–9.

42. Silverman ML, Eyre RC, Zinman LA, Crosson AW. Mixed mucinous and papillary adenocarcinoma involving male urethra, probably originating in periurethral glands. Cancer 1981;47:1393–402.

43. Small JD, Albertsen PC, Graydon RJ, Ricci A, Sarofila WV. Adenoid cystic carcinoma of Cowper's gland. J Urol 1992;147:699–701.

44. Taylor RN, Lacey CG, Shuman MA. Adenocarcinoma of Skene's duct associated with a systemic coagulopathy. Gynecol Oncol 1985;22:250 6.

45. Tobisu KI, Tanaka Y, Mizutani T, Kakizoe T. Transitional cell carcinoma of the urethra in men following cystectomy for bladder cancer: multivariate analysis for risk factors. J Urol 1991;146:1551–4.

46. Tran KP, Epstein JI. Mucinous adenocarcinoma of urinary bladder type arising from the prostatic urethra. Distinction from mucinous adenocarcinoma of the prostate. Am J Surg Pathol 1996;20:1346–50.

47. Vadmal MS, Steckel J, Teichberg S, Hajdu SI. Primary neuroendocrine carcinoma of the penile urethra. J Urol 1997;157:956–7.

48. Yachia D, Turani H. Colonic-type adenocarcinoma of male urethra. Urology 1991;37:568–70.

Malignant Melanoma

49. Gupta TD, Grabstald H. Melanoma of the genitourinary tract. J Urol 1965;93:607–14.

50. Manivel JC, Fraley EE. Malignant melanoma of the penis and male urethra: 4 case reports and literature review. J Urol 1988;139:813–6.

51. Oldbring J, Mikulowski P. Malignant melanoma of the penis and male urethra. Report of nine cases and review of the literature. Cancer 1987;59:581–7.

51a. Oliva E, Quinn TR, Amin MB, et al. Primary malignant melanoma of the urethra. A clinicopathologic analysis of 15 cases. Am J Surg Pathol 2000;24:785–96.

52. Pow-Sang JM, Klimberg IW, Hackett RL, Wajsman Z. Primary malignant melanoma of the male urethra. J Urol 1988;139:1304–6.

52a. Radhi JM. Urethral malignant melanoma closely mimicking urothelial carcinoma. J Clin Pathol 1997;50:250–2.

53. Salm R, Rutter TE. A double primary malignant melanoma of the fossa navicularis. Br J Urol 1964;36:91–6.

54. Sanders TJ, Venable DD, Sanusi ID. Primary malignant melanoma of the urethra in a black man: a case report. J Urol 1986;135:1012–4.

55. Stein BS, Kendall AR. Malignant melanoma of the genitourinary tract. J Urol 1984;132:859–68.

Miscellaneous Rare Malignant Primary Tumors

56. Bailey OT. Fibrosarcoma of the male urethra. J Urol 1932;32:103.

57. D'Avanzo M, Savanelli A, Tolone C, et al. Unusual course of a urethral rhabdomyosarcoma in a 10-year-old boy. Ped Med E Chirug 1986;8:721–3.

58. Hatcher PA, Wilson DD. Primary lymphoma of the male urethra. Urology 1997;49:142–4.

59. Kahn DG, Rothman PJ, Weisman JD. Urethral T-cell lymphoma as the initial manifestation of the acquired immune deficiency syndrome. Arch Pathol Lab Med 1991;115:1169–70.

60. Kitamura H, Umehara T, Miyake M, Shimizu T, Kohda K, Ando M. Non Hodgkin's lymphoma arising in the urethra of a man. J Urol 1996;156:175–6.

61. Lopez AE, Latiff GA, Ciancio G, Antun R. Lymphoma of urethra in patient with acquired immune deficiency syndrome. Urology 1993;42:596–8.

62. Mark JA, Pais VM, Chong FK. Plasmacytoma of the urethra treated with transurethral resection and radiotherapy. J Urol 1990;143:1010–1.

63. Rajan N, Allman D, Scaglia B, et al. Non-Hodgkin's lymphoma of the male urethra. J Urol 1995;153;1916–7.

64. Ro J, Dexeus F, Logothetis C, Ayala A. Pure yolk sac tumors in adults: a clinicopathologic study in 18 patients [Abstract]. Mod Pathol 1991;4:50a.

65. Sylora HO, Diamond HM, Kaufman M, Straus F II, Lyon ES. Primary carcinoid tumor of the urethra. J Urol 1975;114:150–3.

66. Witjes JA, DeVries JD, Schaafsma HE, Bogman MJ, Barentsz JO, Corten RL. Extramedullary plasmacytoma of the urethra: a case report. J Urol 1991;145:826–8.

67. Xu YM, Cai RX, Wu P, Jin NT. Urethral carcinosarcoma following total cystectomy for bladder carcinoma. Urol Int 1993;50:104–7.

Secondary Tumors

68. Begin LR, Deschenes J, Mitmaker B. Pagetoid carcinomatous involvement of the penile urethra in association with high-grade transitional cell carcinoma of the urinary bladder. Arch Pathol Lab Med 1991;115:632–5.

69. Cordonnier JJ, Spjut HJ. Urethral occurrence of bladder carcinoma following cystectomy. J Urol 1962;87:398–403.

70. Hardeman SW, Soloway MS. Urethral recurrence following radical cystectomy. J Urol 1990;144:666–9.

71. Lieber MM, Malek, RS, Farrow GM, McMutry J. Villous adenocarcinoma of the male urethra. J Urol 1983;130:1191–3.

71a. Lowe LH, Banks WJ, Allen TD. Urethral metastasis of Wilms tumor. J Urol 1998;160:165.

72. Melicow MM, Roberts MM. Pathology and natural history of urethral tumors in males. Review of 142 cases. Urology 1978;11:83–9.

73. Nurmi M, Puntala P, Ekfors T. Urethral recurrence after cystoprostatectomy for bladder carcinoma. Scand J Urol Nephrol 1989;23:1–2.

74. Powell FC, Bjornsson J, Doyle JA, Cooper AJ. Genital Paget's disease and urinary tract malignancy. J Am Acad Dermatol 1985;13:84–90.

75. Salazar G, Frable WJ. Extramammary Paget's disease: a case involving the prostate urethra. Am J Clin Pathol 1969;52:607–12.

76. Subudhi CL, Panda SN, Pangirami KK. Urethral metastases from carcinoma of the prostate. Int J Cancer 1994;31:31–3.

77. Taylor GB, McNeal JE, Cohen RJ. Intraductal carcinoma of the prostate metastatic to the penile urethra: a rare demonstration of two morphologic patterns of tumor growth. Pathology 1998;30:218–21.

78. Tomaszewski JE, Korat OC, LiVolsi VA, Connor AM, Wein A. Paget's disease of the urethral meatus following transitional cell carcinoma of the bladder. J Urol 1986;135:368–70.

79. Turner AG. Pagetoid lesions associated with carcinoma of the bladder. J Urol 1980;123:124–6.

80. Wolinska WH, Melamed MR, Schellhammer PF, Whitmore WF. Urethral cytology following cystectomy for bladder carcinoma. Am J Surg Pathol 1977;1:225–33.

81. Woodhead DM, Gigax JH, Wahle WH, Holcomb TM. Urothelial implantation of Wilms' tumor. Ann Surg 1968; 167:127–31.

82. Xu YM, Cai RX, Wu P, Jin NT. Urethral carcinosarcoma following total cystectomy for bladder carcinoma. Urol Int 1993;50:104–7.

83. Young RH. Carcinosarcoma of the urinary bladder. Cancer 1987;59:1333–9.

Transitional Cell Papillomas

84. Eble JN, Young RH. Benign and low-grade papillary lesions of the urinary bladder: a review of the papilloma-papillary carcinoma controversy, and a report of five typical papillomas. Semin Diagn Pathol 1989;6:351–71.

85. Heaton ND, Kadow C, Yates-Bell AJ. Inverted papilloma of the penile urethra. Br J Urol 1990;66:661–2.

86. Kunze E, Schauer A, Schmitt M. Histology and histogenesis of two different types of inverted urothelial papilloma. Cancer 1983;51:348–58.

87. Renfer LG, Kelley J, Belville WD. Inverted papilloma of the urinary tract: histogenesis, recurrence and associated malignancy. J Urol 1988;140:832–4.

88. Walsh IK, Keane PE, Herron B. Benign urethral polyps. Br J Urol 1993;72:937–8.

Villous Adenoma

89. Algaba F, Matias-Guiu X, Badia F, Sole-Balcells F. Villous adenoma of the prostatic urethra. Eur Urol 1988; 14:255–7.

89a. Cheng L, Montironi R, Bostwick DG. Villous adenoma of the urinary tract: a report of 23 cases, including 8 with adenocarcinoma. Am J Surg Pathol 1999;23:764–71.

90. Foot NC. Glandular metaplasia of the epithelium of the urinary tract. South Med J 1944;37:137–44.

91. Tran KP, Epstein JI. Mucinous adenocarcinoma of urinary bladder type arising from the prostatic urethra. Distinction from mucinous adenocarcinoma of the prostate. Am J Surg Pathol 1996;20:1346–50.

Benign Mesenchymal Tumors

92. Begley BJ. Hemangioma of the male urethra: treatment by Johanson-Denis Browne technique. J Urol 1960;84:111–2.

93. Hayashi T, Igarashi K, Sekine H. Urethral hemangioma: case report. J Urol 1997;158:539–40.

94. Paci KD, Dolezel J, Skoumal R, Bucek J, Kladensky J. Very rare angioleiomyoma of the male urethra. Int Urol Nephrol 1993;25:479–84.

95. Tilak GH. Multiple hemangiomas of the male urethra—treatment by Denis Browne-Swinney-Johanson urethroplasty. J Urol 1967;97:96–7.

Von Brunn's Nests, Urethritis Glandularis, Urethritis Cystica, and Papillary-Polypoid Urethritis

96. Kiernan M, Gaffney EF. Brunn's nests and glandular metaplasia: normal urothelial variants in the supramontanal prostatic urethra. J Urol 1987;137:877–9.

97. Maung R, Kelly JK, Grace DA. Intestinal metaplasia and dysplasia of prostatic urethra secondary to stricture. Urology 1988;32:361–3.

98. Player LP, Mathe CP. A study of tumors of the vesical neck and the prostatic urethra and their relation to the treatment of chronic prostatitis. J Urol 1921;5:177–205.

99. Posso MA, Berg GA, Murphy AI, Totten RS. Mucinous adenocarcinoma of the urethra: report of a case associated with urethritis glandularis. J Urol 1961;85:944–8.

100. Schinella R, Thurm J, Feiner H. Papillary pseudotumor of the prostatic urethra: proliferative papillary urethritis. J Urol 1974;111:38–40.

101. Weinberger HW, Ropes MW, Kulka JP, Bauer W. Reiter's syndrome, clinical and pathologic observations. A long term study of 16 cases. Medicine 1962;41:35–91.

102. Zaher MF, el-Deeb AA. Bilharzial urethritis cystica. J Urol 1969;101:870–3.

Nephrogenic Adenoma

103. Bhagavan BS, Tiamson EM, Wenk RE, Berger BW, Hamamoto G, Eggleston JC. Nephrogenic adenoma of the urinary bladder and urethra. Hum Pathol 1981;12:907–16.

104. Daroca PJ, Martin AA, Reed RJ, Krenger SS, Hellstrom WJ. Nephrogenic adenoma of the prostatic urethra. A report of these cases including a case with infiltration of the prostatic stroma. J Urol Pathol 1993;1:157–72.

105. Ingram EA, Depauw P. Adenocarcinoma of the male urethra with associated nephrogenic metaplasia. Case report and review of the literature. Cancer 1985;55:160–4.

106. Malpica A, Ro JY, Troncoso P, Ordonez NG, Amin MB, Ayala AG. Nephrogenic adenoma of the prostatic ure-thra involving the prostate gland: a clinicopathologic and immunohistochemical study of eight cases. Hum Pathol 1994;25:390–5.

107. Oliva E, Young RH. Nephrogenic adenoma of the urinary tract: a review of the microscopic appearance of 80 cases with emphasis on unusual features. Mod Pathol 1995;8:722–30.

108. Young RH. Nephrogenic adenomas of the urethra involving the prostate gland: a report of two cases of a lesion that may be confused with prostatic adenocarcinoma. Mod Pathol 1992;5:617–20.

Fibroepithelial Polyps

109. Carter MF. Polypoid granuloma pyogenicum of the posterior urethra. J Urol 1974;111:616–7.

110. De Castro R, Campobasso P, Belloli G, Pavanello P. Solitary polyp of posterior urethra in children: report of seventeen cases. Eur J Pediatr Surg 1993;3:92–6.

111. Foster RS, Garrett RA. Congenital posterior urethral polyps. J Urol 1986;136:670–2.

Prostatic Type Polyps

112. Baroudy AC, O'Connell JP. Papillary adenoma of the prostatic urethra. J Urol 1984;132:120–2.

113. Butterick JD, Schnitzer B, Abell MR. Ectopic prostatic tissue in urethra: a clinicopathological entity and a significant cause of hematuria. J Urol 1971;105:97–104.

114. Chan JK, Chow TC, Tsui MS. Prostatic-type polyps of the lower urinary tract: three histogenetic types? Histopathology 1987;11:789–801.

115. Craig JR, Hart WR. Benign polyps with prostatic-type epithelium of the urethra. Am J Clin Pathol 1975;63:343–7.

116. Glancy RJ, Gaman AJ, Rippey JJ. Polyps and papillary lesions of the prostatic urethra. Pathology 1983;15:153–7.

117. Hara S, Horie A. Prostatic caruncle: a urethral papillary tumor derived from prolapse of the prostatic duct. J Urol 1977;117:303–5.

118. Nesbit RM. The genesis of benign polyps in the prostatic urethra. J Urol 1962;87:416–8.

119. Stein AJ, Prioleau PG, Catalona WJ. Adenomatous polyps of the prostatic urethra: a cause of hematospermia. J Urol 1980;124:298–9.

120. Walker AN, Mills SE, Fechner RE, Perry JM. Epithelial polyps of the prostatic urethra. A light-microscopic and immunohistochemical study. Am J Surg Pathol 1983;7:351–6.

121. Walker AN, Mills SE, Fechner RE, Perry JM. "Endometrial" adenocarcinoma of the prostatic urethra arising in a villous polyp. A light microscopic and immunoperoxidase study. Arch Pathol Lab Med 1982;106:624–7.

122. Zeid M, Gaeta JF, Asirwatham JE, Suffrin G. Papillary adenoma of the prostatic urethra. Prostate 1986;9:9–14.

Condyloma Acuminatum and Squamous Papilloma

123. Bissada NK, Cole AT, Fried FA. Extensive condylomas acuminata of the entire male urethra and the bladder. J Urol 1974;112:201–3.

124. Culp OS, Kaplan IW. Condylomata acuminata. Two hundred cases treated with podophyllin. Ann Surg 1944;120:251–6.

125. DeBenedictis TJ, Marmar JL, Praiss DE. Intraurethral condylomas acuminata: management and review of the literature. J Urol 1977;118:767–9.

126. Del Mistro A, Braunstein JD, Halwer M, Koss LG. Identification of human papillomavirus types in male urethral condylomata acuminata by in situ hybridization. Hum Pathol 1987;18:936–40.

127. Fralick RA, Malek RS, Goellner JR, Hyland KM. Urethroscopy and urethral cytology in men with external genital condyloma. Urology 1994;43:361–4.

128. Gartman E. Intraurethral verruca acuminata in men. J Urol 1956;75:717–8.

129. Gersh I. Condylomata acuminata of the male external genitalia: an effective method of surgical treatment. Urol Cutan Rev 1945;49:432–45.

129a. Glancy RJ, Gaman AJ, Rippey JJ. Polyps and papillary lesions of the prostatic urethra. Pathology 1983;15:153–7.

130. Haas EN, Roth AA. Benign squamous tumors of the entire male urethra. J Urol 1963;89:836–8.

131. Hartwick RW, Swanson DB, Kandel RA. Human papillomavirus DNA in male urethral condyloma acuminatum. Detection by in situ hybridization with biotinylated DNA probes. J Urol Pathol 1993;1:365–75.

132. Huvos A, Grabstald H. Urethral meatal and parameatal tumors in young men: a clinicopathologic and electron microscopic study. J Urol 1973;110:688–92.

133. Iwasawa A, Hiltunen-Back E, Reunala T, Nieminen P, Paavonen J. Human papillomavirus DNA in urine specimens of men with condyloma acuminatum. Sexually Transm Dis 1997;24:165–8.

134. Lindner HJ, Pasquier CM Jr. Condylomata acuminata of the urethra. J Urol 1954;72:875–9.
135. Morrow RP, McDonald JR, Emmett JL. Condylomata acuminata of the urethra. J Urol 1952;68:909–17.

136. Murphy WM, Fu YS, Lancaster MD, Jenson AB. Papillomavirus structural antigen in condyloma acuminatum of the male urethra. J Urol 1983;130:84–5.
137. Noronha RF, Sundaram M. Are intraurethral condylomata premalignant? Br J Urol 1984;56:546–7.

Transitional Cell Hyperplasia

138. Gardner WA, Culberson DE. Atrophy and proliferation in the young adult prostate. J Urol 1987;137:53–6.
139. Yantiss RK, Young RH. Transitional cell "metaplasia" in the prostate gland: a survey of its frequency and features based on over 100 consecutive prostatic biopsy specimens. J Urol Pathol 1997;7:71–80.

Malakoplakia

140. McClure J. Malakoplakia. J Pathol 1983;140:275–330.

141. Sharma TC, Kagan HN, Sheils JP. Malacoplakia of the male urethra. J Urol 1981;125:885–6.

Amyloidosis

142. Bodner H, Retsky MI, Brown G. Primary amyloidosis of glans penis and urethra: resection and reconstruction. J Urol 1981;125:586–8.
143. Christie AJ, Weingarten CJ. Amyloidosis presenting in the urethra. J Roy Soc Med 1988;81:174–5.
144. Madersbacher S, Maier U. Localized amyloidosis of the urethra. Br J Urol 1995;75:245–6.
145. Mani S, Flynn SD, Duffy TP, Morgan W. Isolated amyloidosis of the penile urethra and corpus spongiosum: a case report. J Urol 1993;150:1915–6.

146. Rosenbaum TP, Nicholas DS, Rundle JS. Localised amyloidosis of the urethra. Br J Urol 1987;60:183–4.
147. Stillwell TJ, Segura JW, Farrow GM. Amyloidosis of the urethra. J Urol 1989;141:52–3.
148. Ullmann AS, Fine G, Johnson AJ. Localized amyloidosis (amyloid tumor) of the urethra. J Urol 1964;92:42–4.
149. Vasudevan P, Stein AM, Pinn VW, Roa CN. Primary amyloidosis of urethra. Urology 1981;17:181–3.
150. Williams OE, Kynaston H, Dixon G, Arya OP. Amyloid tumour of the urethra presenting as non-specific urethritis. Genitourin Med 1992;68:332–3.

Verumontanum Gland Hypertrophy

151. Herbut P. Urological pathology, vol I. Philadelphia: Lea & Febiger, 1952:51–2.

10

THE PENIS

ANATOMY AND HISTOLOGY

The phallus originates from the genital tubercle, which is located at the cranial end of the cloacal membrane. Due to androgenic hormonal stimuli from the fetal testes, the phallus increases in size to form the penis, which pushes both the urogenital folds and the urethral sulcus ventrally. The glandular plaque, an ectodermal group of cells, forms the glans and distal urethral epithelium. Occasionally, misplaced endodermal cells from the proximal urethra are located in the parameatal region of glans epithelium. The foreskin and coronal sulcus are also ectodermal (fig. 10-1).

The penis is composed of three parts: the body or shaft, which forms the central portion, and the two ends, anterior and posterior (the root). The anterior portion of the penis is composed of the glans, coronal (balanopreputial) sulcus, and foreskin (prepuce) (1,2,5,7,9).

The glans is a conical extension of the urethral corpus spongiosum. There is a vertical cleft, the meatus, in the apex, which measures from 5 to 8 mm in length and is attached to the foreskin by a ventral triangular plicature of the mucosa, known as the frenulum (fig. 10-2). The base of the cone, whose diameter is greater than that of the corpus, is represented by the corona, a slightly elevated, circular ridge surrounding the glans which is more prominent in the dorsal aspect. The coronal sulcus, which is behind or below the corona, separates the glans from the foreskin (fig. 10-3).

The glans is composed of the following layers: epithelium, lamina propria, corpus spongiosum, tunica albuginea, and corpora cavernosa (fig. 10-4) (1); the latter is present in the glans to a variable degree from case to case (see below). The stratified squamous epithelium is thin and nonkeratinized in uncircumcised males and keratinized

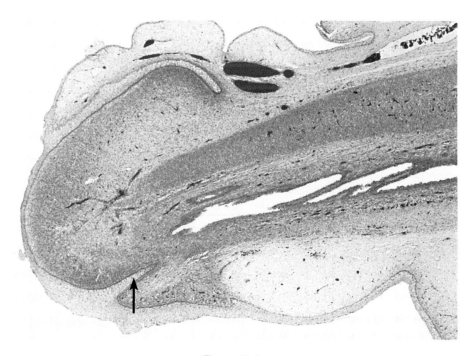

Figure 10-1

FETAL PENIS

The penis in a 20-week fetus shows almost complete development of the foreskin and phallus. Note in the lower part of the glans (arrow) the ectodermal invagination which will become the meatal or distal urethra. The space of the endodermal (urothelial) urethra is seen in its central location. (Courtesy of Dr. G. Ayala, Houston, TX.)

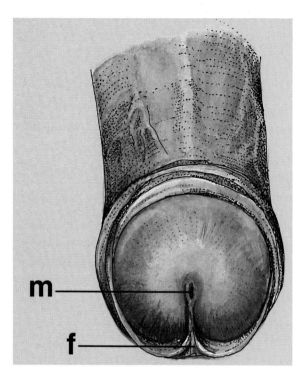

Figure 10-2
ANATOMY OF MEATUS AND FRENULUM
The vertical cleft or meatus (m) is attached to the foreskin by a triangular shaped frenulum (f). The glans is covered by smooth pink mucosa.

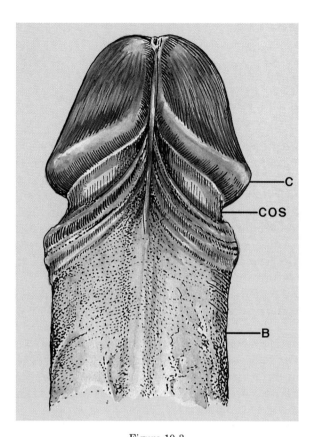

Figure 10-3
ANATOMY OF CORONA AND CORONAL SULCUS
The glans is a cone whose base, the corona (C), is a circular ridge with a diameter greater than that of the body (B) (shaft). Between the corona and the foreskin, which is retracted in the picture, lies the coronal sulcus (COS).

Figure 10-4
ANATOMY OF CUT
SECTION OF PENIS

The drawing is not through the center so the urethra is not demonstrated. From the surface to deep tissues the following layers are schematically demonstrated: mucosa of glans and foreskin (m), lamina propria of glans and foreskin (lp), corpus spongiosum (cs), and corpus cavernosum (cc). The white tissue that encases the corpus cavernosum, the tunica albuginea (a), is dense fibroelastic tissue separating the corpus spongiosum from the corpus cavernosum. The foreskin (f) has four layers: mucosa (m), lamina propria (lp), dartos (dt), and skin (s). The body (left) shows similar layers and, additionally, Buck's fascia (bf) which separates the dartos (dt) from the tunica albuginea (a) and terminates at the coronal sulcus.

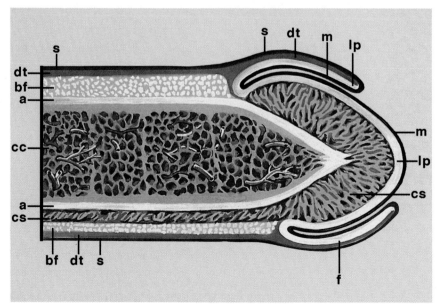

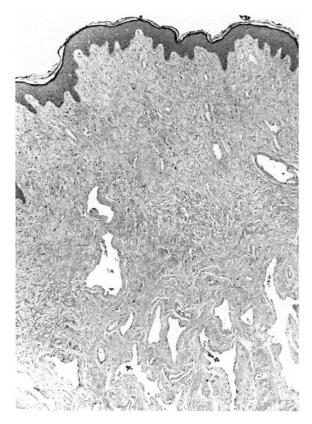

Figure 10-5
GLANS

Three histologic levels are present: slightly keratinized squamous epithelium (in a circumcised man), lamina propria, and the richly vascular erectile tissue of the corpus spongiosum.

in circumcised males (fig. 10-5). In both situations, there is a granular cell layer and a well-developed basal cell layer, with a limiting basement membrane. Melanocytes are normally absent. Most epithelial neoplasms of the penis originate in this epithelium. The lamina propria is a loose connective tissue layer, 1 to 3 mm thick, which separates the epithelium from the corpus spongiosum. It contains lymphatics, peripheral nerves, and occasional Vater Paccini corpuscles (2).

The corpus spongiosum is the main component of the glans and is composed of specialized erectile tissues, with numerous anastomosing venous sinuses of varying caliber having multiple peripheral nerves between them (7). The transition between the lamina propria and the corpus spongiosum is not sharp and sometimes is difficult to determine (fig. 10-5). The glans corpus spongiosum is about 8 to 10 mm thick.

The tunica albuginea is a very dense, white, fibrous and elastic membrane which terminates distally, in or near the glans, in a conical, ">" shaped manner, separating the corpus spongiosum from the corpora cavernosa (fig. 10-4). It is 1 to 2 mm thick in the flaccid state and is thinner during erection. It completely encases the corpora cavernosa and constitutes an important barrier to the spread of cancer to it.

The coronal sulcus is a narrow and circumferential "cul de sac" located just below the glans corona, and represents the reflection of glans squamous epithelium over the foreskin (fig. 10-3). The coronal sulcus is a common site of recurrence of carcinoma or of a positive margin in cases of primary foreskin carcinoma. Microscopically, the coronal sulcus is composed of squamous epithelium and lamina propria, identical to that of the glans. There is a close relationship between the connective tissue of the lamina propria, smooth muscle fibers of the penile dartos muscle, and multiple, large vessels and nerves from the insertion of Buck's fascia. There has been confusion in the literature with regard to the presence of sebaceous glands in the corona, in part due to the use of the term "Tyson's glands" and a failure to recognize for many years that Tyson actually described the structures subsequently identified as pearly penile papules or hirsutoid papillomas (see page 468). In numerous sections from over 200 surgical penectomy specimens studied by one of us (ALC), we have seen only two cases in which there were isolated but well-developed small sebaceous glands located in the mucosa of the foreskin, just above the coronal sulcus; sebaceous glands rarely have been documented by others (7). Smegma is histologically composed of keratinous debris, desquamated epithelium, and mucinous material secreted by the periurethral glands of Littré.

The foreskin (fig. 10-6, top) is a double membrane which encases the glans and from which it is separated by a potential space (fig. 10-4). It ends distally in the preputial ring. The length of the foreskin is variable: it covers two thirds, one half, or only the posterior third of the glans. Before puberty it is redundant, and the preputial ring is very narrow; in the adult, the ring is behind the meatus. Rarely, it is even shorter, the ring being reduced to a short collar behind the corona with a completely uncovered glans.

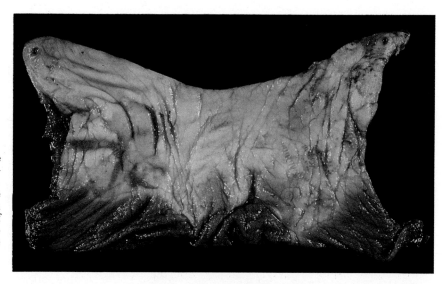

Figure 10-6
NORMAL FORESKIN
Top: The mucosal portion of the foreskin (top), merges with the wrinkled hyperpigmented skin (bottom).
Bottom: Histologically the squamous epithelium of the skin (bottom) is undulating and that of the mucosa (top) is flat. The lamina propria and dartos separate the mucosa and skin.

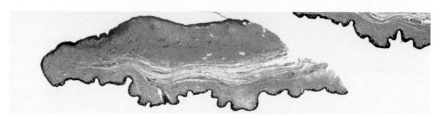

Wynder's review (10) of the types of foreskin in North American males showed a marked variation: A, completely covers the glans; B, covers one half of the glans; C, covers one fourth of the glans; D, absence of foreskin. Microscopically, the foreskin has five histologic layers: 1) the mucosal epithelium, which is similar to that of the glans and coronal sulcus epithelium; 2) the 2 to 3 mm thick lamina propria; 3) the 6 to 10 mm thick dartos muscle composed of a double layer of smooth muscle fibers situated within loose connective tissue; 4) the dermis; and 5) the epidermis, which is outermost, thin and wrinkled (fig. 10-6). The latter feature and a scant component of adnexal structures, enables distinction of foreskin epidermis from mucosal epithelium.

The central portion of the penis is the body or shaft. It is composed of three cylinders of firmly adherent erectile tissues: a ventral corpus spongiosum with a centrally located urethra, and two corpora cavernosa, which are separated by a median raphe that is continuous with the tunica albuginea (figs. 10-7, 10-8) (9). Both the corpora cavernosa and corpus spongiosum are covered by the albuginea and encased in Buck's fascia.

Microscopically, the cut surface at the mid-level of the body shows the following layers: 1) a thin, wrinkled, pigmented epidermis with very few adnexal structures; 2) dermis; 3) dartos muscle; 4) adipose tissue; 5) Buck's fascia, with numerous vessels and nerves; 6) tunica albuginea; and 7) erectile tissue of the corpora cavernosa and corpus spongiosum, the latter encasing the urethra (figs. 10-8, 10-9). The erectile tissue of the corpora cavernosa and corpus spongiosum is composed of numerous vascular spaces surrounded by a latticework of interconnected smooth muscle fibers that become tense as the cylinder expands during erection (7). The corpora cavernosa cylinders are separated from each other by the dense connective tissue of the raphe. The periurethral corpus spongiosum is also surrounded by Buck's fascia and incompletely by the albuginea. The albuginea is a thick sheath of partially hyalinized collagen fibers, and Buck's fascia is a fibroelastic membrane containing blood vessels (fig. 10-10).

The posterior part or root of the penis is deeply embedded in the perineum. It is fixed to the anterior wall of the pelvis by a ligamentous

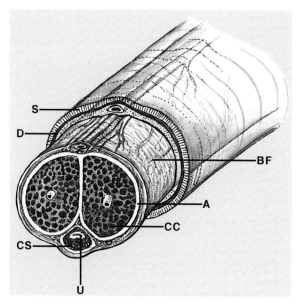

Figure 10-7
ANATOMY OF BODY (SHAFT) OF PENIS

Cross section showing from outer to inner: skin (S), dartos (D), fibroadipose tissue (in yellow), Buck's fascia (BF) with numerous vessels and nerves, tunica albuginea (A), and corpora cavernosa (CC). Ventrally, the urethra (U) is surrounded by corpus spongiosum (CS) and tunica albuginea, seen in white.

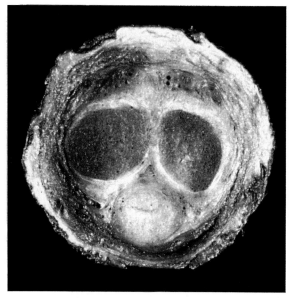

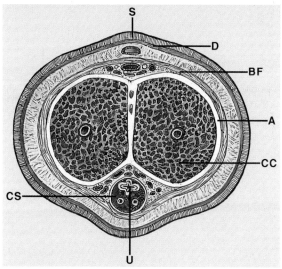

Figure 10-8
ANATOMY OF BODY (SHAFT) OF PENIS

Top: Cross section of the body from a case in which carcinoma envelops the urethra (bottom). Note the paired corpora cavernosa.

Bottom: A drawing depicting the normal cross sectional anatomy of the body. The dartos (D) is closely attached to the skin (S); Buck's fascia (BF) covers the inferior of the urethra (U); the corpus spongiosum (CS) and the urethra are located in the groove between the corpora cavernosa (CC) and Buck's fascia. The tunica albuginea (A) encases the corpora cavernosa.

insertion of the corpora cavernosa in the ischium and pubic bones.

A rich network of lymphatics of the glans and corpora cavernosa courses along the dorsal vein to the symphysis pubis and drains into superficial and deep inguinal lymph nodes. Lymphatics of the foreskin and skin of the shaft course along the dorsal aspect of the penis to its root and drain into superficial inguinal lymph nodes (4).

The inguinal lymph nodes are divided into superficial and deep nodes by a horizontal line crossing the point where the greater saphenous vein enters the femoral vein. The superficial nodes (approximately 12 to 15) are above the cribriform fascia and are subdivided into four groups or quadrants, outlined by horizontal and vertical lines drawn at the saphenofemoral junction (8). The sentinel lymph node group (1 to 3 nodes) is located in the upper inner quadrant, at the anterior or medial aspect of the superficial epigastric vein; this is the most common site for lymph node metastasis in penile carcinoma (3). The deep inguinal nodes (2 to 3 nodes) are beneath the cribriform fascia, forming a small chain in the adipose tissue within the femoral sheath and surrounding the femoral vessels. The most conspicuous member of this group is the node of Cloquet. The next level of drainage is the pelvic (iliac) nodes. They are located external or

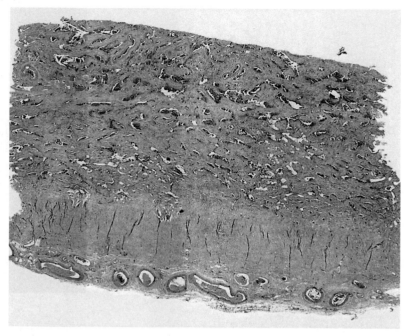

Figure 10-9
BODY (SHAFT)
Longitudinal section of midportion after removal of the skin and dartos. Buck's fascia, with numerous vessels, is seen at the bottom. Above is the dense tunica albuginea and above that the highly vascular corpus cavernosum.

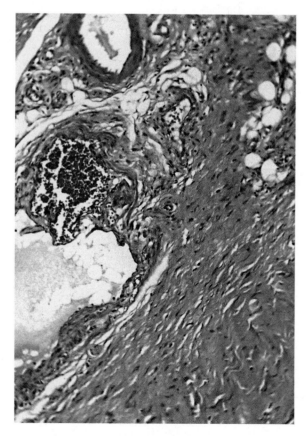

Figure 10-10
BODY (SHAFT)
Loose connective tissue, arteries, and veins of Buck's fascia and adjacent dense collagen of the tunica albuginea.

medial to the iliac vessels. The hypogastric and common iliac nodes are situated next to their homonymous blood vessels.

EPITHELIAL ABNORMALITIES AND PRECANCEROUS SQUAMOUS LESIONS INCLUDING PENILE HORN, MICACEOUS BALANITIS, AND BOWENOID PAPULOSIS

Our classification of tumors and tumor-like lesions of the penis is presented in Table 10-1.

Squamous Hyperplasia

General Features. In our experience, squamous hyperplasia is associated with approximately 90 percent of squamous cell carcinomas. It is present in the mucosa of the glans, coronal sulcus, and foreskin, adjacent to, distant from, or in continuity with the carcinoma. It is found with all histologic subtypes of squamous cell carcinoma, but is particularly frequent and prominent in association with carcinomas with verruciform growth patterns (see page 423).

Gross Findings. The epithelium is thickened, smooth, and white. The boundaries between squamous hyperplasia and normal mucosa are irregular. The lesion may be visualized on cut surface as a pearly, bright, linear condensation of mucosa,

Table 10-1
TUMORS AND TUMOR-LIKE LESIONS OF THE PENIS

I. Primary Tumors
  A. Epithelial
    1. Premalignant
      a. Carcinoma in situ (includes erythroplasia of Queyrat and Bowen's disease)
    2. Other
      a. Bowenoid papulosis
      b. Other
    3. Malignant
      a. Squamous cell carcinoma
        1) Usual type
        2) Basaloid
        3) Warty (condylomatous)
        4) Verrucous
        5) Papillary, not otherwise specified
        6) Sarcomatoid (spindle cell) carcinoma*
      b. Adenosquamous carcinoma
      c. Other rare pure primary carcinomas
      d. Mixed carcinomas
      e. Basal cell carcinoma
      f. Paget's disease
  B. Melanocytic
    1. Nevi and other benign melanocytic proliferations
    2. Malignant melanoma
  C. Mesenchymal
    1. Benign
      a. Hemangioma
      b. Angiokeratoma
      c. Leiomyoma
      d. Other
    2. Malignant
      a. Kaposi's sarcoma
      b. Angiosarcoma
      c. Leiomyosarcoma
      d. Rhabdomyosarcoma
      e. Epithelioid sarcoma
      f. Other

  D. Hematopoietic
    1. Malignant lymphoma
    2. Other
  E. Miscellaneous rare primary tumors

II. Secondary Tumors
  A. Bladder
  B. Prostate
  C. Colon
  D. Kidney
  E. Other

III. Tumor-Like Lesions
  A. Cysts
  B. Infectious or inflammatory lesions
    1. Balanitis/posthitis/balanoposthitis
    2. Zoon's balanitis
    3. Condyloma acuminatum
    4. Syphilis
    5. Granuloma inguinale
    6. Lymphogranuloma venereum
    7. Chancroid
    8. Molluscum contagiosum
    9. Bacillary angiomatosis
    10. Other
  C. Balanitis xerotica obliterans
  D. Peyronie's disease
  E. Verruciform xanthoma
  F. Pearly papules
  G. Lipogranulomas
  H. Tancho's nodules
  I. Melanosis-lentiginosis
  J. Fournier's gangrene - Corbus' disease
  K. Wegener's granulomatosis
  L. Os penis
  M. Other (includes sarcoidosis, Crohn's disease, amyloidosis, sebaceous hyperplasia, inflammatory pseudotumor)

---

*Carcinosarcoma is included with sarcomatoid carcinoma for purposes of this work. These tumors are also designated metaplastic carcinoma by some authors.

---

which rarely is slightly papillary, sometimes merging with an adjacent neoplasm.

In our opinion, two particular lesions that have received specific designations in the literature, penile horn and micaceous balanitis, are best considered specific examples of florid epithelial hyperplasia with striking hyperkeratosis. It is crucial to be aware that these grossly impressive processes may overlie benign epithelium, premalignant lesions including carcinoma in situ, or

invasive carcinoma. The literature on penile horns (22) contains striking examples in which the underlying lesion has been a neoplasm (17,36). The second of these two lesions, micaceous balanitis (13,15a,19,25,26,29), is even more controversial because some have postulated that this lesion may be synonymous in some cases with carcinoma, particularly verrucous carcinoma (13). It is our opinion that the process is particularly common in association

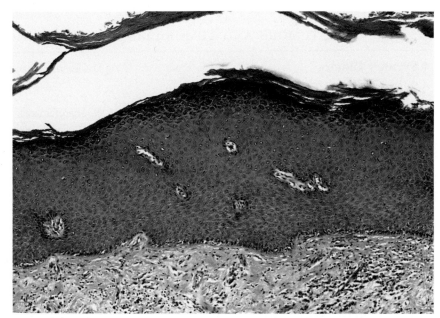

Figure 10-11
SQUAMOUS CELL
HYPERPLASIA, FLAT
There is hyperkeratosis and acanthosis.

with tumors of that type which are prone to produce large amounts of keratin, but is not specific for them, and the entity may be seen in any case with massive keratin formation, whether the underlying lesion is benign or malignant.

Microscopic Findings. The lesion may be flat or papillary. In our experience, flat lesions account for approximately 60 percent of the cases, papillary lesions for about 10 percent, and mixed patterns for the remainder. Flat squamous hyperplasia shows acanthosis and hyperkeratosis, with normal maturation of squamous cells (figs. 10-11, 10-12). Parakeratosis is rare, and cytologic atypia is absent by definition. The interface between the basal layer and stroma is usually linear but elongation of rete ridges or a downward proliferation of basal cells may be seen. Papillary hyperplasia has a serrated appearance at low-power microscopy (fig. 10-13). The papillae are low, with hyperkeratosis or parakeratosis, and they may be pointed or rounded at their surface (fig. 10-13). Cytologic atypia is again absent. Pseudoepitheliomatous hyperplasia may be seen in both types of hyperplasia, but more commonly in papillary hyperplasia. Squamous aggregates in the lamina propria that appear detached from the overlying epithelium (fig. 10-14) may simulate squamous cell carcinoma. This differential is discussed on page 427 and in the Fascicle, Nonmelanocytic Tumors of the Skin (31a).

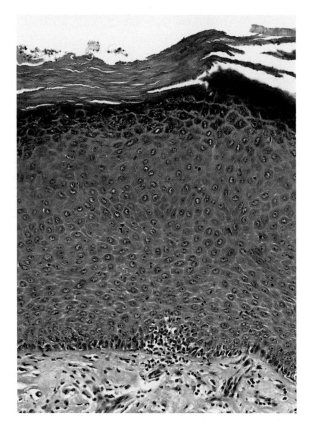

Figure 10-12
SQUAMOUS CELL HYPERPLASIA, FLAT

High-power view of case in prior illustration showing normal maturation without atypia.

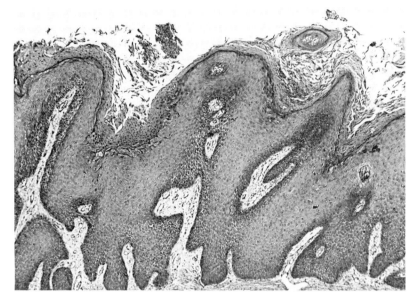

Figure 10-13
SQUAMOUS CELL
HYPERPLASIA, PAPILLARY
There is hyperkeratosis, papillomato-
sis, and acanthosis.

Figure 10-14
PSEUDOEPITHELIOMATOUS
SQUAMOUS CELL HYPERPLASIA
There is a downward proliferation of
mature, nonatypical squamous epithelium
forming nests with focal keratinization.

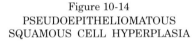

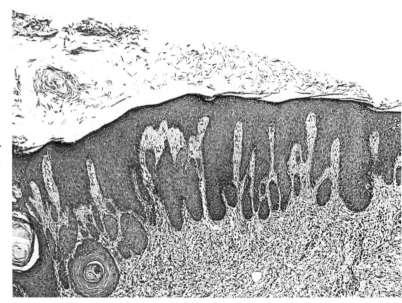

In cases of penile horn and micaceous balanitis, massive keratin production dominates the microscopic picture. Individual biopsy specimens may procure little or no underlying epithelium and if minimal tissue of this type is available for evaluation, this should be recorded, including a comment stating that the possibility of an underlying malignant process cannot be excluded. As noted above, the underlying epithelium may be benign, atypical, or carcinomatous in cases that have borne the diagnosis of penile horn or micaceous balanitis, terms that, in our opinion, are more appropriately descriptive of the clinical appearance. This view is in accordance with at least some who have written on this topic (26), although this issue remains controversial.

Precancerous Lesions

General Features. There is a spectrum of atypical intraepithelial squamous lesions characterized by abnormalities in maturation, polarity, and nuclear atypia (11,12,18,20,21,24,28,31). Various designations such as squamous intraepithelial

Table 10-2

COMPARISON BETWEEN ERYTHROPLASIA OF QUEYRAT, BOWEN'S DISEASE, AND BOWENOID PAPULOSIS*

Feature	Erythroplasia of Queyrat	Bowen's Disease	Bowenoid Papulosis
Site	glans, prepuce	shaft	shaft
Age	4th - 6th decade	4th - 6th decade	3rd and 4th decade
Lesion	erythematous plaque	scaly plaque	papules
Hyperkeratosis	–	+	+
Maturation	–	–	+
Sweat gland involvement	–	–	+
Pilosebaceous involvement	–	+	–
Progress to carcinoma	10 percent	5 to 10 percent	–
Spontaneous regression	–	–	+
Association with cutaneous or visceral malignancy	+/–	+	–

*Modified from Table 13-1 in Bostwick DG, Eble JN, eds. Urologic surgical pathology. St. Louis: Mosby, 1997:694.

lesion, low and high grade; mild, moderate, and severe dysplasia; penile intraepithelial neoplasia I, II, and III; and carcinoma in situ have been used. We use the term squamous intraepithelial lesion for purposes of this discussion, in accord with that used in the female genital tract (30). Erythroplasia of Queyrat (35) and Bowen's disease are both synonymous with *high-grade squamous intraepithelial lesion* or *squamous cell carcinoma in situ,* the former term usually used clinically for lesions of the glans and foreskin mucosa, the latter predominantly for lesions of the body (shaft).

Squamous intraepithelial lesions may be solitary but are more frequently associated with adjacent invasive squamous cell carcinoma of typical type. They are rare in cases of verrucous carcinoma or papillary carcinoma, not otherwise specified. If untreated, 5 to 10 percent of cases of erythroplasia of Queyrat and Bowen's disease progress to invasive squamous cell carcinoma. Patients with high-grade squamous intraepithelial lesions are typically in the middle to later years of life, with a peak frequency of occurrence in the early sixth decade (33), but the process may be seen in early adult life. These lesions occur, on average, at a later age than cases of Bowenoid papulosis (Table 10-2) (14,16, 32,34) (see page 415).

Gross Findings. Erythroplasia of Queyrat is typically moist and erythematous (fig. 10-15A); Bowen's disease may be erythematous or white (fig. 10-15B). The lesions may appear as a papule or plaque, and may be focal and discrete, usually measuring 0.5 to 1 cm, or diffuse with irregular borders. Multicentricity may be seen. Lesions with lesser cytologic atypia (low- or moderate-grade squamous intraepithelial lesion) may not be clinically apparent or appear as white patches of "leukoplakia."

Microscopic Findings. Low- and moderate-grade squamous intraepithelial lesions have atypical cells restricted to the lower or middle third of an often acanthotic epithelium (fig. 10-16), the surface of which is often hyperkeratotic. The nuclei are enlarged, pleomorphic, and hyperchromatic, with irregular nuclear membranes and occasional normal or abnormal mitotic figures. Koilocytosis may be present. High-grade squamous intraepithelial lesions show similar nuclear changes, but are usually more cytologically atypical and involve two thirds or more of the thickness of the epithelium (fig. 10-15C).

The histologic appearance of squamous intraepithelial lesions is variable and can be classified into three main groups: usual squamous intraepithelial lesion (fig. 10-15C), basaloid type

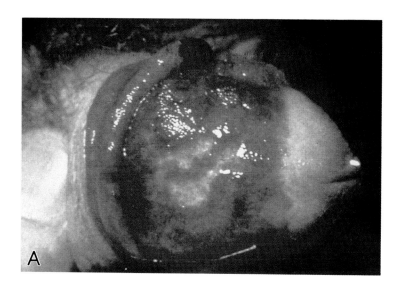

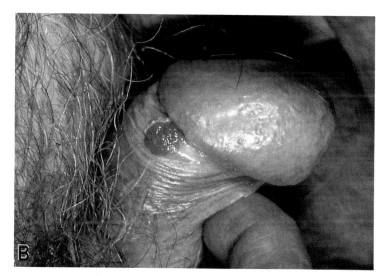

Figure 10-15
ERYTHROPLASIA OF QUEYRAT
AND BOWEN'S DISEASE

The former is a moist red lesion involving most of the glans (A) and the latter a circumscribed, raised, granular red lesion involving the distal shaft and extending to the coronal sulcus (B). Typical microscopic features of squamous cell carcinoma in situ are seen in C.

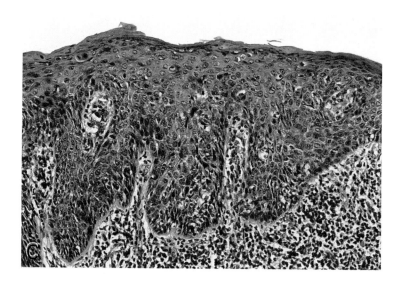

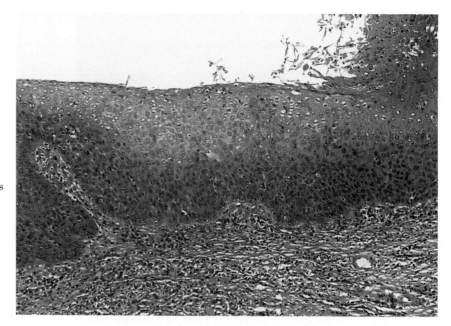

Figure 10-16
SQUAMOUS
INTRAEPITHELIAL
LESION, KERATINIZING
There is moderate squamous dysplasia.

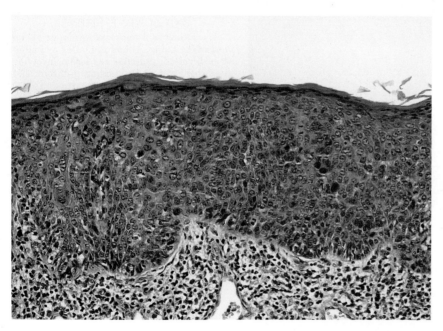

Figure 10-17
HIGH-GRADE SQUAMOUS
INTRAEPITHELIAL LESION,
BASALOID TYPE
Most of the epithelium is replaced by small hyperchromatic atypical cells.

(fig. 10-17), and warty type (condylomatous) (fig. 10-18). The appearance of the in situ process usually corresponds to that of the associated carcinoma but there are occasional exceptions. High-grade basaloid intraepithelial lesions (fig. 10-17) are similar to the lesion reported in the vulva (30) and are associated with about 60 percent of invasive basaloid carcinomas and oc-

casionally with other subtypes of squamous cell carcinoma. The epithelium is replaced by immature, atypical basal-type cells; individual cell necrosis may be prominent, resulting in a "starry sky" pattern. The surface is usually flat and the base may be flat or irregular, with the rete pegs showing downward proliferation. High-grade warty intraepithelial lesions are hyperkeratotic or

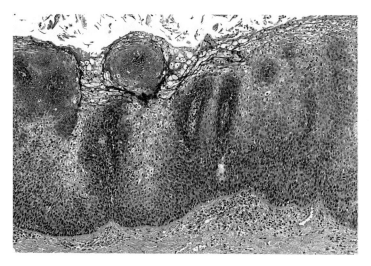
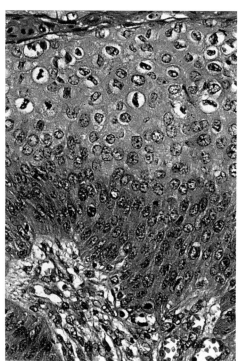

Figure 10-18
HIGH-GRADE SQUAMOUS INTRAEPITHELIAL
LESION, WARTY TYPE
There is hyperkeratosis, parakeratosis, papillomatosis, acanthosis, and koilocytotic atypia. Note mitotic figures near the surface and cytoplasmic clearing in the figure on the right.

parakeratotic, with marked nuclear pleomorphism, abnormal mitotic figures, and koilocytotic atypia (fig. 10-18). A slightly elevated papillary or "spiky" pattern is characteristic (fig. 10-18), but the surface may be flat. The base usually shows widened rete pegs. In a given case admixtures of different types of squamous intraepithelial lesions may be present.

Differential Diagnosis. Various diseases may produce penile lesions that are difficult or impossible to distinguish from erythroplasia of Queyrat and Bowen's disease, particularly the former, on gross inspection. For example, the gross manifestations of Zoon's balanitis (see page 461) closely mimic those of erythroplasia of Queyrat; benign dermatoses also may enter the clinical differential to varying degrees. On microscopic examination the interpretation should be straightforward. On histologic grounds alone distinguishing Bowenoid papulosis from erythroplasia of Queyrat and Bowen's disease is usually impossible (see below), although subtle differences are suggestive in certain cases (Table 10-2). Squamous cell carcinoma in situ of the glans epithelium must be distinguished from urethral transitional cell carcinoma in situ which may secondarily involve the glans mucosa.

Bowenoid Papulosis

This is a human papilloma virus (HPV)-related condition that affects young males (15,23, 24,27,32,37–40), whose mean age in one large series was 29.5 years (33). The process is evident as multiple soft papules, most commonly on the skin of the shaft (fig. 10-19) but occasionally on the glans or foreskin. The lesions usually regress spontaneously, leaving no sequelae. The histologic features are similar to those of usual squamous or basaloid in situ carcinoma. There is, however, in general, a more spotty distribution of atypical cells than seen in Bowen's disease or erythroplasia of Queyrat and greater maturation of keratinocytes (fig. 10-20). Other differences are summarized in Table 10-2. HPV types 16 and 18 have been associated with Bowenoid papulosis (24). The diagnosis can usually be suspected clinically because of the patient's age, location of the lesion, presence of multicentricity, and papular morphology. On microscopic examination, the only differential diagnosis is with unequivocal precursor lesions in the erythroplasia of Queyrat and Bowen's disease categories. As noted already, morphologic similarities between these are such that microscopic distinction may

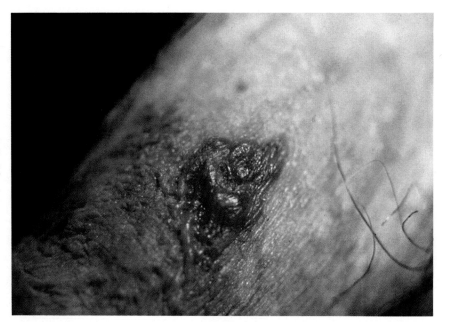

Figure 10-19
BOWENOID PAPULOSIS
Two small papules with irregular margins are present on the shaft. (Fig. 19.4 from Weiss MA, Mills SE. Atlas of genitourinary tract disorders. Philadelphia: J.B. Lippincott, 1988:19.5.)

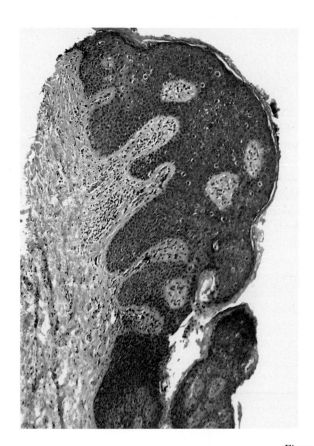

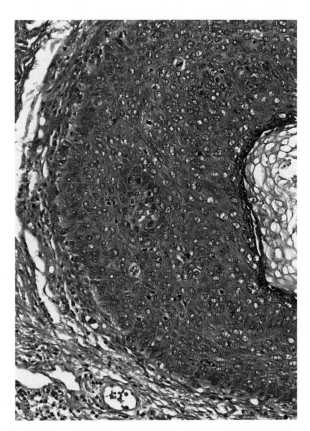

Figure 10-20
BOWENOID PAPULOSIS
There is acanthosis (left) and a spotty distribution of atypical cells within the epithelium (right). (Fig. 19.5 from Weiss MA, Mills SE. Atlas of genitourinary tract disorders. Philadelphia: J.B. Lippincott, 1988:19.5.)

be difficult, and the diagnosis usually depends on the clinical background.

SQUAMOUS CELL CARCINOMA

The overwhelming majority of neoplasms of the penis are squamous cell carcinomas (46,51, 56,57,63–66,73,74,79,80,82–87,89,92,93,96,109– 111,114,116,139). These cancers have a wide variety of growth patterns, resulting in diverse gross and microscopic appearances, influenced additionally by the site of origin and number of penile compartments involved (figs. 10-21–10-47). Evaluation of penile cancer by the surgical pathologist includes: 1) determining whether biopsy material is adequate for correct pathologic classification, including the distinction of hyperplastic lesions, with or without atypia, from carcinoma (70,76), and determining the histologic grade and depth of invasion; 2) distinguishing between entities in the category of verruciform lesions (condyloma, warty [condylomatous] carcinoma, verrucous carcinoma, and low-grade papillary carcinoma, not otherwise specified); 3) accurately assessing the surgical margins of resection; and 4) identifying the pertinent prognostic parameters in resected specimens. The pathologist's opinion is important for patient management since it influences the extent of surgical resection and whether or not a bilateral inguinal lymph node dissection should be performed (41, 52,53,67,106,107,118,119,121,130,131,137, 138,142). A comprehensive understanding of penile anatomy and histology, and knowledge of the wide spectrum of pathologic features of squamous cell carcinoma of the penis are essential so that appropriate information is conveyed to the urologist and oncologist.

Clinical Features

Carcinoma of the penis is rare in the United States and Europe, but has a much higher frequency in Latin America, Africa, and Asia, with the exception of Japan (65,116,120,127). Environmental factors appear to be more important in the pathogenesis of penile cancer than genetic factors (50,97) but occasional cases are familial (123). Epidemiologic studies have identified several risk factors (50,68,97,120,127,134). The strongest predisposing factors are poor hygiene and phimosis (126), seen in about one quarter of

the cases in a recent series (137) and more frequently in older reports (63). Other risk factors are: a history of genital warts, difficulty in retracting the foreskin, accumulation of smegma, lack of circumcision at birth or late circumcision (47,129), cigarette smoking (75,129), and a history of penile rash or trauma. A history of venereal disease is common in the older literature, but whether venereal disease is an independent risk factor is controversial. In a relatively contemporary series, a history of venereal disease was present in 7 percent of patients (137). A possible role of HPV in the pathogenesis of penile carcinoma is supported by its presence in preneoplastic and neoplastic squamous penile lesions of sexual partners of women with HPV-related lesions and HPV-associated cervical carcinoma; also there is an overall association between penile and cervical squamous cell carcinoma in sexual partners (44,48,54,71,77,81,87, 98,102). One third of penile squamous cell carcinomas contain HPV-DNA, usually type 16, less frequently type 18, and occasionally other types (44,49,54,60,81,88,105,132,145,147,149). One study suggested that HPV may be related to specific subtypes of penile cancer, such as the warty and basaloid carcinomas (72) rather than the usual squamous cell carcinoma, similar to vulvar cancer. An association between immunosuppression and penile cancer has been reported in transplant patients and those with psoriasis treated with psoralens and ultraviolet A (PUVA) (140). A relationship with lichen planus has been documented but may be coincidental (42). A definite association with balanitis xerotica obliterans (see page 466) remains unproven although sporadic cases of cancer associated with the former are documented (45,122).

Some patients with penile carcinoma treated by radiation therapy (131) have developed an apparently independent second neoplasm as a complication of the therapy. One center reported five cases of this type which arose in the radiation field at a mean of 158 months after treatment of the initial tumor (125). In another large series of 102 patients with penile carcinoma, 2 had received prior radiation which included the penis in the field (137). The second neoplasms in these cases are usually of higher grade and more invasive than the first neoplasms (125).

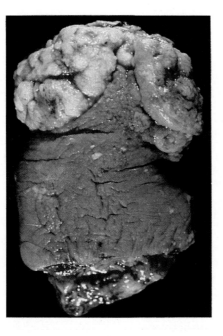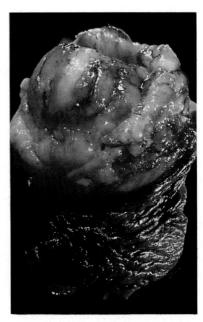

Figure 10-21
SQUAMOUS CELL
CARCINOMA OF GLANS
Left: An exophytic cauliflower-like mass has effaced the glans.
Right: The glans is extensively involved by a multinodular mass with focal ulceration.

The average age of patients with squamous cell carcinoma of the penis is about 58 years, but the tumor is occasionally seen in young adults; in one series 22 percent were under 40 years (63). It is exceptionally rare in children (109). Usually, the patient seeks medical attention because of a self-appreciated gross abnormality. Pain is infrequent and seen in 12 percent of the cases in a contemporary series (137). The gross abnormality is usually a discrete mass (approximately two thirds of the cases) but presentation as an ulcer or area of erythema is seen in 30 to 40 percent of cases (137). Bleeding and dysuria are relatively infrequent (5 percent of the cases [137]). In some cases (12 percent in one series [137]) the disease may be recognized secondary to identification of metastatic disease, usually due to enlarged inguinal nodes (121). Rare neoplasms have occurred in patients with human immunodeficiency virus (HIV) infection (137,151). Hypercalcemia occurs occasionally (146). When there is severe phimosis, a submucosal mass may be palpated but not visualized clinically. As a result, a primary foreskin carcinoma, usually treatable by circumcision, may be confused with a lesion of the glans, potentially leading to an unnecessary partial penectomy. Gross infiltration of the epidermis of the foreskin may be a presenting sign in uncircumcised patients (fig. 10-26). Involvement of the skin of the shaft often correlates with infiltration of the corpora cavernosa.

In a clinicopathologic study of 100 patients with squamous cell carcinoma of the penis done by one of the authors (ALC), 18 had primary neoplasms in other organs; 16 patients had two primaries and 2 had three primaries. Three were synchronous and 15 were metachronous, with an interval of from 9 months to 18 years (median, 10 years) between the penile and subsequent neoplasms in 13 cases; in 2 cases the other tumors preceded the penile neoplasm by 10 years. In another study, 31 of 175 patients (17.7 percent) had multiple primaries (86). The most common of the other primary tumors are tobacco-related cancers in the lung, larynx, mouth, and bladder. A causal relationship between smoking and penile carcinoma is well established (78). A number of patients, in the experience of one of us (ALC), have had colorectal carcinoma, an enigmatic association.

Classification

Squamous cell carcinomas of the penis are classified here according to their site of origin, growth pattern, and histologic appearance.

Site of Origin. The majority of penile carcinomas originate in the squamous epithelium of the mucosa covering the glans (fig. 10-21), foreskin (fig. 10-22), and coronal sulcus (fig. 10-23). Tumors of one compartment often spread to involve others

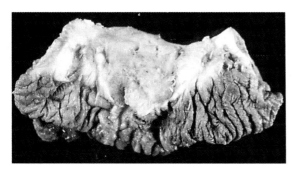
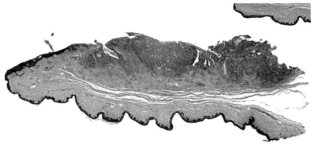

Figure 10-22
SQUAMOUS CELL CARCINOMA OF FORESKIN
A circumcision specimen (left) shows a flat, granular, beige neoplasm involving mucosa of the foreskin but not the skin. Histologic appearance of another case (right) with the mucosa involved by carcinoma at the top and uninvolved epidermis at the bottom.

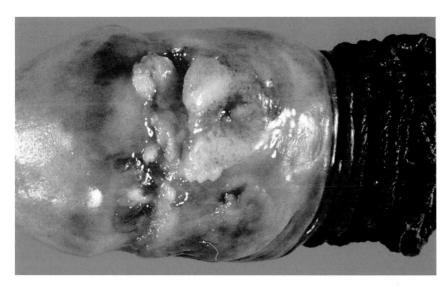

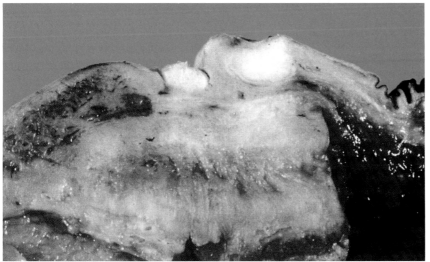

Figure 10-23
SQUAMOUS CELL CARCINOMA OF CORONAL SULCUS

Nodular white tumor extensively involves the sulcus (top). Cut section (bottom) shows two discrete nodules of tumor. The glans is to the left and the foreskin to the right. The nodule to the left is in the sulcus, the one on the right involves the foreskin. (Fig. 19.10 from Weiss MA, Mills SE. Atlas of genitourinary tract disorders. Philadelphia: J.B. Lippincott, 1988:19.8.)

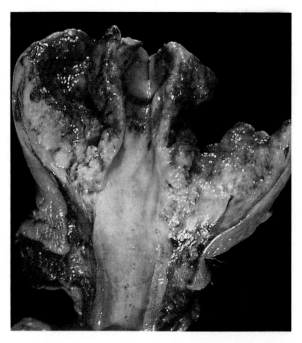

Figure 10-24
SQUAMOUS CELL CARCINOMA
There is massive involvement of the glans, coronal sulcus, and foreskin with complete effacement of the corpus spongiosum. The urethra is spared.

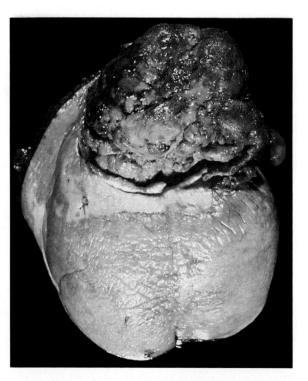

Figure 10-25
SQUAMOUS CELL CARCINOMA
Massive involvement has resulted in autoamputation of the penis. This patient had a penile lesion for at least 11 years but declined treatment until his penis had been destroyed by the cancer, necessitating an emasculating surgical procedure.

(fig. 10-24), particularly when the patient has delayed seeking medical attention, and massive local growth may be striking (figs. 10-25, 10-26). Carcinomas of the glans are most common, followed by those of the foreskin mucosa and coronal sulcus, representing about 80, 15, and 5 percent of the cases, respectively, in our experience. Squamous cell carcinomas arising in the skin of the foreskin (57) or skin of the shaft are rare. In cases with bulky disease, it may be impossible to know where the tumor arose. Foreskin mucosal lesions appear to have the best prognosis because the tumors are usually low grade and infiltrate only superficial anatomic layers. Carcinomas of the coronal sulcus are relatively uncommon and experience with them is limited, but from our observations it appears that due to early invasion of the fibrovascular Buck's fascia, the frequency of metastasis is higher than for tumors arising in other sites.

Growth Patterns. The morphologic patterns of penile squamous cell carcinoma are as follows and have prognostic significance: *superficial spreading,* a flat tumor growing horizontally that typically just superficially invades the anatomic layers of the penis, is usually moderately to well differentiated, and is associated with a low rate of nodal spread; *vertical growth,* a tumor that spreads vertically down, usually deeply, is often of high grade, and has a high rate of inguinal lymph node metastasis; and *verruciform,* several subtypes of well- to occasionally moderately differentiated papillary neoplasms, with, collectively, a low frequency of nodal metastasis. In this category are verrucous carcinoma, warty (condylomatous) carcinoma, and papillary carcinoma, not otherwise specified. Mixtures of the above patterns may occur. Occasionally, multicentric, independent primary neoplasms in various penile anatomic compartments are seen (56).

Superficial Spreading. These slowly growing neoplasms typically widely involve the mucosa and superficial layers of glans, coronal sulcus, and foreskin (figs. 10-22, right, 10-27, 10-28). They account for approximately one third of carcinomas of the glans and foreskin. More than one epithelial compartment (glans, sulcus, or foreskin) is involved in 60 percent of the cases. Tumors confined either to the glans or foreskin occur in only approximately 25 and 15 percent of the cases, respectively. In later stages a vertical growth phase may develop, with invasion of corpus spongiosum (fig. 10-28), corpora cavernosa, or skin.

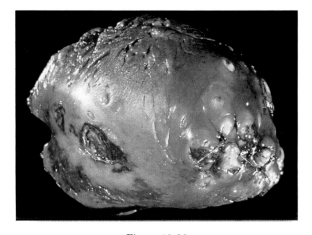

Figure 10-26
SQUAMOUS CELL CARCINOMA
Massive involvement has caused multiple foci of ulceration of the foreskin in an uncircumcised patient.

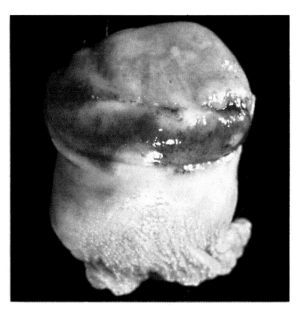

Figure 10-27
SUPERFICIAL SPREADING
SQUAMOUS CELL CARCINOMA

The tumor involves the glans with extension to the coronal sulcus. There is an abnormal geographic, white to erythematous abnormality of the glans mucosa which on microscopic examination was extensive squamous cell carcinoma in situ with minor foci of invasion.

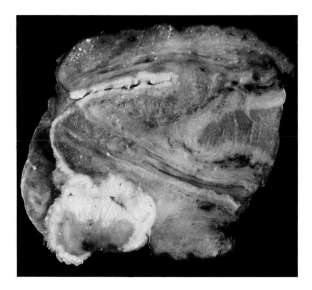

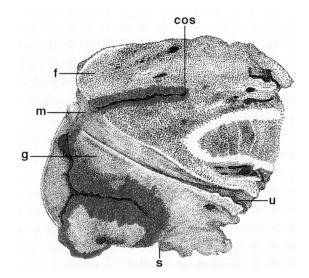

Figure 10-28
SUPERFICIAL SPREADING SQUAMOUS CELL CARCINOMA

Left: The tumor is white and involves the mucosa of foreskin and coronal sulcus, and completely covers the glans. There is focal infiltration of the corpus spongiosum. Deep corpus spongiosum and tunica albuginea are not involved.

Right: The diagram shows in red the widespread involvement of epithelial compartments: mucosa of the foreskin (f), glans (g), and coronal sulcus (cos). Urethra (u), meatus (m), and skin of shaft (s) are not involved.

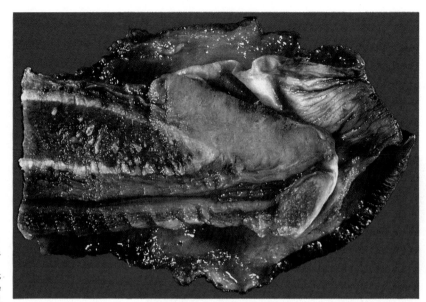

Figure 10-29
VERTICAL GROWTH
SQUAMOUS CELL CARCINOMA

Top: A solid yellow-tan neoplasm in the dorsal half of the glans.

Bottom: The diagram shows that the neoplasm (in red) replaces the corpus spongiosum of the dorsal glans and is present at the interface with the tunica albuginea (a). Foreskin (f), meatus(m), urethra (u), and corpus cavernosum (cc) are not compromised.

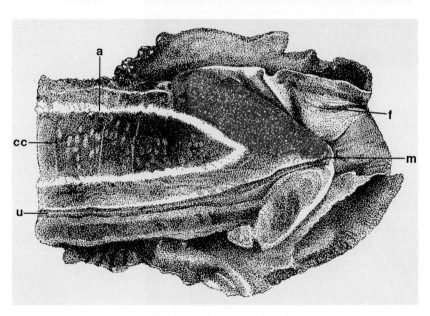

Most commonly there is a slightly elevated, white, granular or firm neoplasm, involving most of the epithelial surfaces (fig. 10-28). The cut surface characteristically shows white or gray-white firm tissue that may be ulcerated, involving much of the surface of the specimen in a band-like fashion (fig. 10-28). In approximately one third of the cases there is additionally a nodular component (fig. 10-28). The thickness of the neoplasm typically varies from 1 to 10 mm and measures 2 to 3 cm in lateral extent. On microscopic examination there is often squamous car-cinoma in situ with an associated invasive tumor of variable differentiation; occasionally, carcinoma in situ predominates (fig. 10-27).

Vertical Growth. Approximately 20 percent of penile carcinomas are of this type. A large, fungating, often ulcerated, white-gray or hemorrhagic mass is typical. The cut surface shows tumor deeply invading corpus spongiosum or corpora cavernosa (fig. 10-29). Cystic changes due to necrosis rarely may be extensive. The tunica albuginea is usually penetrated by the neoplasm, and the urethra may be replaced or surrounded by the carcinoma (fig. 10-8, top). Occasionally, rounded, well-demarcated, "satellite" nodules of tumor are present away from the main mass, either in the corpus spongiosum or more commonly in the corpora cavernosa. Direct extension to preputial or shaft skin may occur.

Verruciform. These exophytic tumors account for approximately 25 percent of penile carcinomas. The duration of the disease prior to the diagnosis is longer than for superficial spreading or vertical growth phase tumors. The glans is the most commonly involved site, but the foreskin and rarely the coronal sulcus may be affected.

Grossly, these are large, granular, white to gray, exophytic neoplasms (fig. 10-30). The cut surface shows a papillary lesion, often with a relatively well-defined base. There are three histologically distinctive microscopic patterns: verrucous, warty (condylomatous), and papillary, not otherwise specified, whose features are schematically contrasted with those of a giant condyloma acuminatum in figure 10-31 (Table 10-3). Many tumors are low grade, with no invasion or only invasion of superficial anatomic levels (lamina propria), but deeper invasion may be seen in some cases.

Mixed. About 10 to 15 percent of penile squamous cell carcinomas have multiple (mixed) patterns of growth, composed of superficial spreading, vertical growth, or verruciform components (figs. 10-32). The gross appearance is variable and there is often a combination of low- and high-grade histology.

Multicentric. Multicentric carcinoma is defined as two or more independent foci of carcinoma separated by benign tissue. The tumors may be synchronous or metachronous. The whole organ section technique may facilitate identification of these cases (56), which account for up to 5 percent of penile carcinomas. Multicentric carcinomas typically affect several epithelial compartments (fig. 10-33), and are usually of superficial spreading type. The mucosa between the neoplastic foci may be normal or hyperplastic. Microscopic examination may show carcinoma in situ and variable grades of infiltrating carcinoma.

Histologic Subtypes. The majority of penile squamous cell carcinomas are histologically similar to squamous cell neoplasms of other organs. The greatest similarities are found with carcino-

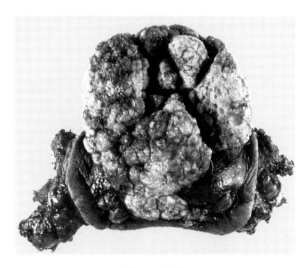

Figure 10-30
VERRUCOUS CARCINOMA

A large, destructive, cauliflower-like mass has extensively replaced the penis. (Fig. 19.11 (right) from Weiss MA, Mills SE, eds. Atlas of genitourinary tract disorders. Philadelphia: J.B. Lippincott, 1988:19.9.)

mas of the oral mucosa and vulva, particularly the latter. About 70 percent of squamous cell carcinomas of the penis are nonpapillary, usually focally keratinizing, and are classified as squamous cell carcinoma of the usual type. The remaining 30 percent have a predominant (arbitrarily defined as being more than 80 percent) histologic appearance that is different, and classified as basaloid (about 10 percent of all the cases) or verruciform (about 20 percent of all the cases). Minor foci of the other patterns are occasionally found in tumors that are predominantly of the usual type.

Squamous Cell Carcinoma, Usual Type

Clinical Features and Gross Findings. As the majority of penile carcinomas fall in this category, the age distribution, clinical features, and gross findings are those presented in the general discussion of penile carcinoma above.

Microscopic Findings. Most of these tumors are well to moderately differentiated, with variable amounts of keratin production, but occasional examples are poorly differentiated (fig. 10-34). The relative rarity of poorly differentiated tumors, which is our own personal experience, is supported by one large study in which not a single example was considered poorly differentiated;

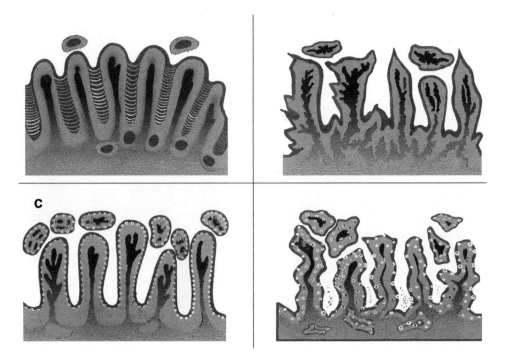

Figure 10-31
VERRUCIFORM LESIONS: PATTERNS OF GROWTH

A: Verrucous carcinoma: regular papillae with broad bulbous bases and prominent hyperkeratosis (red). Keratinized cysts are present (seen on cross section at base).

B: Papillary carcinoma, not otherwise specified: papillae that are more irregular than in A, many with fibrovascular cores. Infiltration is present at the base and koilocytosis is absent.

C: Giant condyloma: arborescent hyperkeratotic papillae with broad bases and koilocytosis (indicated by the white dots) at the surface.

D: Warty (condylomatous) carcinoma: papillae are more irregular than in C, koilocytosis is diffuse, and the interface between tumor and stroma is irregular.

Table 10-3

COMPARISON OF VERRUCIFORM LESIONS

	Giant Condyloma	Warty Carcinoma	Verrucous Carcinoma	Papillary Carcinoma, NOS
Papillae	arborizing, non-undulating, rounded	long and undulating, condylomatous, complex	straight	variably complex
Fibrovascular Cores	prominent	prominent	rare	present
Base	regular, broad, and pushing	rounded or irregular and jagged	regular, broad, and pushing	irregular and jagged
Grade	I	I/II	I	I/II
Koilocytotic Atypia	present at surface	prominent and diffuse	absent	absent
Metastasis	no	yes	no	yes

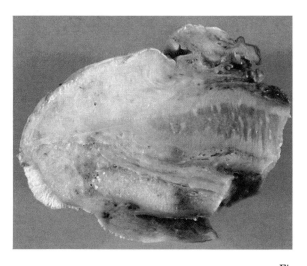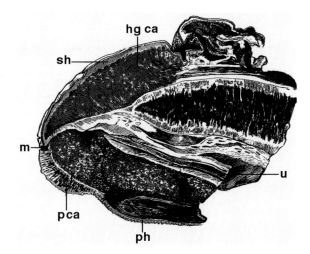

Figure 10-32
MIXED LOW- AND HIGH-GRADE SQUAMOUS CELL CARCINOMA

Gross picture (left) and diagram (right) of a neoplasm showing superficial, white, serrated papillary and tan, solid, deeply invasive components. In the diagram, the glans surface is completely covered dorsally by a thickened solid tissue (dark blue), which corresponds to squamous hyperplasia (sh); a papillary exophytic appearance just below the meatus (in mixed blue-red-black colors), which corresponds to a low-grade papillary carcinoma (pca); and a serrated benign papillary hyperplasia (ph) (lower part). Most of the corpus spongiosum, including its periurethral and meatal (m) components, is replaced by a high-grade carcinoma (red). Surgical margins are positive ventral to the urethra (u).

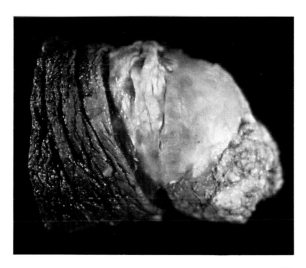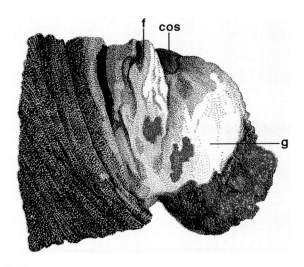

Figure 10-33
MULTICENTRIC CARCINOMA

Four separate foci of carcinoma are present (red in diagram on right). The larger neoplasm is located in the ventral portion of the glans (g) and is exophytic. Three smaller, flat lesions involve the glans, coronal sulcus (cos), and mucosa of the foreskin (f).

73 percent of the tumors were considered well differentiated, and 27 percent moderately differentiated (96). Similarly, in another series (137) in which a four-grade system was used, 71 percent of the tumors were grade 1, 10 percent grade 2, 5 percent grade 3 and only 1 percent grade 4.

Occasional neoplasms have foci that, viewed in isolation, are undifferentiated, but uniformly undifferentiated carcinomas of the penis are exceptionally rare. Associated dysplasia or carcinoma in situ is often present in adjacent epithelium as mentioned earlier. Irregularly shaped

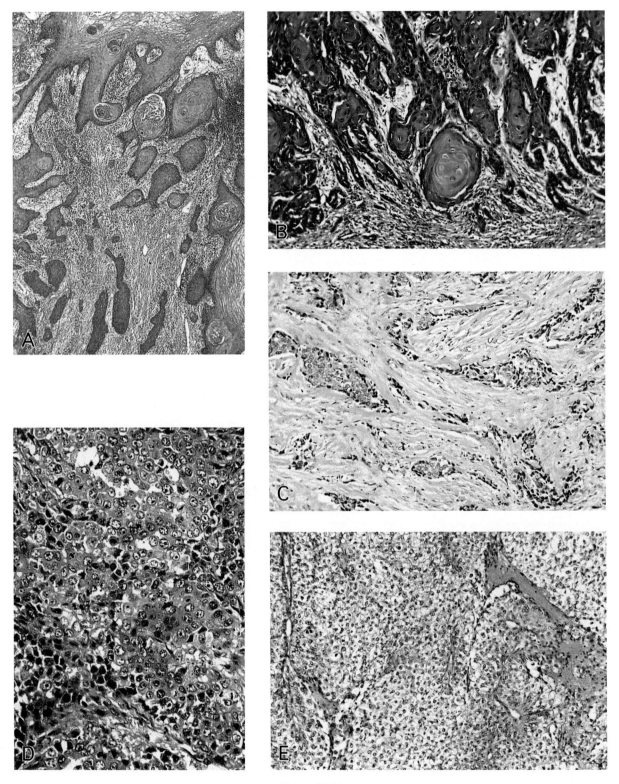

Figure 10-34
SQUAMOUS CELL CARCINOMA, USUAL TYPE
Examples of low-grade keratinizing (A,B), moderate to high-grade nonkeratinizing (C), high-grade nonkeratinizing (D) tumors, and carcinoma with a prominent component of glycogenated clear cells (E).

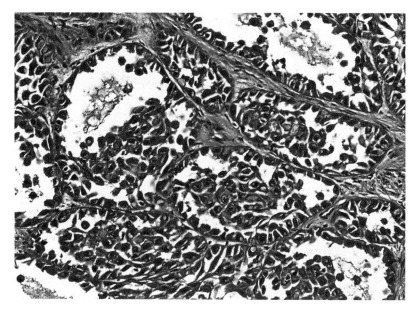

Figure 10-35
SQUAMOUS CELL CARCINOMA
WITH PSEUDOGLANDULAR
FEATURES
(Fig. 19.9 from Weiss MA, Mills SE.
Atlas of genitourinary tract disorders.
Philadelphia: J.B. Lippincott, 1988:19.8.)

nests of cells with appreciable eosinophilic cytoplasm irregularly infiltrate into the lamina propria or beyond. As may be encountered in squamous cell carcinomas elsewhere, there may be a component of cells with abundant clear glycogenated cytoplasm. We have seen an extensive change of this type in two cases of squamous cell carcinoma of the penis (fig. 10-34E). In early invasive carcinomas the neoplastic cells may be seen to bud from the overlying epithelium. Many tumors are associated with a stromal reaction and a modest to occasionally intense chronic inflammatory cell infiltrate. Minor degrees of spindle cell growth may be seen in occasional poorly differentiated tumors, and rare neoplasms are predominantly or purely spindle cell-sarcomatoid carcinomas (see page 435). Neoplasms that are usually high grade may exhibit prominent acantholysis resulting in a pseudoglandular (adenoid) appearance (fig. 10-35)(148). The spaces are either empty or contain keratin or inflammatory and necrotic debris, and are lined by squamous cells that may be flattened. We have seen one penile carcinoma in a 40-year-old man that resembled inflammatory carcinoma of the breast. There was massive lymphatic permeation by tumor in the lamina propria without identifiable invasive carcinoma; the overlying epithelium showed squamous cell carcinoma in situ. Clinically, the glans was red and firm without ulceration or a discrete mass.

Differential Diagnosis. The differential diagnosis of squamous cell carcinoma is primarily with pseudoepitheliomatous hyperplasia and metastasis or extension from transitional cell carcinoma. In pseudoepitheliomatous hyperplasia, the acanthotic epithelium has long, slender, often angulated rete ridges which, when cut tangentially, appear as nests "infiltrating" the stroma. These nests have an orderly disposition and are composed of bland-appearing squamous cells, often with peripheral palisading. The invasive nests of carcinoma are more irregular than those of pseudoepitheliomatous hyperplasia. Additionally, the cells in carcinoma are cytologically more atypical, especially at the periphery, and lack palisading; also, there is often a desmoplastic and inflammatory reaction around the nests with associated dysplasia or carcinoma in situ in the overlying squamous epithelium. Pseudoepitheliomatous hyperplasia and superficially invasive squamous cell carcinoma may coexist in the same specimen, and the finding of the former alone should prompt one to consider whether the biopsy is representative of the lesion.

Extensively glycogenated squamous cell carcinoma may resemble a clear cell adenocarcinoma, particularly if there are pseudoglandular spaces. However, clear cell carcinoma primary in the penis (as opposed to the urethra), is not described. A transitional cell carcinoma may also be in the differential because that neoplasm, like squamous cell carcinoma, can have cells with abundant clear cytoplasm and may show squamous differentiation. The search for more typical foci of squamous cell neoplasia, continuity with squamous cell carcinoma in situ, and lack of unequivocal gland differentiation are helpful in this differential. Direct extension of a poorly differentiated transitional cell carcinoma of the urethra to the glans may pose a difficult diagnostic problem, particularly in cases of advanced disease. In one retrospective review of cases at a large cancer hospital, 2 of 78 penile carcinomas were considered probably to represent transitional cell carcinomas of the urethra (46). The anatomic location in the ventral penis, absence of squamous intraepithelial changes, presence of transitional cell carcinoma in situ in the urethral epithelium, and history of bladder cancer facilitate the diagnosis. Cytokeratin 20 negativity in penile squamous cell carcinoma and positivity in transitional cell carcinoma may aid in the differential (57a). Metastatic transitional cell carcinoma from the bladder to the penis (see page 457) primarily affects vascular spaces of the corpora cavernosa; the history of a previously treated transitional cell carcinoma of the urinary bladder and the prominence of tumor in vascular spaces aid in the diagnosis.

There is one reported case of invasive squamous cell carcinoma of the penis that was associated with xanthoma cells in the stroma, leading to initial misdiagnosis as a verruciform xanthoma (141). Retrospective review of the initial misinterpreted material showed architectural and cytologic atypicality that in hindsight was a clue to the diagnosis of carcinoma. This rare pitfall in diagnosis should be remembered when evaluating hyperplastic squamous lesions of the penis with stromal xanthoma cells.

BASALOID CARCINOMA

Basaloid carcinoma, which accounts for approximately 10 percent of penile cancers, is an HPV-related (58), often deeply invading, penile neoplasm composed of solid nests or sheets of small, poorly differentiated basaloid cells. It has a high frequency of recurrence and lymph node metastasis, and a poor prognosis.

Clinical Features. The patients range from 33 to 84 years (average, 55 years) and usually present with a large mass in the glans. Secondary involvement of the coronal sulcus and foreskin is common. Less frequently, there is infiltration of the skin of the shaft. Two thirds of patients have enlarged, positive inguinal lymph nodes at the time of diagnosis. In a follow-up study of 16 patients, 9 were dead of disease in less than 3 years, and 3 were alive with disease up to 38 months after diagnosis. Three of the remaining 4 patients were free of disease at an average of 54 months, and 1 died of other causes (58).

Gross Findings. An ulcerated, irregular, gray to reddish mass with an average diameter over 4 cm is typical. The cut surface typically shows deeply invasive, solid tumor, with a rounded or slightly lobulated contour (fig. 10-36). Focal necrosis is common.

Microscopic Findings. The most frequent pattern is vertical growth (fig. 10-37A), although a superficial spreading pattern may also be present; multicentricity is rare. Closely packed solid nests of cells, many showing central comedonecrosis (fig. 10-37A,C), are characteristic. The nests may be surrounded by a clear space due to retraction artifact. The nests are composed of uniform, small, poorly differentiated basophilic cells (fig. 10-37D), with mostly inconspicuous nucleoli and numerous mitoses (fig. 10-37C,D). Peripheral palisading is rare and when present is not prominent. Focal keratinization is present in the majority of the cases, usually in the center of the nests; other microscopic findings are a "starry sky" appearance due to frequent individual cell necrosis (fig. 10-37B) and stromal hyalinization. The tumors are usually deeply invasive, frequently extending into corpus spongiosum or corpora cavernosa. Perineural and vascular invasion are frequent.

Differential Diagnosis. Basaloid carcinoma differs from the usual squamous cell carcinoma by having smaller, more regular cells compared to the large, more pleomorphic cells with appreciable eosinophilic cytoplasm of the latter. Keratinization in basaloid carcinomas is usually abrupt and focal within the center of a solid nest and does not have the irregular distribution typical of a usual squamous carcinoma. Although transitional cell carcinomas occasionally are composed of relatively small cells and may have a nesting pattern similar to that of basaloid carcinoma, a transitional character to the neoplastic nuclei is often appreciable

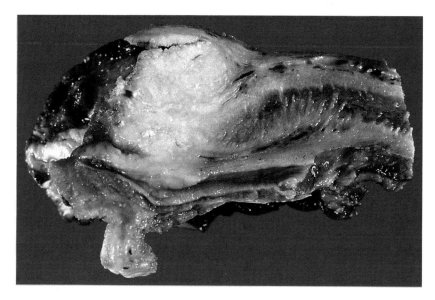

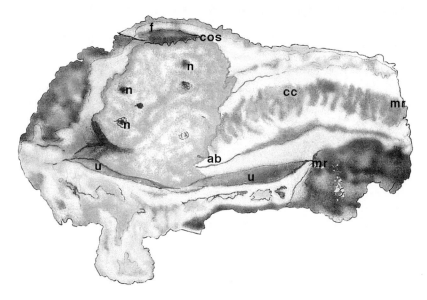

Figure 10-36
BASALOID CARCINOMA
Top: The distal penis is extensively involved by a yellowish white neoplasm that exhibits the typical vertical growth of this variant. The mucosal aspect of the foreskin and the glans, corpus spongiosum, corpus cavernosum and tunica albuginea, and urethra are involved.

Bottom: A diagrammatic representation showing the tumor in yellow with foci of necrosis (n) and other landmarks (cos-coronal sulcus, cc-corpus cavernosum, ab-tunica albuginea, u-urethra, mr-margin of resection).

and, as with the squamous tumors, there is usually more pleomorphism than in the basaloid tumors. In most cases the association with a papillary or in situ transitional cell neoplasm of the urothelial mucosa, or history of the same, are helpful. Basaloid carcinomas are more malignant in appearance than basal cell carcinomas, and the latter characteristically occur in the skin of the shaft in contrast to the typical glans location of basaloid carcinoma. The basaloid carcinomas usually lack the peripheral palisading common in basal cell carcinoma.

WARTY (CONDYLOMATOUS) CARCINOMA

This is a low-grade, verruciform, malignant penile neoplasm, similar to its vulvar counterpart, that has undulating papillae, HPV-related changes, and cytologic and architectural features of carcinoma (59). Dissecting out bona fide cases of warty carcinoma from the literature is very difficult because of inconsistent classification of verruciform neoplasms (59,61,62,94,124, 128,133). In our opinion, many cases of giant

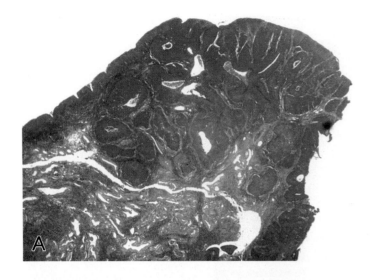

Figure 10-37
BASALOID CARCINOMA

A low-power view (A) shows closely packed nests with focal, central, comedo type necrosis infiltrating deeply into the corpus spongiosum of the glans. Basaloid features are more conspicuous on higher power (B) which also shows the "starry sky" appearance. A focus of necrosis is present in C. The typical cytologic features (small cells with hyperchromatic, mitotically active nuclei) are seen on high power (D).

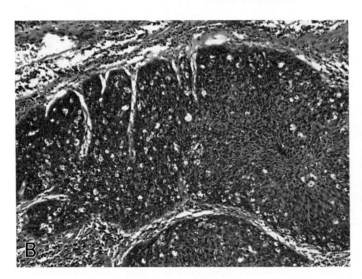

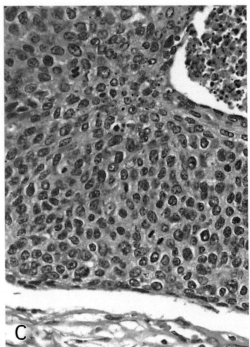

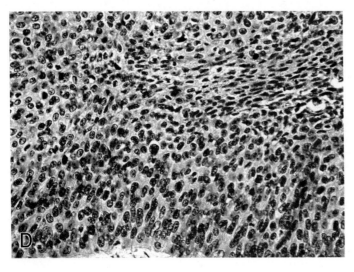

condyloma acuminatum probably represent warty carcinoma, particularly when "invasion" is referred to. Additionally, many tumors reported as "verrucous carcinoma" probably represent warty carcinoma, particularly if koilocytotic changes are referred to and irregular stromal invasion is present.

Clinical Features. These are slow-growing lesions that are frequently present several years prior to pathologic diagnosis (59,61). The median patient age is 61 years. They account for about 6 percent of all penile carcinomas and for 35 percent of verruciform neoplasms. The most common site is the glans, but multiple sites are frequently involved. Inguinal node metastases are infrequent.

Gross Findings. A cauliflower-like, firm, white-gray granular mass measuring up to 7 cm (average, 4 cm) is typical (fig. 10-38A). The cut surface shows a papillary neoplasm with exophytic and endophytic growth patterns (fig. 10-38B,C). The interface between tumor and underlying tissues often appears grossly to be well demarcated, although examination with a magnifying lens shows a jagged or serrated appearance at the base. There is usually gross involvement of the lamina propria and corpus spongiosum, but the corpora cavernosa are rarely invaded.

Microscopic Findings. Long papillae with a central fibrovascular core (fig. 10-39) and a characteristic complex undulating appearance, burrowing into underlying lamina propria and corpus spongiosum (fig. 10-39, left), are characteristic. The tips of the papillae may be spiky (fig. 10-39, above) or blunt, with a striking similarity to benign condylomas, which may be associated with the lesion. Prominent hyperkeratosis and parakeratosis are usual. The most conspicuous microscopic finding is the presence of obvious nuclear pleomorphism of koilocytotic type (fig. 10-39, above), which is not present in other verruciform penile carcinomas. The nuclei are increased in size, wrinkled, and hyperchromatic, with frequent binucleation or multinucleation; perinuclear clear halos and individual cell necrosis are prominent. Most of these changes, which may be seen even in deeply invasive foci, are morphologically compatible with the koilocytotic atypia of HPV-related lesions. Mitoses are usually conspicuous. Most tumors are grade 1 or 2.

Differential Diagnosis. Warty carcinomas should be distinguished from other verruciform neoplasms (Table 10-3). Giant condyloma may be histologically similar but the koilocytotic changes are most conspicuous at the interface between the keratin and granular layers, the pleomorphism is not as marked, and most importantly, the base of the tumor is broad and "pushing" rather than irregular as in warty carcinomas (59). Verrucous and papillary carcinomas, not otherwise specified, show no HPV-related changes, and the former is not irregularly invasive.

VERRUCOUS CARCINOMA

These are extremely well-differentiated, exophytic, papillary neoplasms with hyperkeratosis and broad-based, pushing margins. As with warty carcinoma, it is difficult to consistently identify in the literature cases of "verrucous carcinoma" that meet our strict criteria; cases with irregular infiltration at the base and associated koilocytotic changes should be placed in the category of papillary squamous cell carcinoma, not otherwise specified, or warty carcinoma, respectively. In our opinion, true verrucous carcinoma is rare, certainly rarer than the reported cases of "verrucous carcinoma" of the penis might suggest. Others have pointed out that many cases of "verrucous carcinoma" can be reclassified as other verruciform neoplasms (128).

Clinical Features. Based on the literature, verrucous carcinoma accounts for approximately 3 percent of all penile cancers and 20 percent of the verruciform neoplasms, although, as noted above, it is difficult to ascertain the true frequency because of misinterpretation of condylomas and warty or papillary squamous cell carcinomas, not otherwise specified, as verrucous carcinoma (42, 62,91,95,99,104,108,115,135,136). We suspect their true frequency is lower than the numbers just given. They are slowly growing and often present for some years prior to histologic diagnosis.

Gross Findings. An exophytic, white to gray, firm neoplasm measuring about 3 cm in diameter is typical, but huge destructive lesions may be encountered (figs. 10-30, 10-40). The glans is the most common site, but the foreskin and coronal sulcus may also be involved. The tumor is usually unicentric.

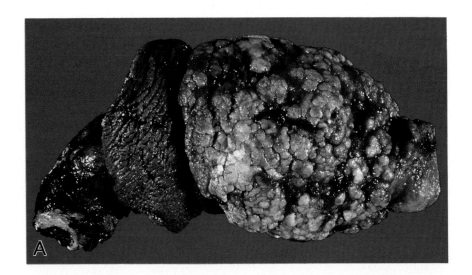

Figure 10-38
WARTY (CONDYLOMATOUS)
CARCINOMA

Exophytic, cauliflower-like white to tan tissue replaces the glans (A). Cut section (B) shows an exophytic neoplasm that covers the entire glans and extends to the foreskin. Note the characteristic undulating appearance of the neoplastic papillae. The base of the lesion is ragged and infiltrates the corpus spongiosum. In the diagram (C) the tumor is in yellow. The corpus spongiosum is effaced by tumor (ca) which also involves the coronal sulcus (cos), tunica albuginea (alb), and foreskin (ca-f). The corpus cavernosum (cc) is spared.

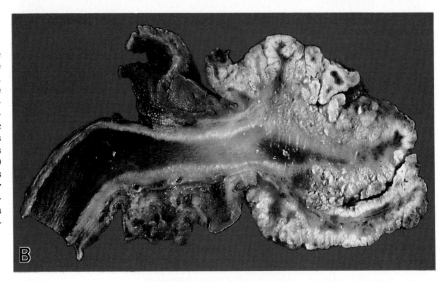

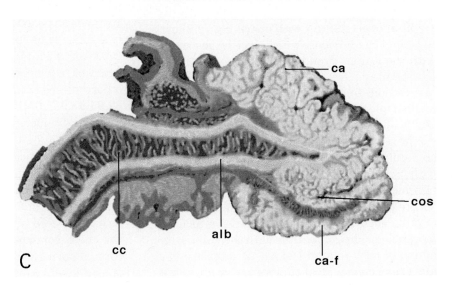

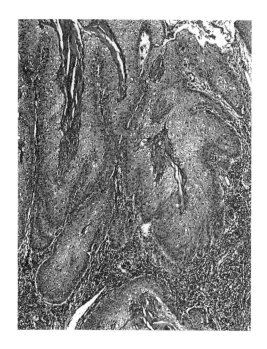

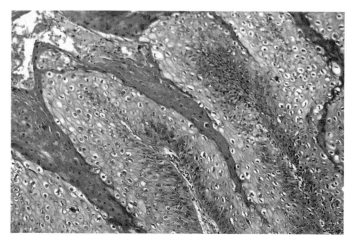

Figure 10-39
WARTY (CONDYLOMATOUS) CARCINOMA
Undulating, complex, hyperkeratotic papillae with infiltration at the base (left). High-power view of papillae with hyperkeratosis, parakeratosis, and koilocytotic atypia (above).

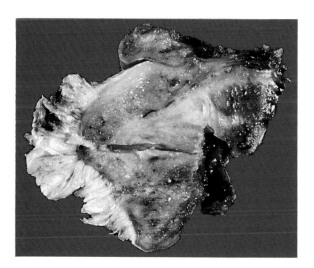

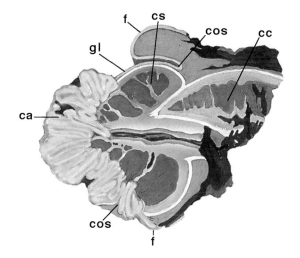

Figure 10-40
VERRUCOUS CARCINOMA
Cut section of the penis (left) shows a papillary lesion involving the glans with extension to coronal sulcus and foreskin. In the diagram (right) the tumor is represented in yellow and landmarks are indicated as follows: f-foreskin, cos-coronal sulcus, ca-carcinoma, gl-glans, cs-corpus spongiosum, cc-corpus cavernosum. Note the bulbous, pushing contour of the tumor base.

Microscopic Findings. Papillomatosis, hyperkeratosis, and acanthosis are prominent (fig. 10-41). The papillae usually do not have a central fibrovascular core, although exceptions occur. Cross section of the tips of the papillae shows a central keratin plug, with neoplastic cells at the periphery. Keratohyaline granules are present, as is parakeratosis, and vacuolated cells, distinct from the koilocytotic cells of warty carcinoma, are noted at the surface. The tumors are extremely well differentiated, with prominent intercellular bridges and minimal atypia; rare

433

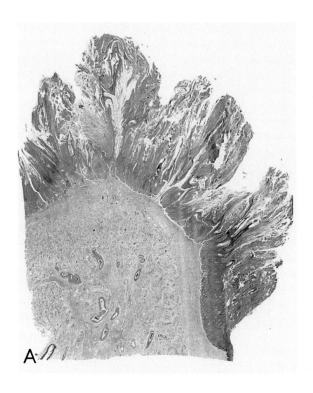

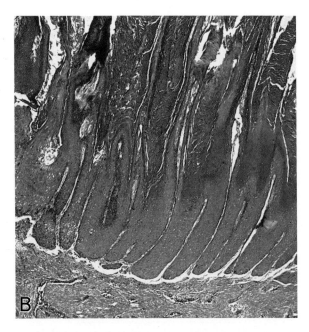

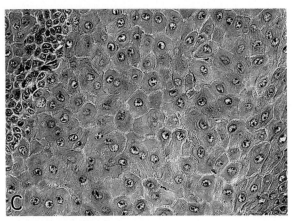

Figure 10-41
VERRUCOUS CARCINOMA

Whole mount of tumor in figure 10-40 showing the pronounced exophytic nature of the neoplasm. The lesion is well differentiated with hyperkeratosis, papillomatosis, and acanthosis. The interface between the neoplasm and the lamina propria is sharp, and the bases of the squamous tongues are broad and blunt (B). The tumor cells have bland cytologic features (C).

mitotic figures may be present in the basal layer. The base of the tumor is broad in all cases, with pushing, regular borders composed of broad bulbous projections (fig. 10-41B), which are usually restricted to the lamina propria but may extend deeper. A dense inflammatory cell infiltrate may be present at the interface between tumor and stroma, and may occasionally obscure it. One third of verrucous carcinomas recur due to insufficient surgery or because multicentric neoplasia was not identified at original presentation. Regional or distant metastasis is not seen in pure verrucous carcinoma of the penis. Verrucous carcinomas associated with carcinoma of another type have been referred to as "hybrid" carcinomas (see below).

Differential Diagnosis. There has been much confusion in the literature concerning the distinction between giant condyloma and verrucous carcinoma, as already stated. It is our opinion that if strict morphologic criteria are applied, the two entities can be separated (Table 10-3). Verrucous carcinomas lack the HPV-related cellular changes characteristically seen in giant condyloma and warty carcinoma. Also, the papillae are shorter and most lack a central fibrovascular core, unlike giant condyloma. Verrucous carcinomas are not causally related to HPV, unlike giant condyloma. Papillary squamous cell carcinoma, not otherwise specified, exhibits more cytologic atypia than verrucous carcinoma and has an irregular invasive front.

PAPILLARY CARCINOMA, NOT OTHERWISE SPECIFIED (NOS)

These are exophytic squamous cell carcinomas that have papillae lined by atypical cells lacking HPV-related features and with irregular infiltrative margins.

Clinical Features. Papillary carcinoma, NOS is the most common of the verruciform cancers. The average patient age is 60 years. Although it may occur at all sites, the most common are the glans and foreskin; rarely, the coronal sulcus alone is involved. The 5-year survival rate is approximately 90 percent.

Gross Findings. These are large, cauliflower-like, firm, white-gray, granular tumors measuring up to 14 cm (fig. 10-42A). The cut surface shows pearly white neoplastic tissue with a serrated surface and a poorly delineated interface between tumor and stroma (fig. 10-42B). Gross invasion is usually noted into the dartos muscle, corpus spongiosum, and rarely, corpora cavernosa or skin; the urethra is seldom invaded.

Microscopic Findings. The low-power appearance is that of a well- to moderately differentiated papillary squamous cell lesion, with acanthosis and hyperkeratosis (fig. 10-42C,D). The papillae may be short or elongated and spiky or blunt, with or without a central fibrovascular core reaching the top. Irregular wide areas of keratinization ("keratin lakes") are present between adjacent papillae, sometimes reaching to their tip (fig. 10-42D). The base of the lesion is characteristically jagged, with irregular nests of infiltrating squamous cell carcinoma spreading into subjacent tissue (fig. 10-42E). Invagination of the bases of papillae into the stroma in a pushing manner should be distinguished from true invasion. In the former the nests are well defined, with palisading at the periphery, often with a central keratin plug and without a stromal reaction. Invasive nests are irregular, with cytologically atypical cells and associated reactive stroma. Other findings may include microabscesses, acantholysis, and focal clear cell changes at the surface of the papillae.

Differential Diagnosis. Papillary squamous cell carcinoma, NOS should be differentiated from other verruciform neoplasms (Table 10-3). Warty carcinomas have distinctive HPV-related cellular changes in the majority of the cells. Verrucous carcinomas are cytologically less atypical than papillary carcinomas, NOS, and the bulbous rete pegs have a "pushing" smooth interface with the stroma in contrast to the jagged and irregular base of most of the latter.

SARCOMATOID CARCINOMA

Sarcomatoid carcinomas are unusual, aggressive, bulky neoplasms predominantly composed of spindle cells and sometimes giant cells; they have little or no component of conventional squamous cell carcinoma. In accord with the approach used in coverage of the prostate gland (see page 238), the exceptionally rare penile neoplasms that are carcinosarcomas are considered here under "sarcomatoid carcinoma" because their rarity does not merit separate coverage, even though in our practice some of the authors of this work separately categorize them. Some prefer to designate these tumors "metaplastic carcinoma" when elements of chondrosarcoma or osteosarcoma are present.

Clinical Features. Sarcomatoid carcinomas account for about 1 percent of penile carcinomas. The average patient age is 60 years. They most commonly affect the glans (101,150). Recurrences are common. The one tumor reported as a carcinosarcoma occurred in a 65-year-old man (113).

Gross Findings. These are large (5 to 7 cm), irregular, white-gray or reddish, fungating or polypoid masses (fig. 10-43A,B). The cut surface characteristically shows deep invasion into corpus spongiosum and corpora cavernosa (fig. 10-43A,B). Contiguous growth along Buck's fascia and extension to the skin of the shaft may occur. Frequently, there are small white or gray-white, round satellite nodules of tumor deep in the corpora cavernosa or in the skin of the penis. The reported carcinosarcoma (113) was a large polypoid mass that measured almost 5 cm and was present on the glans. It had a stony hard consistency.

Microscopic Findings and Differential Diagnosis. The appearance is that of a neoplasm with a prominent component of malignant spindle cells (fig. 10-43C) arranged in fascicles and bundles (resembling fibrosarcoma, leiomyosarcoma, or malignant fibrous histiocytoma), sometimes admixed with pleomorphic epithelioid cells. Giant cells or markedly atypical "bizarre" cells may be present in variable amounts. Necrosis is often prominent,

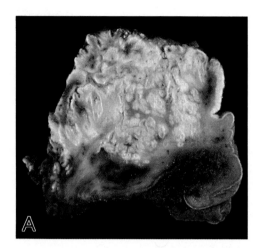

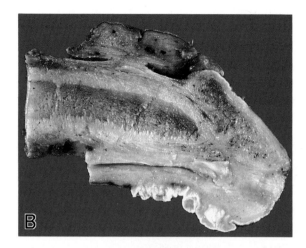

Figure 10-42
PAPILLARY SQUAMOUS
CELL CARCINOMA,
NOT OTHERWISE SPECIFIED

A papillary carcinoma (A) involves the foreskin. B shows a longitudinal section after removal of the foreskin. Note a pearly white superficial neoplasm involving the ventral portion of the glans. C shows surface papillarity and focal invasion. Note well-differentiated papillae and lack of koilocytosis in another case (D) which had invasion at the base (E).

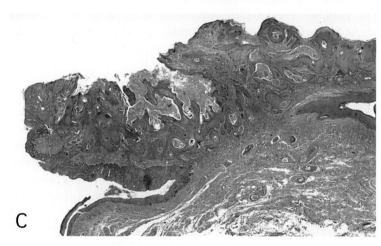

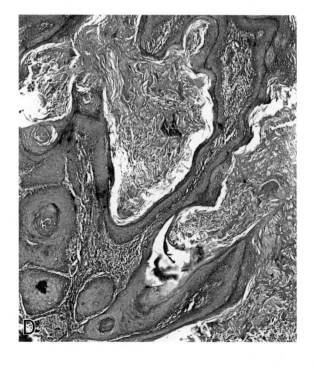

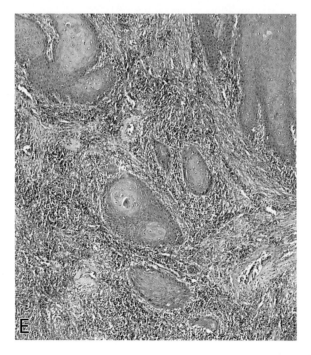

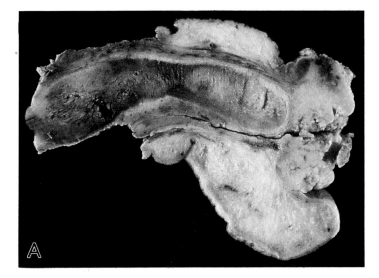

Figure 10-43
SARCOMATOID (SPINDLE CELL)
CARCINOMA
A polypoid solid mass (A) replaces the glans
and surrounds the urethra. In the diagram (B) the
tumor (red) spares the urethra (u) and meatus (m)
but there is extensive involvement of the glans (g)
and corpus cavernosum (cc). Nodules of tumor are
deep in the shaft of the penis (red), with positive
resection margins (rm). The foreskin (f) is edematous. Histologic examination (C) shows an aggregate of rounded carcinoma cells (top right) and
highly atypical spindled carcinoma cells. (A: Fig.
49 from Cubilla AL, Barreto JE, Ayala G. The
penis. In: Sternberg SS, ed. Diagnostic surgical
pathology, 2nd ed. New York: Raven Press,
1994:1966.)

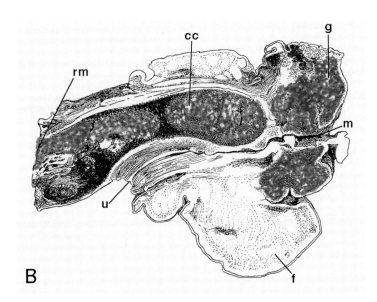

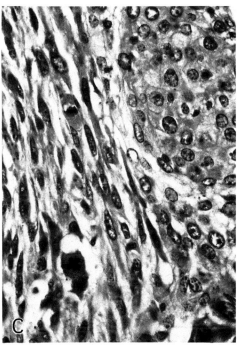

and mitoses are numerous. The presence or history of conventional squamous cell carcinoma or the
presence of dysplasia or carcinoma in situ in the
adjacent epithelium help to establish the diagnosis
of spindle cell carcinoma; immunohistochemical
positivity for cytokeratin is supportive. Spindle cell
melanoma may be in the differential diagnosis; the
finding of melanosis or lentiginous mucosal
changes are helpful, as are immunostains for S-
100 and HMB-45. Ultrastructural features (102),
including poorly developed desmosomes and
cytoplasmic bundles of filaments and the absence
of specific ultrastructural features for leiomyosarcoma or melanoma, also aid in the diagnosis.

The reported case of carcinosarcoma was composed of conventional, moderately differentiated
squamous cell carcinoma and foci of osteosarcoma,
with merging of the two components (113). One of
us (ALC) has seen a similar tumor which also
contained foci of chondrosarcoma. One spindle cell
carcinoma in the literature may have had non-neoplastic bone and cartilage in the reactive stroma,
based on the published description (112). Sarcomatoid carcinoma can be seen in cases of recurrent
penile carcinoma in which the primary neoplasm
did not have sarcomatoid characteristics (68a).
In one case exemplifying this phenomenon, the
primary tumor, according to our criteria, was a

papillary squamous cell carcinoma, NOS; the recurrent tumor developed after 2 years and followed initial treatment by both excision and radiation therapy (68a).

ADENOSQUAMOUS CARCINOMA

Only five tumors have been reported under this designation, two in men over 70 years old and three in younger men of 30, 37, and 50 years of age (55, 90,103). An additional tumor reported as an adenocarcinoma (144) may be best interpreted as an adenosquamous carcinoma with dominant glandular differentiation because of the documentation of "carcinoma with squamous features" in the initial biopsy material. The tumor in that case occurred on the glans penis of a 54-year-old man. The glandular component of adenosquamous carcinoma may be related to embryologically misplaced mucous cells which are occasionally encountered in the perimeatal squamous epithelium of the glans, to goblet cells in the squamous epithelium of the foreskin, or simply to aberrant differentiation of neoplastic squamous epithelium. Inguinal node metastasis was present in one patient who was well 8.5 years after radical surgery (55); a second patient died with widespread metastases (103); one patient was alive and well 12 months after diagnosis; one was lost to follow-up (55); and one patient initially treated by radiation therapy had tumor recurrence at 2 years but no further follow-up was available (90). The patient with "adenocarcinoma" was well at 5 months (144).

Gross Findings. The gross appearance is that of a granular white-gray, firm, large neoplasm, which on cut section replaces most of the glans, sometimes extending to the coronal sulcus and foreskin. Deep infiltration is common (fig. 10-44).

Microscopic Findings. The squamous cell component usually predominates over the glandular. Both components are usually discrete, admixtures being present only rarely (fig. 10-44C). The glandular portion of the tumor is frequently present just below the squamous epithelium at the perimeatal region of the glans. The squamous component may be of the warty (condylomatous) type or the deeply invasive, usual type. The glands are lined by cuboidal or cylindrical epithelium and have intraluminal and intracellular mucin. Solid areas punctuated by mucinous cells may also be present. Squamous dysplasia is usu-

ally present in mucosa adjacent to the invasive carcinoma. Immunostains for carcinoembryonic antigen are typically positive in the glandular component (fig. 10-44D).

Differential Diagnosis. Adenosquamous carcinomas of the urethra have been described, but they are restricted to periurethral tissues and corpora cavernosa without involvement of the glans. Secondary invasion of Littre's glands by squamous cell carcinoma of the penis can simulate an adenosquamous carcinoma. In such cases the glands appear benign. Adenoid or pseudoglandular squamous cell carcinoma of the penis with prominent acantholysis may have a gland-like appearance but the spaces are lined by acantholytic squamous cells and contain an admixture of keratin and necrotic debris. Transitional cell carcinoma of the anterior urethra may show glandular differentiation but the frequent presence of transitional cell carcinoma in situ of the urethra is a helpful finding in the differential diagnosis, as is the transitional appearance of the invasive component. Adenocarcinoma of Littre's glands is usually located in the ventral portion of the penis and rarely has squamous elements. In adenocarcinoma metastatic to the penis, the metastatic foci are usually present predominantly in the corpora cavernosa, and only rarely affect the corpus spongiosum or lamina propria.

OTHER RARE PURE PRIMARY CARCINOMA

A small number of rare neoplasms in this category have been documented with varying degrees of completeness in the literature (43), including a small cell carcinoma of neuroendocrine type (69), a Merkel cell carcinoma (143), an adenocarcinoma (96), and a sebaceous carcinoma (117).

MIXED CARCINOMAS

The most common mixed pattern of neoplasia is the focal presence of moderate- to high-grade squamous cell carcinoma of the usual type in an otherwise typical verruciform carcinoma (figs 10-32, 10-45). These have been referred to in the literature as *hybrid carcinomas* (91). The frequency of node metastasis in such cases is related to the grade and extent of the invasive component. Other mixed components encountered

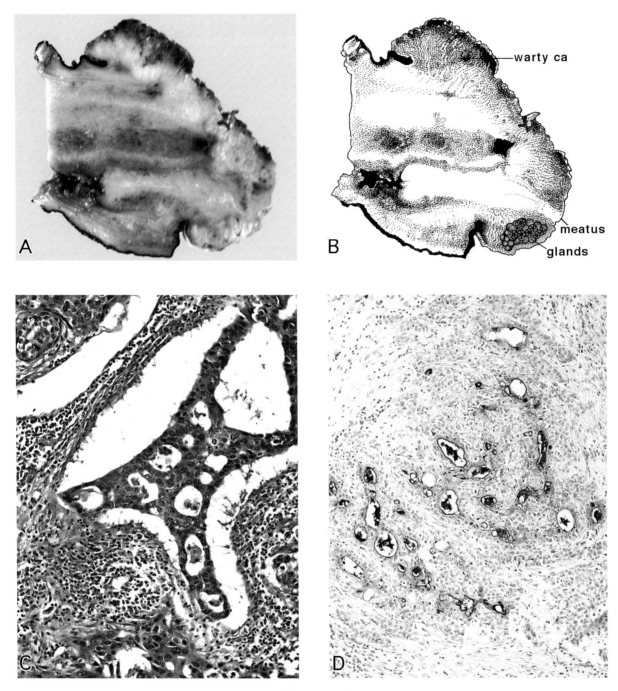

Figure 10-44
ADENOSQUAMOUS CARCINOMA
There is deep invasion of the lamina propria and corpus spongiosum (A). A diagram of the tumor (B) shows in red a neoplasm that was mostly squamous but had focal glandular differentiation (green). Infiltrating carcinoma shows both squamous and glandular features (C). Carcinoembryonic antigen positivity is seen in the glandular component (D).

occasionally include typical or warty squamous cell carcinoma and basaloid carcinoma (fig. 10-46). We have seen one case of composite infiltrat-

ing squamous cell and neuroendocrine small cell carcinoma of the glans, with the small cells arranged in nests, trabeculae, and ribbons (fig. 10-47).

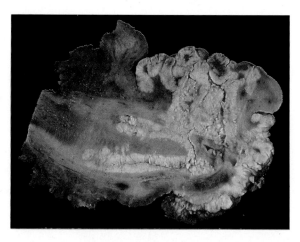
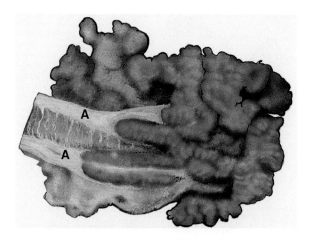

Figure 10-45
MIXED CARCINOMA
Left: Most of the glans is covered by white-tan granular neoplastic tissue.
Right: The diagram shows extensive burrowing (purple) into the tunica albuginea (left) and the corpus spongiosum is effaced. Areas of this tumor were verrucous carcinoma, but other foci were deeply invasive and showed the irregular infiltration and cytologic atypia of conventional squamous cell carcinoma.

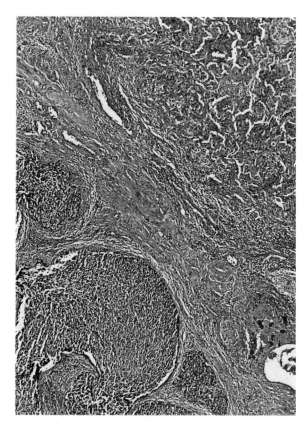

Figure 10-46
MIXED CARCINOMA
Conventional high-grade squamous cell carcinoma is seen at the top right and basaloid carcinoma at the bottom left.

PROGNOSTIC FACTORS

Pathologic factors that help predict regional or systemic metastasis are: size and site of primary tumor, morphologic patterns of growth, histologic subtypes, grade of tumor, anatomic level and depth of infiltration (figs. 10-48–10-51), mitotic rate, and presence of vascular invasion (152,153,155,156). For nonverruciform neoplasms there is a correlation between large size and aggressive behavior. Tumors of the foreskin tend to be less aggressive than those of the glans or coronal sulcus. This may be due to the high frequency of verruciform, superficially spreading, and multicentric cancers of the foreskin and the better prognosis of these types. The aggressive nature of carcinomas of the coronal sulcus is related to their propensity to invade the dartos muscle and Buck's fascia which have numerous vascular spaces, facilitating spread. The prognosis of patients with tumors of the glans, based only on location, is intermediate between that of those with tumors of the foreskin and coronal sulcus in our experience.

Patients with tumors with a verruciform growth pattern have the best prognosis, those with a superficial spreading pattern an intermediate prognosis, and those with vertical growth pattern, the worst prognosis.

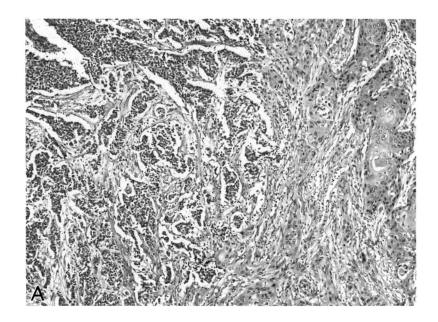

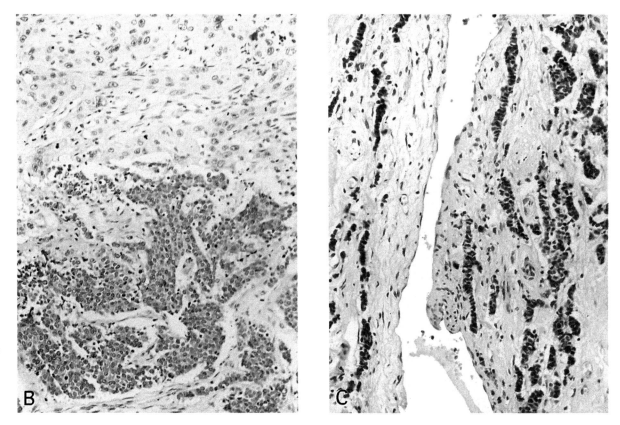

Figure 10-47
COMPOSITE SQUAMOUS–NEUROENDOCRINE CARCINOMA

Biphasic infiltrating neoplasm (A) composed of a grade 2 keratinizing squamous cell carcinoma (right) and small cell carcinoma (left). Immunostain for neuron-specific enolase (B) is positive in the small cell component (bottom) and negative in the squamous component (top). Deep in the corpus spongiosum the small cell carcinoma shows a ribbon-like arrangement (C). (Courtesy of Dr. G. Ayala, Houston, TX.)

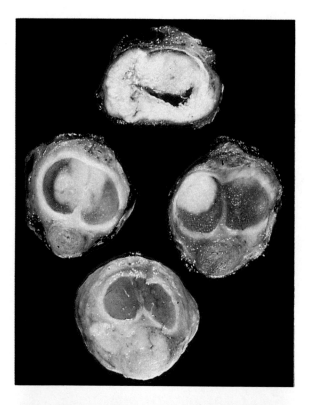

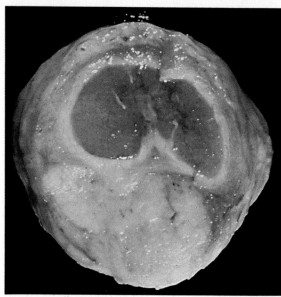

Figure 10-48
ASSESSMENT OF DEPTH OF INVASION
OF TUMOR IN RESECTED SPECIMEN

Top: Penile carcinoma that has been transversely sectioned at intervals showing differing depths of invasion of crucial anatomic compartments. Note involvement of corpora cavernosa (central two slices), urethra and periurethral corpus spongiosum (top), and Buck's fascia (top and bottom).

Bottom: A close-up of the bottom portion of the top specimen is seen.

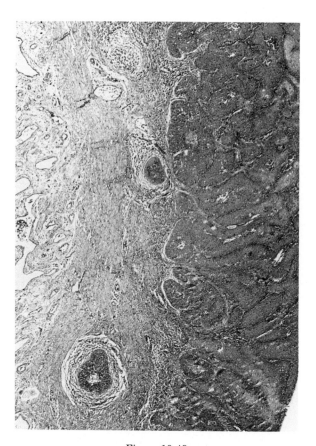

Figure 10-49
SQUAMOUS CELL CARCINOMA
There is invasion of the lamina propria with sparing of the corpus spongiosum (left).

The histologic subtype associated with the best prognosis is verrucous carcinoma, when strictly defined. Patients with warty carcinomas and papillary squamous cell carcinomas, NOS have a relatively good prognosis but one that is worse than that of verrucous carcinoma; those with squamous cell carcinoma of usual type, nonpapillary, have an intermediate prognosis; and those with basaloid and sarcomatoid carcinomas have the worst prognosis.

The degree of histologic differentiation is also of prognostic significance. In one series the percentage of node metastases in the well, moderately, and poorly differentiated carcinoma categories was 24, 46, and 82 percent, respectively (157). About half of patients with vascular invasion develop lymph node metastasis and two thirds of patients with lymph node metastasis show vascular invasion in their primary tumor. The most significant

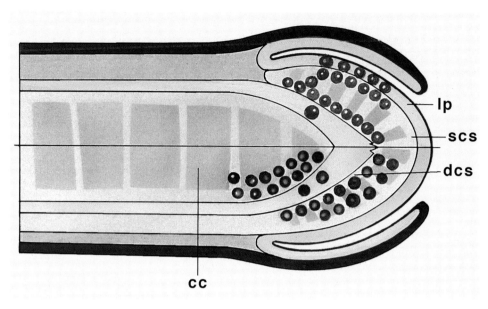

Figure 10-50

SCHEMATIC REPRESENTATION OF EFFECT OF ANATOMIC LEVEL OF INVASION
ON RISK OF LYMPH NODE METASTASIS IN CARCINOMA OF THE GLANS

Each dot represents an individual case in a series of 51 cases, the green representing cases without lymph node metastasis and the red, cases with lymph node metastasis. Note the propensity for the latter cases to spread into the deep corpus spongiosum or corpus cavernosum. The converse is true for the cases represented by the green dots. (lp-lamina propria, scs-superficial corpus spongiosum, dcs-deep corpus spongiosum, cc-corpus cavernosum.)

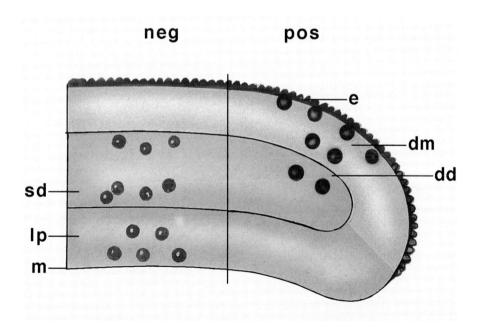

Figure 10-51

SCHEMATIC REPRESENTATION OF EFFECT OF ANATOMIC DEPTH OF INVASION ON RISK OF
LYMPH NODE METASTASIS IN CARCINOMA ARISING FROM THE MUCOSA OF THE FORESKIN

Each dot represents an individual case in a series of 20 cases, the green dots representing cases without lymph node metastasis and the red dots, cases with lymph node metastasis. Note the tendency for most of the former to invade no deeper than the superficial dartos and the spread to deep dartos or beyond of all cases with lymph node metastasis. (m-mucosa, lp-lamina propria, sd-superficial dartos, dd-deep dartos, dm-dermis, e-epidermis.)

Table 10-4

SCORING SYSTEM FOR SQUAMOUS CELL CARCINOMA OF PENIS*

Degree of keratinization
  Points
  0: No keratin pearls. Keratin in < 25 percent of cells
  1: No keratin pearls. Keratin in 25 to 50 percent of cells
  2: Keratin pearls incomplete or keratin in 50 to 75 percent of cells
  3: Keratin pearls complete or keratin in > 75 percent of cells

Mitotic activity
  Points
  0: 10 or more mitotic cells/field
  1: 6–9 mitotic cells/field
  2: 3–5 mitotic cells/field
  3: 0–2 mitotic cells/field

Cellular atypia
  Points
  0: All cells atypical
  1: Many atypical cells/field
  2: Moderate number of atypical cells/field
  3: Few atypical cells/field

Inflammatory cells
  Points
  0: No inflammatory cells present
  1: Inflammatory cells (lymphocytes) present

Grade 1: 8–10 points
Grade 2: 5–7 points
Grade 3: 3–4 points
Grade 4: 0–2 points

*Data from reference 159.

Table 10-5

PROGNOSTIC INDEX FOR SQUAMOUS CELL CARCINOMA OF PENIS

A: Numerical Values of Histologic Grade

Grade	Value
I	1
II	2
III	3

B: Numerical Values of Anatomic Levels of Invasion

Site	Level	Value
Glans	Epithelium	0
	Lamina propria	1
	Corpus spongiosum	2
	Corpora cavernosa (CC)	3
Foreskin	Epithelium	0
	Lamina propria	1
	Dartos	2
	Skin	3
Coronal Sulcus	Epithelium	0
	Lamina propria	1
	Dartos	2
	Buck's fascia-CC	3

pathologic parameters in predicting lymph node metastasis and mortality are the combination of histologic grade and anatomic level of invasion.

Maiche et al. (159) have proposed a scoring system for grading squamous cell carcinoma of the penis based on the degree of keratinization, mitotic activity, cellular atypia, and inflammatory cell infiltrate (Table 10-4). They arrived at a four-grade system by giving points for various features in the above categories and found a good correlation with stage. McDougal (160,161) has emphasized the importance of depth of invasion, in addition to grade, in determining prognosis.

One of us (ALC) has in his own practice utilized a so-called prognostic index in an attempt to predict regional lymph node metastasis and overall prognosis (Table 10-5). This expands upon the observations of McDougal by further stratifying the cases according to depth of invasion with regard to the three main sites of disease (Table 10-5B), with particular emphasis on tumors of the glans (the most common), which in our opinion should be separately classified with regard to invasion of the corpus spongiosum or corpora cavernosa. The prognostic index (Table 10-5) is represented by numbers from 1 to 6, arrived at by adding numerical values given to the histologic grade and anatomic level of invasion. Each histologic grade is given a number equal to the grade (Table 10-5A). In the glans, the numerical values of the anatomic levels are as follow: lamina propria, 1; corpus spongiosum, 2; corpora cavernosa, 3 (Table 10-5B). In the foreskin, the values for lamina propria, dartos muscle, and skin are 1, 2, and 3, respectively (Table 10-5B). Patients with indices of 1, 2, and 3 have a very low risk of developing metastases or of dying of

Table 10-6

DEFINITION OF TNM STAGING SYSTEM*

Primary Tumor (T)

TX   Primary tumor cannot be assessed
T0   No evidence of primary tumor
Tis   Carcinoma in situ
Ta   Noninvasive verrucous carcinoma
T1   Tumor invades subepithelial connective tissue
T2   Tumor invades corpus spongiosum or cavernosum
T3   Tumor invades urethra or prostate
T4   Tumor invades other adjacent structures

Regional Lymph Nodes (N)

NX   Regional lymph nodes cannot be assessed
N0   No regional lymph node metastasis
N1   Metastasis in a single superficial inguinal lymph node
N2   Metastasis in multiple or bilateral superficial inguinal lymph nodes
N3   Metastasis in deep inguinal or pelvic lymph node(s), unilateral or bilateral

Distant Metastasis (M)

MX   Presence of distant metastasis cannot be assessed
M0   No distant metastasis
M1   Distant metastasis

*From: AJCC Cancer Staging Manual, 5th Edition, Lippincott-Raven, Philadelphia, 1997:215-6, and International Union Against Cancer (UICC). TNM classification of malignant tumors. 5th ed. New York: Wiley-Liss 1997:167–9.

cancer. Index 4 is the most commonly encountered value in resected specimens and is associated with lymph node metastasis in about 10 to 20 percent of cases. Indices 5 and 6 correlate with frequent nodal metastasis and poor survival. In an unpublished study, we found that the risk of dying from cancer with prognostic indices 1 to 3 was 0.064 (adjusted relative risk), whereas the risk for indices 5 or 6 was 391.8. It is useful, therefore, to group the indices into low (prognostic index 1 to 3), intermediate (prognostic index 4), and high (prognostic index 5 or 6) risk categories for metastasis. In carcinomas of the glans, indices 4 to 6 are more common than 1 to 3, but in the foreskin lower indices are more frequent, reflecting their overall better prognosis. The prognostic index should be the result of a careful pathologic evaluation of the resected specimen. This method is only applicable to resected specimens; elective groin dissection, based on this risk assessment, must be performed separately. The greatest predictive value is for the low indices (1 to 3). In our personal experience with over 200 patients we found only one error in predicting negative inguinal nodes on the basis of a low prognostic index. The prediction for intermediate and high indices (4 to 6) is accurate in about 80 percent of cases.

Staging

The staging of cancer of the penis published in the Cancer Staging Manual, sponsored by the American Joint Committee on Cancer, is shown in Table 10-6. We believe there is merit in future staging systems to subcategorize T2 into T2a (invasion of corpus spongiosum only) and T2b (invasion into corpora cavernosa). Other staging systems have been proposed (154,158).

FROZEN SECTION EVALUATION OF PENILE CANCER

Circumcision Specimen. The treatment for primary carcinoma of the foreskin is complete resection of the foreskin. The entire circumference and thickness of the mucosal margin of resection should be submitted for frozen section evaluation. Three or four "shave margins" are

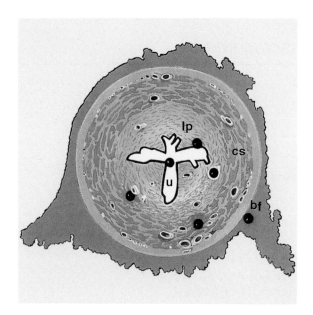 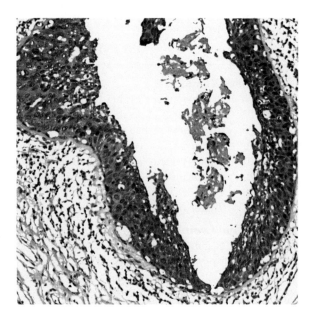

Figure 10-52
POSSIBLE SITES OF RESECTION MARGIN INVOLVEMENT AT TIME OF FROZEN SECTION
Left: Diagrammatic representation of possible sites of involvement. The purple dots indicate the usual sites of positive margins (u-urethra, lp-lamina propria, cs-corpus spongiosum, bf-Buck's fascia).
Right: Urethral mucosal involvement is illustrated microscopically.

enough to study the entire circumference. The specimen should be oriented with the coronal sulcus borders up. The most common finding is subclinical carcinoma in situ in superficially spreading carcinoma. The rate of recurrence of this tumor in the foreskin is 40 percent, usually due to inadequate pathologic sampling at the time of operation. If carcinoma in situ is present in the surgical margin, some surgeons perform a partial penectomy while others prefer a more conservative approach such as observation, local resection, cryosurgery, laser techniques, the Mohs' procedure, or radiation therapy. When infiltrating carcinoma is present at the margin, partial penectomy is the preferable therapy.

Partial Penectomy Specimen. In this situation, the surgical margins are all the anatomic structures of the shaft. The most common site of involvement by carcinoma is the cylinder composed of the periurethral corpus spongiosum, lamina propria, and urethra (figs. 10-52, 10-53), involvement of the spongiosum being less common than that of the lamina propria or urethra. The involvement may occur as invasive tumor or carcinoma in situ in the urethral urothelium (fig. 10-52, right), periurethral mucinous glands of Littré, or ducts, which may be deeply located in the lamina propria or corpus spongiosum. The entire urethral lumen may be occluded by invasive carcinoma extending from the glans. Infiltrating cancer can involve the lamina propria, especially lymphatics or perineural spaces. When the corpus spongiosum is involved, tumor nests are present in vascular spaces or in intervascular fibrous stroma. One frozen section usually suffices to study all these periurethral structures. Buck's fascia may be involved by carcinoma in the shaft at the time of surgery (fig. 10-54). Two to four sections are needed to study the cut surface of the shaft.

Total Penectomy Specimen. Only the urethra and the periurethral tissues should be frozen for margin evaluation during the operation. Occasionally, the skin of the shaft is involved by tumor, especially the superficial spreading type. In these cases, or when the lesion is grossly near the skin margin, frozen sections of the entire skin circumference may be appropriate.

Lymph Nodes. The "sentinel" lymph nodes are supposed to be the first site of metastasis of squamous cell carcinoma of the penis, although skip metastasis to other superficial or deep inguinal

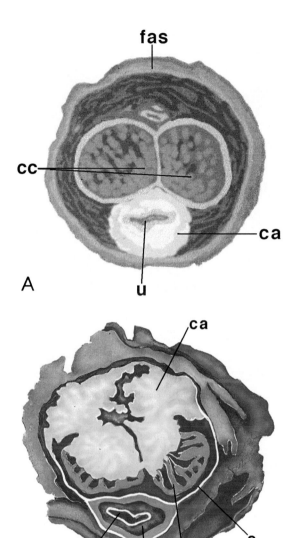

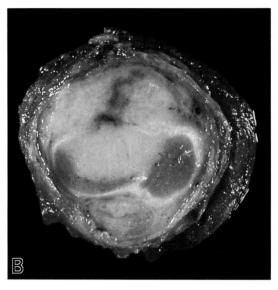

Figure 10-53
FROZEN SECTION EVALUATION
OF SURGICAL MARGINS

A: Diagrammatic representation of periurethral corpus spongiosum involvement by carcinoma (ca-yellow, u-urethra, cc-corpora cavernosa, fas-Buck's fascia).

B: Squamous cell carcinoma involves the corpora cavernosa, with the left more involved than the right. The urethra (bottom) is uninvolved.

C: Diagram of B showing tumor involvement in yellow (ca-carcinoma, a-tunica albuginea, cc-corpus cavernosum, cs-corpus spongiosum, u-urethra).

nodes may occur. We have identified only one case of widespread dissemination of basaloid carcinoma of the penis after a negative pathologic evaluation of inguinal lymph nodes. In some institutions, when the sentinel nodes are bilaterally negative, an inguinal dissection is not performed.

GUIDELINES FOR HANDLING THE RESECTED SPECIMEN

The various anatomic components of the penis should be examined as any of these may be the site of involvement, to varying degrees in individual cases (figs. 10-24, 10-48).

Foreskin. Stretch and pin the specimen to a rectangular shape (fig. 10-6, top). Fix for several hours or overnight in formalin (unless special studies requiring fresh tissue are to be done). Include the entire mucosal and skin margin of resection and make serial vertical sections, labeling 1 to 12, clockwise. The tissue on the slide should show the skin, the mucocutaneous junction, and all five histologic layers (fig. 10-6, bottom).

Foreskin, Coronal Sulcus, and Glans. Remove the foreskin, leaving a 2 to 3 mm redundant edge of foreskin around the sulcus. This permits a better evaluation of the coronal sulcus. If the primary tumor appears grossly to originate

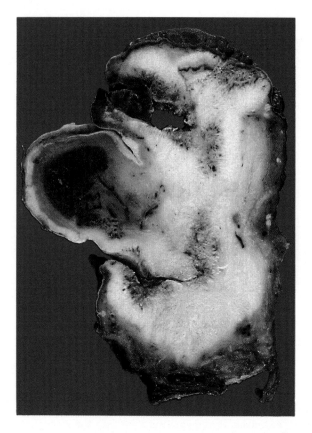
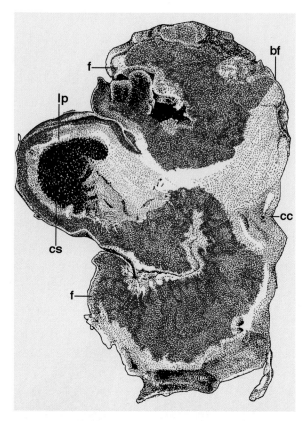

Figure 10-54
PARTIAL PENECTOMY SPECIMEN
Left: There is extensive involvement by carcinoma, including Buck's fascia, at the resection margin (top right).
Right: This is seen diagrammatically in this figure (top right). (bf-Buck's fascia, f-foreskin, lp-lamina propria, cs-corpus spongiosum, cc-corpus cavernosum.)

in the coronal sulcus, a wider margin of foreskin may be left. Proceed with the foreskin as indicated above. Even if the primary tumor is located in the glans, it is important to submit the foreskin serially and in orderly fashion, labeled with numbers or letters.

Urethral Margin. A transverse section, margin up, should include the mucosal surface, surrounding lamina propria, and corpus spongiosum. The cylinder composed of the urethra and above listed anatomic layers is usually shorter than the penile shaft in partial penectomy specimens because most surgical techniques use a long urethral stump for reconstruction. The skin of the shaft and penile dartos muscle are not included in the specimen. In larger specimens it is important to submit two or three additional sections of the more distal urethral cylinder to

ensure the adequacy of the resection margin, ruling out urethral or periurethral involvement by carcinoma. Microscopic evidence of lymphatic invasion, which is associated with a high incidence of local recurrence and regional node metastasis, may be seen.

Shaft Margin. This is usually a large specimen. Divide it in two, from dorsal to ventral, along the central septum or median raphe, and submit the cut surface entirely. Each half should be labeled left or right. One section of each half is sufficient, and the cut surface should include the skin of the shaft (epidermis and subcutaneous adipose tissue), the penile dartos muscle, Buck's fascia, the thick tunica albuginea, and the corpus cavernosum. Within the fascia at the dorsal dome, both superficial and deep dorsal veins should be present as well as other minor vessels and nerves. Often the skin, after adequate orientation, is submitted as a separate section; at times it may be difficult to obtain a complete section of the cut surface because of the usual shrinkage of the skin over the albuginea. If the specimen has a long shaft, cut two or three additional sections distal to the margins.

Glans. Several sagittal (longitudinal) sections should be taken (fig. 10-4). Cut first at the central area (use the meatus and proximal urethra as reference points), separating the specimen into two halves, and label them left and right. Then cut three to six serial sections, 2 to 3 mm in width, from each half. The central section should include from surface to deep areas: the five foreskin layers in the short stump; the intact coronal sulcus with its epithelium, lamina propria, dartos muscle, and fascial point of insertion; in the glans, the epithelium, lamina propria, corpus spongiosum, tunica albuginea, and corpora cavernosa; the meatus, urethral mucosa, urethral lamina propria, and surrounding coronal sulcus. This method of sectioning permits easy orientation of the complex anatomy of the penis, and facilitates the reconstruction of the lesion in a diagram. Superficially spreading tumors can be distinguished from vertical growth, unicentric and multicentric carcinomas can be identified, and all in situ and other associated epithelial lesions can be located in their precise anatomic sites.

REPORTING OF RESECTED SPECIMENS OF PENILE CARCINOMA

The pathology report of carcinoma of the penis should contain the following information: 1) tumor size; 2) patterns of growth and histologic type; 3) grade; 4) anatomic sites of involvement and site of origin; 5) anatomic levels and depth of invasion; 6) comment on vascular and perineural invasion; 7) margins of resection; 8) associated lesions. In our experience, the prognostic index also provides valuable information and may be included in the report. An example of a complete report is: "2 cm superficial spreading, moderately differentiated (grade 2/3), infiltrating squamous cell carcinoma of the glans penis, with secondary involvement of the coronal sulcus and foreskin. The tumor infiltrates lamina propria and superficial corpus spongiosum in the glans to a depth of 4 mm. No vascular or perineural

invasion is seen. Prognostic index (grade=2, anatomic level=2) of 4. Foreskin, urethra, and shaft margins of resection are free of tumor. Carcinoma in situ is seen in coronal sulcus and foreskin, contiguous with main tumor mass. Squamous hyperplasia and balanitis xerotica obliterans are present in glans and foreskin mucosa."

BASAL CELL CARCINOMA

Basal cell carcinoma is exceptionally rare as a primary tumor of the penis (162–166,168,169). The majority have involved the shaft, but apparently valid cases involving the glans and foreskin are described. Some cases in the older literature reported under this designation and with a rapidly malignant course may represent examples of basaloid carcinoma. The patients have all been adults, typically elderly, and on gross examination the lesion has had the features seen elsewhere: a small, frequently ulcerated mass. Microscopic features are also as seen in other areas (see the Fascicle on non-melanocytic tumors of the skin [167]). The differential diagnosis primarily involves basaloid carcinoma (see page 428). The latter typically involves the glans, exhibits much more atypicality and mitotic activity than basal cell carcinoma, and does not have its regular architecture.

PAGET'S DISEASE

This is a very rare penile lesion (170,173). The penis is sometimes involved as part of widespread disease of the inguinal and scrotal region (171,172). Isolated primary penile disease is exceptional, less common than that of the scrotum. The patients have usually been in the sixth and seventh decades and have presented with a scaly eczematous lesion characterized microscopically by an intraepithelial proliferation of atypical cells, with vacuolated, mucin-rich cytoplasm and vesicular nuclei (fig. 10-55).

Paget's disease primary in the penis must be distinguished from pagetoid spread of carcinoma, usually from the urothelium, a more common occurrence than true primary Paget's disease of the penis. The clinical history and allied clinical findings are crucial in this distinction, as is awareness of the propensity for urothelial carcinoma to spread in this way. The differential diagnosis

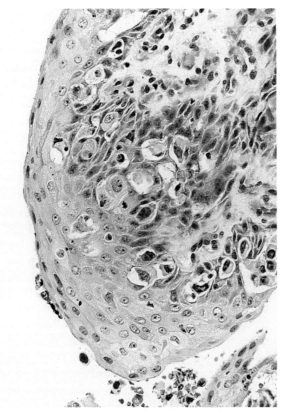

Figure 10-55
PAGET'S DISEASE
Note the typical, basally located, atypical cells with abundant vacuolated cytoplasm.

with squamous cell carcinoma in situ and melanocytic lesions is evaluated using criteria applicable in the skin and may be confirmed by appropriate immunohistochemical stains.

MALIGNANT MELANOMA

Malignant melanoma of the penis is rare, with just over 100 cases reported in the literature, mostly as case reports or small series (174–194). Penile melanoma makes up about 0.1 percent of all primary skin and mucosal melanomas. It is more common in whites and usually occurs between the ages of 50 and 70 years, an older population than cutaneous melanoma. The duration of the disease prior to pathologic diagnosis is reported to be longer than for squamous cell carcinoma and melanoma of other sites. The most common site of involvement is the glans,

but it may occur on the foreskin or the skin of the shaft, coronal sulcus, or meatus. Sometimes melanoma involves both penis and urethra, with an extensive in situ component extending seamlessly between both. Preexisting or coexisting melanosis, melanotic nevi, or lentiginous melanosis is occasionally found (180,183). Four patients with penile melanomas and von Recklinghausen's disease were reported in Japan (185).

Grossly, a flat dark macule, ulcer, or black or bluish nodule may be seen, usually with irregular edges (fig. 10-56, left). Histologically, all the usual types of malignant melanoma, such as superficial spreading, nodular (fig. 10-56, right), and lentiginous have been described. The depth of invasion (Breslow level) correlates with lymph node metastasis and survival.

At the time of diagnosis, most patients with penile melanoma have inguinal lymph node metastases. In contrast to squamous cell carcinoma of the penis, in which infiltration to a depth of 5 to 6 mm is usually necessary for regional metastasis, melanoma may metastasize with lesions as superficial as 1 or 2 mm and, accordingly, has a much worse prognosis than squamous cell carcinoma. For tumors infiltrating deeper than 1 mm a prophylactic inguinal dissection is recommended. Spindle cell melanomas may be confused with either spindle cell carcinoma or leiomyosarcoma. Appropriate immunohistochemical stains aid in the distinction in most cases. The differential with metastatic melanoma is usually aided by the clinical background.

MESENCHYMAL TUMORS

Benign Tumors

Benign soft tissue neoplasms such as leiomyoma, hemangioma (including the epithelioid variant), schwannoma, neurofibroma, lymphangioma, glomus tumor, fibrous histiocytoma, and granular cell tumor, have been reported in the penis but are exceedingly rare, and their features are as seen elsewhere (202,204,206,210, 211,218,221–223,227,228,235,237–239,242). In the experience of the Armed Forces Institute of Pathology (AFIP), benign soft tissue tumors were seen most often on the glans and malignant tumors in the shaft (202). In that series of 46

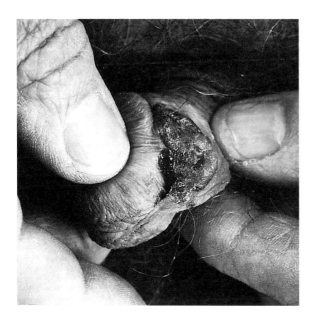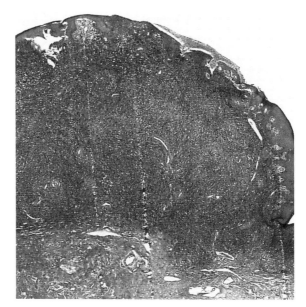

Figure 10-56
MALIGNANT MELANOMA
Left: An ulcerated dark mass involves the prepuce and coronal sulcus.
Right: Deeply invasive nodular tumor on the glans from another case. (Courtesy of Dr. P. Mikulowski, Malmo, Sweden.)

tumors, only 13 percent involved the foreskin; two thirds of those neoplasms were benign.

Angiokeratoma

One distinctive benign vascular lesion of particular relevance to the penis is the angiokeratoma (215). Although the angiokeratoma of Fordyce characteristically involves the scrotum, it may occasionally involve the penis. The penis may also be involved in patients with Fabry's disease (angiokeratoma corporis diffusum) in which angiokeratomas involve the penis as part of widespread involvement of the skin. The lesions are grossly similar in these two conditions, although those in patients with Fabry's disease tend to be smaller and more numerous (fig. 10-57). Microscopic examination shows similar features in each circumstance: many dilated capillaries forming irregular telangiectatic channels occasionally containing thrombi are present in the superficial dermis (fig. 10-58). Those of Fabry's disease also show deposits of periodic acid–Schiff (PAS)-positive material, glycolipoprotein, in endothelial cells, pericytes, and fibroblast cytoplasm. Although these lesions have often been confused clinically with melanoma (215) this is not an issue on microscopic examination.

Malignant Tumors

The most common sarcomas of the penis are those of vascular origin (202): angiosarcoma (207, 212,232,243), epithelioid hemangioendothelioma (203,225), and Kaposi's sarcoma (198,200, 201,214,219,220,234,240,241,246,247). The majority of patients with malignant vascular tumors are over 40 years of age (196,202). A noteworthy aspect of the clinical presentation is the greater frequency of priapism in patients with vascular sarcomas as compared to patients with nonvascular sarcomas (196,202); of patients with vascular sarcomas other than Kaposi's in the older literature, 25 percent had that presentation (196). Kaposi's sarcoma was formerly considered an unusual penile lesion, although certainly well described. For example, in the review of cases seen at the AFIP (202) from the pre-AIDS (acquired immunodeficiency syndrome) era, four of seven malignant vascular tumors of the penis were Kaposi's sarcoma. With the increasing frequency of AIDS, Kaposi's sarcoma of the penis has become more common. Genital involvement by Kaposi's sarcoma has a prevalence of about 20 percent in AIDS patients, and in about 3 percent the initial lesion is in the penis (220,240). The disease typically presents (either singly or, more

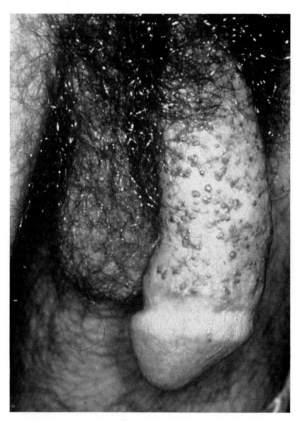

Figure 10-57
ANGIOKERATOMAS IN FABRY'S DISEASE
Multiple, small, dark brown, shiny lesions in the skin of the shaft.

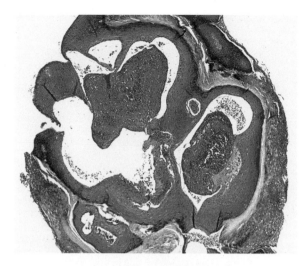

Figure 10-58
ANGIOKERATOMAS IN FABRY'S DISEASE
Dilated vascular spaces in the dermis. (Fig. 18.3, top, from Weiss MA, Mills SE, eds, Atlas of genitourinary tract disorders. Philadelphia: J. B. Lippincott Co., 1988:18.3.)

commonly, multifocally) as small bluish, black, or wine red, smooth-surfaced or ulcerated papules or nodules, usually on the glans or coronal sulcus (fig. 10-59). Histologically, the appearance is as seen elsewhere (fig. 10-60).

The most common site of other miscellaneous sarcomas is the shaft, usually involving the corpora cavernosa. The tumors are typically large with apparent circumscription. The majority of other reported sarcomas of the penis have been interpreted as leiomyosarcomas (195,196,209, 216,224,229,236) or fibrosarcomas (196,244), with rare examples of other subtypes including epithelioid sarcoma (fig. 10-61) (208,213,226), malignant fibrous histiocytoma (fig. 10-62) (245), osteosarcoma (197,205), chondrosarcoma (fig. 10-63) (199), rhabdomyosarcoma (230,231), clear cell sarcoma (233), and Ewing's sarcoma (217). Most of these tumors have occurred in adults, but subtypes, such as rhabdomyosar-

coma, prone to occur in younger patients in other parts of the body, have occurred in children when seen in the penis (230,231). Leiomyosarcomas probably arise in the smooth muscle of the walls of the numerous vascular structures of the erectile tissues, both in the corpus spongiosum and corpora cavernosa. Tumors originating in the glans, corpus spongiosum, or shaft dermis are usually superficial; neoplasms arising in the corpora cavernosa are deep, metastasize earlier, and have a worse prognosis than superficial tumors (195). Microscopically, the appearance of the leiomyosarcoma is as seen at other sites. The distinction between leiomyoma and leiomyosarcoma is usually straightforward and depends on the assessment of mitotic activity, pleomorphism, infiltrative growth, and necrosis. Rigid criteria for the diagnosis of sarcoma, however, have not been established in this location. The other major differential diagnosis is with two malignant tumors: sarcomatoid carcinoma and malignant melanoma. In the former, foci of unequivocal carcinomatous differentiation, including overlying intraepithelial neoplasia, or positive epithelial immunostains are usually helpful. In the latter, HMB-45 or S-100 protein immunohistochemical markers are usually positive. Embryonal rhabdomyosarcoma is usually located in the shaft or near the root of the penis (230,231).

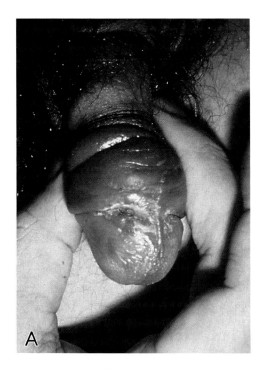

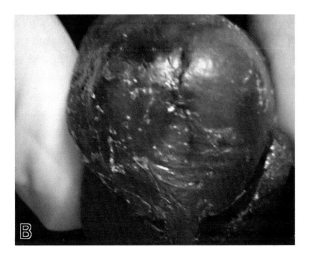

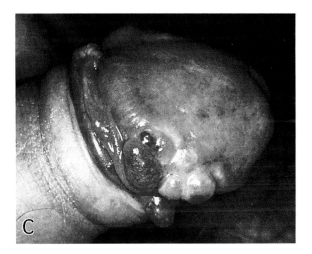

Figure 10-59
KAPOSI'S SARCOMA

A: Ulcerated plaque in coronal sulcus of a 42-year-old homosexual. (Courtesy of Dr. Harry L. Ioachim, New York, NY.)

B: Extensive involvement of glans with resultant meatal stricture. The patient was a 36-year-old male with AIDS. (Courtesy of Dr. S. J. Swierzewski, Ann Arbor, MI.)

C: The tumor in this case is forming discrete nodules. (Fig. 1 from Andriole GL, Macher AM, Reichert CM, Masur H, Gelmann E, Linehan WM. AIDS case for diagnosis. Mil Med 1996;151:M49-M56.)

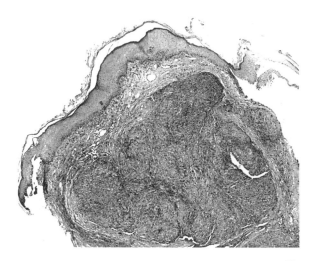

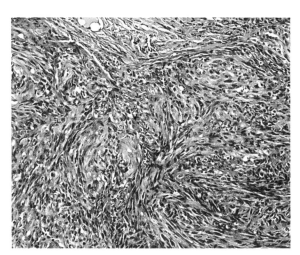

Figure 10-60
KAPOSI'S SARCOMA, LOW- AND HIGH-POWER VIEWS

Note the slit-like blood vessels. (From the teaching collection of the Pathology Department, Memorial Sloan Kettering Cancer Center, New York. Courtesy of Dr. P. Gaudin.)

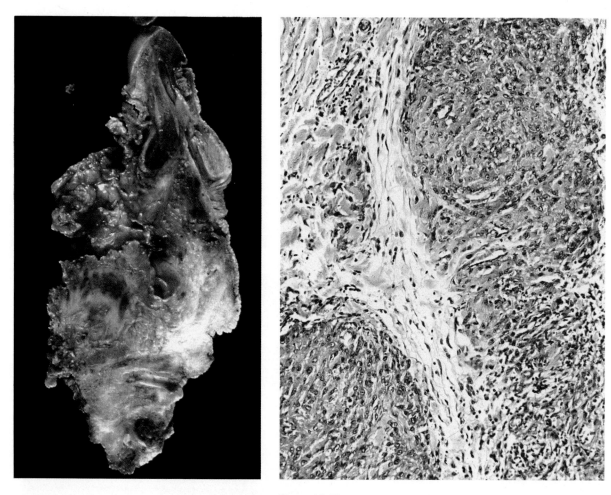

Figure 10-61
EPITHELIOID SARCOMA OF PENIS
Left: There is massive destruction of the body of the penis.
Right: Characteristic nodular growth of tumor cells with abundant eosinophilic cytoplasm. (Courtesy of Dr. F. Algaba, Barcelona, Spain.)

Microscopic features are as seen at other sites. We have seen a case of low-grade superficial leiomyosarcoma that was clinically and pathologically confused with Peyronie's disease, and a similar error has been documented in the literature in a case of epithelioid sarcoma (226).

MALIGNANT LYMPHOMA AND RELATED LESIONS

A relatively recent literature review uncovered less than a dozen examples of lymphoma involving the penis (251). Grossly, a fleshy white neoplasm or nonspecific appearing ulcer may be encountered (figs. 10-64, 10-65A). Most tumors have been of the diffuse large cell type, but other subtypes may occur (fig. 10-58B) (251–255,257–260). The differential diagnosis with other tumors and tumor-like lesions is made using criteria applied elsewhere in the body and, despite the rarity of the condition, diagnosis should be straightforward in most instances. Therapy may be effective cosmetically (fig. 10-65C).

Rarely, the penis is involved in cases of leukemia (248,258) or histiocytosis X (250,256), as a primary manifestation of disease or a significant clinical component of established disease. One example of a neoplasm interpreted as representing "polymorphic reticulosis" with involvement of the penis, scrotum, and perineum has been

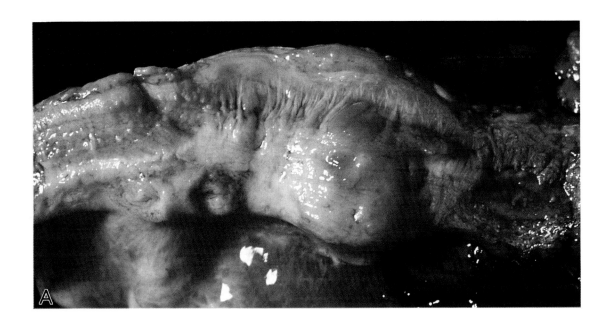

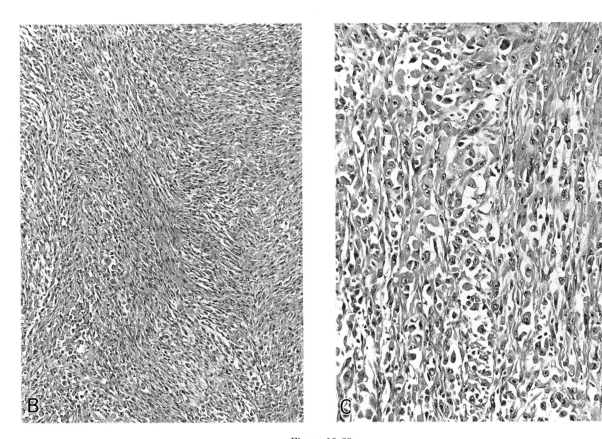

Figure 10-62
MALIGNANT FIBROUS HISTIOCYTOMA OF PENIS

A tan, ovoid neoplasm in the central portion of the midshaft (A). Low-power microscopic view shows a vague storiform pattern (B) and a high-power view (C) shows spindled and epithelioid cells with abundant eosinophilic cytoplasm.

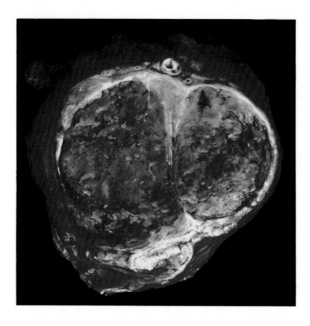

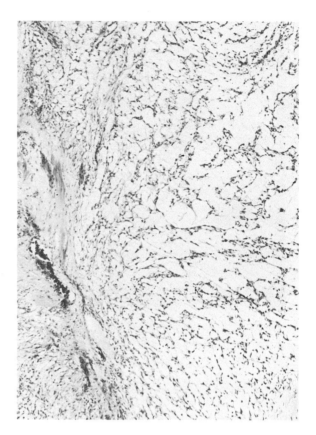

Figure 10-63
MYXOID CHONDROSARCOMA
Above: The corpora cavernosa are replaced by bulging lobulated, myxoid masses.
Right: Photomicrograph showing a prominent myxoid background. (Courtesy of Dr. S. Blasius, Westfalia, Germany.)

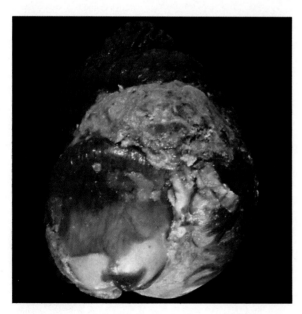

Figure 10-64
MALIGNANT LYMPHOMA OF PENIS
An irregular, shaggy, white-gray mass involves the dorsal aspect of the foreskin and extensively involves the glans. This lesion accounted for the clinical presentation. (Courtesy of Dr. L. Duncan, Boston, MA.)

described (249). That patient was free of disease 7 years after primary surgical therapy. The features of these rare entities on the penis are as seen elsewhere.

MISCELLANEOUS OTHER RARE PRIMARY TUMORS

Other primary tumors of the penis are of such rarity as to frequently merit a case report. Rare dermoid cysts of the penis have been reported (263), as has a single case of yolk sac (endodermal sinus) tumor that occurred in a 17-month-old child (262). The yolk sac tumor was a 1.5 cm nodule, associated with elevation of the alpha-fetoprotein level, and had typical microscopic features including Schiller-Duval bodies. The alpha-fetoprotein level returned to normal following chemotherapy but extended follow-up was unavailable. A peculiar unclassified tumor of probable epithelial type which contained structures resembling thyroid follicles has been described in the glans of a 30-year-old man (261).

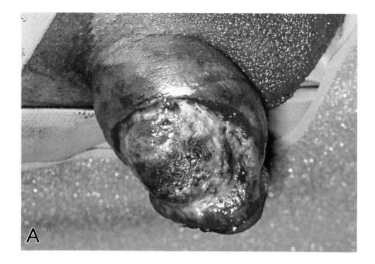

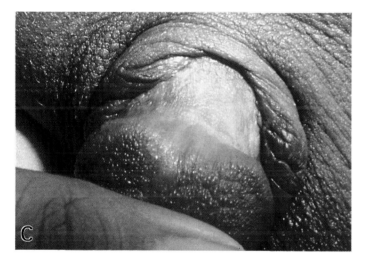

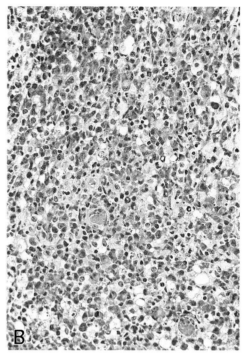

Figure 10-65
MALIGNANT LYMPHOMA OF PENIS
A: An ulcer measuring up to 5 cm involves the dorsum of the penis.
B: Biopsy of lesion showing large cell lymphoma.
C: Site of ulcer seen in A 4 months after chemotherapy shows striking resolution. Further follow-up of almost 2 years showed no evidence of recurrence.

SECONDARY NEOPLASMS

Despite its rich vascularity, secondary involvement of the penis by tumors of other organs, even those relatively close, is rare. The urogenital organs, particularly the urinary bladder and prostate which in combination account for about 70 percent of the cases with a slight predominance for bladder cases, are the most common sources of secondary tumors of the penis (264–267,269,275, 277–279,281,282,286,287). The majority of the remaining tumors of genitourinary tract origin emanate from the kidney, with occasional examples from the testis or rarely other sites (271,274,276, 283). The majority of the remaining tumors originate in the gastrointestinal tract, usually the rectosigmoid, and account for about 15 percent of

cases overall (268). A great number of tumors primary in other locations have sporadically been documented to spread to the penis, perhaps the most noteworthy of which is the rare spread of gastric cancer to the penis (272) compared to the frequent spread of this tumor to the female genital tract, and the rare spread of melanoma, in contrast to the frequent spread of this tumor to various other locations.

As expected, given the usual occurrence of the primary neoplasms in the middle to later years of life, the majority of the patients are in those age groups. The most noteworthy clinical finding is priapism, which has been documented in almost half of the cases. The frequency of priapism correlates with the tendency for the metastatic disease to be centered in the corpora cavernosa,

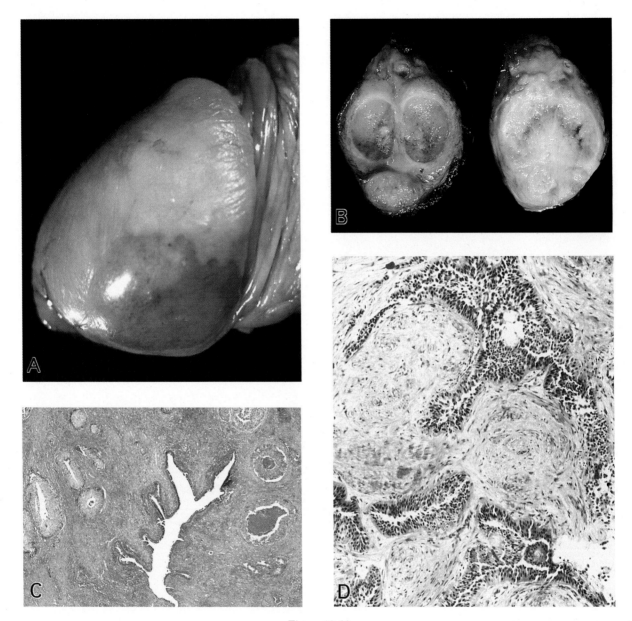

Figure 10-66
METASTATIC TRANSITIONAL CELL CARCINOMA FROM URINARY BLADDER
The ventral glans mucosa is slightly elevated and discolored reflecting metastatic carcinoma in the lamina propria (A). Transverse sections through the penis from another case (B) show involvement of both corpora cavernosa on the left, as well as periurethral involvement, and on the right, massive obliteration of the penile compartments. Tumor cells plug periurethral blood vessels in C and line the vessels of the corpus cavernosum in D.

but occasionally, solitary metastases to the penile skin, mucosa of the glans, or corpus spongiosum are seen, and a diverse array of gross and microscopic appearances may be encountered (figs. 10-66–10-69). Involvement of the foreskin is rare (285).

Most cases of secondary spread to the penis occur as the terminal event of a known cancer, but striking exceptions are seen, usually in patients with known cancer, but exceptionally as the presentation of disease. In most cases the clinical findings, the prominent involvement of

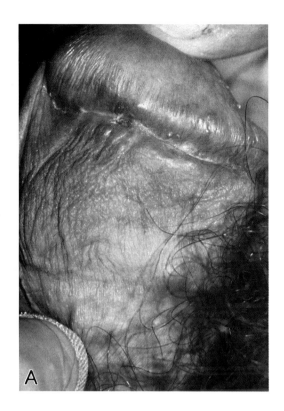

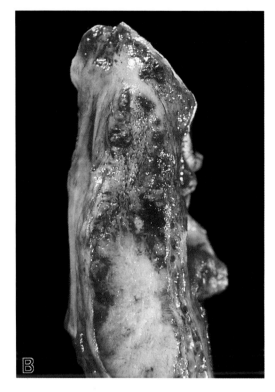

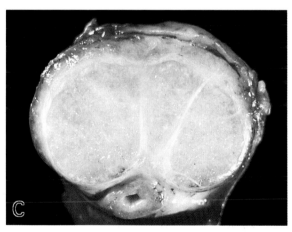

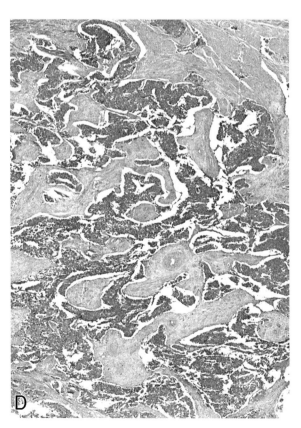

Figure 10-67

METASTATIC ADENOCARCINOMA
FROM THE PROSTATE

A: Small nodules are seen in the coronal sulcus. (Fig. 17.27 from Ro JY, Grignon DG, Amin MB, Ayala AG. Atlas of surgical pathology of the male reproductive tract. Philadelphia: W.B. Saunders, 1997:218).

B: Longitudinal section of penile shaft in another case showing replacement of corpora cavernosa by tan-white solid tumor tissue. The glans is uninvolved.

C: Transverse section through the shaft in a third case shows massive replacement of the corpora cavernosa by tumor with distortion of the tunica albuginea.

D: Microscopic examination in another case shows massive involvement of erectile tissue.

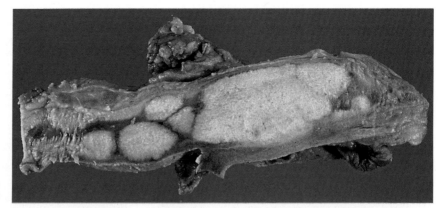

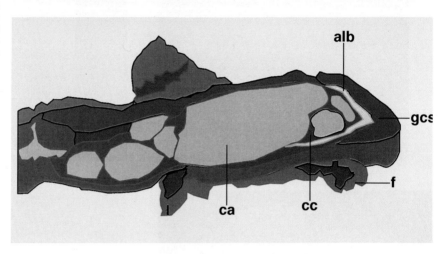

Figure 10-68
METASTATIC CARCINOMA
FROM THE PROSTATE

Top: There are multiple discrete tumor masses involving the corpus cavernosum.

Bottom: The diagram shows the relationship of the tumor to various anatomic landmarks (gcs-glans corpus spongiosum, alb-tunica albuginea, f-foreskin, cc-corpus cavernosum, ca-carcinoma).

the corpora cavernosa, and the lack of resemblance of the neoplasm to the usual carcinoma of the penis facilitate the diagnosis. One particular form of microscopic involvement which is seen especially in patients with transitional cell neoplasia of the urinary tract, is involvement of the penis in a pagetoid manner (270,273,280,284). It is important that this be distinguished from the rare primary Paget's disease of the penis (see page 449). Clinical findings are crucial in this regard.

TUMOR-LIKE LESIONS

A wide variety of dermatoses and infectious disorders can involve the penis (288,289,291–293), but their features are essentially as seen elsewhere, and they generally do not mimic a tumor, either clinically or pathologically; when they do, the pathologic differential diagnosis with carcinoma is almost invariably straightforward. From the clinical viewpoint, it is important that

problematic penile lesions be evaluated in concert with abnormalities in other areas of the body which may be key in establishing the diagnosis (290). The following review of tumor-like lesions is selective for lesions that may potentially be mistaken for a neoplasm, clinically or pathologically, or for those we have deemed especially important for the general surgical pathologist. A lavishly illustrated survey of numerous inflammatory and other non-neoplastic lesions of the penis has recently been published (289) and the interested reader is referred to this for more extensive coverage of non-neoplastic penile lesions than is indicated in this work, which emphasizes neoplasia and pseudoneoplasia.

Cysts

Epidermal cysts account for most penile cysts and typically occur on the shaft (295). They exceed 1 cm in maximum dimension only occasionally

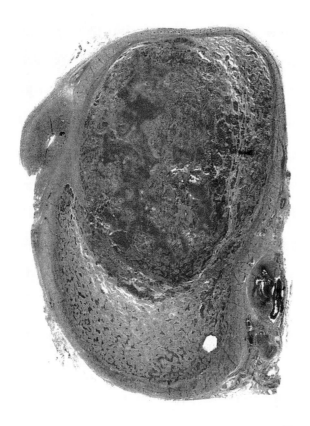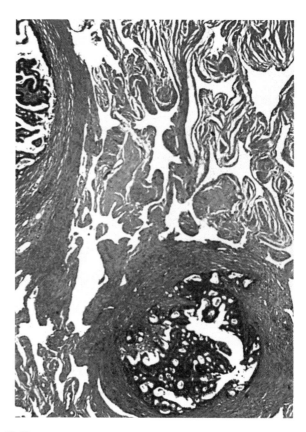

Figure 10-69
METASTATIC COLON CARCINOMA
Left: A large focus of tumor replaces much of the corpora cavernosa at autopsy.
Right: Two nodules of metastatic colonic adenocarcinoma are present in the corpus cavernosum of another patient. The patient had a sigmoid carcinoma resected 1 year previously and presented with multiple nodules in the penis on this occasion.

(299) and have the usual microscopic features. Median raphe cysts are also relatively common, accounting for most of the cysts in one series of penile tumors and tumor-like lesions (297). They may be unilocular or multilocular and are lined by pseudostratified columnar epithelium (294, 298). Rare unilocular mucous cysts of the penis arise from ectopic urethral mucosa and are lined by stratified columnar mucinous epithelial cells (296). They are usually located in the prepuce or glans and range up to 2 cm.

Infectious or Inflammatory Lesions

Balanitis - Posthitis - Balanoposthitis. Inflammation of the glans (balanitis), the foreskin (posthitis), or both (balanoposthitis) is a common inflammatory condition of the penis, without a specific etiologic agent identified in most cases.

Although the non-neoplastic nature of the lesion is generally evident, examples are encountered in which a biopsy may be indicated to exclude malignancy because of a gross appearance which is consistent with neoplasia (fig. 10-70).

Plasma Cell Balanitis (Zoon's Balanitis). This relatively common entity may clinically resemble erythroplasia of Queyrat (fig. 10-71). The disorder predominantly affects uncircumcised males and typically presents as a solitary, large, bright red, moist patch on the glans or inner prepuce of elderly men (fig. 10-71) (300,301). Rarely multiple lesions are present. Microscopic examination shows a band-like infiltrate of plasma cells in the upper dermis, which may show other inflammatory changes such as dilated capillaries. The differential diagnosis with carcinoma in situ is straightforward on microscopic examination.

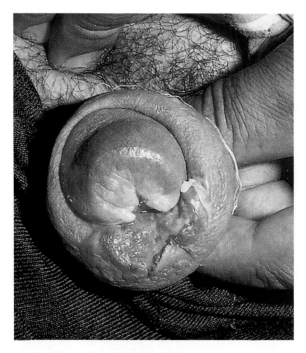

Figure 10-70
BALANOPOSTHITIS
There is marked ulceration, with tissue destruction causing concern for neoplasia. A biopsy from this patient, who was a paraplegic with incontinence, showed no evidence of malignancy. (Fig. 6.2 from Fisher BK, Margesson LJ. Genital skin disorders, diagnosis and treatment. St. Louis: Mosby, 1998:41.)

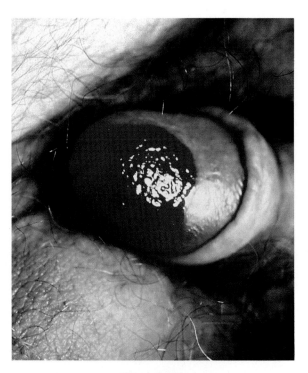

Figure 10-71
ZOON'S BALANITIS
The glans mucosa is extensively involved by a erythematous lesion mimicking erythroplasia of Queyrat. (Fig. 13.8 from Ro JY, Amin MB, Ayala AG. Penis and scrotum. In: Bostwick DG, Eble JN, eds. Urologic surgical pathology. St. Louis: C.V. Mosby, 1997:680.)

Condyloma Acuminatum. The locations of penile condyloma acuminata, in decreasing order of frequency, are: glans, foreskin, meatus, and shaft (304). Small or flat lesions may be clinically inconspicuous or inapparent (303) and, hence, topical acetic acid and urethroscopy are necessary for their detection (310). The typical papillary, warty, cauliflower-like appearance associated with this lesion elsewhere in the body is usual (fig. 10-72, left). Varying degrees of papillomatosis, acanthosis, parakeratosis, and hyperkeratosis are seen (fig. 10-72, above), with prominent to inconspicuous koilocytes with cytoplasmic vacuolization, wrinkled nuclei, and binucleation. The most common types of HPV found by immunohistochemistry, in situ hybridization, or polymerase chain reaction procedures are 6 and 11 (308,309).

Giant Condyloma Acuminatum. This lesion, sometimes referred to as *Buschke-Lowenstein tumor* (302,306), affects slightly older patients than typical condylomata acuminata. In our opinion, the majority of the cases of so called giant condyloma and Buschke-Lowenstein tumor reported in the literature are most likely warty or verrucous carcinomas. Bona fide examples of giant condyloma are very rare, but we have encountered occasional examples. The lesion is often present for a long time prior to diagnosis and appears as a white to gray, firm, cauliflower-like growth (fig. 10-73, left) with an average diameter of 5 cm. The cut surface is pearly white, solid, and gyriform. The base is well circumscribed, with a characteristic endophytic growth pattern that results in deep burrowing into underlying tissues and erosion or ulceration of adjacent skin. Microscopic examination shows essentially similar features to those seen in typical condylomata acuminatum (fig. 10-73, right), with the exception that the papillomatosis is particularly exuberant, and bulbous expansion into underlying tissue is conspicuous.

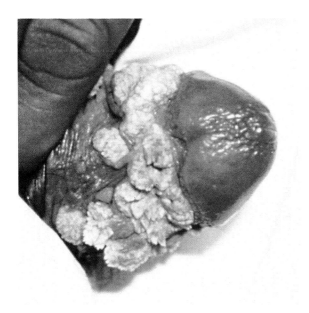

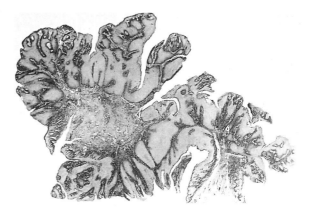

Figure 10-72
CONDYLOMA ACUMINATUM

Left: The coronal sulcus and distal shaft are involved by numerous exophytic, small, white, cauliflower-like lesions.

Above: A well-developed lesion shows prominent acanthosis and papillarity on microscopic examination.

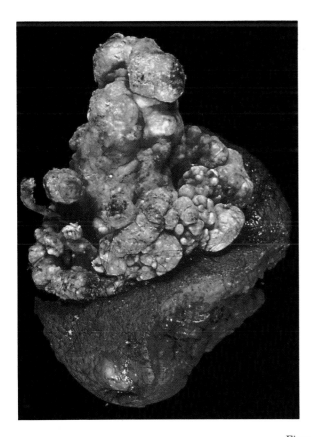

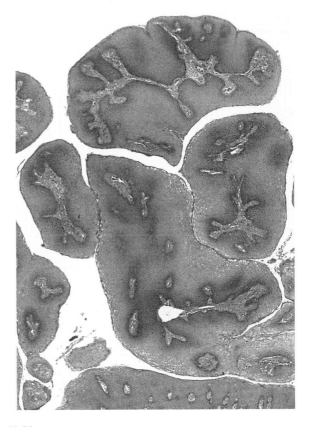

Figure 10-73
GIANT CONDYLOMA ACUMINATUM

Left: A massive, multinodular, exophytic mass involves the penis and extends to pubic skin.

Right: Microscopic depiction of tumor on the left showing typical features of condyloma acuminatum and bland cytologic features.

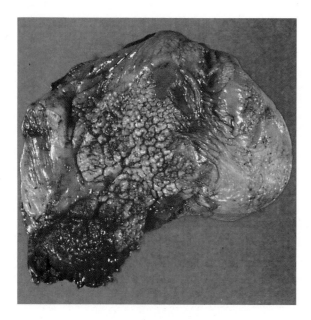

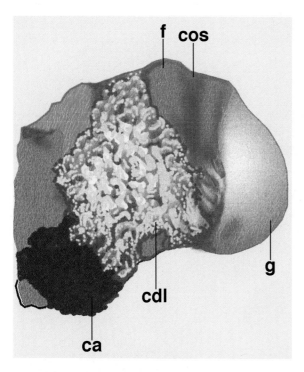

Figure 10-74
TYPICAL SQUAMOUS CELL CARCINOMA
ASSOCIATED WITH CONDYLOMA ACUMINATUM

Lateral view of penectomy specimen showing lesion with a cobblestone appearance beneath the corona representing the condyloma (top). More ventrally near the surgical margin is an elevated, reddish, strawberry-like mass representing the carcinoma. Diagrammatic representation in the bottom figure. (f-foreskin, cos-coronal sulcus, g-glans, cdl-condyloma, ca-carcinoma.)

The major differential diagnosis is with warty carcinoma because of the shared koilocytotic features of the two lesions. However, warty carcinomas show greater cytologic atypia than that allowable for the conventional koilocytotic atypia of giant condyloma. Additionally, the carcinomas exhibit mitotic figures and unequivocal stromal invasion. Despite the confusion in the literature because of lack of consistent criteria for the diagnosis of giant condyloma and verrucous carcinoma, we believe the two lesions have distinctly different features as discussed already under the latter neoplasm on page 434. A similar comment pertains to papillary carcinoma, NOS which has unequivocal malignant features, albeit sometimes low grade, and definite invasion.

Both typical and giant condyloma acuminatum may be associated with carcinoma (305, 307), in some instances warty carcinoma (see page 429), in other instances squamous cell carcinoma of the usual type (fig. 10-74).

Syphilis. The classic lesion of primary syphilis, the chancre, is unusual nowadays. It is a single, round, painless ulcer with well-defined margins and an indurated base (fig. 10-75). It is preceded by a small papule which progresses to the classic ulcerated chancre. Condyloma latum and gumma are most characteristic of secondary and tertiary syphilis, respectively (311–315). The former is a gray maculopapule characterized microscopically by papillary projections of edematous connective tissue containing plasma cells and lymphocytes, with a perivascular predilection. The endarteritis can be superficial or deep. Pseudoepitheliomatous hyperplasia can be seen, and neutrophilic exocytosis also may be present. The gumma is a mass represented microscopically by a zone of coagulative necrosis, surrounded by epithelioid histiocytes and multi- nucleated giant cells. There also is an obliterative endarteritis surrounded by a dense plasma cell infiltrate. The causative agent, *Treponema pallidum,* can be visualized with any of the silver impregnation stains (Steiner, Dieterle, Warthin-Starry). The blackened spirochetes are present in the dermis, around and within the walls of dermal blood vessels, and between epidermal cells, especially in areas of neutrophilic exocytosis.

Granuloma Inguinale. This sexually transmitted infection may present as a small, painless, nodular lesion on the penis or an ulcer with

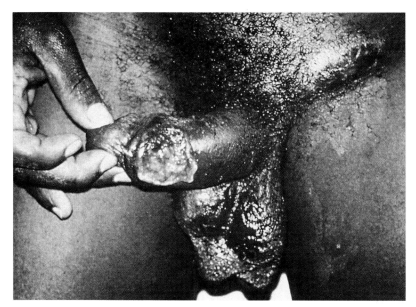

Figure 10-75
SYPHILITIC CHANCRE
A sharply delineated ulcerated lesion with granulation tissue at the base and slightly elevated borders is present on the distal shaft. There is associated lymph node enlargement. (Courtesy of Dr. F.V. Chandler, Augusta, GA.)

abundant granulation tissue in the base (fig. 10-76, top) (316–320). In advanced cases, large, destructive, tumor-like nodules may be seen (fig. 10-76, bottom). Satellite lesions called pseudobuboes can be present. Microscopically, an extensive plasma cell infiltrate is present in the granulation tissue as well as a diffuse infiltrate of neutrophils, which may form microabscesses. Large mononuclear histiocytes with cytoplasmic vacuoles contain dark particulate inclusions, Donovan bodies, which are large, encapsulated, bipolar bacilli that are better seen in smears and with special stains such as Giemsa. The causative agent, *Calymmatobacterium granulomatis,* can be demonstrated in tissue sections with any of the silver impregnation stains (Steiner, Dieterle, Warthin-Starry).

Lymphogranuloma Venereum. This sexually transmitted disease, caused by the obligate intracellular microorganism, *Chlamydia trachomatosis,* is characterized by penile and inguinal lymph node infections. A painless nodule or ulcer may be seen on the penis. A flat base of granulation tissue with zonal marginal necrosis and neutrophilic infiltration is present. Plasma cells and lymphocytes also are visible, as are non-necrotizing granulomas surrounded by plasma cells (321–323). Pseudoepitheliomatous hyperplasia affects the skin. Inguinal lymph nodes initially show small neutrophilic microabscesses that eventually coalesce, forming the typical stellate lesion. Lymphoid hyperplasia and an intense plasma cell infiltrate may be seen. In longstanding cases, suppurative granulomas may develop, with burrowing sinuses, fistulae, and fibrosis.

Chancroid. Chancroid or soft chancre is a sexually transmitted disease caused by *Haemophilus ducreyi,* a gram-negative bacterium (325). The lesion is a painful, soft-based penile ulcer (fig. 10-77). Histologically, there is characteristic zonation consisting of superficial necrosis, and deposition of fibrin and leukocytes, and underlying granulation tissue bordered by plasmacytic and lymphocytic infiltrates (324).

Molluscum Contagiosum. The lesion, caused by a pox virus, is a 3 to 6 mm dome-shaped papule that often shows central umbilication and is usually on the shaft (fig. 10-78, left). Microscopic examination of hematoxylin and eosin–stained sections is diagnostic, showing the cup-shaped invagination of acanthotic epidermis into the dermis and characteristic cytoplasmic inclusions (fig. 10-78, right) (326–329).

Bacillary Angiomatosis. The penis may be involved by this lesion, usually in immunocompromised individuals such as those with AIDS. The penile manifestations, like those of the skin in general, usually take the form of red papulonodular lesions (fig. 10-79) which, particularly when the patient has AIDS, clinically resemble Kaposi's sarcoma. Microscopic examination

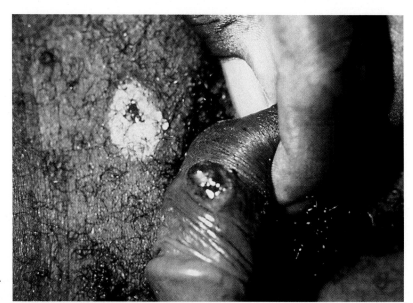

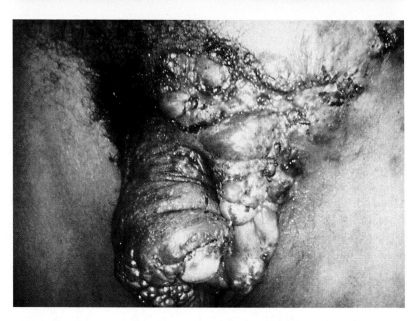

Figure 10-76
GRANULOMA INGUINALE

Top: A nummular ulcerated lesion is present in the mucocutaneous region of the foreskin. The base shows red granulation tissue. Another whitish lesion is present in the skin of the pubis.

Bottom: There is massive nodular destruction of the penis, adjacent scrotum, and lower abdominal wall in another case.

shows lobular proliferations of capillaries in an edematous stroma; there is a neutrophilic infiltrate associated with the blood vessels. Spirochetes of the *Bartonella* family can be identified by the appropriate special stains, such as Warthin-Starry (330).

Others. Potentially, a number of miscellaneous other infectious diseases could, on rare occasions, produce a clinical picture that would cause some suspicion for neoplasia, but such processes are usually correctly interpreted clinically. This has occurred in the older literature (331) in cases of tuberculosis (334). Microscopic examination, including the use of appropriate special stains, should facilitate the differential diagnosis in this situation and others (331–335).

Noninfectious Lesions

Balanitis Xerotica Obliterans. This condition affects mainly the foreskin or glans and is identical to vulvar lichen sclerosis et atrophicus (336–339). It may produce phimosis, with severe narrowing of the preputial orifice or the urethral

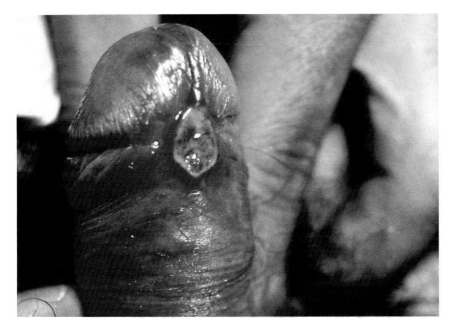

Figure 10-77
CHANCROID
A slightly raised flat disc with central ulceration is present near the frenulum.

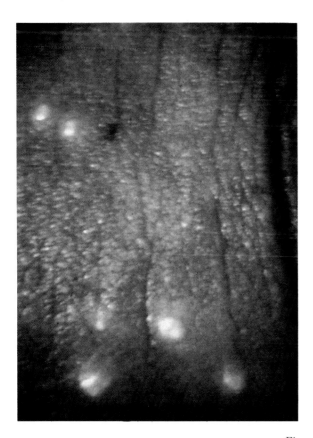

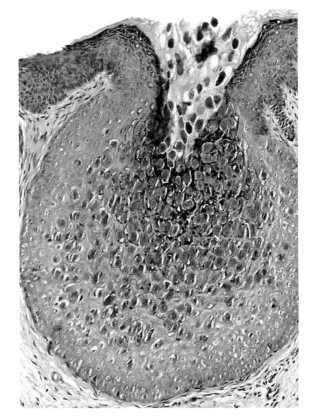

Figure 10-78
MOLLUSCUM CONTAGIOSUM

Left: Multiple lesions are present on the penile shaft of a 30-year-old drug abuser. (Courtesy of Dr. H.L. Ioachim, New York, NY.)

Right: Typical cup-shaped invagination with numerous characteristic inclusions.

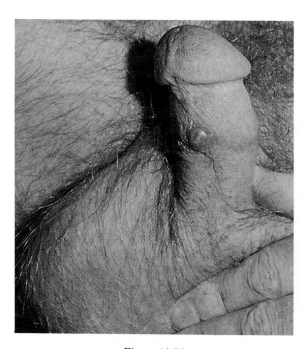

Figure 10-79
BACILLARY ANGIOMATOSIS
A smooth, pink, slightly eroded papule is present on the shaft of the penis in a patient with AIDS. (Fig. 4-20 from Fisher BK, Margesson LJ. Genital skin disorders, diagnosis and treatment. St. Louis: Mosby, 1998:32.)

meatus. In some cases the process is associated with squamous cell carcinoma. Gray-white, irregular, atrophic areas are seen in the foreskin or glans, especially around the meatus (fig. 10-80A). In more advanced cases, the mucosal folds of the foreskin disappear due to replacement of elastic fibers by fibrous tissue. Microscopically, hyperkeratosis with marked atrophy of the epithelium and vacuolization of the basal cells are seen. The characteristic finding is dense eosinophilic fibrosis in the lamina propria with an associated nonspecific lymphocytic infiltrate (fig. 10-80B,C). The lesion is superficial, measuring no more than 3 to 4 mm in depth, and usually spares the dartos muscle and the corpus spongiosum.

Peyronie's Disease. This disease affects men who are usually over 20 years of age, with a median of about 53 years (346). The patients typically complain of painful erection or "penile bending" (fig. 10-81, left). Typically, a firm area or plaque is detected on the dorsal surface of the erect penis, examination in the flaccid state usually being unremarkable. The process is often diffuse but a plaque-like lesion potentially causing

concern for a neoplasm may be present. This is an unusual variant of superficial fibromatosis in which the process affects mainly the tunica albuginea (fig. 10-82, top) (341,342). An association of Peyronie's disease and the carcinoid syndrome has been reported (340), and it also has been related to coital trauma, urethral instrumentation, use of beta blockers, hypertension, diabetes, and immune reactions. Microscopically, the appearance is similar to that of fibromatosis at other sites although it tends to be less cellular and more sclerotic than most other types of superficial fibromatosis (figs. 10-81, right, 10-82, bottom). A perivascular lymphoid infiltrate may be seen in early stage disease. Rarely, calcification or ossification occurs (fig. 10-82, bottom) (343, 345). The clinical and resultant microscopic picture of Peyronie's disease has been simulated in cases in which patients have injected themselves with pharmacological agents (344).

Verruciform Xanthoma. This process is rarely seen in the penis (347–352) and is similar to the lesion of the oral cavity; it is a warty tumor-like lesion (fig. 10-83A) characterized by acanthosis, hyperkeratosis, and parakeratosis. A distinctive feature is the presence of a prominent xanthomatous dermal infiltrate between elongated rete ridges (fig. 10-83B,C), sometimes associated additionally with neutrophils. This distinctive xanthomatous infiltrate should facilitate the diagnosis and help avoid confusion with a carcinoma, although, exceptionally, carcinomas have a similar infiltrate (see page 428). In these cases architectural and cytologic features should point towards carcinoma.

Papillomatosis of Corona (Pearly Penile Papules, Hirsutoid Papilloma). This is a very common hyperplastic condition, present in 20 to 30 percent of normal males, and has an association with marked sexual activity. The lesions are multiple, asymptomatic, pearly gray to white papillomas characteristically arranged in two to three rows on the dorsal aspect of the glans corona (fig. 10-84, left) (353–356,358). Rarely, they cover much of the glans (357). They are frequently diagnosed by peniscopy and often confused with HPV-related lesions. The diagnosis is easily established clinically by the uniformity of the lesion, the arrangement in rows, and the location on the dorsal aspect of the glans corona. We have rarely seen histologically identical, multiple small lesions on

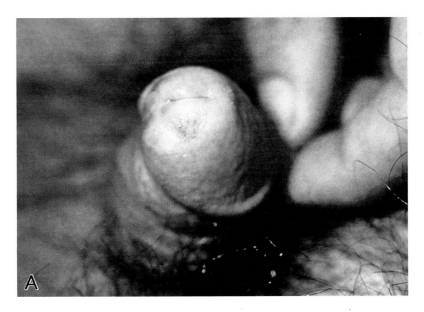

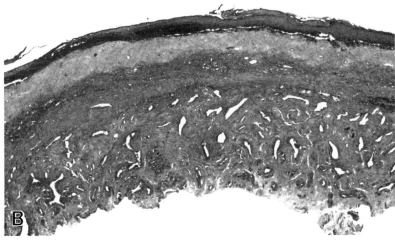

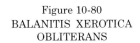

Figure 10-80
BALANITIS XEROTICA
OBLITERANS

The perimeatal glans is pearly white
(A). A band-like subepithelial zone of
dense fibrous tissue is seen. The corpus
spongiosum is uninvolved (B). The lamina propria is edematous to focally
hyalinized. Inflammatory cells are present (C). (A: Fig. 18.4 from Weiss MA,
Mills SE, eds. Atlas of genitourinary tract
disorders. Philadelphia: J. B. Lippincott
Company, 1988:18.3.)

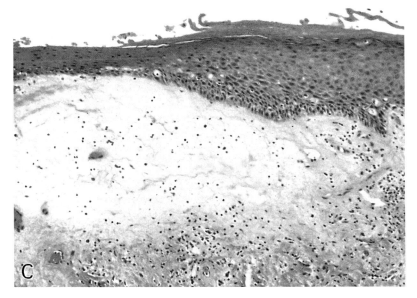

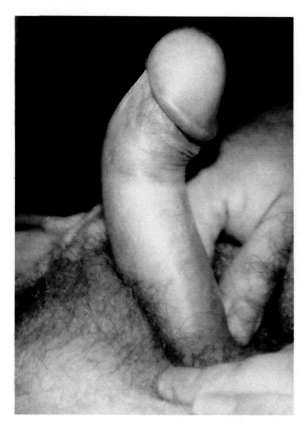
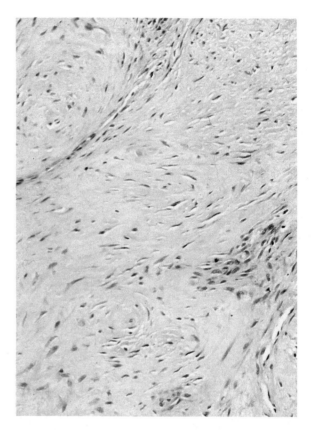

Figure 10-81
PEYRONIE'S DISEASE

Left: There is distortion of the penile contour ("penile bending"). (Fig. 13.12 from Ro JY, Amin MB, Ayala AG. Penis and scrotum. In: Bostwick DG, Eble JN, eds, Urologic surgical pathology, St. Louis: C.V. Mosby, 1997:683.)

Right: Typical microscopic features.

the foreskin. Microscopic examination shows features of an angiofibroma (fig. 10-84, right) but as noted above the lesions appear to be of hyperplastic rather than neoplastic nature.

Lipogranulomas. Foreign substances injected into the penis, such as paraffin, silicone, or wax, produce a characteristic foreign body inflammatory reaction (359–363). Of 23 cases of genital lipogranulomas in males from the AFIP the penis was involved in 10 (361). The penile lesion was solitary in 6 of the cases; in the remaining 4 there was involvement of adjacent structures, usually the scrotum. In these cases there may be marked gross abnormalities of the penis which may cause significant distortion of the organ (fig. 10-85, left) and potential confusion with a neoplasm, although in the majority of cases the picture is sufficiently unusual as to suggest the possibility of a rare non-neoplastic process; in others an appropriate

history may suggest the diagnosis. The excised tissues have no specific gross features. Occasionally cysts may be detected.

Microscopic examination shows numerous, variably sized vacuoles, some tiny, some large and cystically dilated, separated by a stroma that may be markedly sclerotic and typically contains an inflammatory cell component and foreign body giant cells (fig. 10-85, right). The cysts are devoid of an epithelial lining. Because of the marked sclerosis that is sometimes present the designation *sclerosing lipogranuloma* is often appropriate. The differential diagnosis with adenomatoid tumor, sclerosing liposarcoma, or lymphangioma may arise (361). The vacuoles are much more variable in size than those of the adenomatoid tumor and contain lipid. In contrast to the spaces of lymphangioma endothelial cells are absent from the lining of the vacuoles and cysts. The

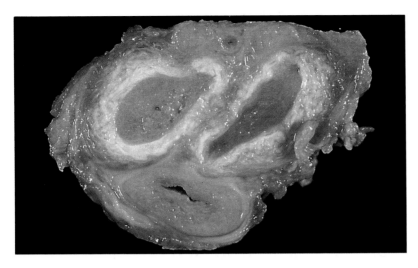

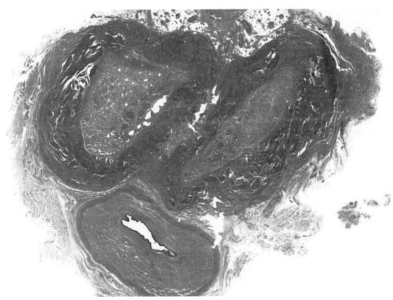

Figure 10-82
PEYRONIE'S DISEASE

Top: The tunica albuginea surrounding both corpora cavernosa is thickened. (Fig. 1B from Narita T, Kudo H, Matsumoto K. Circumferential Peyronie's disease involving both the corpora cavernosa. Pathol Int 1995;45:383–7.)

Bottom: Whole mount section showing thickened tunica albuginea with focal calcification. (Courtesy of Dr. T. Narita, Hirosaki, Japan.)

foreign body giant cells of sclerosing lipogranuloma are not seen in the other entities and, in contrast to sclerosing liposarcoma, lipoblasts are absent. There is typically a more striking inflammatory infiltrate in the lipogranuloma than in any of the neoplasms.

Tancho's Nodules. This is another factitious condition (the other being lipogranuloma) which may cause considerable clinical confusion, although less confusion is engendered for the pathologist compared to cases of lipogranuloma. This disorder, which has been primarily reported in the Far East, arises when individuals implant glass spheres in their penis with the intent of increasing stimulation of the sexual partner (364–367). Discrete penile nodules may be encountered which when incised are hard and discovered to be marble-like spheres. The foreign nature of the material is self-evident, and the pathologic differential diagnosis is less problematic than the clinical one.

Melanosis-Lentiginosis. Penile melanosis is usually a large, often single, flat, pigmented macule with irregular borders (fig. 10-86, left) (368,369). Microscopic examination discloses variable melanocytic hyperplasia with prominent hyperpigmentation of the basal layers of a normal epidermis (fig. 10-86, right).

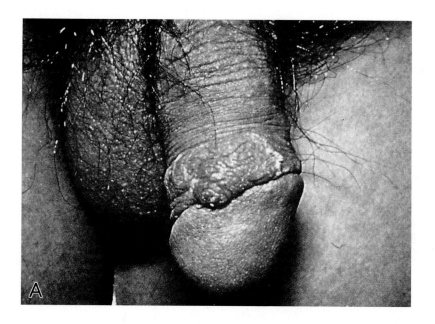

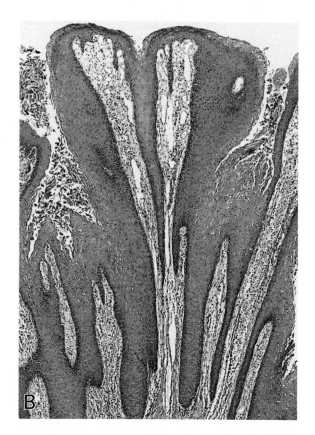

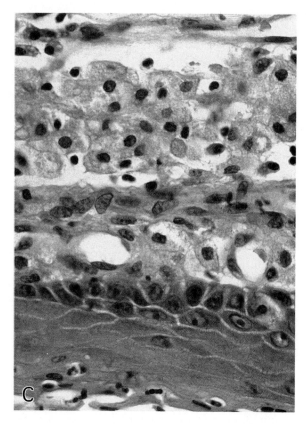

Figure 10-83
VERRUCIFORM XANTHOMA

A granular, elevated, tan-white mass involves the distal shaft and the coronal sulcus (A). (Fig. 1 from Kraemer BB, Schmidt WA, Foucar E, Rosen T. Verruciform xanthoma of the penis. Arch Dermatol 1981;117:516-8.) Microscopic examination shows papillary epithelial hyperplasia (B) and stromal histiocytes with foamy cytoplasm in the papillary cores (B and C).

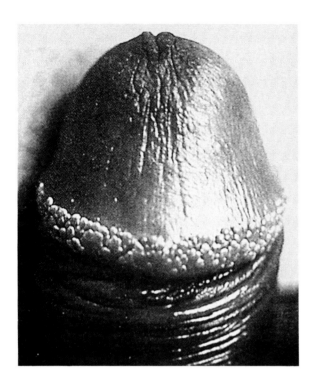
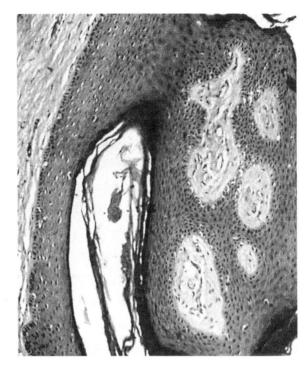

Figure 10-84

PAPILLOMATOSIS OF CORONA

Regular rows of small papules form a ring around the corona (left). (Fig. 7-35A from Hasmat AI, Das S. The penis. Baltimore: Waverly Press, 1993:94). Microscopic examination shows benign epithelial hyperplasia with a vascular, fibrous stroma (right).

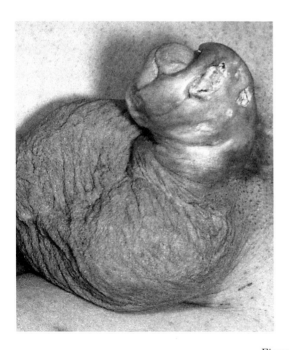
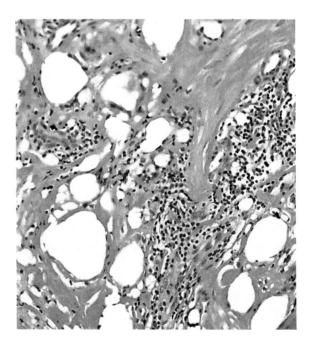

Figure 10-85

LIPOGRANULOMA

There is marked deformity of the penis (left). Characteristic vacuoles, sclerotic stroma, and occasional foreign body giant cells are seen on microscopic examination (right).

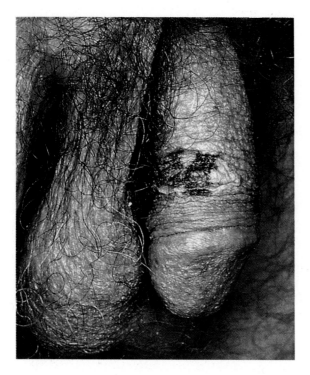
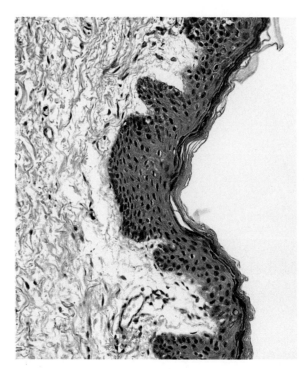

Figure 10-86
MELANOSIS
Left: An irregular darkly pigmented patch is present on the skin of the shaft. (Fig. 8.3 from Fisher BK, Margesson LJ. Genital skin disorders, diagnosis and treatment. St. Louis: Mosby, 1998:73.)
Right: Hyperpigmentation of the basal cell layer is seen on microscopic examination from another case. There is focal elongation of the rete pegs.

Penile lentigines are small, 2 to 3 mm, oval, uniformly hyperpigmented, macular lesions scattered on the shaft, glans, or both. Microscopically, they show elongate rete with benign melanocytic hyperplasia and hyperpigmentation.

Fournier's Gangrene and Corbus' Disease. Fournier's gangrene is characterized by necrotizing fasciitis centered on the male genital region but may extend to involve adjacent skin of the anterior abdomen. The disease may be idiopathic or associated with various conditions including debilitating diseases and HIV infection (370–377). The disease is usually more striking in the scrotum, but involvement of the penis may also be seen, the latter manifestation sometimes being referred to as Corbus' disease (balanitis gangrenosa, necrotizing balanitis) (fig. 10-87). The necrotizing nature of the process is usually evident clinically, and confusion with a neoplasm is not an issue on microscopic examination.

Wegener's Granulomatosis. Rare cases of Wegener's granulomatosis affecting the penis or distal urethra have been reported. Typical features include granulomatous inflammation, tissue necrosis, and vasculitis (378–382,385). Massive destruction of the penis may result (fig. 10-88), and the gross appearance of a carcinoma may be simulated, with resultant inappropriate treatment (381). The penis is rarely involved in other rare conditions in which vasculitis is present (383,384), and exceptionally, nodular lesions have been described (383).

Os Penis. Most mammals have penile bones (priapi or bacula), except for chimpanzees and humans. Ossification of the human penis is a rare acquired phenomenon produced by metaplasia, usually associated with an underlying condition such as trauma, Peyronie's disease, diabetes, gout, venereal disease, or neoplasia (387–390). It is usually seen in the elderly, but a case of congenital os penis has been described (386).

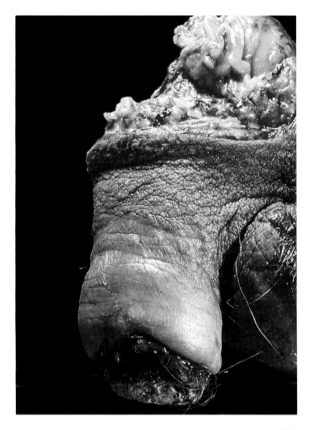 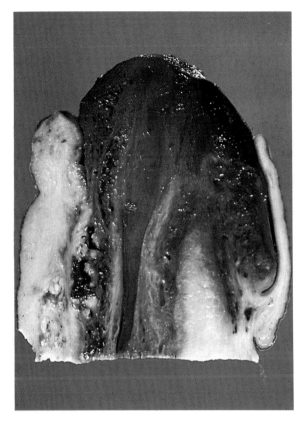

Figure 10-87
FOURNIER'S GANGRENE (BALANITIS GANGRENOSA, CORBUS' DISEASE)
There is complete necrosis of the glans with preservation of the foreskin and skin of the shaft (left). Cut surface of the glans shows massive necrosis of the glans and urethra (right). Note the hemorrhage in Buck's fascia consistent with spread of the process via the fascia. The foreskin is uninvolved.

Miscellaneous Other Rare Tumor-Like Lesions

Granulomatous diseases other than those already considered rarely may involve the penis (411). These include sarcoidosis and Crohn's disease (392–394,397,402,404,408,409); at least one patient with sarcoid was initially thought to have a malignant lesion on clinical evaluation (406). In a case of necrobiosis lipoidica consideration was apparently given to the diagnosis of epithelioid sarcoma (396). Cases of juvenile xanthogranuloma with penile involvement are documented (399), and a young boy with a painless nodule on the glans had a process interpreted microscopically as an angiocentric myofibroblastic tumor of questionable neoplastic or reactive nature (407). A case of primary amyloidosis with a mass on the penile shaft is documented

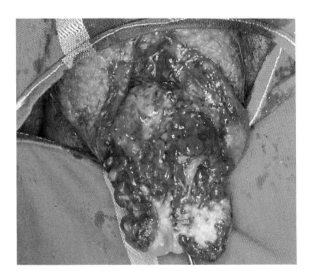

Figure 10-88
WEGENER'S GRANULOMATOSIS
The penis is replaced by an ulcerating destructive process with partial involvement of the scrotal skin. (Courtesy of Dr. R. Piazza, Padova, Italy.)

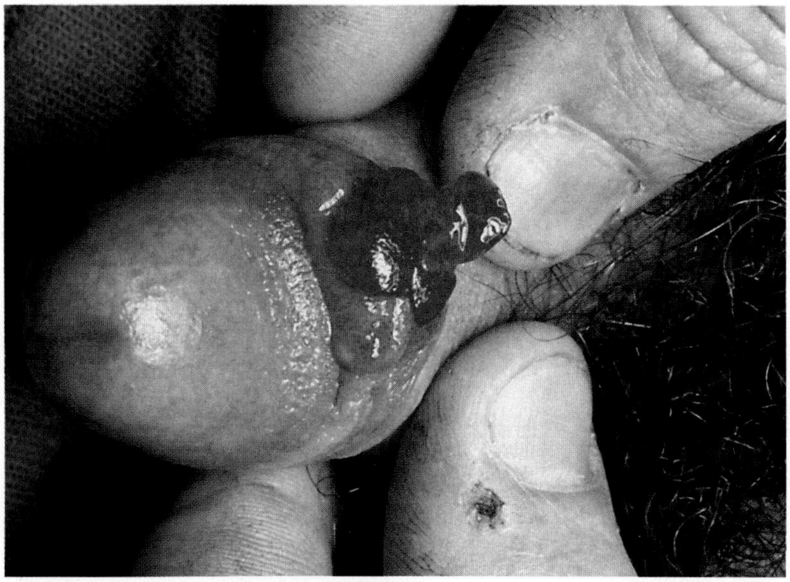

Figure 10-89
PYOGENIC GRANULOMA
A strawberry colored, lobulated polypoid mass involves a portion of the coronal sulcus. (Courtesy of Dr. M. Walzman, Coventry, United Kingdom.)

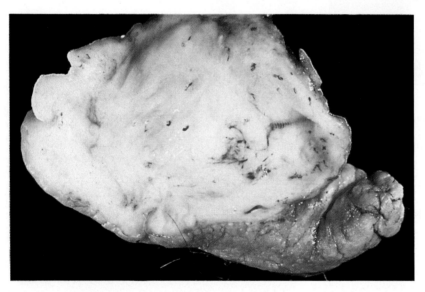

Figure 10-90
INFLAMMATORY
PSEUDOTUMOR
The dorsal aspect of the penis is replaced by a 5 cm, tan-pink, slightly lobulated mass with a fish-flesh consistency. Microscopic examination showed sparsely cellular dense collagen with scattered chronic inflammatory cells and rare foreign body type granulomas. (Fig. 1 from Nielsen GP, Rosenberg AE, Dretler SP, Young RH. An unusual pseudotumor of the penis. J Urol Pathol 1996;4:79–84.)

(400). Vascular lesions of the penis other than those considered already are exceptionally rare. One case of pyogenic granuloma produced a striking gross abnormality (fig. 10-89) (410). One case of intravascular papillary endothelial hyperplasia of the penis is documented (395). Occasionally, lymphangitis of the penis, usually involving the shaft, can form a gross abnormality; although the cord-like nature of the lesion usually does not lend itself to misdiagnosis as a neoplasm (398,401), rarely, consideration is given to such a diagnosis (391). Preputial seba-

ceous glands have mimicked molluscum contagiosum (405). Finally, one unusual case has been reported in which a man who had been on chronic "condom" catheterization developed a 5 cm, tan-pink, lobulated solid mass on the dorsal aspect of the penis (fig. 10-90) (403). Microscopic examination showed paucicellular dense collagen with scattered chronic inflammatory cells and rare foreign body granulomas that had replaced the corpus cavernosum. This lesion was interpreted as due to longstanding chronic irritation and a variant of inflammatory pseudotumor.

REFERENCES

Anatomy and Histology

1. Barreto J, Caballero C, Cubilla AL. Penis. In: Sternberg SS, ed. Histology for pathologists, 2nd. ed. Philadelphia: Lippincott-Raven, 1997:1039–50.
2. Bloom W, Fawcett DW. A textbook of histology. 11th ed. Philadelphia: WB Saunders, 1991:802.
3. Cabañas RM. Anatomy and biopsy of sentinel lymph nodes. Urol Clin North Am 1992;19:267–76.
4. Crawford ED, Daneshgari F. Management of regional lymph drainage in carcinoma of the penis. Urol Clin North Am 1992;19:305–17.
5. Hricak H, Marotti M, Gilbert TJ, et al. Normal penile anatomy and abnormal penile conditions: evaluation with MR imaging. Radiology 1988;169:683–90.
6. Hyman AB, Brownstein MH. Tyson's "glands." Ectopic sebaceous glands and papillomatous penis. Arch Derm 1969;99:31–6.
7. Maximow AA, Bloom W. The penis. In: A textbook of histology, 3rd ed. Philadelphia: WB Saunders Co, 1941:519–23.
8. Rouviere H. Anatomy of the human lymphatic system. Edwards Broders, ed. Ann Arbor, 1938.
9. Testut L, Latarjert A. Tratado de Anatomia Humana. Salvat eds. Barcelona, 1979.
10. Wynder EL. Some epidemiological observations on cancer of the penis. Revista del Instituto Nacional de Cancerología 1964;15:273–85.

Epithelial Abnormalities and Precancerous Squamous Lesions
(Including Penile Horn, Micaceous Balanitis, and Bowenoid Papulosis)

11. Andersson L, Jonsson G, Brehmer-Andersson E. Erythroplasia of Queyrat-carcinoma in situ. Scand J Urol Nephrol 1967;1:303–6.
12. Aynaud O, Ionesco M, Barrasso R. Penile intraepithelial neoplasia. Specific clinical features correlate with histologic and virologic findings. Cancer 1994;74:1762–7.
13. Beljaards RC, Van Dijk E, Hausman R. Is pseudoepitheliomatous, micaceous and keratotic balanitis synonymous with verrucous carcinoma? Br J Dermatol 1987;117:641–6.
14. DeVillez RL, Stevens CS. Bowenoid papules of genitalia. A case progressing to Bowen's disease. J Am Acad Dermatol 1980;3:149–52.
15. Eisen RF, Bhawan J, Cahn TH. Spontaneous regression of bowenoid papulosis of the penis. Cutis 1983;32:269–72.
15a. Ganem JP, Steele BW, Creager AJ, Carson CC. Pseudoepitheliomatous keratotic and micaceous balanitis. J Urol 1999;161:217–8.
16. Gimeno E, Vilata JJ, Sanchez JL, Lloret A, Fortea JM. Bowenoid papulosis: clinical and histological study of eight cases. Geniturin Med 1987;63:109–13.
17. Goldstein HH. Cutaneous horns of the penis. J Urol 1933;30:367–74.
18. Graham JH, Helwig EB. Erythroplasia of Queyrat. A clinicopathologic and histochemical study. Cancer 1973;32:1396–414.
19. Gray MR, Ansell ID. Pseudo-epitheliomatous hyperkeratotic and micaceous balanitis: evidence for regarding it as pre-malignant. Br J Urol 1990;66:103–4.
20. Grossman B. Premalignant and early carcinomas of the penis and scrotum. Urol Clin North Am 1992;19:221–6.
21. Haneke E. Skin diseases and tumors of the penis. Urol Int 1982;37:172–82.
22. Hassan AA, Orteza AM, Milam DF. Penile horn: review of literature with 3 case reports. J Urol 1967;97:315–7.
23. Hurwitz RM, Egan WT, Murphy SH, Pontius EE, Forster ML. Bowenoid papulosis and squamous cell carcinoma of the genitalia: suspected sexual transmission. Cutis 1987;39:193–6.
24. Ikenberg H, Gissmann L, Gross G, Grussendorf-Conen EI, Zur-Hausen H. Human papillomavirus type-16-related DNA in genital Bowen's disease and in Bowenoid papulosis. Int J Cancer 1983;32:563–5.
25. Irvine C, Anderson JR, Pye RJ. Micaceous and keratotic pseudoepitheliomatous balanitis and rapidly fatal fibrosarcoma of the penis occurring in the same patient. Br J Dermatol 1987;116:719–25.
26. Jenkins D Jr, Jakubovic HR. Pseudoepitheliomatous, keratotic, micaceous balanitis. A clinical lesion with two histologic subsets: hyperplastic dystrophy and verrucous carcinoma. J Am Acad Dermatol 1988;18:419–22.
27. Katz HI, Posalaky Z, McGinley D. Pigmented penile papules with carcinoma in situ changes. Br J Dermatol 1978;99:155–62.
28. Kaye V, Zhang G. Dehner LP, Fraley EE. Carcinoma in situ of penis. Is distinction between erythroplasia of Queyrat and Bowen's disease relevant? Urology 1990;36:479–82.
29. Krunic AL, Djerdj K, Starcevic-Bozovic A, et al. Pseudoepitheliomatous, keratotic and micaceous balanitis. Case report and review of the literature. Urol Int 1996;56:125–8.
30. Kurman RJ, Norris HJ, Wilkinson E. Tumors of the cervix, vagina and vulva. Atlas of Tumor Pathology, 3rd Series. Fascicle 4. Washington D.C.: Armed Forces Institute of Pathology 1992:202–3.
31. Lucia MS, Miller GJ. Histopathology of malignant lesions of the penis. Urol Clin North Am 1992;19:227–46.
31a. Murphy GF, Elder DE. Non-melanocytic tumors of the skin. Atlas of Tumor Pathology, 2nd Series, Fascicle 1. Washington D.C.: Armed Forces Institute of Pathology, 1991.
32. Obalek S, Jablonska S, Beadenon S, Walczak L, Orth G. Bowenoid papulosis of the male and female genitalia: risk of cervical neoplasia. J Am Dermatol 1986;14:433–44.
33. Patterson JW, Kao GF, Graham JH, Helwig EB. Bowenoid papulosis. A clinicopathologic study with ultrastructural observations. Cancer 1986;57:823–36.
34. Peters MS, Perry HO. Bowenoid papules of the penis. J Urol 1981;126:482–4.
35. Queyrat L. Erythroplasie du gland. Bull Soc Franc Dermatol Syph 1911;22:378–82.
36. Raghavaiah NV, Soloway MS, Murphy WM. Malignant penile horn. J Urol 1977;118:1068–9.
37. Su CK, Shipley WU. Bowenoid papulosis: a benign lesion of the shaft of the penis misdiagnosed as squamous carcinoma. J Urol 1997;157:1361–2.
38. Taylor DR, South DA. Bowenoid papulosis: a review. Cutis 1981;27:92–8.

39. Wade TR, Kopf AW, Ackerman AB. Bowenoid papulosis of the genitalia. Arch Dermatol 1979;115:306–8.

40. Wade TR, Kopf AW, Ackerman AB. Bowenoid papulosis of the penis. Cancer 1978;42:1890–903.

Squamous Cell Carcinoma and Its Variants

41. Adeyoju AB, Thornhill J, Corr J, Grainger R, McDermott TE, Butler M. Prognostic factors in squamous cell carcinoma of the penis and implications for management. Br J Urol 1997;80:937–9.

42. Bain L, Geronemu S. The association of lichen planus of the penis with squamous cell carcinoma in situ and with verrucous squamous carcinoma. J Dermatol Surg Oncol 1989;15:413–7.

43. Barney JD, Gall EA. Unusual tumor of penis: case report. J Urol 1939;42:623–8.

44. Barraso R, De Brux J, Croissant O, Orth G. High prevalence of papilloma virus associated penile intraepithelial neoplasia in sexual partners of women with cervical intraepithelial neoplasia. N Engl J Med 1987;317:916–23.

45. Bart RS, Kopft AW. Squamous cell carcinoma arising in balanitis xerotica obliterans. J Dermatol Surg Oncol 1978;4:556–8.

46. Bassett JW. Carcinoma of the penis. Cancer 1952;5:530–8.

47. Bissada NK, Morcos RR, El-Senoussi M. Post-circumcision carcinoma of the penis. I. Clinical aspects. J Urol 1986;135:283–5.

48. Boon ME, Schneider A, Hogewoning CJ, Van der Kwast TH, Bolhuis P, Kok LP. Penile studies and heterosexual partners. Peniscopy, cytology, histology and immunocytochemistry. Cancer 1988;61:1652–9.

49. Boon ME, Susanti I, Torsche MJ, Kok LP. Human papilloma virus (HPV) associated male and female genital carcinomas in a Hindu population. The male as vector and victim. Cancer 1989;64:559–65.

50. Brinton LA, Yao LJ, Shou-de R, et al. Risk factors for penile cancer: results from a case control study in China. Int J Cancer 1991;47:504–9.

51. Buddington WT, Kickham CJ, Smith WE. As assessment of malignant disease of the penis. J Urol 1963;89:442–9.

52. Caballero C, Cubilla AL, Barreto J, Riveros M. Factores patológicos relacionados con metastasis inguinal en carcinoma epidermoide del glande peneal. Patología (Spain) 1991;24:1137–41.

53. Cabañas RM. An approach for the treatment of penile carcinoma. Cancer 1977;39:456–66.

54. Campion MJ, McCance DJ, Mitchell HS, Jenkins D, Singer A. Subclinical penile human papillomavirus infection and dysplasia in consorts of women with cervical neoplasia. Genitourin Med 1988;64:90–9.

55. Cubilla AL, Ayala MT, Barreto JE, Bellasai JG, Nöel JC. Surface adenosquamous carcinoma of the penis. A report of three cases. Am J Surg Pathol 1996;20:156–60.

56. Cubilla AL, Barreto JE, Caballero C, Ayala G, Riveros M. Pathologic features of epidermoid carcinomas of the penis. A prospective study of 66 cases. Am J Surg Pathol 1993;17:753–63.

57. Cubilla AL, Bray C, Barreto J, Caballero C. Carcinoma epidermoide del prepucio. Estudio clinico-patológico de 40 casos. Anales de la Facultad de Ciencias Médicas. Asunción 1992; XXIV(Nos.1–2):187–208.

57a.Cubilla AL, Philip AT, Amin MB, et al. Cytokeratin subset distribution in histologic variants of squamous cell carcinoma of the penis. Mod Pathol 1999;12:92A.

58. Cubilla AL, Reuter V, Ayala G, Ocampos S, Fair W. Basaloid squamous cell carcinoma of the penis: a distinctive human papilloma virus-related penile neoplasm. Am J Surg Pathol 1998;22:755–61.

59. Cubilla AL, Velazquez EF, Reuter VE, Oliva E, Mihm MC Jr, Young RH. Warty (condylomatous) squamous cell carcinoma of the penis. A report of 11 cases and proposed classification of "verruciform" penile tumors. Am J Surg Pathol 2000;24:505-12.

60. Cupp MR, Malek RS, Goellner JR, Smith TF, Espy MJ. The detection of human papillomavirus deoxyribonucleic acid in intraepithelial, in situ, verrucous and invasive carcinoma of the penis. J Urol 1995;154:1024–9.

61. Davies SW. Giant condyloma acuminata: incidence among cases diagnosed as carcinoma of the penis. J Clin Pathol 1965;18:142–9.

62. Dawson DF, Duckworth JK, Bernhardt H, Young JM. Giant condyloma and verrucous carcinoma of the genital area. Arch Pathol 1965;79:225–31.

63. Dean AL Jr. Epithelioma of the penis. J Urol 1935;33:252–83.

64. Derrick FC Jr, Lynch KM, Kretkowski C, Yarbrough WJ. Epidermoid carcinoma of the penis: computer analysis of 87 cases. J Urol 1973;110:303–5.

65. Dodge OG, Linsell CA. Carcinoma of the penis in Ugandan and Kenyan Africans. Cancer 1963;16:1255–63.

66. Ekstrom T, Edsmyr F. Cancer of the penis. A clinical study of 229 cases. Acta Chir Scand 1958;115:25–45.

67. Fraley EE, Zhang G, Manivel C, Niehans GA. The role of ilioinguinal lymphadenectomy and significance of histological differentiation in the treatment of carcinoma of the penis. J Urol 1989;142:1478–82.

68. Franco EL, Filho NC, Villa LL, et al. Correlation patterns of cancer relative frequencies with some socioeconomic and demographic indicators in Brazil: an ecologic study. Int J Cancer 1988;41:24–9.

68a.Fukunaga M, Yokoi K, Miyazawa Y, Harada T, Ushigome S. Penile verrucous carcinoma with anaplastic transformation following radiotherapy. A case report with human papillomavirus typing and flow cytometric DNA studies. Am J Surg Pathol 1994;18:501–5.

69. Galanis E, Frytak S, Lloyd RV. Extrapulmonary small cell carcinoma. Cancer 1997;79:1729–36.

70. Goldstein AM, Reynolds WF, Terry R. Diagnostic problems of epithelial tumor of penis. Urology 1977;9:79–82.

71. Graham S, Priore R, Graham M, Browne R, Burnett W, West D. Genital cancer in wives of penile cancer patients. Cancer 1979;44:1870–4.

72. Gregoire L, Cubilla AL, Reuter VE, Haas G, Lancaster WD. Preferential association of virus with high grade histologic variants of penile-invasive squamous cell carcinoma. JNCI 1995;87:1705–9.

73. Hanash KA, Furlow WL, Utz DC, Harrison EG Jr. Carcinoma of the penis: a clinicopathologic study. J Urol 1970;104:291–7.

74. Hardner GJ, Bhanalaph T, Murphy GP, Albert DJ, Moore RH. Carcinoma of the penis: analysis of therapy in 100 consecutive cases. J Urol 1972;108:428–30.

75. Harish K, Ravi R. The role of tobacco in penile carcinoma. Br J Urol 1995;75:375–7.

76. Hayashi T, Tsuda N, Shimada O, et al. A clinicopathologic study of tumors and tumor-like lesions of the penis. Acta Pathol Jpn 1990;40:343–51.

77. Hellberg D, Nilsson S. Genital cancer among wives of men with penile cancer. A study between 1958–1982. Br J Obstet Gynaecol 1989;96:221–5.

78. Hellberg D, Valentin J, Eklund T, Nilsson S. Penile cancer: is there an epidemiological role for smoking and sexual behaviour? Br Med J 1987;295:1306–8.

79. Heyns CF, van Vollenhoven P, Steenkamp JW, Allen FJ. Cancer of the penis—a review of 50 patients. S Afr J Surg 1997;35:120–4.

80. Heyns CF, van Vollenhoven P, Steenkamp JW, Allen FJ, van Velden DJ. Carcinoma of the penis—appraisal of a modified tumour-staging system. Br J Urol 1997;80:307–12.

81. Hippellainen M, Ylykoski M, Saarikiske S, Syrjanen S, Syrjanen K. Genital human papillomavirus lesions of the male sexual partners: the diagnostic accuracy of peniscopy. Genitourin Med 1991;67:291–6.

82. Hoppmann HJ, Fraley EE. Squamous cell carcinoma of the penis. J Urol 1978;120:393–8.

83. Horenblas S, Van Tinteren H. Squamous cell carcinoma of the penis. IV. Prognostic factors of survival: analysis of tumor, nodes and metastasis classification system. J Urol 1994;151:1239–43.

84. Horenblas S, Van Tinteren H, Delemarre JF, Moonen LM, Lustig V, Kröger R. Squamous cell carcinoma of the penis: accuracy of tumor, nodes and metastasis classification system, and role of lymphangiography, computerized tomography scan and fine needle aspiration cytology. J Urol 1991;146:1279–83.

85. Horenblas S, Van Tinteren H, Delmarre JF, Moonen LM, Lustig V, van Waardenberg EW. Squamous cell carcinoma of the penis. III. Treatment of regional nodes. J Urol 1993;149:492–7.

86. Hubbell CR, Rabin VR, Mora RG. Cancer of the skin in blacks. V. A review of 175 black patients with squamous cell carcinoma of the penis. J Am Acad Dermatol 1988;18:292–8.

87. Iversen T, Tretli S, Johansen A, Holte T. Squamous cell carcinoma of the penis and of the cervix, vulva and vagina in spouses: is there any relationship? An epidemiological study from Norway, 1960–1992. Br J Cancer 1997;76:658–60.

88. Iwasawa A, Kumamoto Y, Fujinaga K. Detection of human papillomavirus deoxyribonucleic acid in penile carcinoma by polymerase chain reaction and in situ hybridization. J Urol 1993;149:59–63.

89. Jackson SM. The treatment of carcinoma of the penis. Br J Surg 1966;53:33–5.

90. Jamieson NV, Bullock KN, Barker TH. Adenosquamous carcinoma of the penis associated with balanitis xerotica obliterans. Br J Urol 1986;58A:730–1.

91. Johnson DE, Lo RK, Srigley J, Ayala AG. Verrucous carcinoma of the penis. J Urol 1985;133:216–8.

92. Jones WG, Fossa SD. Hamers H, VanDen Bogaert W. Penis cancer: a review by the Joint Radiotherapy Committee of the European Organization for Research and Treatment of Cancer (EORTC) Genitourinary and Radiotherapy Groups. J Surg Oncol 1989;40:227–31.

93. Kamat MR, Kulkarni JN, Tongaonkar HB. Carcinoma of the penis: the Indian experience. J Surg Oncol 1993;52:50–5.

94. Kovi J, Tillman RL, Lee SM. Malignant transformation of condyloma acuminatum. Am J Clin Pathol 1974;61:702–10.

95. Kraus FT, Perez-Mesa C. Verrucous carcinoma: clinical and pathologic study of 105 cases involving oral cavity, larynx and genitalia. Cancer 1966;19:26–38.

96. Lenowitz H, Graham AP. Carcinoma of the penis. J Urol 1946;56:458–84.

97. Maden C, Sherman KJ, Beckman AM, et al. History of circumcision, medical conditions and sexual activity and risk of penile cancer. JNCI 1993;85:19–24.

98. Maiche AG, Pyrhonen S. Risk of cervical cancer among wives of men with carcinoma of the penis. Acta Oncol 1990;29:569–71.

99. Maiche AG, Pyrhonen S. Verrucous carcinoma of the penis: three cases treated with interferon–alpha. Br J Urol 1997;79:481–3.

100. Maiche AG, Pyrhonen S, Karkinen M. Histological grading of squamous cell carcinoma of the penis: a new scoring system. Br J Urol 1991;67:522–6.

101. Manglani KS, Manaligod JR, Ray B. Spindle cell carcinoma of the glans penis: a light and electron microscopic study. Cancer 1980;46:2267–72.

102. Martinez I. Relationship of squamous cell carcinoma of the cervix uteri to squamous cell carcinoma of the penis among Puerto Rican women married to men with penile carcinoma. Cancer 1969;24:777–80.

103. Masera A, Ovcak Z, Volavsek M, Bracko M. Adenosquamous carcinoma of the penis. J Urol 1997; 157:2261.

104. Masih AS, Stoler MH, Farrow GM, Wooldridge TN, Johansson SL. Penile verrucous carcinoma: a clinicopathologic human papillomavirus typing and flow cytometric analysis. Mod Path 1992;5:48–55.

105. McCance DJ, Kalache A, Ashdown K, et al. Human papillomavirus types 16 and 18 in carcinoma of the penis from Brazil. Int J Cancer 1986;37:55–9.

106. McDougal WS. Carcinoma of the penis: improved survival by early regional lymphadenectomy based on the histologic grade and depth of invasion of the primary lesion. J Urol 1995;154:1364–6.

107. McDougal WS, Kirchner FK Jr, Edwards RH, Killion LT. Treatment of carcinoma of the penis: the case for primary lymphadenectomy. J Urol 1986;136:38–41.

108. McKee PH, Lowe D, Haigh J. Penile verrucous carcinoma. Histopathology 1983;7:897–906.

109. Melicow MM, Ganem EJ. Cancerous and precancerous lesions of the penis: a clinical and pathological study based on twenty-three cases. J Urol 1946;55:486–514.

110. Merrin CE. Cancer of the penis. Cancer 1980;45:1973–9.

111. Micali G, Innocenzi D, Nasca MR, Musumeci ML, Ferrati F, Greco M. Squamous cell carcinoma of the penis. J Am Acad Dermatol 1996;35:432–51.

112. Morgan C Jr. Bone formation in the penis associated with neoplasm. J Urol 1966;96:229–34.

113. Morinaga S, Nakamura S, Moro K, Moteki K. Carcinosarcoma (carcinoma with sarcomatous metaplasia) of the penis. J Urol Pathol 1995;3:369–76.

114. Narayana AS, Olney LE, Loening SA, Weimar GW, Culp DA. Carcinoma of the penis: analysis of 219 cases. Cancer 1982;49:2185–91.

115. Nöel JC, Vanderbossche M, Peny MO, et al. Verrucous carcinoma of the penis: importance of human papillomavirus typing for diagnosis and therapeutic decision. Eur Urol 1992;22:83–5.

116. Oota K. Cancer of the penis in Japan. Rev Inst Nac Cancer 1964;15:289–92.

117. Oppenheim AR. Sebaceous carcinoma of the penis. Arch Dermatol 1981;117:306–7.

118. Ornellas AA, Seixas AL, de Moraes JR. Analyses of 200 lymphadenectomies in patients with penile carcinoma. J Urol 1991;146:330–2.

119. Ornellas AA, Seixas AL, Marota A, Wisnescky A, Campos F, deMoraes JR. Surgical treatment of invasive squamous cell carcinoma of the penis: retrospective analysis of 350 cases. J Urol 1994;151:1244–9.

120. Persky L. Epidemiology of cancer of the penis. Recent results. Cancer Res 1977;60:97–109.

121. Pizzocaro G, Piva L, Bandieramonte G, Tana S. Up-to-date management of carcinoma of the penis. Eur Urol 1997;32:5–15.

121a. Poblet E, Alfaro L, Fernander-Segoviano P, Jimenez-Reyes J, Salido EC. Human papillomavirus-associated penile squamous cell carcinoma in HIV-positive patients. Am J Surg Pathol 1999;23:1119–23.

122. Pride HB, Miller F III, Tyler WB. Penile squamous cell carcinoma arising from balanitis xerotica obliterans. J Am Acad Dermatol 1993;29:469–73.

123. Raney AM, Jhavari DD. Familial carcinoma of the penis. N Y State J Med 1981;81:1786–8.

124. Rathigan RM, Jimenez S, Chopskie EJ. Condyloma acuminatum and carcinoma of the penis. South Med J 1972;65:423–8.

125. Ravi R. Radiation-induced carcinoma of the penis. Urol Int 1995;54:147–9.

126. Reddy CR, Devendranath V, Pratap S. Carcinoma of penis—role of phimosis. Urology 1984;24:85–8.

127. Riveros M, Lebron RF. Geographical pathology of cancer of the penis. Cancer 1963;16:798–811.

128. Robertson DI, Maung R, Duggan MA. Verrucous carcinoma of the genital tract: is it a distinct entity? Can J Surg 1993;36:147–51.

129. Ross BS, Levine VJ, Dixon C, Ashinoff R. Squamous cell carcinoma of the penis in a circumcised man: a case for dermatology and urology, and review of the literature. Cutis 1998;61:41–3.

130. Rubio-Briones J, Villavicencio H, Regalado R, et al. Squamous cell carcinoma of the penis: treatment protocol according to our 14 years of experience. Archivos Españoles de Urologia 1997;50:473–80.

131. Sarin R, Norman AR, Steel GG, Horwich A. Treatment results and prognostic factors in 101 men treated for squamous carcinoma of the penis. Int J Radiation Oncol Biol Phys 1997;38:713–22.

132. Sarkar FH, Miles BJ, Plieth DH, Crissman JD. Detection of human papillomavirus in squamous neoplasms of the penis. J Urol 1992;147:389–92.

133. Schmauz R, Findlay M, Lalwak A, Katsumbira N, Buxton E. Variation in the appearance of giant condyloma in an Ugandan series of cases of carcinoma of the penis. Cancer 1977;40:1686–96.

134. Schrek R, Lenowitz H. Etiologic factors in carcinoma of the penis. Cancer Research 1947;7:180–7.

135. Schwartz RA. Buschke-Lowenstein tumor: verrucous carcinoma of the penis. J Am Acad Dermatol 1990;23:723–7.

136. Seixas AL, Ornellas AA, Marota A, Wisnescky A, Campos F, de Moraes JR. Verrucous carcinoma of the penis: retrospective analysis of 32 cases. J Urol 1994;152:1476–8.

137. Soria JC, Fizazi K, Piron D, et al. Squamous cell carcinoma of the penis: multivariate analysis of prognostic factors and natural history in a monocentric study with a conservative policy. Ann Oncol 1997;8:1089–98.

138. Srinivas V, Morse MJ, Herr JW, Sogani PC, Whitmore WF Jr. Penile cancer: relation of extent of nodal metastasis to survival. J Urol 1987;137:880–2.

139. Staubitz WJ, Lent MH, Oberkircher OJ. Carcinoma of the penis. Cancer 1955;8:371–8.

140. Stern RS. Genital tumors among men with psoriasis exposed to psoralens and ultraviolet A radiation (PUVA) and ultraviolet B radiation. The photochemotherapy follow up study. N Engl J Med 1990;322:1149–51.

141. Takiwaki H, Yokota M, Ahsan K, Yokota K, Kurokawa Y, Ogawa I. Squamous cell carcinoma associated with verruciform xanthomas of the penis. Am J Dermatol Pathol 1996;18:551–4.

142. Theodorescu D, Russo P, Zhang SF, Morash C, Fair WR. Outcomes of initial surveillance of invasive squamous cell carcinoma of the penis and negative nodes. J Urol 1996;155:1626–31.

143. Tomic S, Warner TF, Messing E, Wilding G. Penile Merkel cell carcinoma. Urology 1995;45:1062–5.

144. Van Savage JG, Carson CC. Primary adenocarcinoma of the penis. J Urol 1994;152:1555–6.

145. Varma VA, Sanchez-Lanier M, Unger ER, et al. Association of human papillomavirus with penile carcinoma: a study using polymerase chain reaction and in situ hybridization. Hum Pathol 1991;22:908–13.

146. Videtic GM, Ago CT, Winquist EW. Hypercalcemia and carcinoma of the penis. Med Pediatr Oncol 1997;29:576–7.

147. Villa LL, Lopes A. Human papillomavirus DNA sequences in penile carcinomas in Brazil. Int J Cancer 1986;37:853–5.

148. Watanabe K, Mukawa A, Miyazaki K, Tsukahara K. Adenoid squamous cell carcinoma of the penis. Report of a surgical case clinically manifested with rapid lung metastasis. Acta Pathol Jpn 1983;33:1243–50.

149. Weaver MG, Abdul Karin FW, Dale G, Sorensen K, Huang YT. Detection and localization of human papillomavirus in penile condylomas and squamous cell carcinomas using in situ hybridization with biotinylated DNA viral probes. Mod Pathol 1989;2:94–100.

150. Wood EW, Gardner WA, Brown FM. Spindle cell squamous carcinoma of the penis. J Urol 1972;107:990–1.

151. Yoganathan K, Patel RN, Maitland N, McManus TJ, Calman FM, Pozniak A. Carcinoma of the penis in a HIV positive patient. Genitourin Med 1995;71:41–2.

Prognostic Factors

152. Caballero C, Cubilla AL, Barreto J, Riveros M. Factores patológicos relacionados con metastasis inguinal en carcinoma epidermoide del glande peneal. Patología (Spain) 1991;24:1137–41.

153. Fraley EE, Zhang G, Manivel C, Niehans GA. The role of ilioinguinal lymphadenectomy and significance of histological differentiation in the treatment of carcinoma of the penis. J Urol 1989;142:1478–82.

154. Heyns CF, van Vollenhoven P, Steenkamp JW, Allen FJ, van Velden DJ. Carcinoma of the penis—appraisal of a modified tumour-staging system. Br J Urol 1997;80:307–12.

155. Horenblas S, Van Tinteren H. Squamous cell carcinoma of the penis. IV. Prognostic factors of survival: analysis of tumor, nodes and metastasis classification system. J Urol 1994;151:1239–43.

156. Horenblas S, Van Tinteren H, Delemarre JF, Moonen LM, Lustig V, Kröger R. Squamous cell carcinoma of the penis: accuracy of tumor, nodes and metastasis classification system, and role of lymphangiography, computerized tomography scan and fine needle aspiration cytology. J Urol 1991;146:1279–83.

157. Horenblas S, Van Tinteren H, Delmarre JF, Moonen LM, Lustig V, van Waardenberg EW. Squamous cell carcinoma of the penis. III. Treatment of regional nodes. J Urol 1993;149:492–7.

158. Jackson SM. The treatment of carcinoma of the penis. Br J Surg 1966;53:33–5.

159. Maiche AG, Pyrhonen S, Karkinen M. Histological grading of squamous cell carcinoma of the penis: a new scoring system. Br J Urol 1991;67:522–6.

160. McDougal WS. Carcinoma of the penis: improved survival by early regional lymphadenectomy based on the histologic grade and depth of invasion of the primary lesion. J Urol 1995;154:1364–6.

161. McDougal WS, Kirchner FK Jr, Edwards RH, Killion LT. Treatment of carcinoma of the penis: the case for primary lymphadenectomy. J Urol 1986;136:38–41.

Basal Cell Carcinoma

162. Goldminz D, Scott G, Klaus S. Penile basal cell carcinoma. Report of a case and review of the literature. J Am Acad Dermatol 1989;20:1094–7.

163. Greenbaum SS, Krull EA, Simmons EB. Basal cell carcinoma at the base of the penis in a black patient. J Am Acad Dermatol 1989;20:317–9.

164. Kim ED, Kroft S, Dalton DP. Basal cell carcinoma of the penis: case report and review of the literature. J Urol 1994;152:1557–9.

165. Ladocsi LT, Siebert CF Jr, Rickert RR, Fletcher HS. Basal cell carcinoma of the penis. Cutis 1998;61:25–7.

166. McGregor DH, Tanimura A, Weigel JW. Basal cell carcinoma of the penis. Urology 1982;20:320–3.

167. Murphy GF, Elder DE. Non-melanocytic tumors of the skin. Atlas of Tumor Pathology, 2nd Series, Fascicle 1. Washington D.C.: Armed Forces Institute of Pathology, 1991.

168. Peison B, Benisch B, Nicora B. Multicentric basal cell carcinoma of penile skin. Urology 1985;25:322–3.

169. Sulaiman MZ, Polacarz SV, Partington PE. Basal cell carcinoma of penis: case report. Genitourin Med 1988;64:128–9.

Paget's Disease

170. Helwig EB, Graham JH. Anogenital extramammary Paget's disease. A clinicopathological study. Cancer 1963;16:387–403.

171. Kvist E, Osmundsen PE, Sjolin KE. Primary Paget's disease of the penis. Scand J Urol Nephrol 1992;26:187–90.

172. Mitsudo S, Nakanishi I, Koss L. Paget's disease of the penis and adjacent skin. Its association with fatal sweat gland carcinoma. Arch Pathol Lab Med 1981;105:518–20.

173. Urabe A, Matsukuma A, Shimizu N, Nishimura M, Wada H, Hori Y. Extramammary Paget's disease: comparative histopathologic studies of intraductal carcinoma of the breast and apocrine adenocarcinoma. J Cutan Pathol 1990;17:257–65.

Malignant Melanoma

174. Begun FP, Grossman HB, Diokno AC, Sogani PC. Malignant melanoma of the penis and male urethra. J Urol 1984;132:123–5.

175. Castineiras J, Vilches J, Lopez A, Cabello P, Rodriguez Rubio F. Melanoma of the glans penis: report of a case and review of the literature. Arch Esp Urol 1988;41:880–3.

176. Creagh TA, Murphy DM. Malignant melanoma of the penis. Aust N Z J Surg 1993;63:820–1.

177. Das Gupta T, Grabstald H. Melanoma of the genitourinary tract. J Urol 1965;93:607–14.

178. de Bree E, Sanidas E, Tzardi M, Gaki B, Tsiftsis D. Malignant melanoma of the penis. Eur J Surg Oncol 1997;23:277–9.

179. Fenn NJ, Johnson RC, Sharma AK, Attanoos RL, Horgan K. Malignant melanoma of the penis. Eur J Surg Oncol 1996;22:548–9.

180. Jaeger N, Wirtler H, Tschubel K. Acral lentiginous melanoma of penis. Eur Urol 1982;8:182–4.

181. Johnson DE, Ayala AG. Primary melanoma of penis. Urology 1973;2:174–7.

182. Khezri AA, Dounis A, Roberts JB. Primary malignant melanoma of the penis. Two cases and a review of the literature. Br J Urol 1979;51:147–50.

183. Konigsberg HA, Gray GF. Benign melanosis and malignant melanoma of penis and male urethra. Urology 1976;7:323–6.

184. Manivel JC, Fraley EE. Malignant melanoma of the penis and male urethra: 4 case reports and literature review. J Urol 1988;139:813–6.

185. Miyauchi T, Marouka M, Nagayama T. Malignant melanoma of the penis associated with Von Recklinghausen's neurofibromatosis: report of a case. Hinyokika Kiyo 1988;34:710–3.

186. Myskow MW, Going JJ, McLaren KM, Inglis JA. Malignant melanoma of penis. J Urol 1988;139:817–8.

187. Oldbring J, Mikulowski P. Malignant melanoma of the penis and male urethra. Report of nine cases and review of the literature. Cancer 1987;59:581–7.

188. Primus G, Soyer HP, Smolle J, Mertl G, Pummer K, Kerl H. Early "invasive" malignant melanoma of the glans penis and the male urethra. Report of a case and review of the literature. Eur Urol 1990;18:156–9.

189. Rashid AM, Williams RM, Horton LW. Malignant melanoma of penis and male urethra. Is it a difficult tumor to diagnose? Urology 1993;41:470–1.

190. Schneiderman C, Simon MA, Levine RM. Malignant melanoma of the penis. J Urol 1965;93:615–7.

191. Shanik GD, Jagoe SW. Case report: malignant melanoma of the penis. Ir J Med Sci 1976;145:207–8.

192. Stillwell TJ, Zincke H, Gaffey TA, Woods JE. Malignant melanoma of the penis. J Urol 1988;140:72–5.

193. Talerman A. Malignant melanoma of the penis. Urol Int 1972;27:66–80.

194. Zurrida S, Bartoli C, Clemente C, De Palo G. Malignant melanoma of the penis. A report of four cases. Tumori 1990;76:599–602.

Mesenchymal Neoplasms

195. Amin M, Srigley JR, Ro JY, et al. Leiomyosarcoma of the penis: a study of 7 cases [Abstract]. Mod Pathol 1997;10:68A.

196. Ashley DJ, Edwards EC. Leiomyosarcoma of the penis. Report of a case and review of the literature. Br J Surg 1957;45:170–9.

197. Bacetic D, Knezevic M, Stojsic Z, Atanackovic M, Vujanic GM. Primary extraskeletal osteosarcoma of the penis with a malignant fibrous histiocytoma-like component. Histopathology 1998;33:184–94.

198. Bayne D, Wise G. Kaposi sarcoma of penis and genitalia: a disease of our times. Urology 1988;31:22–5.

199. Blasius S, Brinkschmidt C, Bier B, et al. Extraskeletal myxoid chondrosarcoma of the penis. J Urol Pathol 1995;3:73–80.

200. Casado M, Jimenez F, Borburjo J, et al. Spontaneous healing of Kaposi's angiosarcoma of the penis. J Urol 1988;139:1313–5.

201. Conger K, Sporer A. Kaposi's sarcoma limited to glans penis. Urology 1985;26:173–5.

202. Dehner LP, Smith BH. Soft tissue tumors of the penis. A clinico-pathologic study of 46 cases. Cancer 1970; 25:1431–47.

203. Deutsch M, Lee RL, Mercado R. Hemangioendothelioma of the penis with late appearing metastases: report of a case with review of the literature. J Surg Oncol 1973;5:27–34.

204. Dwosh J, Mininberg DT, Schlossberg J, Peterson P. Neurofibroma involving the penis in a child. J Urol 1984;132:988–9.

205. Edwards AT, Somerville JJ. Primary osteosarcoma of the penis. Br J Urol 1990;66:552–3.

206. Fletcher CD, Lowe D. Inflammatory fibrous histiocytoma of the penis. Histopathology 1984;8:1079–84.

207. Ghandur-Mnaymneh L, Gonzalez MS. Angiosarcoma of the penis with hepatic angiomas in a patient with low vinyl chloride exposure. Cancer 1981;47:1318–24.

208. Gower RL, Pambakian H, Fletcher CD. Epithelioid sarcoma of the penis: a rare tumour to be distinguished from squamous carcinoma. Br J Urol 1987;59:592–3.

209. Greenwood N, Fox H, Edwards EC. Leiomyosarcoma of the penis. Cancer 1972;29:481–3.

210. Hemal AK, Goswani AK, Sharma SK, Radotra BD, Malik N. Penile venous hemangioma. Aust NZ J Surg 1989;59:814–6.

211. Hermann RN, Fletcher RR. Congenital penile tumor: a case report. J Urol 1962;87:701–4.

212. Hodgins TE, Hancock RA. Hemangio-endothelial sarcoma of the penis: report of a case and review of the literature. J Urol 1970;104:867–70.

213. Huang DJ, Stanisic TH, Hansen KK. Epithelioid sarcoma of the penis. J Urol 1992;147:1370–2.

214. Humes KB, Greence JB, Marcus A, et al. Kaposi's sarcoma in homosexual men. A report of eight cases. Lancet 1981;1:598–600.

215. Imperial R, Helwig EB. Angiokeratoma. A clinicopathologic study. Arch Dermatol 1967;95:166–75.

216. Isa SS, Almaraz R, McGovern J. Leiomyosarcoma of the penis. Case report and review of the literature. Cancer 1984;54:939–42.

217. Jimenez-Verdejo J, Fernandez PL, Haddad A, Garcia-Carriazo A, Zuluaga A, Nogales F. Extraskeletal Ewing's sarcoma metastatic to penis. Br J Urol 1992;70:206–7.

218. Kinoshita H, Okada K, Nagata Y, Kawamura N. Fibrous histiocytoma of penis. Urology 1985;25:544–6.

219. Lands RH, Ange D, Hartman DL. Radiation therapy for classic Kaposi's sarcoma presenting only on the glans penis. J Urol 1992;147:468–70.

220. Lowe FC, Lattimer DG, Metroka CE. Kaposi's sarcoma of the penis in patients with acquired immunodeficiency syndrome. J Urol 1989;142:1475–7.

221. Macaluso JN, Sullivan JW, Tomberlin S. Glomus tumor of glans penis. Urology 1985;25:409–10.

222. Maher JD, Thompson GM, Loening J, Platz CE. Penile plexiform neurofibroma: case report and review of the literature. J Urol 1988;139:1310–2.

223. Mathur P, Porwal KK, Pendse AK, Parihar US, Chittora R. Hemangiomatous penile horn. J Urol 1996;155:1738.

224. McDonald MW, O'Connell JR, Manning JT, Benjamin RS. Leiomyosarcoma of the penis. J Urol 1983;130:788–9.

225. Mentzel T, Behman A, Calonje E, Katenkamp D, Fletcher CD. Epithelioid hemangioendothelioma of skin and soft tissues: clinicopathologic and immunohistochemical study of 30 cases. Am J Surg Pathol 1997;21:363–74.

226. Moore SW, Wheeler JE, Hefter LG. Epithelioid sarcoma masquerading as Peyronie's disease. Cancer 1975;35:1706–10.

227. Mortensen H, Murphy L. Angiomatous malformations of the glans penis. J Urol 1950;64:396–9.

228. Ogawa A, Watanabe K. Genitourinary neurofibromatosis in a child presenting with an enlarged penis and scrotum. J Urol 1986;135:755–7.

229. Pack GT, Trinidad SS, Humphreys GA. Primary leiomyosarcoma of the penis. Report of a case. J Urol 1963;89:839–41.

230. Pak K, Sakaguchi N, Takayama H, Tomoyoshi T. Rhabdomyosarcoma of the penis. J Urol 1986;136:438–9.

231. Ramos JZ, Pack GT. Primary embryonal rhabdomyosarcoma of the penis in a 2-year-old child. J Urol 1966;96:928–32.

232. Rasbridge SA, Parry JR. Angiosarcoma of the penis. Br J Urol 1989;63:440–1.

233. Saw D, Tse CH, Chan J, Watt CY, Ng CS, Poon YF. Clear cell sarcoma of the penis. Hum Pathol 1986;17:423–5.

234. Seftel AD, Sadick NS, Waldbaum RS. Kaposi's sarcoma of the penis in a patient with the acquired immune deficiency syndrome. J Urol 1987;136:673–5.

235. Senoh K, Miyazaki T, Kikuchi J, Sumivoshe A, Kohga A. Angiomatous lesions of the glans penis. Urology 1981;17:194–6.

236. Smart RH. Leiomyosarcoma of the penis. J Urol 1984;132:356–7.

237. Srigley JR, Ayala AG, Ordonez NG, van Nostrand P. Epithelioid hemangioma of the penis. A rare and distinctive vascular lesion. Arch Pathol Lab Med 1985;109:51–4.

238. Stone NN, Sun CC, Brutscher S, Zein T. Granular cell tumor of penis. J Urol 1983;130:575.

239. Suarez GM, Lewis RW. Granular cell tumor of the glans penis. J Urol 1986;135:1252–3.

240. Swierzewski SJ III, Wan J, Boffini A, Faerber GJ. The management of meatal obstruction due to Kaposi's sarcoma of the glans penis. J Urol 1993;150:193–5.

241. Vapnek JM, Quivey JM, Carroll PR. Acquired immunodeficiency syndrome-related Kaposi's sarcoma of the male genitalia: management with radiation therapy. J Urol 1991;146:333–6.

242. Waguespack RL, Fair KP, Svetec DA, Rozanski TA. Glomangioma of the penile and scrotal median raphe. J Urol 1996;156:179.

243. Williams JJ, Mouradian JA, Hagopian BA, Gray GF. Hemangioendothelial sarcoma of penis. Cancer 1979;44:1146–9.

244. Wilson LS, Lockhart JL, Bergman H, et al. Fibrosarcoma of the penis: case report and review of the literature. J Urol 1983;129:606–7.

245. Yantiss RK, Althausen AF, Young RH. Malignant fibrous histiocytoma of the penis. Report of a case and review of the literature. J Urol Pathol 1998;9:171–80.

246. Zambolin T, Simeone C, Baronchelli C, Cunico SC. Kaposi's sarcoma of the penis in a patient with acquired immunodeficiency syndrome. J Urol 1989;142:1475–7.

247. Zambolin T, Simeone C, Baronchelli C, Cunico SC. Kaposi's sarcoma of the penis. Br J Urol 1989;63:645–6.

Malignant Lymphoma and Related Lesions

248. Begun FP, Derus J, Toorkey B, Almagro U. Leukemia of the penis. J Urol 1989;142:123–4.

249. Bostwick DG, Guthman DA, Letendre L, Banks PM, Texter JH Jr, Lieber MM. Polymorphic reticulosis (idiopathic midline destructive disease) of the penis, scrotum, and perineum. J Urol Pathol 1996;5:57–63.

250. Caputo R, Gianotti R, Monti M. Nodular "pure" mucocutaneous histiocytosis X in an adult. Arch Dermatol 1987;123:1274–5.

251. Fairfax CA, Hammer CJ, Dana BW, Hanifin JN, Barry JM. Primary penile lymphoma presenting as a penile ulcer. J Urol 1995;153:1051–2.

252. Gonzalez-Campora R, Nogales FF Jr, Lerma E, Navarro A, Matilla A. Lymphoma of the penis. J Urol 1981;126:270–1.

253. Gough J. Primary reticulum cell sarcoma of the penis. Br J Urol 1970;42:336–9.

254. Hashine K, Akiyama M, Sumiyoshi Y. Primary diffuse large cell lymphoma of the penis. Int J Urol 1994;1:189–90.

255. Lopez Muñoz A, Castineiras Fernandez J, Vilches Troya J, Varo Solis C, Cabello Torres P, Rodriguez Rubio Vidal F. Lymphoma of the penis. Arch Esp Urol 1990;43:186–9.

256. Myers DA. Strandjord SE, Marcus RB Jr, Pierson KK, Walker RD. Histiocytosis X presenting as a primary penile lesion. J Urol 1981;126:268–9.

257. Scott GC, Ungaro PC, Cashman J, Gonzalez JJ. Large cell lymphoma presenting as a coronal penile lesion. Mod Med 1989;86:278–9.

258. Steinbach F, Essbach U, Florschütz A, Gruss A, Allhoff EP. Ulcerative balanoposthitis as the initial manifestation of acute promyelocytic leukemia. J Urol 1998;160:1430–1.

259. Stewart AL, Grieve RJ, Banerjee SS. Primary lymphoma of the penis. Eur J Surg Oncol 1985;11:179–81.

260. Yu GS, Nseyo UO, Carson JW. Primary penile lymphoma in a patient with Peyronie's disease. J Urol 1989;142:1076–7.

Miscellaneous Other Rare Primary Tumors

261. Barney JD, Gall EA. Unusual tumor of penis: case report. J Urol 1939;42:623–8.

262. Kennedy R, Lacson A. Congenital endodermal sinus tumor of the penis. J Pediatr Surg 1987;22:791–2.

263. Tomasini C, Aloi F, Puiatti P, Caliendo V. Dermoid cyst of the penis. Dermatology 1997;194:188–90.

Secondary Tumors

264. Abehouse BS, Abehouse GA. Metastatic tumors of the penis: a review of the literature and a report of two cases. J Urol 1961;86:99–112.

265. Adjiman S, Flam TA, Zerib M, et al. Delayed nonurothelial metastatic lesions of the penis: a report of two cases. Eur Urol 1989;16:391–2.

266. Belville WD, Cohen JA. Secondary penile malignancies: the spectrum of presentation. J Surg Oncol 1992;51:134–7.

267. Haddad FS. Penile metastases secondary to bladder cancer. Review of the literature. Urol Int 1984;39:125–42.

268. Haddad FS, Manne RK. Involvement of the penis by retrocolic adenocarcinoma. A report of a case and review of literature. Dis Colon Rectum 1987;30:123–9.

269. Haddad FS, Manne RK. Prostatic tumors with penile secondaries: review of the literature with a case report. Urol Int 1986;41:465–70.

270. Hayes MC, Meehan CJ, Ratan P, Theaker JM, Smart CJ. Extramammary Paget's disease of the penis is associated with long-standing transitional cell carcinoma and radiotherapy. Br J Urol 1997;80:673–4.

271. Hsieh JT, Liu SP, Shun CT, Lai MK. Metastatic yolk sac tumor of the corpus cavernosum of the penis. J Urol 1998;160:833–4.

272. Karanjie ND, King H, Schweitzer FA. Metastasis to the penis from carcinoma of the stomach. Br J Urol 1987;60:368–75.

273. Metcalf JS, Lee RE, Maize JC. Epidermotropic urothelial carcinoma involving the glans penis. Arch Dermatol 1985;121:532–4.

274. Ordoñez NG, Ayala AB, Bracken RB. Renal cell carcinoma metastatic to penis. Urology 1982;19:417–9.

275. Paquin AJ Jr, Roland SI. Secondary carcinoma of the penis. A review of the literature and a report of nine cases. Cancer 1956;9:626–31.

276. Perez LM, Shumway RA, Carson CC, Fischer SR, Hudson WR. Penile metastases secondary to supraglottic squamous cell carcinoma: review of the literature. J Urol 1992;147:157–60.

277. Perez-Mesa C, Oxenhandler R. Metastatic tumors of the penis. J Surg Oncol 1989;42:11–5.

278. Philip AT, Amin MB, Cubilla AA, Young RH. Secondary tumors of the penis: a study of 16 cases. Mod Pathol 1999;12:104A.

279. Powell BL, Craig JB, Muss HB. Secondary malignancies of the penis and epididymis: a case report and review of the literature. J Clin Oncol 1985;3:110–6.

280. Powell FC, Bjornsson J, Doyle JA, Cooper AJ. Genital Paget's disease and urinary tract malignancy. J Am Acad Dermatol 1985;13:84–90.

281. Powell FC, Venecie PY, Winkelmann RK. Metastatic prostate carcinoma manifesting as penile nodules. Arch Dermatol 1984;20:1604–6.

282. Robey EL, Schellhammer PF. Four cases of metastases to the penis and a review of the literature. J Urol 1984;132:992–4.

283. Saltzman B, Srinivas V, Morse MJ, Hajdu SI. Sacrococcygeal chordoma metastatic to penis. Urology 1985;25:541–3.

284. Smith DJ, Hamdy FC, Evans JW, Falzon M, Chapple CR. Paget's disease of the glans penis: an unusual urological malignancy. Eur Urol 1994;25:316–9.

285. Tan HT, Vishniavsky S. Carcinoma of the prostate with metastases to the prepuce. J Urol 1971;106:588–9.

286. Ucar FJ, Robles JE, Sanchez de la Muela P, De Castro F, Zudaire JJ, Besrian JM. Secondary carcinoma of the penis. A report of three new cases. Eur Urol 1989;16:308–9.

287. Valadez RA, Wheeler JJ, Canning JR, Moylan DJ. Metastatic transitional cell carcinoma to penis. Urology 1987;29:394–7.

Tumor-Like Lesions

General References

288. Connor DH, Chandler FW, Schwartz DA, Manz HJ, Lack EE. Pathology of infectious diseases. Stamford, CT: Appleton and Lange, 1997.

289. Fisher BK, Margesson LJ. Genital skin disorders. Diagnosis and treatment. St. Louis: Mosby, 1998.

290. Horan DB, Redman JF, Jansen GT. Papulosquamous lesions of glans penis. Urology 1984;23:1–4.

291. Margolis DJ. Cutaneous diseases of the male external genitalia. In: Walsh PC, Retik AB, Vaughan ED, Wein AJ, eds. Campbell's urology, 7th ed. Philadelphia: WB Saunders Co, 1998.

292. Varghese M, Kindel S. Pigmentary disorders and inflammatory lesions of the external genitalia. Urol Clin Am 1992;19:111–21.

293. Wise GJ. Fungal infections of the external genitalia. Urol Clin Am 1992;19:103–9.

Cysts

294. Asarch RG, Golitz LE, Sausker WF, et al. Median raphe cysts of the penis. Arch Dermatol 1979;115:1084–6.

295. Claudy AL, Dutoit M, Boucheron S. Epidermal and urethroid penile cyst. Acta Dermatol Venereol 1991;71:61–2.

296. Cole LA, Helwig EB. Mucoid cysts of the penile skin. J Urol 1976;115:397–400.

297. Hayashi T, Tsuda N, Shimada O, et al. A clinicopathologic study of tumors and tumor-like lesions of the penis. Acta Pathol Jpn 1990;40:343–51.

298. Quiles DR, Betlcoh Mas Y, Jimenez A, Verdeguer J, Botella R, Castells A. Gonococcal infection of the penile raphe cyst. Int J Dermatol 1987;26:242–3.

299. Rattan J, Rattan S, Gupta DK. Epidermoid cyst of the penis with extension into the pelvis. J Urol 1997;158:593.

Nonspecific Inflammatory Lesions

300. Davis DA, Cohen PR. Balanitis circumscripta plasmacellularis. J Urol 1995;153:424–6.

301. Yoganathan S, Bohl TG, Mason G. Plasma cell balanitis and vulvitis (of Zoon). A study of 10 cases. J Reprod Med 1994;39:939–44.

Specific Inflammatory Lesions
Condyloma Acuminatum Including Giant Condyloma

302. Ananthakrishnan N, Ravindran R, Veliath AJ, Parkash S. Löwenstein-Buschke tumour of penis—a carcinoma mimic. A report of 24 cases with review of the literature. Br J Urol 1981;53:460–5.

303. Arumainayagam JT, Sumathipala AH, Smallman LA, Shahmanesh M. Flat condylomata of the penis presenting as patchy balanopostitis. Genitourin Med 1990;66:251–3.

304. Gersh I. Condylomata acuminata of the male external genitalia: an effective method of surgical treatment. Urol Cutan Review 1945;49:432–45.

305. Loning T, Riviere A, Henke RP, Von Preyss S, Dorner A. Penile-anal condylomas and squamous cell cancer. A HPV DNA hybridization study. Virchows Arch 1988;413:491–8.
306. Lowenstein LW. Carcinoma-like condylomata acuminata of the penis. Med Clin North Am 1939;23:789–95.
307. Milburn PB, Brandsma JL, Goldsman CI, Teplitz DE, Heilman EL. Disseminated warts and evolving squamous cell carcinoma in a patient with acquired immuno-deficiency syndrome. J Acad Dermatol 1988;1:401–5.

308. Nuovo GI, Hochman HA, Ellezri YD, Lastarria D, Comite SL, Silvers DN. Detection of human papillomavirus DNA in penile lesions histologically negative for condylomata. Analysis for in situ hybridization and the polymerase chain. Am J Surg Pathol 1990;14:829–36.
309. Schultz RE, Miller JW, McDonald GR, et al. Clinical and molecular evaluation of acetowhite genital lesions in men. J Urol 1990;143:920–3.
310. Schultz RE, Skelton HG. Value of acetic acid screening for flat genital condylomata in men. J Urol 1988;139:777–9.

Syphilis

311. Chapel TA. Primary and secondary syphilis. Cutis 1984;33:47–53
312. Fitzgerald F. The great imitator, syphilis. West J Med 1982;134:424–32.
313. Hay PE, Tam FW, Kitchen VS, Horner S, Bridger J, Weber J. Gummatous lesions in men infected with human immunodeficiency virus and syphilis. Genitourin Med 1990;66:374–9.
314. Hutchinson CM, Hook EW III. Syphilis in adults. Med Clin North Am 1990;74:1389–416.
315. Olansky S. Late benign syphilis (gumma). Med Clin North Am 1964;48:653–65.

Granuloma Inguinale

316. Beerman H, Sonck CE. The epithelial changes in granuloma inguinale. Am J Syphilis 1952;36:501–10.
317. Davis CM. Granuloma inguinale. A clinical, histological and ultrastructural study. JAMA 1970;211:632–6.
318. Fritz GS, Hubler WR Jr, Dodson RF, Rudolph A. Mutilating granuloma inguinale. Arch Dermatol 1975;111:1464–5.

319. Richens J. The diagnosis and treatment of donovanosis (granuloma inguinale). Genitourin Med 1991;67:441–52.
320. Sayal SK, Kar PK, Anand LC. A study of 255 cases of granuloma inguinale. Indian J Dermatol 1987;32:91–7.

Lymphogranuloma Venereum

321. Kleine W. Granuloma venereum. Z Hautkr 1985; 60:100–2.
322. Sheldon WH, Heyman A. Lymphogranuloma venereum. Am J Path 1947;23:653–64.

323. Smith MJ, Custer RP. The histopathology of lymphogranuloma venereum. J Urol 1950;63:546–63.

Chancroid

324. McCarley ME, Cruz PD Jr, Sontheimer RD. Chancroid: clinical variants from an epidemic in Dallas County 1986–1987. J Am Acad Dermatol 1988;19:330–7.

325. Sheldon WH, Heyman A. Studies on chancroid: observations of the histology with an evaluation of biopsy as a diagnostic procedure. Am J Pathol 1946;22:415–25.

Molluscum Contagiosum

326. Brown ST, Nally JF, Kraus SJ. Molluscum contagiosum. Sex Trans Dis 1981;8:227–34.
327. Epstein WL. Molluscum contagiosum. Semin Dermatol 1992;11:184–9.

328. Gordon SK, Stearns DB. Molloscum contagiosum of the penis: case report. J Urol 1960;84:738–9.
329. Lewis EJ, Lam M, Crutchfield CE III. An update on molluscum contagiosum. Cutis 1997;60:29–34.

Bacillary Angiomatosis

330. LeBoit PE. Bacillary angiomatosis. In: Connor DH, Chandler FW, Schwartz DA, Manz HJ, Lack EE, eds. Pathology of infectious diseases, Stamford, CT: Appleton and Lange, 1997.

Other Specific Infectious Diseases

331. Lazarus JA, Rosenthal AA. Primary tuberculosis of the penis. J Urol 1936;35:361–77.
332. Meyer R, Nosanchuk J. Parasitic infection of the penis. J Urol 1996;155:2030–1.
333. Preminger B, Gerard PS, Lutwick L, Frank R, Minkowitz S, Plotkin N. Histoplasmosis of the penis. J Urol 1993;149:848–50.

334. Ramesh V, Vasanthi R. Tuberculosis cavernositis of the penis: case report. Genitourin Med 1989;65:58–9.
335. Walker D, Jordan WP Jr. Tuberculosis ulcer of the penis. J Urol 1968;100:36–7.

Balantitis Xerotica Obliterans

336. Chalmers RJ, Burton PA, Bennett R, et al. Lichen sclerous et atrophicus: a common distinctive cause of phimosis in boys. Arch Dermatol 1984;120:1025–7.
337. Garat JM, Chechile G, Algaba F, Santaularia JM. Balantitis xerotica obliterans in children. J Urol 1986;136:436–7.
338. Rheinschild GW, Olsen BS. Balanitis xerotica obliterans. J Urol 1970;104:860–3.
339. Ridley CM. Lichen sclerosus et atrophicus. Arch Dermatol 1989;123:457–60.

Peyronie's Disease

340. Bivens CH, Marecek RL, Feldman JM. Peyronie's disease: a presenting complaint of the carcinoid syndrome. N Engl J Med 1973;289:844–5.
341. Brock G, Hsu GL, Nunes L, Von Heyden B, Lue TF. The anatomy of the tunica albuginea in the normal penis and Peyronie's disease. J Urol 1997;157:276–81.
342. Davis CJ Jr. The microscopic pathology of Peyronie's disease. J Urol 1997;157:282–4.
343. Gelbard MK. Dystrophic penile calcification in Peyronie's disease. J Urol 1988;139:738–40.
344. Hu KN, Burks C, Christy WC. Fibrosis of tunica albuginea: complication of longterm intracavernous pharmacological self-injection. J Urol 1987;138:404–5.
345. Narita T, Kudo H, Matsumoto K. Circumferential Peyronie's disease involving both the corpora cavernosa. Pathol Int 1995;45:383–7.
346. Smith BH. Peyronie's disease. Am J Clin Pathol 1966;45:670–8.

Verruciform Xanthoma

347. Cuozzo DW, Vachher P, Sau P, Frishberg DP, James WD. Verruciform xanthoma: a benign penile growth. J Urol 1995;153:1625–7.
348. Geiss DF, Del Rosso JQ, Murphy J. Verruciform xanthoma of the glans penis: a benign clinical simulant of genital malignancy. Cutis 1993;51:369–72.
349. George WM, Azadeh B. Verruciform xanthoma of the penis. Cutis 1989;44:167–70.
350. Kraemer BB, Schmidt WA, Foucar E, Rosen T. Verruciform xanthoma of the penis. Arch Dermatol 1981;117:516–8.
351. Mohsin SK, Lee MW, Amin MB, et al. Cutaneous verruciform xanthomas: a report of five cases investigating the etiology and nature of xanthomatous cells. Am J Surg Pathol 1998;22:479–87.
352. Requena L, Sarasa JL, Martin L, et al. Verruciform xanthoma of the penis with acantholytic cells. Clin Exp Dermatol 1995;20:504–8.

Pearly Penile Papules, Hirsutoid Papillomas

353. Ackerman AB, Kornberg R. Pearly penile papules. Acral angiofibromas. Arch Dermatol 1973;108:673–5.
354. Hyman AB, Brownstein MH. Tyson's "glands." Ectopic sebaceous glands and papillomatous penis. Arch Dermatol 1969;99:31–6.
355. Magid M, Garden JM. Pearly penile papules: treatment with the carbon dioxide laser. J Dermatol Surg Oncol 1989;15:552–4.
356. Tanenbaum MH, Becker SW. Papillae of the corona of the glans penis. J Urol 1965;93:391–5.
357. Vesper JL, Messina J, Glass LF, Fenske NA. Profound proliferating pearly penile papules. Int J Dermatol 1995;34:425–6.
358. Winer JH, Winer LH. Hirsutoid papillomas of the coronal margin of the glans penis. J Urol 1955;74:375–8.

Lipogranuloma

359. Arduino LJ. Sclerosing lipogranuloma of male genitalia. J Urol 1959;82:155–61.
360. Lee T, Choi HR, Lee YT, Lee YH. Paraffinoma of the penis. Yonsei Med J 1994;35:3440–8.
361. Oertel YC, Johnson FB. Sclerosing lipogranuloma of male genitalia. Review of 23 cases. Arch Pathol Lab Med 1977;101:321–6.
362. Smetana HF, Bernhard W. Sclerosing lipogranuloma. Arch Pathol 1950;50:296–325.
363. Soyer HP, Petritsch P, Glavanovitz P, Kerl H. Sclerosing lipogranuloma (paraffin-inducted granuloma) of the penis with a clinical picture of carcinoma. Hautarzt 1988;39:174–6.

Tancho's Nodules

364. Gilmore WA, Weigand DA, Burgdorf WH. Penile nodules in Southeast Asian men. Arch Dermatol 1983;119:446–7.
365. Lim KB, Seow CS, Tulip T, Daniel M, Vijayasingham SM. Artificial penile nodules: case reports. Genitourin Med 1986;62:123–5.
366. Norton SA. Fijian penis marbles: an example of artificial penile nodules. Cutis 1993;51:295–7.
367. Serour F. Artificial nodules of the penis. Report of six cases among Russian immigrants in Israel. Sex Transm Dis 1993;20:192–3.

Melanosis/Lentiginosis

368. Barnhill RL, Albert LS, Shama SK, Goldenhersh MA, Rhodes AR, Sober AJ. Genital lentiginosis: a clinical and histopathologic study. J Am Acad Dermatol 1990;22:453–60.

369. Revuez J, Clerici T. Penile melanosis. J Am Acad Dermatol 1989;20:567–70.

Fournier's Gangrene

370. Bahlmann JC, Fourie JH, Arndt TC. Fournier's gangrene: necrotising fasciitis of the male genitalia. Br J Urol 1983;55:85–8.

371. Basoglu M, Gul O, Yildigran I, Balik AA, Ozbey I, Oren D. Fournier's gangrene: review of fifteen cases. Am Surg 1997;63:1019–21.

372. DeWire DM, Bergstein JM. Carcinoma of the sigmoid colon: an unusual cause of Fournier's gangrene. J Urol 1992;147:711–2.

373. Elem B, Ranjan P. Impact of immunodeficiency virus (HIV) on Fournier's gangrene: observations in Zambia. Ann R Coll Surg Engl 1995;77:283–6.

374. Gerber GS, Guss SP, Pielet RW. Fournier's gangrene secondary to intra-abdominal processes. Urology 1994;44:779–82.

375. Haddad FS. Subcutaneous abscess and gangrene of the penis. Report of four cases. J Urol Pathol 1997;5:223–7.

376. Levy V, Jaffabey J, Aouad K, Zittoun R. Fournier's gangrene during induction treatment of acute promyelocytic leukemia, a case report. Ann Hematol 1998;76:91–4.

377. Theiss M, Hofmockel G, Frohmüller HG. Fournier's gangrene in a patient with erectile dysfunction following use of a mechanical erection aid device. J Urol 1995;153:1921–2.

Wegener's Granulomatosis

378. Davenport A, Downey SE, Goel S, Maciver AG. Wegener's granulomatosis involving the urogenital tract. Br J Urol 1996;78:354–7.

379. Dore B, Duriez P, Grange P, Aubert J. Wegener's granulomatosis with urethral–penile location. Apropos of a case. Ann Urol Paris 1990;24:256–8.

380. Matsuda S, Mitsukawa S, Ishii N, Shirai M. A case of Wegener's granulomatosis with necrosis of the penis. Tohoku J Exp Med 1976;118:145–51.

381. Nielsen GP, Pilch BZ, Black-Schaffer WS, Young RH. Wegener's granulomatosis of the penis clinically stimulating carcinoma. Report of a case. J Urol Pathol 1996;4:265–72.

382. Piazza R, Altavilla G, Aragona F, Zattoni F, Tavolini IM, Piazza M. Granulomatosis of external genitalia: a new disease or part of the spectrum? J Urol 1996;153:1231–3.

383. Rubenstein M, Wolff SM. Penile nodules as a major manifestation of subacute angiitis. Arch Intern Med 1961;114:449–52.

384. Tripp BM, Chu F, Halwani F, Hassouna MM. Necrotizing vasculitis of the penis in systemic lupus erythematosus. J Urol 1995;154:528–9.

385. Vella EJ, Waller DG. Granulomatous vasculitis of the penis with glomerulonephritis. Postgrad Med J 1981;57:262–4.

Os Penis

386. Champion RH, Wegrzyn J. Congenital os penis. J Urol 1964;91:663–4.

387. Elliott JP Jr, Fischman JL. Os penis. J Urol 1962;88:655–6.

388. Milad M, Zein T. Large bony lesions of the penis. Ann Saudi Med 1996;16:568–9.

389. Sarma DP, Weilbaecher TG. Human os penis. Urology 1990;35:349–50.

390. Vahlensieck WK Jr, Schaefer HE, Westenfelder M. Penile ossification and acquired penile deviation. Eur Urol 1995;27:252–6.

Miscellaneous Other Tumor–Like Lesions

391. Ball TP Jr, Pickett JD. Traumatic lymphangitis of penis. Urology 1975;6:594–7.

392. Chiba M, Iizuka M, Horie Y, Masammune O. Metastatic Crohn's disease involving the penis. J Gastroenterol 1997;32:817–21.

393. Cockburn AG, Krolikowski J, Balogh K, Roth RA. Crohn disease of penile and scrotal skin. Urology 1980;15:596–8.

394. Coldiron BM, Jacobson C. Common penile lesions. Urol Clin North Am 1988;15:671–85.

395. Dekio S, Tsujino Y, Jidoi J. Intravascular papillary endothelial hyperplasia on the penis: report of a case. J Dermatol 1993;20:657–9.

396. España A, Sanchez-Yus E, Serna MJ, Redondo P, Robledo A, Quintanilla E. Chronic balanitis with palisading granuloma: an atypical genital localization of necrobiosis lipoidica responsive to pentoxifylline. Dermatology 1994;188:222–5.

397. Goh M, Tekchandani AH, Wojno KJ, Faerber GJ. Metastatic Crohn's disease involving penile skin. J Urol 1998;159:506–7.

398. Greenberg RD, Perry TL. Nonvenereal sclerosing lymphangitis of the penis. Arch Dermatol 1972;105:728–9.

399. Hautmann RE, Bachor R. Juvenile xanthogranuloma of the penis. J Urol 1993;150:456–7.

400. Leal SM, Novsam N, Zacks SI. Amyloidosis presenting as a penile mass. J Urol 1988;140:830–1.

401. Mor Y, Zaidi SZ, Rose DS, Ransley PG, Mouriquand PD. Granulomatous lymphangitis of the penile skin as a cause of penile swelling in children. J Urol 1997;158:591–2.

402. Neri I, Bardazzi F, Fanti PA, Guidetti MS. Penile Crohn's disease: a case report. Genitourin Med 1995;71:45–6.

403. Nielsen GP, Rosenberg AE, Dretler SP, Young RH. An unusual pseudotumor of the penis. Report of a case associated with chronic catheterization. J Urol Pathol 1996;4:79–84.

404. Phillips SS, Baird B, Joshi V, Rosenberg AJ, Janosko EO. Crohn's disease of the prepuce in a 12-year-old boy: a case report and review of the literature. Pediatr Pathol Lab Med 1997;17:497–502.

405. Piccinno R, Carrel CF, Menni S, Brancaleon W. Preputial ectopic sebaceous glands mimicking molluscoum contagiosum. Acta Derm Venereol (Stockh) 1990;70:344–5.

406. Rubinstein I, Baum GL, Hiss Y. Sarcoidosis of the penis: report of a case. J Urol 1986;135:1016–7.

407. Schwartz SL, Perkins PL, Ritchey ML. Angiocentric myofibroblastic tumor of the penis in a child: case report and literature review. J Urol 1993;149:1114–5.

408. Slaney G, Muller S, Clay J, Sumathipala AH, Hillenbrand P, Thompson H. Crohn's disease involving the penis. Gut 1986;27:329–33.

406. Vitenson JH, Wilson JM. Sarcoid of the glans penis. J Urol 1972;108:284–6.

410. Walzman M, Kundu A, Fraser I. Pyogenic granuloma of the penis—a rare entity? Genitourin Med 1995;71:43–4.

411. Westermark P, Henriksson TG. Granulomatous inflammation of the vulva and penis—a genital counterpart to cheilitis granulomatosa. Dermatologica 1979;158:269–74.

✧✧✧

Prostate Gland

---

*Numbers in boldface indicate table and figure pages.

Seminal Vesicle

Male Urethra

Penis